Radiology Imaging Words and Phrases

Second Edition

Diagnostic Imaging
Interventional Radiology
Therapeutic Radiology
Nuclear Medicine
Ultrasonography
Computed Tomography (CT)
Positron Emission Tomography (PET)
Single Photon Emission Computed
Tomography (SPECT)
Magnetic Resonance Imaging (MRI)

Health Professions Institute • Modesto, California • 2005

Radiology Imaging Words and Phrases
2nd Edition

Published by

Health Professions Institute
P. O. Box 801
Modesto, CA 95353
Phone (209) 551-2112
Fax (209) 551-0404
Web Site: http://www.hpisum.com
E-mail: hpi@hpisum.com

Sally Crenshaw Pitman, M.A.
Editor & Publisher

Printed by
Parks Printing & Lithograph
Modesto, California

ISBN 0-934385-85-8

Last digit is the print number: 9 8 7 6 5 4 3 2 1

To

Lori Laraine Pitman Sookhoo

Preface

Radiology Imaging Words and Phrases, second edition, is an update of the 1997 edition. This new book has over 60,000 entries from the specialties of diagnostic imaging, therapeutic radiology, nuclear medicine, ultrasonography, computed tomography (CT), magnetic resonance imaging (MRI), positron emission tomography (PET), single photon emission computed tomography (SPECT), and the latest technological advances in interventional radiology and neuroradiology.

Our research to update an eight-year-old book in this fast-moving field led us to many new words and phrases in all new imaging modalities. From diagnostic imaging (MRI and CT scans) to interventional radiology (IR), we've added thousands of new terms to our lexicon.

Interventional radiology is hailed as the new frontier for many life-threatening conditions which in the past required invasive surgery. As the quality of medical imaging has improved, it is necessary to add a highly technical vocabulary to this publication. Terminology in the field of radiology imaging crosses all body systems and medical specialties, thus challenging us to cover all the bases with a minimum amount of redundancy. With so many new developments in medicine, surgery, and technology in the past eight years, our research yielded thousands of new terms. We added scores of imaging agents currently in use and deleted outdated ones, thanks to Ellen and Randy Drake and their research for the pharmaceutical database they update annually for *Saunders Pharmaceutical Word Book*.

To streamline the book and make it most useful to medical transcriptionists and other healthcare professionals, we deleted hundreds of obsolete terms and outdated products while adding over 12,000 new entries not found in other word books. We've culled abbreviations, coined words, medical slang, and words and phrases from hundreds of transcripts of radiology imaging dictation, as well as medical databases, scholarly journals, textbooks, and other electronic and printed references, and we added dozens of phonetic renderings for otherwise hard-to-find terms.

This new edition was made possible by the fine scholarly research of Ellen Drake, CMT, and Linda Campbell, CMT. Invaluable assistance in verifying the accuracy of entries and reconciling discrepancies from various authoritative references was provided by John H. Dirckx, M.D.

Sally Crenshaw Pitman, M.A.
Editor & Publisher

How to Use This Book

The words and phrases in this book are alphabetized letter by letter of all words in the entry, ignoring puntuation marks and words in parentheses. The possessive form (*'s*) is omitted from eponyms for ease in alphabetizing. Numbers are alphabetized as if written out, with the exception of subscripts and superscripts which are ignored.

Eponyms may be located alphabetically as well as under the nouns they modify; for example, *Batten disease* may also be found under *disease*. A list of over 1500 subentries under *imaging* includes trademarked scans and scanners and other imaging devices. Hundreds of contrast media are listed under *imaging agents*. A separate short list of *medications* includes bowel prep pharmaceuticals.

The names of hundreds of imaging agents (generic and brand names) used in radiology imaging and radiotherapeutic modalities are included. The main entries *artery, muscle,* and *vein* include many phrases and descriptive terms related to arteries, muscles, and veins as they are dictated in patient reports, rather than only the names of anatomical terms readily available in medical dictionaries. Physicians dictate many abbreviations, especially for anatomical groups, and those terms frequently abbreviated in medical dictation are listed as main entries with their translations and as subentries.

In medical dictation physicians arbitrarily refer to a diagnostic, therapeutic, or interventional procedure (both invasive and noninvasive) as an *approach*, *method, operation, procedure, repair,* or *technique*, or by the type of procedure, such as *angioplasty*. Thus, procedures and imaging studies are listed alphabetically by the eponym or noun as well as under the type of procedure and under the main entry.

Instruments used in interventional, therapeutic, and diagnostic procedures may also be referred to variously as a *device, system*, or a particular type of device, such as *catheter* or *coil*. Thus, instruments are listed under the type when there are many examples given, and those devices or instruments or machines that do not fit neatly under their own categories are listed under the general term *device* or *imaging* or *system*.

A few main entries with extensive subentries include the following:

aneurysm	fistula	muscle	syndrome
angle	fracture	node	system
artery	image	position	test
bone	imaging	pressure	therapy
canal	imaging agent	projection	tumor
carcinoma	lesion	radiotherapy	tomography
catheter	ligament	scanner	ultrasound
classification	lung	sign	vein
disease	MRI	stent	view

A, a

A (ampere)
AA (ascending aorta)
AAA (abdominal aortic aneurysm)
AAA (anterior apical aneurysm)
AAL (anterior axillary line)
AAS (acute abdominal series)
AAST (American Association for the
    Surgery of Trauma) criteria
ABBI (advanced breast biopsy instru-
    mentation) system
Abbott artery
Abbreviated Injury Scale (AIS)
ABC (aneurysmal bone cyst)
abdomen
    acute
    acute surgical
    boat-shaped
    distended
    nondistended
    postlymphangiography
    postsurgical
    scaphoid
    surgical
abdominal abscess
abdominal aneurysm
abdominal angina
abdominal aorta

abdominal aorta thrombosis
abdominal aortic aneurysm (AAA)
abdominal aortic coarctation
abdominal aortography
abdominal carcinosis
abdominal circumference (AC)
abdominal contents
abdominal distention
abdominal ectopic pregnancy locations
abdominal endometriosis
abdominal hernia
abdominal iron deposition
abdominal mass
abdominal MRI/magnetic resonance
    cholangiopancreatography (MRCP)
abdominal paracentesis, ultrasonic
    guidance for
abdominal part of ureter
abdominal pregnancy
abdominal situs inversus
abdominal vascular accident
abdominal wall abscess
abdominis rectus muscle
abdominopelvic actinomycosis
abdominopelvic CT imaging
abdominopelvic CT scan
abdominopelvic mass

1

abducens (or abducent) nucleus
abducens nerve (sixth cranial nerve)
abduction fracture
abduction stress test
abductor muscle of little finger
abductor muscle of little toe
abductor digiti quinti (ADQ) muscle
abductor hallucis muscle
abductor mechanism
abductor pollicis brevis (APB)
   muscle
abductor pollicis longus (APL)
   muscle
abductovalgus, hallux
ABER (abduction and external rotation)
   position
aberrant
aberrant micturition phenomenon
aberrant right subclavian artery
aberrations, intersegmental
ABI (ankle/brachial index)
ablate
Ablatherm HIFU (high intensity
   focused ultrasound) system
ablation
   direct current (DCA)
   heat
   intraoperative laser
   laser thermal
   open heart endocardial radio-
     frequency
   percutaneous radiofrequency
   percutaneous radiofrequency
     catheter
   percutaneous transluminal septal
     myocardial
   radiofrequency (RF)
   radiofrequency thermal
   radiopharmaceutical
   renal cyst
   saline-enhanced RF tissue
   stereotactic or stereotaxic
   surgical

ablation *(cont.)*
   thermal
   total
   transaortic radiofrequency
   transapical endocardial
   transmural cryoablation
   transseptal radiofrequency
   ultrasound-guided percutaneous
     interstitial laser
ablation lesion
ablation of myocardium
ablative laser therapy
abnormal bowel wall enhancement
abnormal concentration
abnormal intestinal transit time
abnormality
   accumulation
   acral
   Alder-Reilly morphological
   arch of aorta
   augmentation
   bony
   bulbar
   cranial nerve
   cytoarchitectonic
   definitive
   fetal
   figure of 8
   focal
   frontal plane growth
   functional
   gestational sac
   gray matter
   obstructive
   perfusion
   restrictive
   screening-detected
   soft tissue
   subtle
   subtle mural
   torsional
   tracer
   ultrastructural

abnormality *(cont.)*
    white matter
    vasculature
    vessel wall
abnormal mammographic findings
abnormal tubular function
aboral direction
ABR (American Board of Radiology)
Abrikosov tumor
abrupt vessel closure
abruptio placentae (abruption of
    placenta)
abscess (pl. abscesses)
    abdominal
    abdominal wall
    actinomycotic brain
    acute
    adrenal
    amebic liver
    anaerobic lung
    anorectal
    aortic root
    appendiceal
    areolar
    arthrifluent
    Aspergillus cerebral
    atheromatous
    Bartholin gland
    Bezold
    bilateral tubo-ovarian
    bladder
    bone
    brain
    breast
    broad ligament
    Brodie
    Brodie metaphyseal
    bulbourethral gland
    cerebral
    coalescent multiple intrarenal
    collar button
    corpus cavernosum
    Cowper gland

abscess *(cont.)*
    cuff
    daughter
    deep interloop
    deep pelvic
    Douglas
    encapsulated brain
    enteroperitoneal
    epidural
    extradural
    fallopian tube
    fluctuant
    frontal
    gallbladder wall
    gas-forming liver
    growth plate
    hepatic
    horseshoe (in the hand)
    iliopsoas
    interloop
    intermesenteric
    intersphincteric
    intra-abdominal
    intradural
    intrahepatic
    intramesenteric
    intraosseous
    intraperitoneal
    ischiorectal
    kidney
    lesser sac
    Littré gland
    liver
    lung
    mammary
    medullary
    meningeal
    metaphyseal
    midpalmar
    mycobacterial psoas
    nipple
    nonpuerperal breast
    orbital

abscess *(cont.)*
  ovarian
  Paget
  pancreatic
  paracolic
  parametrial
  parametric
  parapharyngeal space
  pararectal
  pararenal
  pelvic
  penile
  perianal
  periappendiceal
  pericecal
  pericolic
  pericolonic
  perinephric
  perirectal
  perirenal
  peritoneal cavity
  peritonsillar
  periurethral
  phoenix
  pituitary
  postoperative
  Pott
  pouch of Douglas
  premammary
  prostatic
  psoas
  pulmonary
  pyogenic liver
  rectal
  retroperitoneal
  retroperitoneal iliopsoas
  retropharyngeal
  scrotal
  serous
  soft tissue
  sperm
  spinal epidural (SEA)
  splenic

abscess *(cont.)*
  subaponeurotic
  subareolar
  subdiaphragmatic
  subdural
  subgaleal
  subhepatic
  submammary
  subperiosteal
  subperiosteal orbital
  subphrenic
  subungual
  suture
  syphilitic
  testicular
  thecal
  thenar space
  tubal rugae
  tubo-ovarian
  urethral
  urethral gland
  vulvar
abscess formation
Abscession fluid drainage catheter
absence
  adenoidal
  congenital
  left liver lobe
  limb
  partial pericardial
  pericardial
  right liver lobe
absence of kidney
absence of right common carotid artery
absence of rugal folds
absence of uptake
absence ("ab-sahnz") seizure
absent aortic knob
absent bow-tie sign
absent pericardium
absent thymus
absolute artery dimensions
absolute emission probability

absolute peak efficiency calibration
absolute scotomata
absorbance
  discrete
  measured
absorbance level
absorbed dose per unit
absorbed dose range
absorbed fraction
absorbed fraction method
absorbency
absorber
absorptiometer
absorptiometry
  double photon (DPA)
  dual x-ray
  single photon (SPA)
  single energy x-ray (SXA)
  x-ray
absorption
  actinide
  bony
  broad beam
  impaired
  linear
  lysosomal (of cartilage in
    rheumatoid arthritis)
  x-ray
absorption cavity
absorption coefficient
absorption of radionuclide
absorptive capacity
absorptive pathways
absorptive pertubation
absorptivity
  dynamic
  molar
abstraction
abut, abutted
abutment
abutment of implant
abutting
AC (abdominal circumference)

AC (acromioclavicular) joint separation
AC (anterior commissure)
AC-PC (anterior commissure-
  posterior commissure)
  AC-PC line
  AC-PC plane
ACA (anterior cerebral artery)
ACA (anterior choroidal artery)
ACAD (atherosclerotic carotid artery
  disease)
acalculous cholecystitis
acanthopelvis
acanthotic lesion
ACAT (automated computed [comput-
  erized] axial tomography)
ACB (asymptomatic carotid bruit)
ACBE (air contrast barium enema)
accelerated acute rejection
accelerated fractionation
accelerated hyperfractionated
  radiotherapy
accelerated peristalsis
acceleration time
accelerator
  alpha particle
  dual energy
  electron linear
  linear
  medical linear
  particle
  Philips linear
  Siemens Mevatron 74 linear
accelerator mass spectrometry (AMS)
accentuation of markings
access
  blind
  transpedicular
  vascular
accessible lesion
accessory atlantoaxial ligament
accessory bones
accessory cardiac bronchus
accessory fallopian tube

accessory hemiazygos vein
accessory hepatic artery
accessory lobe, hepatic
accessory lung
accessory nerve
accessory organ
accessory ossification centre
accessory ovary
accessory pancreatic duct
accessory renal artery
accident
  cardiovascular
  cerebrovascular (CVA)
  vascular
accidental correction
accordion sign on CT scan of colon
accidental hemorrhage
Accucore II core biopsy needle used in
  ultrasound
accuDEXA bone densitometry
accuDEXA bone mineral density
  assessment device
Accu-Flo CSF reservoir
Accu-Flo ventricular catheter
accumulation
  abnormal tracer
  dependent extracellular fluid
  fluid
  gas
  noninflammatory fluid (in pleural
    cavity)
  parenchymal tracer
  residual urine
  tracer
accumulation of air in interlobar
  spaces
accumulation of gas
Accu-Vu sizing catheter
ACE (angiotensin-converting enzyme)
  inhibitor
ACE fixed-wire balloon catheter
ACE inhibition scintigraphy
ace of spades sign on angiogram

acetabular angle of Sharp
acetabular bone
acetabular cup
  cemented Lubinus
  cemented Reflection
  uncemented Reflection
  uncemented Trilogy
acetabular depth to femoral head
  diameter (AD/FHD)
acetabular dysplasia
acetabular fossa
acetabular fracture
  anterior column
  anterior column with posterior
    hemitransverse
  anterior wall
  both column
  posterior column
  posterior column with posterior wall
  posterior wall
  transverse
  transverse with posterior wall
  T-shaped
acetabular head index (AHI)
acetabular index
acetabular labrum
acetabular line
acetabular notch
acetabular osteolysis
acetabular rim
acetabular roof
acetabular roof obliquity angle
acetabular teardrop figure
acetabuli, os
acetabulum (pl. acetabula)
  cup-shaped
  deep-shelled
  dish-shaped
  dysplastic
  egg-shaped congruous
  saucer-shaped
acetazolamide (Diamox) challenge test
acetazolamide-enhanced SPECT

acetylation
acetylcholine receptor antibody
(AChRab)
ACF (anterior cervical fusion)
ACG (angiocardiogram)
ACG (apexcardiogram, apexcardiography)
ACh (acetylcholine) receptor
achalasia
classic
cricopharyngeal
esophageal
pelvirectal
sphincteral
ureteral
vigorous
Achiever balloon dilatation catheter
Achilles bulge sign
Achilles bursa
Achilles+ ultrasound bone densitometer
Achilles tendon (tendo Achillis)
achillodynia
achlorhydria, gastric
achlorhydric
acholic stool
achondrogenesis
achondroplasia
achondroplastic dwarfism
AChR (acetylcholine receptor)
antibody
AChRab (acetylcholine receptor
antibody)
acid
DTPA (diethylenetriamine
pentaacetic)
low dose folinic
acid aspiration
acid aspiration pneumonitis
acidophilic pituitary tumor
acinar cell carcinoma
acinar-like
acinus, pulmonary

ACIS (adenocarcinoma in situ)
ACJ (acromioclavicular joint)
Ackerman criteria for osteomyelitis
Ackrad balloon-bearing catheter
ACL (anterior cruciate ligament)
ACM (automated cardiac flow measurement) ultrasound technology
ACMI ulcer measuring device
ACoA (anterior communicating artery)
Acolysis ultrasound intravascular
thrombolysis system
Acoma scanner
acoprosis
acoprous
acorn catheter tip
acorn-tipped catheter
acoustically induced rupture of
membranes
acoustical shadowing (in ultrasonography)
acoustic artifact
acoustic backscatter characteristics of
blood
acoustic crest
acoustic cyst
acoustic impedance
acoustic interface
acoustic microscope, scanning
acoustic nerve
acoustic nerve tumor
acoustic neurinoma
acoustic neuroma
acoustic papilla
acoustic quantification, left ventricular
ejection fraction
acoustic radiation
acoustic reflection method
acoustic schwannoma
acoustic shadow
acoustic trauma
acoustic tubercle
acoustic vesicle
acoustic window

acquired disease
acquired diverticulum
acquired lesion
acquired toxoplasmosis
acquired tracheobronchomalacia
acquired unilateral hyperlucent lung
acquired ventricular septal defect
(AVSD)
acquisition
  automated data
  data
  double helix
  ECT
  image
  multiphase
  multiple gated (MUGA)
  multisection multirepetition
  multislice
  segmented volume
  sequential image
  spirometric
  volume
acquisition matrix
acquisition technique
acquisition time
acral abnormality
Acrel ganglion
acrocephalopolysyndactyly
acrocephalosyndactyly
acrodysostosis
acrodysplasia
acrofacial dysostosis
acromegaly
acromelic dysplasia
acromesomelic dysplasia
acromial angle
acromial bone
acromioclavicular (AC) joint (ACJ)
acromiocoracoid ligament
acromiohumeral interval (AHI)
acromiothoracic artery
acro-osteolysis
  idiopathic phalangeal
  mutilating

acropachy
acropectorovertebral dysplasia
acrosyndactyly
ACR teleradiology standard
ACS (Advanced Cardiovascular
  Systems)
  ACS anchor exchange device
  ACS Endura coronary dilation
    catheter
  ACS Hi-Torque Balance middle-
    weight guidewire
  ACS JL4 (Judkins left 4) French
    catheter
  ACS Mini catheter
  ACS Multilink coronary stent
  ACS OTW (over the wire) Photon
    coronary dilatation catheter
  ACS OTW Lifestream coronary
    dilatation catheter
  ACS RX (rapid exchange) Comet
    coronary dilatation catheter
  ACS RX Multi-Link stent
  ACS SULP II balloon
  ACS Tourguide II guiding catheter
ACTH (adrenocorticotrophic
  hormone) antibody
  ACTH independent hyperplasia
  ACTH-producing pituitary
    adenoma
  ACTH-producing pituitary tumor
actinium
actinomycosis
  abdominopelvic
  retroperitoneal
actinomycotic brain abscess
active biplanar MR imaging guidance
active emptying fraction (left atrium)
active tracking
activity
  focal epileptiform
  interhemispheric tracer
  specific
AcuNav ultrasound catheter

Acuson Aspen ultrasound system
Acuson computed sonography
Acuson linear array transducer
Acuson 128EP imager
Acuson 128XP ultrasound system
Acuson transvaginal sonography
acutance, image edge profile
acute abdominal series
acute abscess
acute avulsion fracture
acute basilar artery thrombosis
acute cholecystitis
acute compartment syndrome
acute coronary insufficiency
AcuTect (technetium Tc 99m apcitide)
acute fibrinous pleurisy
acute inhalational injury
acute interstitial pneumonitis
acute lung injury (ALI)
acute mesenteric artery occlusion
acute myocardial infarction (AMI)
acute phase gene expression
acute pneumonia
acute pyelonephritis
acute renal failure (ARF)
acute respiratory distress syndrome,
   asymmetric
acute tubular necrosis (ATN)
acute urethral edema
AD (Alzheimer disease)
AD (aortic diameter)
adactyly (adactylia)
adamantinoma of the long bones
adamantinoma, pituitary
adamantinomatous craniopharyngioma
Adamkiewicz artery
Adams modification of Hermodsson
   view
adaptive array detector
adaptive frame averaging
ADC (analog to digital) conversion
   quantization error
ADC (apparent diffusion coefficient)
   mapping

Addison point
additive white gaussian noise distortion
Add-On Bucky digital x-ray image
   acquisition system
Add-On Bucky imaging device
adduct
adduction fracture
adduction to neutral
adductor canal
adductor hiatus
adductor magnus
adductor sweep of thumb
adductor tubercle
adductus
   metatarsus (MTA)
   true metatarsus (TMA)
adenocarcinoma
   annular
   colloid
   exophytic
   giant cell
   infiltrating
   metastatic
   papillary
   peripheral lung
   scirrhous
   ulcerating
adenocarcinoma in situ (ACIS; AIS)
adenocarcinoma of the urachus
adenocyst
adenohypophysial
adenohypophysis
adenoidal absence
adenolymphoma, Warthin
adenoma
   acidophilic
   acinous
   ACTH-producing pituitary
   adrenal
   aldosterone-producing
   basophilic
   benign liver
   bile duct (BDA)

adenoma *(cont.)*
  breast
  bronchial
  carcinoma ex pleomorphic
  chromophobic
  colonic
  colorectal
  cutaneous
  duodenal
  eosinophilic
  esophageal
  fibroid
  gallbladder
  gastric
  glycoprotein-secreting
  gonadotropin-secreting
  hepatic
  hepatocellular (HCA)
  intraspinal
  lactating
  liver cell
  malignant pleomorphic
  moderately differentiated
  mucinous
  nephrogenic
  null cell
  pancreatic
  papillary
  parotid pleomorphic
  pituitary
  pleomorphic
  poorly differentiated
  prolactin-producing
  prolactin-secreting
  prostatic
  renal
  renal cortical
  sebaceum
  sessile
  small bowel
  suprasellar
  toxic
  tubular

adenoma *(cont.)*
  tubulovillous
  undifferentiated
  villoglandular
  villous
  well-differentiated
adenoma sebaceum
adenomatoid malformation
adenomatoid metaplasia, urethral
adenomatoid oviduct tumor
adenomatoid (adenomatous) tumor
  bladder
  testicular
  urethral
adenomatoid tumor of the epididymis
adenomatosis
  multiple endocrine
  pancreatic
adenomatous hyperplasia (AH)
  hepatic
  prostatic
adenomatous hyperplasia of the gallbladder
adenomatous polyposis coli
adenomyoma, polypoid
adenomyomatosis
adenomyosis
  diffuse
  uterine
adenomyotic cyst
adenopapillomatosis, gastric
adenopathy
  associated
  carcinomatous
  groin
  intramammary
  intrathoracic
  mediastinal
  mesenteric
  peripancreatic
  peripheral
  periportal
  retroperitoneal
  subcarinal

adenosarcoma
  ovarian
  uterine
Adenoscan (adenosine injection) imaging agent
adenosine echocardiography
adenosine-induced stress
adenosine triphosphate (ATP)-sensitive potassium channel openers
adenosis
  blunt duct
  florid
  sclerosing
adenovirus, enteric
AD/FHD (acetabular depth to femoral head diameter)
adherent thrombus
adhesed
adhesio interthalamica
adhesion
adhesive endometriosis
adhesive, pleurisy
ADI (atlanto-dens interval)
adiabatic demagnetization
adiabatic fast passage
adiabatic off-resonance spin-locking
adiabatic RF (radiofrequency) pulses
adiabatic slice selective RF pulses
adiadochokinesia
adipose ligament
adipose tissue
adiposis dolorosa
adiposogenital dystrophy
aditus pelvis
adjacent soft tissue mass
adjacent structure
adjacent voxels
adjunct hypnosis with sedation
adjunctive test
adjunctive therapy
adjuvant hypofractionated conformal radiation therapy
adjuvant radiation therapy

adjuvant therapy
adnexa (*not* adnexae)
adnexal masses
adnexal space
adnexa uteri inflammation
adolescent hallux valgus
adolescent idiopathic scoliosis (AIS)
ADQ (abductor digiti quinti) muscle
ADR ultrasound
adrenal abscess
adrenal adenoma
adrenalectomy, laparoscopic
adrenal hemorrhage
adrenal cortical adenoma
adrenal gland
adrenal hyperandrogenism
adrenal hyperplasia
adrenal imaging MIBG (meta-iodobenzylguanidine)
adrenal medulla
adrenal medullary hyperplasia
adrenal scintiscanning
adrenal tuberculosis
adrenogenital syndrome
ADR Ultramark 4 ultrasound
adult respiratory distress syndrome (ARDS)
adumbration
advanced breast biopsy instrumentation (ABBI) system
advanced metastasis
advanced real-time motion analysis (ARTMA)
advanced cortical disease
Advanced NMR Systems scanner
Advantx LC+ cardiovascular imaging system
adventitia
adventitious bursa
adynamic ileus
AE (above elbow) amputation
AE (angiographic embolization)
AEG (acute erosive gastritis)

Aeon vascular access port
Aestiva/5 MRI anesthesia machine
AER (apical ectodermal ridge)
aerate, aerated
aeration
aerophagia
aerosol ventilation study
aerosolized technetium Tc 99m DTPA
   evaluation
aerosolized technetium Tc 99m PYP
AF (arcuate fasciculus)
A-FAIR (arrhythmia-insensitive flow-
   sensitive alternating inversion
   recovery) imaging
AFBG (aortofemoral bypass graft)
afferent digital nerve
afferent loop
afferent vessels of kidney
afferent view
affix, affixed
AFI (amniotic fluid index)
afterglow
afterloader
afterloading (see also *brachytherapy*)
   high dose rate
   192I high dose rate remote
   remote
afterloading brachytherapy
AFV (amniotic fluid volume)
AG (angular gyrus)
aganglionic segment of colon
AGC (anatomically graduated
   component)
age
   bone
   chronologic
   gestational
   menstrual
AGE (acute gastroenteritis)
AGE (angle of greatest extension)
age-based standards
agenesis
   callosal
   corpus callosum

agenesis *(cont.)*
   lung
   renal
   sacral
   uterine
   vaginal
agenetic fracture
agent (see also *imaging agent;*
      implant; radiotherapy agent)
   cardioselective
   cyanocobalamin radioactive
   Eaton agent pneumonia
   effervescent
   Embol-78 liquid embolic
   ethylene vinyl alcohol copolymer
      thrombotic
   glomerular filtration
   inhaled oxygen brain MR contrast
   intra-arterial injection of water-
      soluble iodinated contrast
   intratumoral
   magnetic resonance receptor
   neurotropic MR imaging contrast
   oral contrast
   perfusion
   radioactive cancer-specific targeting
   radiotherapeutic
   radiotherapy
   renal cortical isotope scanning
   reticuloendothelial contrast
   rose bengal sodium 131I radioactive
      biliary
   time activity curve of contrast
AGF (angle of greatest flexion)
Agfa CR system
Agfa Medical scanner
Agfa PACS system
aggregated albumin with technetium
   Tc 99m (albumin, aggregated [with
   technetium Tc 99m])
aggregated follicle
aggregated iodinated 131I serum
   albumin (albumin, iodinated I 131
   human serum)

aggregated lymphatic follicle
aggressive angiomyxoma
aggressive angiomyxoma tumor
aglutition
agonist muscle groups
agyria
ahaustral
AHI (acetabular head index)
AHI (acromiohumeral interval)
Ahlback method (weightbearing knee
   in full extension)
Ahlback view of knee in full extension
AH (adenomatous hyperplasia) nodule
AHO (acute hematogenous osteomyelitis)
AICA (anterior inferior cerebellar
   artery)
AICA (anterior inferior cerebral
   artery)
AICA ("i'-ka") (anterior inferior
   communicating artery)
Aicardi syndrome
AICS (artery of inferior cavernous
   sinus)
AIDS dementia complex (ADC)
AI 5200 diagnostic ultrasound system
air
   bowel loop
   colonic
   free
   intracranial
   intramural colonic
   intraorbital
   intraperitoneal
   pleural cavity
   subcutaneous
air arthrography
air block syndrome
air bolus
air bronchogram
air bronchogram sign
air bubble filling defect
air cavity

air cisternography
air column, corrugated
air conditioner lung
air-containing microbubbles
air contrast barium enema (ACBE)
air crescent sign
air cyst
air cystogram
air density
air embolism
AIREN (Association Internationale
   pour la Recherche et l'Enseigne-
   ment en Neurosciences)
air encephalography
air enema
air enema fluoroscopic imaging
air exchange
air-filled lungs
air-fluid level
Airis II open MRI system
air gap
air hunger
air inflation
air insufflation
air interface on x-ray
air leak
airless lung
airlessness, alveolar
air luminogram
air meniscus sign
air myelogram
air plethysmography
air pocket
air sac
air space
   apical
   terminal
air space consolidation
air space disease
air space opacity
air space pattern metastases
air tissue interface
air trapping, localized

airway fluoroscopy
airway inflammation
airway opening pressure
airway narrowing
airway obstruction
airway opening
airway pressure
airways disease, reversible
airways tuberculosis
airway trees
AIS (Abbreviated Injury Scale)
AIS (adenocarcinoma in situ)
AIS (adolescent idiopathic scoliosis)
Aitken classification of epiphyseal
  fracture
AIUM (American Institute of
  Ultrasound in Medicine)
AJC (ankle joint complex)
Ajmalin liver injury
AK (above knee) amputation (AKA)
Akerlund deformity
akinetic posterior wall
akinetic segmental wall motion
ala (pl. alae)
  nasal
  sacral
ala cerebelli
ala magna
Alagille syndrome
Alanson amputation
ALARA (as low as reasonably achiev-
  able)
alar bone
alar ligament
Albers-Schönberg (Schoenberg)
  disease
Albers-Schönberg marble bones
Albers-Schönberg view (of temporomandibular joint)
Albright-McCune-Sternberg syndrome
Albunex ultrasound imaging agent
  (human albumin, sonicated)

albumin
  aggregated
  aggregated iodinated ^{131}I serum
  chromated ^{51}Cr serum
  human serum
  macroaggregated (MAA)
  normal human serum
  radioactive iodinated serum (RISA)
  sonicated
  technetated aggregated human
  technetium ^{99m}Tc
albumin microspheres
Alcock canal
alcohol embolization
alcoholic cirrhosis of liver
alcoholic liver disease (ALD)
alcoholic pneumonia
alcohol sclerotherapy
ALD (alcoholic liver disease)
Alder-Reilly morphological
  abnormality
aldosterone-producing adenoma
aldosteronoma
Alexander disease
Alexander method for viewing optic
  canal
Alexander stress view (acromioclavicular joint)
algebraic reconstruction technique
  (ART)
algorithm
  annealing
  bioeffects
  block uniform resampling (BURS)
  clustering
  cone-beam reconstruction
  contour-following
  Cooley-Tukey fast Fourier trans-
    form alignment
  correlation (CR)
  decryption
  defuzzification
  DIP

algorithm *(cont.)*
  document-recognition
  dual lookup table
  dynamic range control (DRC)
  edge-enhanced error diffusion
  edge-enhancing
  encryption
  Feldkamp
  Fermi-Eyges-Hogstrom (FEH)
  fringe thinning
  histogram equalization
  image restoration
  interpolation
  iterative
  JPEG (joint photographic experts
    group)
  K-means clustering
  least squares (LS)
  lossy
  mapping
  maximum likelihood
  memory intensive
  mensuration
  MIP (maximum intensity
    projection)
  Monte Carlo
  neural evaluation
  pixel-oriented
  quantizer design
  Ramesh and Pramod
  reconstruction
  SSD (shaded surface display)
  3D elastic subtraction
  wavelet scalar quantization (WSQ)
  word segmentation
  z-interpolation
ALI (acute lung injury)
alias artifact
aliasing (wraparound ghosting)
  artifact
aliasing phenomenon in Doppler studies
aliasing, temporal
alien hand sign

alignment
  anatomic
  angular
  field
  fracture fragment
  integrity and
  leaf
  rotational
  torsional
  transverse-plane
  vertebral body
alignment and registration of 3D
  images
alimentary canal
alimentary system
alimentary tract
alkaline reflux gastritis
ALL (anterior longitudinal ligament)
Allen-Brown shunt
Allen-Brown vascular access shunt
allergic airway inflammation
allergic fungal sinusitis
allergic pneumonia
allergy, latex
Allis sign of fracture of the femoral
  neck
Allman classification of acromioclavicular injury
allocortex
allodynia
alloesthesia
allogenic marrow transplantation
allogenous bone graft
alloy
  cobalt-chromium
  stainless steel
  Ti-Nidium
  Ti6A14V
  Wood
All-Tronics scanner
Aloka color Doppler system for blood
  flow imaging
Aloka echocardiograph machine

Aloka linear scanner
Aloka sector scanner
Aloka SSD ultrasound system
AL-1 catheter
Alouette amputation
Alpers disease
alpha decay
alpha index
alpha motor neuron
alpha particle bombardment
alpha particle emitter
alpha radiation
alpha ray
ALS (amyotrophic lateral sclerosis),
 carcinomatous
ALSVs (arm and lesser saphenous
 veins)
Altaire high-field-performance open
 MR imaging system
alta, patella
alteration in blood-brain barrier
alterations
 bilateral
 hemodynamic
 subtle structural
alternator, film
altitudinal anopsia
altitudinal hemianopsia
Altropane ^{123}I-based radioimaging
 agent
Altschul view
alveolar bone fracture
alveolar clouding
alveolar consolidative process
alveolar echinococcosis
alveolar edema
alveolar hemorrhage
alveolar infiltrate
alveolar opacities
alveolar proteinosis
alveolar rhabdomyosarcoma
alveolar sarcoid
alveolar soft part sarcoma (ASPS)

alveolate
alveoli proliferation
alveolus (pl. alveoli)
 maxillary
 pulmonary
Alzate catheter
Alzheimer disease (AD)
Alzheimer neurofibrillary degeneration
Alzheimer-type, senile dementia
 (SDAT)
AMA-Fab scintigraphy
amaurosis
 central
 cerebral
 uremic
amaurosis fugax
ambient air
ambient cistern
ambilevosity
ambilevous
amblyaphia
ambulant
ambulant venous pressure (AVP)
ambulatory equilibrium angiocardiography
AME (American Medical Electronics)
AME (Austin Medical Equipment)
amebiasis (see *amoebiasis*)
amebic abscess
amebic pneumonia
ameboma
amelia
amenorrhea
amentia
American Association for the Surgery
 of Trauma (AAST)
American Board of Radiology (ABR)
American Institute of Ultrasound in
 Medicine (AIUM)
American Registry of Diagnostic
 Medical Sonographers (ARDMS)
American Roentgen Ray Society
 (ARRS)

American Shared-CuraCare scanner
American Society of Radiologic
   Technologists (ASRT)
americium (Am) radioactive source
ameroid occluder
AMI (acute myocardial infarction)
AMI 121 imaging agent
amine
   basophilic
   macrolytic
AML (amyotrophic lateral sclerosis)
AML (anterior mitral leaflet)
AML (angiomyolipoma) solid renal
   tumor
Ammon horn (mesial temporal)
   sclerosis
amniocentesis, ultrasonic guidance for
amniotic fluid
amniotic fluid index (AFI)
amniotic fluid volume (AFV)
amniotic sac
A-mode echocardiography
A-mode encephalography
A-mode ultrasound
amorphous collection of contrast
amorphous silicon flat-panel detector
Amoss sign
ampere (A)
amphetamine precursor
Amplatz catheter
Amplatzer ductal occluder
Amplatz Teflon-coated guidewire
amplification
   image contrast
   multiscale image contrast
      (MUSICA)
   noise
   signal
amplifier
   linear
   radiofrequency (RF) power
amplitude asymmetry
amplitude image

amplitude limits
amplitude modulation
ampulla of Vater
ampulla, rectal
ampullary carcinoma
ampullar tube ectopic pregnancy
   locations
ampulloma
amputation
   above elbow (AE)
   above knee (AK, AKA)
   Alanson
   Alouette
   Béclard
   below knee (BK, BKA)
   Berger interscapular
   Bier
   Boyd ankle
   Bunge
   Burgess below knee
   button toe
   Callander
   Carden
   chop
   Chopart
   Chopart hindfoot
   circular supracondylar
   closed flap
   complete
   congenital
   digital
   femoral head
   fingertip
   fishmouth
   forearm
   forefoot digital
   forequarter
   Gritti-Stokes distal thigh
   guillotine
   Hey
   hindquarter
   incomplete
   index ray

amputation *(cont.)*
  interinnominoabdominal
  interphalangeal
  interscapular
  interscapulothoracic
  Jaboulay
  Kirk distal thigh
  Le Fort
  Lisfranc
  midthigh
  nonreplantable
  one-stage
  Pirogoff
  ray
  replantable
  supramalleolar open
  Syme
  Syme ankle disarticulation
  Teale
  toe
  transcarpal
  transcondylar
  translumbar
  transmetatarsal (TMA)
  traumatic
  two-stage
  Vladimiroff-Mikulicz
amputation neuroma
amputation stump
AMS (accelerator mass spectrometry)
AMT-25-enhanced MR images
amu (atomic mass unit)
amygdala of cerebellum
amygdala-hippocampal complex
amygdalofugal pathway
amygdaloid area
amygdaloid nuclear complex
amyloid arthropathy
amyloid disease
amyloidoma
amyostatic syndrome
amyotonia congenita
amyotrophic lateral sclerosis (ALS)

anaerobic lung abscess
anaglyph glasses
anal atresia
anal bulging
anal column
anal crypt
anal dilatation
anal endosonography
anal fissure
anal prolapse
anal protrusion
anal sphincter laceration
anal stricture
anal trauma
anal verge
analog
  adenosine
  dysprosium
  L-arginine
  tamoxifen
analog to digital (ADC) conversion
  quantization error
analog to digital converter
analogous
analogue (see *analog*)
analysis
  activation
  advanced real-time motion
    (ARTMA)
  biomechanical
  cephalometric
  Cerenkov scintillation
  clinicopathological
  correlation
  deconvolution
  diagnostic efficacy
  digital frequency
  discriminant
  duplex ultrasound
  eigenvector
  electro-oculographic
  fission track (of urine)
  flow cytometry DNA

analysis *(cont.)*
   focal and diffuse lung texture
   folding-potential
   footprint
   fractal
   Fourier
   fractional volumetric
   gamma spectrometric
   histogram
   kinetic parameter
   late effect
   liquid scintillation
   multi-elemental neuron activation
   multispectral
   neutron activation
   nuclide
   phase
   planimetric
   pole figure texture
   power spectral (PSA)
   prospective
   pulse height spectral
   quantitative
   range-gated Doppler spectral flow
   regression
   residual stress
   risk
   Sassouni
   self-organizing mapping (SOM)
   signal
   sonographic feature
   spectral wave
   spinographic
   stepwise regression
   teboroxime resting washout (TRW)
   thin film
   total body neutron activation
     (TBNAA)
   volume
   volumetric
analyzer
   automated cerebral blood flow
   DMI (Diagnostic Medical
     Instruments)

analyzer *(cont.)*
   Medigraphics
   multichannel
anaplastic astrocytoma
anaplastic glioma
anaplastic Wilms tu mor
anastomosis (pl. anastomoses)
   (anatomical or surgical)
   aorta to vein
   aortic
   aorticopulmonary or aorto-
     pulmonary
   arterio-arterial
   arteriolovenularis
   arteriovenous
   ascending aorta to pulmonary
     artery
   beveled
   bidirectional cavopulmonary
   Billroth II
   cavopulmonary
   cobra-head
   coiling of
   colocolic
   diamond
   diamond-shaped
   dilatation of
   distal
   embryonic
   end to end
   end to side portacaval
   extradural
   extrapericardial
   glomeriform arteriovenous
   heterocladic
   homocladic
   ileal pouch-anal
   ileorectal
   intercavernous
   intercoronary
   internal mammary artery to
     coronary artery
   intradural

anastomosis *(cont.)*
  intrapericardial
  laser-assisted microvascular
    (LAMA)
  left pulmonary artery to
    descending aorta
  LIMA (left internal mammary
    artery)
  mesocaval
  microvascular
  outflow
  portacaval
  portosystemic
  precapillary
  proximal
  pyeloileocutaneous
  right atrium to pulmonary artery
  right internal mammary artery
  right pulmonary artery to
    ascending aorta
  right subclavian to pulmonary
    artery
  Roux-en-Y
  side to end
  side to side
  simple arteriovenous
  splenorenal
  superior vena cava to distal right
    pulmonary artery
  superior vena cava to pulmonary
    artery
  systemic to pulmonary artery
  tendon
  terminoterminal
  tracheal
  transureteroureteral
  ureteroileocutaneous
  ureteroureteral
  uterovaginal
  vascular
anastomotic defect
anastomotic disruption
anastomotic leakage

anastomotic pseudoaneurysm
anastomotic site
anastomotic stoma
anastomotic stricture
anatomic alignment
anatomic distribution
anatomic landmarks
anatomic moment erratum
anatomic neck
anatomic position
anatomic snuffbox
anatomic survey
anatomic variability
anatomic variant
anatomical dead space
anatomical snuffbox
anatomically dominant
anatomy
  anomalous
  distorted
  left-dominant coronary
  medullary venous
  right-dominant coronary
  Saltzman
  sectional
  segmental
Anatrast (barium sulfate) imaging
  agent
anconeal fossa (also anconal fossa)
anconeus
anconoid
Ancure EZ Path catheter sheath
ancyroid cavity (also ankyroid)
Anderson-Hutchins tibial fracture
androgen-secreting tumor
android pelvis
anechoic area
anechoic center
anechoic fluid collection
anemic infarct
anencephaly
anesthesia
anesthetic

aneuploid tumor
aneurysm (also *pseudoaneurysm*)
  abdominal
  abdominal aortic (AAA)
  acquired
  ampullary
  anastomotic
  anterior apical (AAA)
  aortic
  aortic arch
  aortic sinus
  aortic sinusal
  aortoiliac
  arterial
  arteriosclerotic
  arteriovenous
  arteriovenous pulmonary
  ascending
  ascending aortic
  aspergillotic
  atherosclerotic
  atrial septal
  axillary
  bacterial
  basilar artery
  basilar tip
  berry
  berry intracranial
  bland aortic
  brachiocephalic arterial
  brain
  bulge of
  bulging
  calcified wall of
  cardiac
  carotid artery
  cavernous carotid
  cavernous sinus
  cavity of
  cerebral
  cerebral mycotic
  circle of Willis
  circumscript

aneurysm *(cont.)*
  cirsoid
  clinoid
  clip ligation of
  clipping of
  coating of
  coiling of
  compound
  congenital
  congenital aortic sinus
  congenital arteriosclerotic
  congenital cerebral
  contained leak of aortic
  coronary artery
  coronary vessel
  cranial
  cylindroid
  de novo
  debulking of
  descending thoracic
  dilatation of
  dissecting
  dissecting abdominal
  dissecting aortic
  dissecting intracranial
  distal aortic arch
  dome of
  ductal
  ectatic
  eggshell border of
  embolic
  extracerebral
  extracranial
  false
  feeding artery of
  fundus of
  fusiform
  giant
  great cerebral vein of Galen
  hematoma of
  hemorrhage of
  hernial
  hunterian ligation of

aneurysm *(cont.)*
 imperforate
 infected
 infrarenal abdominal aortic
 innominate
 internal carotid artery
 intracerebral
 intracranial
 intramural coronary artery
 isthmus
 juxtarenal
 juxtarenal aortic
 late false
 lateral
 left ventricular
 luetic aortic
 M1 segment
 miliary
 mixed
 mural
 mycotic
 mycotic intracranial
 mycotic suprarenal
 neck of
 neoplastic
 nodular
 orbital
 pararenal aortic
 pelvic
 phthisis of
 PICA (posterior inferior cerebellar
  artery)
 PICA (posterior inferior communicating artery)
 popliteal
 postcatheterization false (PCFP)
 posterior communicating artery
 posterior inferior communicating
  artery (PICA)
 postinfarction ventricular
 precursor sign to rupture of
 prerupture of
 pulmonary arteriovenous

aneurysm *(cont.)*
 pulmonary artery compression
  ascending aorta
 pulmonary artery mycotic
 racemose
 rebleeding of
 renal
 renal artery
 rerupture of
 ruptured
 ruptured atherosclerotic
 ruptured intracranial
 sacciform
 saccular
 sacculated
 sac of
 serpentine
 Shekelton
 sinus of Valsalva
 spindle-shaped
 spontaneous infantile ductal
 spurious
 subclavian
 suprarenal
 suprasellar
 syphilitic
 thoracic
 thoracic aorta
 thoracoabdominal
 thoracoabdominal aortic
 thrombosed
 thrombotic
 trapping of
 traumatic
 traumatic intracranial (TICA)
 true
 tubular
 unruptured
 uterine cirsoid
 Valsalva sinus
 varicose
 varix of
 vein of

aneurysm *(cont.)*
  venous
  ventricular
  ventricular septal
  verminous
  wall of
  wide-neck bifurcation
  windsock
  worm
aneurysmal bone cyst (ABC)
aneurysmal lesion
aneurysmal sac
aneurysmal widening of the aorta
aneurysmectomy, off-pump
angel wing
angel wing sign
AngeLase combined mapping-laser
  probe
Angelchik ring prosthesis
Anger gamma camera
Anger-type scintillation camera
Anghelescu sign
angioarchitecture
angiocardiogram (ACG)
angiocardiographically
angiocardiography (see *angiography*)
angiocatheter (see *catheter*)
angiodysplastic lesion
angiofibroblastic proliferation
angiogenic burden
angiogram (see *angiography*)
angiographically confirmed
angiographically occult intracranial
  vascular malformation (AOIVM)
angiographically occult vessel
angiographically overlapping structures
angiographic catheter
angiographic embolization (AE)
angiographic finding
angiographic gap at site of injury
angiographic string sign
angiographic targeting
angiographic variceal embolization

Angiografin imaging agent
angiogram suite
angiography (also angiogram) (see
  also *angiocardiogram*)
  adrenal
  ambulatory equilibrium
  aortic arch
  aortic root
  balloon occlusion pulmonary
  biplane
  biplane left ventricular
  biplane orthogonal
  black blood magnetic resonance
  blood pool radionuclide
  blush of dye on
  bolus chase three-dimensional MR
    digital subtraction
  Brown-Dodge method for
  cardiac
  cardiac gated MR
  carotid
  celiac
  cerebral
  cine
  cine coronary
  computed tomographic (CTA)
  computerized tomographic hepatic
    (CTHA)
  contrast
  coronary
  CT pulmonary
  cystic duct
  deep-inspiration CT
  diagnostic
  digital subtraction (DSA)
  digital subtraction cerebral
  digital subtraction pulmonary
  digital subtraction rotational
  directional color (DCA)
  dobutamine thallium
  DSA (digital subtraction)
  dynamic tagging MR

angiography *(cont.)*
  ECG-gated reconstructed multi-
    detector row CT coronary
  ECG-synchronized digital subtraction
  elastic subtraction spiral CT
  electrocardiogram-synchronized
    digital subtraction
  electron beam angiography of
    coronary arteries
  elliptic centric contrast-enhanced
    magnetic resonance
  Epistar subtraction
  equilibrium radionuclide
  first pass nuclide rest and exercise
  first pass radionuclide exercise
  fluorescein
  FluoroPlus
  four-vessel cerebral
  free-breathing black-blood coronary
    MR
  free-breathing three-dimensional
  gated blood pool
  gated equilibrium radionuclide
  gated nuclear
  gated radionuclide
  high-spatial-resolution contrast-
    enhanced MR
  ICG (indocyanine green) fluorescein
  IDIS (intraoperative digital
    subtraction)
  indocyanine green
  innominate
  Integris 3-D rotational
  intercostal artery
  internal carotid
  intra-arterial digital subtraction
    (IADSA)
  intra-arterial DSA (digital
    subtraction)
  intravascular signal intensity in MR
  intravenous DSA (digital subtraction)
  intravenous fluorescein (IVFA)
  Judkins coronary

angiography *(cont.)*
  left ventricular
  magnetic resonance (MRA)
  mesenteric
  mesenteric CT
  nonselective
  nontriggered phase-contrast MR
  pancreatic
  multi-injection time-resolved MR
  multislab and cine techniques for
    single breath-hold cardiac-
    synchronized
  multislice computed tomographic
    (MSCTA)
  nonenhanced true FISP MR
  peripheral
  peripheral MR
  phase-contrast
  postangioplasty
  postembolization
  postoperative
  post-tourniquet occlusion
  preoperative
  PTCA coronary
  pulmonary
  pulmonary artery wedge
  pulmonary vein wedge
  pulmonary wedge
  radionuclide (RNA)
  renal
  rest and exercise gated nuclear
  retrograde
  RI (resistive index)
  segmented k-space time of flight
    MR
  Seldinger
  selective
  selective coronary cine
  selective ovarian vein
  selective presaturation MR
  selective renal artery
  shaded-surface display (SSD) CT
  single plane

angiography *(cont.)*
  SIR
  sitting-up view
  small angle-double incidence
    (SADIA)
  spinal
  STAR
  stepping-table gadolinium-enhanced
    digital subtraction MR
  stereotactic cerebral
  superselective
  three-compartment wrist
  three-dimensional (3D or 3-D)
  3D CE (three-dimensional
    contrast-enhanced) magnetic
    resonance
  3D contrast-enhanced MR (3D
    CEMRA)
  3DFT magnetic resonance
  3D gadolinium-enhanced MR
  3D gadolinium-enhanced
    subtracted MR
  3D inflow MR
  3D helical CT
  3D phase contrast MR (3D-PCA)
  time of flight (TOF)
  transseptal
  transvenous digital subtraction
  tumor blush on
  venous
  ventricular
  vertebral
  visceral
  velocity encoding on brain MR
angiography suite
angiolipoma (see also *angiomyolipoma*)
  breast
  littoral cell
  spinal
angioma
  arteriovenous
  cavernous
  cutaneous

angioma *(cont.)*
  intracranial cavernous
  intradermal
  venous
angiomatosis, cystic
Angiomat 6000 contrast delivery system
Angiomedics catheter
angiomyolipoma (AML), multifocal
    (see also *angiolipoma*)
angiomyxoma, aggressive
angiomyxoma tumor
angioparalytic blockade
angioplastic meningioma
angioplasty
  balloon
  boot-strap two-vessel
  color duplex ultrasound-guided
  percutaneous transluminal
  coronary artery
  carotid (with stenting)
  coronary balloon
  cutting balloon percutaneous
    transluminal
  Dotter-Judkins technique for
    percutaneous transluminal
  excimer laser coronary (ELCA)
  femoropopliteal
  Grüntzig (Gruentzig) balloon
    catheter
  iliac artery
  LAIS excimer laser for coronary
    laser
  laser balloon
  laser thermal
  laser thermal coronary
  laser-assisted balloon (LABA)
  microwave thermal balloon
  multilesion
  multivessel
  one-vessel
  patch
  patch-graft
  percutaneous laser

angioplasty *(cont.)*
  percutaneous transluminal (PTA)
  percutaneous transluminal coronary
    (PTCA)
  peripheral
  peripheral laser (PLA)
  single vessel
  supported
  synthetic patch
  transluminal
  transluminal balloon
  transluminal coronary
  transluminal coronary artery
  vein patch
angioplasty catheter, high speed
  rotation dynamic
angioplasty sheath
angiopneumography
AngiOptic microcatheter
angioreticuloendothelioma of heart
angiosarcoma, cavernous
angioscintigraphy
  cerebral
  radionuclide
  red blood cell
  renal
  skeletal
  superselective
  Tc 99m-labeled macroaggregated
    albumin (MAA) selective
Angio-Seal hemostatic puncture
  closure device
angiotensin II (AT-II), AT1 receptor
  imaging
AngioVista angiographic system
angle
  acetabular
  acetabular roof obliquity
  acromial
  anorectal
  antegonial
  anteroposterior talocalcaneal (APTC)
  arch

angle *(cont.)*
  Bauman
  Beatson combined ankle
  bimalleolar
  blunting of costophrenic
  blunting of costovertebral
  Boehler (Böhler)
  Boehler calcaneal
  Boehler lumbosacral
  Bragg
  C
  calcaneal inclination
  calcaneal pitch
  calcaneoplantar
  cardiodiaphragmatic
  cardiohepatic
  cardiophrenic
  carrying
  CE (capital epiphysis)
  central collodiaphyseal (CCD)
  cephalic
  cephalometric
  cerebellopontile (CPA)
  cerebellopontine (CPA)
  Citelli
  Clarke arch
  Cobb lumbar
  Cobb scoliosis
  Codman
  condylar
  costal
  costolumbar
  costophrenic (CP)
  costosternal
  costovertebral (CVA)
  craniofacial
  distal articular
  dorsoplantar talometatarsal
  dorsoplantar talonavicular
  Drennan metaphyseal-epiphyseal
  duodenojejunal
  Ebstein
  epigastric

angle *(cont.)*

fan
femorotibial (FTA)
first fifth intermetatarsal
first metatarsal
first second intermetatarsal
flip
foot-progression (FPA)
Garden
Gissane
gonial
Graf alpha
Graf beta
greater tarsal
hallux abductus
hallux dorsiflexion (DFA)
hallux interphalangeus
hallux valgus (HVA)
hallux valgus interphalangeus
hepatic-renal
hepatorenal
Hibbs metatarsocalcaneal
Hilgenreiner
iliac
IM (intermetatarsal)
increased carrying
infrasternal
intermetatarsal (IMA)
Konstram
lateral plantar metatarsal
lateral talocalcaneal (LTC)
lateral tarsometatarsal
Laurin
Louis
Ludovici
Ludwig
lumbosacral joint
mandibular
Meary metatarsotalar
mediolateral radiocarpal
Merchant
metaphyseal-epiphyseal
metatarsal break

angle *(cont.)*

metatarsocalcaneal
metatarsotalar
metatarsus adductus
metatarsus primus
Mikulicz
navicular to first metatarsal
neck shaft
nutation
obliterated costophrenic
occipitocervical
Pauwels
pelvic femoral
phase
phrenopericardial
Pirogoff
plantar metatarsal
pontine
proximal articular set (PASA)
Q
QRST
radiocarpal
Ranke
resting forefoot supination
sacrohorizontal
sacrovertebral
scapular
scattering
set
Sharp
slip
splenic-renal
splenorenal
sternal
sternoclavicular
subcarinal
subtalar
substernal
sulcus
talar declination
talar-tilt
talocalcaneal
talocrural

angle *(cont.)*
  talometatarsal
  talonavicular
  tarsometatarsal
  TC
  thigh-foot (TFA)
  tibiofemoral (TFA)
  tibiotalar
  TMA-thigh (transmalleolar axis)
  transmetatarsal (TMA)
  urethrovesical
  valgus
  valgus carrying
  varus
  varus metatarsophalangeal (MTP)
  venous
  vesicourethral
  wedge isodose
  Wiberg
  Wiberg center edge (CE)
  Wiltse
  xiphoid
angled pleural tube
angled slice
angle from horizontal plane
angle from vertical plane
angle independent
angle of anteversion
angle of declination of metatarsal
angle of greatest extension (AGE)
angle of greatest flexion (AGF)
angle of inclination of urethra
angle of incongruity
angle of Lequesne and de Seze
angle-tip catheter
Angström unit
angular frequency
angular gyrus (AG)
angular momentum
angular process of orbit
angularis body
angularis sulcus
angulated fracture

angulation
  anterior
  cephalic
  degrees of valgus
  degrees of varus
  forefoot
  post-traumatic
  spinal
angulation of ureter
angulus of stomach
anhaustral colonic gas pattern
anisotropic diffusion
anisotropic effect
anisotropic 3-D or volume study
anisotropy
  curvature
  diffusion
ankle
  disk of
  eversion of
  footballer's
  fractured
  fused
  fusion of
  instability of
  inversion injury of
  mortise of
  neuropathic
  sprained
  swelling of
  syndesmosis sprain of the
  synthetic graft bypass to
  tailor's
  transmalleolar
  twisted
ankle joint complex (AJC)
ankle mortise widening
ankle systolic pressure
ankylosing spondylitis
ankylosis (pl. ankyloses)
  bony
  extracapsular
  false

ankylosis *(cont.)*
　fibrous
　intracapsular
　joint
　ligamentous
　shoulder
　spurious
　vertebral
ankyroid cavity (also *ancyroid*)
anlage (pl. anlagen), cartilaginous
ANMR Insta-scan MR scanner
annealing algorithms
annihilation photons
annotated imaging
annual mammogram
annular abscess
annular array
annular calcification
annular cartilage
annular constriction
annular detector
annular dilatation
annular disruption
annulare, granuloma
annular fibrosis
annular foreshortening
annular fracture
annular hypoplasia
annular ligament
annular pancreas
anococcygeal raphe
anodal block
anode tube reloading
anomalous anatomy
anomalous drainage
anomalous fetuses
anomalous formation
anomalous insertion
anomalous origin
anomalous pathway
anomalous pulmonary venous
　　connection
　partial
　total

anomalous pulmonary venous return
anomalous structure
anomalous topographic pattern
anomalous uterus
anomalous vein of scimitar syndrome
anomalous vessel
anomaly (pl. anomalies)
　aortic arch
　back-angle
　bell clapper (BCA)
　cardiac
　cloacal
　congenital
　congenital cardiac
　conotruncal congenital
　cranial
　Cruveilhier-Baumgarten
　cutaneous vascular
　Ebstein
　extracardiac
　Freund
　May-Hegglin
　migrational
　multiple congenital (MCA)
　radial ray
　Shone
　subtle cerebral and cerebellar
　　morphologic
　subtle dispersion
　Taussig-Bing
　tricuspid valve
　Uhl
　vascular
　vertebral segmentation
　Zahn
anorectal abscess
anorectal ring
anovular ovarian follicle
anoxic ischemia
ansa (pl. ansae)
anserinus, pes
antagonist muscle groups
antebrachial fascia

antebrachium
antecolic anastomosis
antecubital brachial approach for
angiography
antecubital approach for cardiac
catheterization
antecubital fossa (*not* anterior cubital
or anticubital fossa)
antecubital space
antecubital vein
anteflexion
antegonial angle
antegonial notch
antegrade (forward)
antegrade blood flow
antegrade fast pathway
antegrade filling of vessels
antegrade flow
antegrade imaging
antegrade perfusion
antegrade pyelography imaging
antegrade refractory period
antegrade urography
ante mortem orthopantomography
antenna, loopless (dipole) (of catheter
or guidewire)
antepartum hemorrhage
anterior axillary line (AAL)
anterior cardiac vein
anterior cerebellar artery syndrome
anterior cervical pillar of disk
anterior cervical pillar of vertebra
anterior colliculus
anterior column of spine
anterior commissure
anterior communicating artery
anterior compartment syndrome
anterior coronary plexus (of heart)
anterior corpus
anterior corticospinal tract
anterior cruciate ligament (ACL)
anterior cusp
anterior descending artery

anterior descending artery occlusion
anterior fascicular block
anterior feet view
anterior fibular ligament
anterior gray column of cord
anterior head region
anterior horns of spinal cord
anterior hypothalamus
anterior inferior cerebellar artery
(AICA)
anterior inferior cerebral artery
(AICA)
anterior inferior communicating artery
(AICA)
anterior inferior iliac spine
anterior intercostal artery
anterior interhemispheric cistern
anterior interhemispheric fissure
anterior internodal pathway
anterior internodal tract of Bachman
anterior interventricular groove
anterior leaflet prolapse
anterior lip of uterus
anterior lobe
anterior maxillary spine
anterior mediastinum
anterior mitral leaflet (AML)
anterior motion of posterior mitral
valve leaflet
anterior myocardial infarction
anterior oblique band
anterior oblique position
anterior pelvic exenteration
anterior papillary muscle
anterior pillar degeneration
anterior planar image
anterior/posterior (AP)
anterior projection
anterior pulmonary plexus
anterior semilunar valve
anterior septal myocardial infarction
anterior spinal artery
anterior spinocerebellar tract

anterior spinothalamic tract
anterior superior iliac spine (ASIS)
anterior talar dome
anterior talofibular ligament
anterior tibial artery
anterior tibial compartment
anterior tibiofibular ligament
anterior tibiotalar ligament
anterior tricuspid leaflet (ATL)
anterior wall myocardial infarction
anterior wall of urinary bladder
anterior urethra
anterior wall dyskinesis
anterior wall myocardial infarction
anteroapical wall myocardial infarction
anterobasal myocardial infarction
anterofundal placenta
anterograde peristalsis
anterolateral recess of ankle
anterolateral wall
anterolateral wall myocardial infarction
anterolateral white matter of cord
anteroseptal wall myocardial infarction
anterolisthesis
anteromedial
anteroposterior (AP) (also anterior-
    posterior)
antetorsion, femoral
anteversion
    angle of
    femoral
    Magilligan technique for measuring
    neutral
anteversion determination, Budin-
    Chandler
anteverted
Anthonson subtalar joint view
anthracosilicosis
anthrax
anthrax pneumonia
anthrocotic tuberculosis
Anthron heparinized antithrombogenic
    catheter

anthropoid pelvis
anthropometric imaging
anthropometry, 3D surface
anti-AChR (antiacetylcholine receptor)
    antibody
anti-aliasing techniques
antibiotic prophylaxis
antibody (pl. antibodies) (see also
    imaging agent)
AChR (acetylcholine receptor)
ACTH
AE1
AE3
anti-AChR (antiacetylcholine
    receptor)
anti-ACh receptor
anticardiolipin (aCL)
antiglioma monoclonal
antimyosin
antimyosin monoclonal (Fab
    fragment)
antinuclear (ANA)
antiphospholipid
antistriated muscle
beta-endorphin
CAM 5.2
carcinoma-specific monoclonal
CC49 antitumor monoclonal
cytokeratin
EMA (epithelial membrane antigen)
GFAP (glial fibrillary acidic protein)
growth hormone
heterophile
^{125}I-radiolabeled humanized CC49
    monoclonal
IgM anti-human parvovirus
indium
indium-labeled antimyosin
iodine ^{125}I-radiolabeled humanized
    CC49 monoclonal
kinase C
kinase C antiglioma monoclonal
lectin

antibody *(cont.)*
  luteinizing hormone
  lym-1 monoclonal
  Mab-170 monoclonal
  MG (myasthenia gravis)
  monoclonal (MOAB, MoAb)
  neuron-specific enolase (NSE)
  neutralization
  NSE (neuron-specific enolase)
  polyclonal anticardiac myosin
  prealbumin
  precipitating
  prolactin hormone
  RCA (Ricinus communis
    agglutinin 1)
  Re-188 labeled
  7E3 monoclonal antiplatelet
  sheep antidigoxin Fab
  S-100 protein
  SS-A (Ro)
  SS-B (La)
  St. Louis encephalitis
  99mTc-labeled antigranulocyte
  teichoic acid
  thyrotropin hormone
  UE (*Ulex europaeus*)
  vimentin
  VZ (varicella-zoster)
  whole blood monoclonal
antibody-antigen complex
antibody-conjugated paramagnetic
  liposomes (ACPLs)
antibody-labeled circulating
  granulocytes
antibody labeling
anticardiolipin (aCL) antibody
anticoincidence circuit
anti-D-dimer antibodies, radiolabeled
antifibrin (T2G1s) antibodies F(ab)2
antifibrin antibody imaging
antifibrin scintigraphy

antigen
  antiproliferating cell nuclear
  Aspergillus
  autogenous
  CA 15-3
  carcinoembryonic (CEA)
  epithelial membrane (EMA)
  histocompatibility
  HLA-B27
  human leukocyte, B27
  major histocompatibility complex
    class II (MHC-2)
  prostate-specific (PSA)
  serum cryptococcal
anti-estrogen radiologic therapy
antigravity muscles
antimesenteric border of distal ileum
antimesenteric fat pad
antimesocolic side of the cecum
antimony (an element)
antimotility drug
antimyosin antibodies
antimyosin monoclonal antibody, Fab
  fragment
antineoplastic therapy
antinuclear antibody (ANA) test
antiphospholipid antibody syndrome
antiphospholipid anticardiolipin
  antibody
antistreptolysin O (ASO) titer
Antoni-A classification of neurinoma
Anton syndrome
Antopol-Goldman lesion
antral edema
antral gastritis
antral pad sign
antral stasis
antrum
  cardiac
  gastric
  Malacarne
  prepyloric
  pyloric

antrum *(cont.)*
  retained
  Willis
anulus (pl. anuli)
  aortic valve
  atrioventricular
  calcified
  fissure of
  friable
  mitral
  pulmonary valve
  redundant scallop of posterior
  septal tricuspid
  tricuspid valve
  valve
  Vieussens
anulus fibrosus
anulus ovalis
anulus umbilicalis
anus
anvil bone
anvil sign
Ao, AO (aorta)
AO (aortic opening)
AO/AC (aortic valve opening/aortic
  valve closing) ratio
AO classification of ankle fracture
AO-Danis-Weber classification of
  ankle fracture
AOIVM (angiographically occult intracranial vascular malformation)
aorta (Ao, AO)
  abdominal
  aneurysmal widening of
  arch of
  ascending (AA)
  bifurcation of
  biventricular origin of
  biventricular transposed
  calcified
  central
  cervical
  coarctation of

aorta *(cont.)*
  coarcted
  descending
  descending thoracic
  dextroposed
  dextropositioned
  D-malposition of
  double-barreled
  draped
  dynamic
  ectasia of abdominal
  ectasia of thoracic
  elongated
  infrarenal
  infrarenal abdominal
  kinked
  L malposition
  Nikaidoh translocation of
  overriding
  pericardial
  porcelain
  preductal coarctation of
  recoarctation of the
  reconstruction of
  retroesophageal
  root of
  sclerosis of
  small feminine
  stenosis of
  supraceliac
  supradiaphragmatic
  terminal
  thoracic
  thoracoabdominal
  tortuous
  transposed
  unwinding of
  ventral
  wide tortuous
  widening of
aorta-iliac-femoral bypass
aorta-renal bypass
aorta-subclavian-carotid bypass

aorta to vein anastomosis
aortic allograft
aortic anastomosis
aortic aneurysm
aortic angiography
aortic annular region
aortic annulus
aortic arch
  congenital interruption of
  double
aortic arch angiography
aortic arch anomaly
aortic arch atresia
aortic arch calcification
aortic arch hypoplasia syndrome
aortic arch interruption
aortic atherosclerosis
  juxtarenal
  pararenal
aortic atresia
aortic bifurcation
aortic bulb
aortic calcification
aortic cannulation
aortic cartilage
aortic chemoreceptors
aortic closure (AC)
aortic coarctation, juxtaductal
aortic configuration of cardiac shadow
aortic cusp
  perforated
  ruptured
aortic cusp separation
aortic diameter (AD)
aortic dilatation
aortic dissection
  type A
  type B
aortic elongation
aortic fenestration
aortic flush pigtail catheter
aortic flush straight catheter
aortic hiatus

aortic homograft anastomotic dehiscence
aortic impedance
aortic incisura
aortic incompetence
aortic insufficiency (AI)
aortic insult
aortic isthmus, hypoplasia of
aortic knob, blurring of
aortic knob contour
aortic knuckle
aortic leaflets, redundant
aortic-left ventricular pressure
  difference
aortic-left ventricular tunnel
aortic nipple sign
aortic notch
aorticopulmonary anastomosis
aorticopulmonary defect
aorticopulmonary fenestration
aorticopulmonary septal defect
aorticopulmonary shunt
aorticopulmonary trunk
aorticopulmonary window
aortic pseudoaneurysm
aortic root abscess
aortic root reconstruction procedure
aortic valve leaflet
aortic wave velocity
aortic orifice
aortic override
aortic oxygen saturation
aortic paravalvular leak
aortic pressure
aortic pseudoaneurysm
aortic pullback
aortic-pulmonary shunt
aortic regurgitation (AR)
  congenital
  massive
  syphilitic
aortic resection
aortic root angiogram

aortic root dilatation
aortic root homograft
aortic root pressure
aortic root ratio
aortic runoff
aortic rupture
aortic segment
  intradiaphragmatic
  intramuscular
aortic septal defect
aortic shag
aortic sinus aneurysm
aortic sinus to right ventricle fistula
aortic spindle
aortic stenosis (AS)
  calcific
  congenital
  congenital subvalvular
  congenital valvular
  hypercalcemia-supravalvular
  subvalvular
  supravalvular (SAS, SVAS)
  uncomplicated supraclavicular
aortic stiffness
aortic stump blowout (blowout)
aortic subvalvular ring
aortic superior mesenteric bypass
aortic thromboembolism
aortic tract complex hypoplasia
aortic transection, traumatic
aortic tube graft
aortic valve (AVA)
  bicommissural
  bicuspid
  calcified
  composite
  ectatic
  native
  nodules of
  opening of
  prolapse of
  stenosed
  thickened
  unicommissural

aortic valve annulus
aortic valve area
aortic valve atresia
aortic valve calcification
aortic valve endocarditis
aortic valve gradient
aortic valve incompetence
aortic valve insufficiency
aortic valve leaflet prolapse
aortic valve obstruction
aortic valve opening
aortic valve pressure gradient
aortic valve prosthesis
aortic valve regurgitation
aortic valve stenosis
  acquired
  congenital
aortic valve thickening
aortic valvular incompetence
aortic valvular insufficiency
aortic vasa vasorum
aortic vestibule of ventricle
aortic window
aortic window node
aortic wrap
aortobifemoral bypass graft
aortobifemoral reconstruction
aortobiprofunda bypass graft
aortocarotid bypass
aortocaval fistula
aortoceliac bypass
aortocoronary valve
aortoduodenal fistula
aortoenteric fistula
aortoesophageal
aortofemoral arteriography with
  runoff views
aortofemoral bypass graft (AFBG)
aortofemoral runoff
aortogastric
aortogram with distal runoff
aortography (also *aortogram*)
  abdominal
  antegrade

aortography *(cont.)*
  arch
  balloon occlusive
  biplanar
  contrast
  counter-current
  digital subtraction
  digital subtraction supravalvular
  flush
  postangioplasty
  retrograde
  retrograde femoral
  retrograde transaxillary
  retrograde transfemoral
  retrograde translumbar
  selective visceral
  supravalvular
  thoracic
  thoracic arch
  translumbar
  ultrasonic
aortoiliac aneurysm
aortoiliac bypass
aortoiliac disease
aortoiliac inflow assessment
aortoiliac obstructive disease (AIOD)
aortoiliac popliteal bypass
aortoiliac thrombosis
aortoiliofemoral arteries
aortoiliofemoral bypass
aortomegaly, diffuse
aortoplasty
  balloon
  patch-graft
  posterior patch
  subclavian flap
aortoplasty with patch graft
aortopopliteal bypass
aortopulmonary anastomosis
aortopulmonary collaterals
aortopulmonary fistula
aortopulmonary shunt
aortopulmonary window

aortosclerosis
aortoseptal continuity
aortosigmoid fistula
aortovelography, transcutaneous (TAV)
aortoventriculoplasty
AoV (aortic valve)
AOVM (angiographically occult
  vascular malformation)
AP (anteroposterior or anterior-
  posterior)
  AP angle cephalad cervical spine
    x-ray
  AP coccyx, 10-20° caudad x-ray
  AP film
  AP L5-S1, 30-35° cephalad lumbar
    spine x-ray
  AP lordotic view
  AP open-mouth cervical spine x-ray
  AP projection
  AP sacrum, 15-25° cephalad x-ray
  AP supine abdomen x-ray
  AP supine portable view
  AP supine view
  AP 10-15° caudad cystography
  AP upper airway x-ray
  AP upright abdomen x-ray
  AP ureteric compression on intra-
    venous urography
  AP view
AP and PA ribs, above and below
  diaphragm
APB (abductor pollicis brevis) muscle
APC-3 collimator
APC-4 collimator
APCLs (antibody-conjugated paramag-
  netic liposomes)
ape hand (simian griffe)
ape hand of syringomyelia
ape-like hand
aperiodic complex
aperiodic functional MR imaging
aperiodic wave
aperistalsis

aperistaltic distal ureteral segment
Apert disease
aperture, superior thoracic
apex (pl. apices)
    cardiac
    displaced left ventricular
    duodenal bulb
    external ring
    head of femur
    head of fibula
    head of patella
    heart
    horn of spinal cord
    Koch triangle
    left ventricular
    lung
    orbital
    petrous
    systolic retraction of
    uptilted cardiac
    ventricular cardiac
apex beat
apex cordis
apex of petrous portion of temporal
    bone
apex of urinary bladder
apex pneumonia
APEX 409 camera
APEX 415 camera
apexcardiogram, apexcardiography
    (ACG)
apex pneumonia
aphagia
aphalangia
apheresis catheter
aphtha (pl. aphthae)
apical air space on x-ray
apical and subcostal four-chambered
    view
apical cap
apical cap sign
apical capping
apical corn

apical duodenal ulcer
apical four-chamber view
apical granuloma
apical hypoperfusion on thallium scan
apical impulse
apical infiltrate
apical-lateral wall myocardial
    infarction
apical ligament
apical myocardial infarction
apical pneumonia
apical posterior artery
apical posterolateral region of left
    ventricle
apical scar
apical scarring
apical segment
apical short axis slice
apical surface of heart
apical thinning
apical tissue
apical two-chamber view
apical view
apical wall
apical window
apices (pl. of apex)
apicoabdominal bypass
apicoposterior bronchi
apiculate waveform
aPL (antiphospholipid) antibody
APL (abductor pollicis longus) muscle
aplasia, cerebellar
aplasia of deep veins
APM (anterior papillary muscle)
Apogee CX 200 echo system
Apogee ultrasound device
A point
Apomate imaging agent
aponeurosis
    bicipital
    digital
    epicranial
    external oblique

aponeurosis *(cont.)*
  internal oblique
  palmar
  plantar
  tendon
aponeurotic band
aponeurotic triangle
aponeurotic troika
apophyseal fracture
apophyseal joint
apophysis of Rau
apophysitis
  calcaneal
  iliac
apoplexy
  Broadbent
  cerebellar
  delayed
  pineal
  pituitary
  postpartum pituitary
  post-traumatic (of Bollinger)
  pulmonary
  pulmonary artery
  pulmonary vein
APP (average pixel projection)
apparent diffusion coefficient (ADC)
  mapping
appearance (see also *sign*)
  ball-on-spoon
  bat wing
  beading of activity
  beaten silver (of the skull)
  beaver tail (of balloon profile)
  blade of grass
  cauliflower
  Christmas tree
  cobblestone
  cobra head
  cobweb
  coiled spring
  collar-button (in colon)

appearance *(cont.)*
  corkscrew
  cottage loaf
  crazy-paving
  distortions of image
  drooping lily
  feathery
  flame
  froglike
  frondlike
  grainy
  heterogeneous
  homogeneous
  Honda sign
  hooked
  hyperreflectile
  isodense
  licked candy stick
  lobulated saccular
  moth-eaten
  nutmeg (of liver)
  onion peel
  signet ring
  spiral
  string of beads
  super scan
  swirled (on ultrasound)
  target
  targetlike
  trilaminar
  trilayer
  whorled
appendage
  atrial
  cecal
  epiploic
  left atrial (LAA)
  right atrial (RAA)
  truncated atrial
  vermicular
  wide-based blunt-ended
    right-sided atrial

appendagitis
  epiploic
  primary epiploic
appendiceal abscess
appendiceal endometriosis
appendiceal stump
appendices or appendixes (pl.)
appendicitis, acute
appendicolithiasis
appendicular skeleton
appendix (pl. appendixes, appendices)
  cecal
  ensiform
  epiploic
  filiform
  Morgagni
  paracecal
  preileal
  retrocecal
  retroileal
  subcecal
  vermiform
  xiphoid
appendolithiasis
apple core lesion
apple peel syndrome
applicator, nucletron
application-specific integrated circuit
  (ASIC)
appose
apposing articular surfaces
apposition
  bone to bone
  close
  fracture in close
apposition of leaflets
appreciable dilation
approach (see also *method*; *technique*)
  antecubital brachial
  ilioinguinal (of Letournel)
  infracoccygeal
  internal jugular
  transgluteal

approach *(cont.)*
  transiliac
  transosseous
  transsacral
  transsternal
apron
  abdominal
  lead
  quadriceps
APS (air plasma spray) hydroxyapatite
APTC (anteroposterior talocalcaneal)
  angle
apudoma
AquariusNET streaming 2-D/3-D
  medical imaging server
AquaSens FMS 1000 fluid monitoring
  system
aqueduct
  cerebral
  forking of sylvian
  gliosis of
  mesencephalon
  midbrain
  Monro
  Sylvius
  ventricular
aqueduct compression
aqueduct occlusion
aqueduct stenosis
aqueous scintillator
AR (aortic regurgitation)
AR (atrial rate)
AR 2 diagnostic guiding catheter
arachnodactyly
arachnoid canal
arachnoid cyst
arachnoid granulation
arachnoid of uncus
arachnoid villi
Aran-Duchenne amyotrophy
Arani double loop guiding catheter
Arantius canal
arborescens, lipoma

arborescent
arborization of ducts
arborize
arcade
   collateral
   Frohse ligamentous
   mitral
   septal
   Struthers
   superficialis
Arcelin view (of petrous temporal
   region)
arch
   anterior atlas
   anterior metatarsal
   aortic
   articular
   atlas
   carpal
   cervical aortic
   coracoacromial
   deep
   distal aortic
   double aortic
   flat
   flattened longitudinal (of foot)
   Hapad metatarsal
   hemal
   high
   Hillock
   hypoplastic
   interrupted aortic
   longitudinal (of foot)
   lung
   mid aortic
   mural
   neural vertebral
   palmar arterial
   plantar
   plantar arterial
   posterior metatarsal
   pubic
   right aortic

arch *(cont.)*
   right-sided
   Riolan
   subpubic
   superciliary
   superficial palmar arterial
   tarsal
   transverse (of foot)
   transverse aortic
   vertebral
   Zimmerman
   zygomatic
arch and carotid arteriography
Archer syndrome
archicortex
arch index
arching of mitral valve leaflet
architectural alterations of bone
architectural distortion
architecture
   bony
   brain
   foot
   hepatic
   intranodal
   lung
   lobular
   network
arch study (arterial imaging study)
arcitumomab (CEA-Scan) (technetium
   Tc 99m arcitumomab) imaging
   agent
Arcq classification
arcuate artery of kidney
arcuate complex
arcuate eminence
arcuate fasciculus (AF)
arcuate fiber involvement
arcuate ligament
arcuate movement
arcuate nucleus
arcuate uterus
arcuate vessel

ARDMS (American Registry of Diagnostic Medical Sonographers)
ARDS (adult respiratory distress syndrome), asymmetric
area (see also *region*)
  anechoic
  aortic
  arrhythmogenic
  artery
  Bamberger
  body surface (BSA)
  Broca
  Brodmann
  callosal (parolfactory nerve)
  cardiac frontal
  cortical motor
  cross-sectional (CSA)
  denervated
  echo-free
  effective balloon dilated (EBDA)
  Erb
  Haeckerman
  hilar
  hot
  hyperechoic
  hypoechoic
  ischemic
  language
  luminal cross-sectional
  midsternal
  mitral valve (MVA)
  olfactory
  parietal association
  parietotemporal
  perihilar
  peroneal
  premotor
  pulmonic
  rarefied
  sclerotic
  septal
  sonolucent
  stenosis

area *(cont.)*
  subglottic
  suprapubic
  tricuspid
  valve
  watershed (of periventricular white matter)
  Wernicke
area length method for ejection fraction
area of abnormal density
area of asymmetry
area of denudation
area of enhanced contrast
area of high radioactivity
area of increased density
area of increased "radiolabeling"
areola
areolar abscess
areolar lesion
areolar plane
ARF (acute respiratory failure)
argentaffinoma
argon laser
Argyle Medicut R catheter
Argyle umbilical vessel catheter
A ring, esophageal
arm
  abductor lever
  C-
  flail
  Leyla
  linebacker's
  outrigger
  Popeye
arm and lesser saphenous veins (ALSVs)
Armanni-Ebstein kidney
Arnold-Chiari (type II) malformation
array
  annular
  convex
  electrode

array *(cont.)*
  high density
  linear
  linear electrode
  NMRA quadrature detection
  phased
  symmetrical phased
  voxel
array processor (MRI equipment)
arrest
  anoxic
  asystolic cardiac
  bradyarrhythmic cardiac
  cardiac
  cardiopulmonary
  cardiorespiratory
  circulatory
  electrical circulatory
  epiphyseal
  flow
  heart
  hypothermic
  intermittent sinus
  profound hypothermic circulatory
    (PHCA)
  recurrent cardiac
  respiratory
  sinus
  transient sinus
arrested circulation
arrested dilation
arrest reaction
arrhenoblastoma
arrhythmia-insensitive flow-sensitive
  alternating IR
arrhythmogenic area
arrhythmogenic border zone
arrhythmogenic right ventricular
  dysplasia (ARVD) syndrome
arrhythmogenic ventricular activity
  (AVA)
Arrow-Berman balloon angioplasty
  catheter

Arrow-Flex percutaneous sheath introducer
ArrowFlex sheath
ArrowGard Blue Line catheter
ArrowGard Blue Plus catheter
ArrowGard central venous catheter
arrowhead-shaped
arrowhead sign
Arrow-Howes multilumen catheter
Arrow PICC radiology device for
  insertion of central venous lines
Arrow pulmonary artery catheter
ARRS (American Roentgen Ray
  Society)
arterial access site
arterial aneurysm
arterial avulsion
arterial blockage
arterial brachiocephalic trunk
arterial calcification
arterial cannula
arterial cannulation
arterial capillary
arterial circulation
arterial cutoff
arterial deficiency pattern
arterial degenerative disease
arterial dilatation and rupture
arterial dissection
arterial flow phase image
arterial graft
arterial hyperemia
arterial intima
arterial invasion
arterialization of venous blood
arterial line
arterial lumen
arterial malformation (AM)
arterial narrowing
arterial obstruction
arterial occlusion
arterial patency
arterial peak systolic pressure

arterial portography
arterial pressure
arterial pulsation artifact
arterial recoil
arterial return
arterial runoff
arterial rupture
arterial sclerosis
arterial segment
arterial sheath
arterial spasm
arterial spin labeling (ASL)
arterial steal
arterial supply
arterial thrombosis
arterial tonus
arterial topography
arterial tree
arterial varices
arterial wall dynamics
arterial wall thickness
arterio-arterial anastomosis
arteriocapillary sclerosis
arteriogram
arteriography (also *arteriogram*)
   aorta and runoff
   aortofemoral (with runoff views)
   arch and carotid
   balloon occlusion
   biplane pelvic
   biplane quantitative coronary
   brachial
   brachiocephalic
   bronchial
   carotid
   celiac
   cerebral
   cine-
   contrast
   coronary
   CT (computed tomography)
   delayed phase of
   femoral

arteriography *(cont.)*
   four-vessel
   hepatic
   infrahepatic
   intraoperative
   Judkins selective coronary
   left coronary cine-
   longitudinal
   lumbar
   mesenteric
   percutaneous
   percutaneous femoral
   peripheral
   pruned-tree
   pulmonary
   pulmonary artery
   quantitative coronary (QCA)
   renal
   retrograde
   runoff
   selective
   selective cerebral
   selective coronary
   Sones selective coronary
   subclavian
   superior mesenteric
   thrombotic pulmonary (TPA)
   vertebral
   visceral
   wedge
arteriolar sclerosis
arteriole, glomerular
arteriolosclerotic kidney
arterioplasty
arterioportal shunt
arteriorenal
arteriosclerosis
   calcific
   cerebral
   coronary
   generalized
   hyaline
   hypertensive

arteriosclerosis *(cont.)*
  infantile
  intimal
  medial
  Mönckeberg (Moenckeberg)
  obliterative
  peripheral
  presenile
  pulmonary
  senile
arteriosclerosis obliterans (ASO)
arteriosclerotic cardiovascular disease
  (ASCVD)
arteriosclerotic deposits
arteriosclerotic heart disease (ASHD)
arteriosclerotic intracranial aneurysm
arteriosclerotic kidney
arteriosclerotic peripheral vascular
  disease
arteriosclerotic plaque
arteriosclerotic thoracoabdominal
  aortic aneurysm
arteriostenosis
arteriosus, ductus
arteriovenous (AV)
arteriovenous aneurysm
arteriovenous angioma
arteriovenous bovine shunt
arteriovenous fistula (AV, AVF)
arteriovenous interhemispheric
  angioma
arteriovenous malformation (AVM)
arteriovenous pressure gradient
arteriovenous shunt
arteriovenous varix
arteritis, radiation-induced
artery (pl. arteries)
  A1-A5 segments of anterior cerebral
  Abbott
  abdominal aorta
  aberrant
  aberrant coronary
  aberrant left pulmonary

artery *(cont.)*
  aberrant right subclavian
  accessory hepatic
  accessory renal
  acromiothoracic
  Adamkiewicz
  aneurysm of internal carotid
  aneurysm of posterior communi-
    cating
  angular MCA (middle cerebral
    artery)
  anomalous origin of
  anterior cerebral (ACA)
  anterior choroidal (ACA or AChA)
  anterior communicating (ACoA)
  anterior descending branch of
    left coronary
  anterior inferior cerebellar (AICA)
  anterior inferior cerebral (AICA)
  anterior inferior communicating
    (AICA)
  anterior spinal
  anterior spinal canal
  anterior temporal branch of
    posterior cerebral
  aortoiliofemoral
  apical posterior
  arcuate
  ascending frontoparietal (ASFP)
  atrioventricular node
  AV (atrioventricular) nodal
  axillary
  basal perforating
  basilar
  beading of
  bifurcation of anterior
    communicating
  bifurcation of common carotid
  bifurcation of internal carotid
  bifurcation of middle cerebral
  brachial
  brachiocephalic
  branch of

artery *(cont.)*
  calcarine
  calcified
  callosomarginal
  cannulated
  carotid
  celiac
  cerebral
  choroidal branch of internal
    carotid
  choroidal pericallosal
  circumflex (circ, CF, CX)
  circumflex groove
  collateral circulation in
  common carotid (CCA)
  common femoral
  common iliac
  compression of
  C1-C5 segments of internal carotid
  conus
  corduroy
  coronary
  cortical branch of middle cerebral
  costocervical
  course of
  deltoid branch of posterior tibial
  descending septal
  diagonal branch of
  diagonal branch of left anterior
    descending coronary
  diagonal coronary
  dilated
  dissection of
  distal circumflex marginal
  dominant coronary
  dominant left coronary
  dominant right coronary
  dorsal spinal
  Drummond marginal
  dural
  dynamic entrapment of vertebral
  eccentric coronary
  en passage feeder

artery *(cont.)*
  epicardial coronary
  external carotid (ECA)
  external iliac
  extracranial vertebral
  extradural
  familial fibromuscular dysplasia of
  feeder
  femoropopliteal
  first diagonal branch
  first obtuse marginal
  friable
  frontopolar (FPA)
  gastroepiploic
  high left main diagonal
  hilar
  hypogastric
  iliac
  inferior epigastric
  inferior mesenteric
  infragenicular popliteal
  infrageniculate
  innominate
  intercostal
  intermediate coronary
  internal carotid (ICA)
  internal iliac
  internal iliac gluteal
  internal mammary (IMA)
  internal thoracic
  intra-acinar pulmonary
  intracavernous internal carotid
  intracranial vertebral
  ipsilateral downstream
  kinked innominate
  Kugel
  labyrinthine
  LAD (left anterior descending)
  lateral posterior choroidal (LPCh)
  LCA (left coronary)
  LCF or LCX (left circumflex)
  left anterior descending
  left circumflex coronary

artery *(cont.)*
  left common femoral
  left coronary (LCA)
  left internal mammary (LIMA)
  left main coronary (LMCA)
  left pulmonary (LPA)
  lenticulostriate
  leptomeningeal
  LIMA (left internal mammary)
  limb of
  LMCA (left main coronary)
  M1-M5 segments of middle
    cerebral
  main pulmonary (MPA)
  mainstem coronary
  maintenance of flow in
  mammary
  marginal branch of left circumflex
    coronary
  marginal branch of right coronary
  marginal circumflex
  medial plantar
  medial posterior choroidal (MPCh)
  median sacral
  meningeal
  meningohypophyseal trunk (MHT)
  mesencephalic
  mesenteric
  middle cerebral (MCA)
  middle meningeal
  musculophrenic
  narrowing of
  native coronary
  nodular induration of temporal
  nutrient
  obtuse marginal (OM) coronary
  occipital branch of external carotid
  occlusion of
  ophthalmic
  overriding great
  paramalleolar
  paramedian thalamopeduncular
  parietal MCA

artery *(cont.)*
  parieto-occipital branch of
    posterior cerebellar
  patency of
  PDA (posterior descending)
  peduncular segment of superior
    cerebellar
  perforating
  pericallosal
  peripancreatic
  peroneal
  petrous segment of carotid
  phrenic
  pipestem
  plantar metatarsal
  plaque-containing
  P1-P4 segments of posterior
    cerebral
  pontine
  popliteal
  posterior cerebral (PCA)
  posterior choroidal
  posterior communicating (PCA)
  posterior descending (PDA)
  posterior descending branch of
    right coronary
  posterior descending coronary
  posterior inferior cerebellar (PICA)
  posterior inferior communicating
    (PICA)
  posterior intercostal
  posterior parietal
  posterior spinal
  posterior temporal
  posterior tibial
  posterolateral spinal (PLSA)
  post-temporal MCA
  precommunicating segment of
    anterior cerebral
  primitive trigeminal (PTA)
  profunda femoris
  proximal anterior descending
  proximal digital

artery *(cont.)*
proximal left anterior descending
proximal popliteal
pulmonary (PA)
radial digital
radicular
radiculomedullary
radiculospinal
ramus intermedius
ramus medialis
recurrent (of Heubner)
renal
reperfused
resilient
retinal
retroesophageal right subclavian
right coronary (RCA)
right femoral
right inferior epigastric
right internal iliac
right pulmonary (RPA)
right ventricular branch of right
    coronary
scalp branch of external carotid
segmental branch of vertebral
septal perforator
SFA (superficial femoral)
shepherd's crook area of the right
    coronary
sinoatrial node
sinus nodal
splenial branch of posterior
    cerebral
splenic
stenotic coronary
subclavian
subcostal
superficial femoral (SFA)
superficial temporal (STA)
superior cerebellar (SCA)
superior epigastric
superior genicular
superior intercostal

artery *(cont.)*
superior mesenteric
superior thyroid
supraclinoid carotid
takeoff of
temporal
thalamocaudate
thalamogeniculate
thalamoperforating
thyrocervical trunk of subclavian
thyroid
trifurcation of middle cerebral
truncal
twig of
ulnar
ulnar digital
vertebral
vertebral basilar
weakened
artery-vein-nerve bundle
arthrempyesis
arthrifluent abscess
arthritic talonavicular changes
arthritis (pl. arthritides)
    coccidioidomycosis
    juvenile idiopathic
    juvenile rheumatoid
    osteoarthritis
    painful multifocal
    psoriatic
    pyogenic
    rheumatoid (RA)
    septic
    tuberculous
arthritis deformans
arthrogram
arthrography
    air
    Brostrom-Gordon
    coronal computed tomographic
        (CCTA)
    CT (computed tomography)
    direct MR

arthrography *(cont.)*
  double contrast
  Gordon-Brostrom single contrast
  indirect MR
  joint
  MR
  saline-enhanced MR
  single contrast
  temporomandibular joint
arthropathy, amyloid
arthrophyte
arthropyosis
arthroscintigraphy
arthrosis
  crystal-induced
  degenerative
  IRM spiral
arthrosis deformans
arthrotomography of shoulder, double
  contrast
articular capsule
articular cartilage
articular cartilage degeneration
articular cartilage volume
articular cortex
articular disk
articular erosion
articular facet
articular fracture
articular fragment
articular gout
articular process
articular rheumatism
articular surfaces
  apposing
  contiguous
articulate
articulating bone ends
articulation
  acromioclavicular
  atlantoaxial
  body contour orbit
  calcaneocuboid

articulation *(cont.)*
  carpometacarpal
  carporadial
  condylar
  costovertebral
  DIP (distal interphalangeal)
  disturbance of
  humeroradial
  humeroulnar
  intercarpal
  intermetacarpal
  interphalangeal
  metacarpophalangeal (MP)
  occipitocervical
  patellofemoral
  PIP (proximal interphalangeal)
  radiocarpal
  radiohumeral
  radioulnar
  sacroiliac
  scapuloclavicular
  subtalar
  talocalcaneal
  talocalcaneonavicular
  talonavicular
  tarsometatarsal
  thorax
  tibiofibular
  zygapophyseal
artifact
  acoustic
  alias
  aliasing (wrap-around ghosting)
  arterial pulsation
  artifactual
  asymmetric
  attenuation
  barium
  baseline
  beam hardening
  black boundary
  "black comets"
  blooming

artifact *(cont.)*
  bounce point
  braces
  breast
  breathing
  broadband noise detection error
  brown fat
  bulk susceptibility
  calibration failure
  catheter
  catheter impact
  catheter tip motion
  catheter tip position
  catheter whip
  central point
  chemical shift
  chemical shift phenomena
  clothing
  coin
  construction
  corduroy
  crescent
  crinkle
  cross-talk effect
  crown
  CSR fluid flow
  data-clipping detection error
  data spike detection error
  DC (direct current) offset
  developer
  distortion of limitations of image
    reconstruction algorithm
  dog
  double exposure
  double exposure drift
  eddy current
  edge-boundary
  edge misalignment
  edge ringing
  effusion
  end pressure
  entry slice phenomenon
  equipment

artifact *(cont.)*
  faulty RF (radiofrequency)
    shielding
  flow effect
  flow-induced
  flow void
  foreign material
  gaseous oxygen
  geophagia
  ghosting
  Gibbs
  Gibbs phenomenon
  glass eye
  glove phenomenon
  half-moon
  half-moon mark
  hot spot
  image
  image postprocessing errors
  imbalance of phase or gain
  intensifying screen
  iron overload
  kink
  kissing-type
  lettering
  linear
  low attenuation pulsation
  "magic angle" effects
  magnetic susceptibility
  main magnetic field inhomogeneity
  mercury
  mirror image
  misregistration
  mitral regurgitation
    (cineangiography)
  moiré
  moiré fringes
  mosaic
  motion
  movement
  muscle
  muscle uptake PET
  negligible

artifact *(cont.)*
  overlying attenuation
  pacemaker
  pacing
  paramagnetic
  partial volume effect
  patient motion
  pellet
  phase-encoded motion
  pica
  "pseudofracture"
  quadrature phase detector (QPD)
  radiofrequency (RF) spatial distri-
    bution problem reconstruction
  respiration-induced attenuation
  respiratory motion
  reticulation
  RF (radiofrequency) overflow
  screen craze
  skin crease
  skin fold
  skin lesion
  slice-overlap
  slice profile
  stairstep
  stimulated echo
  streak
  subcutaneous injection of contrast
  summation shadow
  superimposition
  susceptibility
  suture
  swallowing
  swamp-static
  temporal instability
  tree
  truncation
  truncation band
  twinkling
  venetian blind
  voluming
  wheelchair
  windmill

artifact *(cont.)*
  wrap-around
  wrap-around ghost (aliasing)
  wrap-around ghosting
  wrinkle
  zebra
  zebra stripes
  zero-fill
  zipper
artifacts mimicking intimal flaps
artifactual
artifactual lesion
artificial cardiac valve
artificial kidney
artificial left ventricular assist device
  (LVAD)
artificial neural network
artificial pneumothorax
Artoscan MRI system
Arvidsson dimension-length method
  for ventricular volume
aryepiglottic fold
arytenoid cartilage
arytenoid sparing
ARTMA (advanced real-time motion
  analysis)
AS (aortic stenosis)
asbestos bodies
asbestos exposure
asbestos-induced pleural fibrosis
asbestos pleural plaques
asbestosis
A-scan ultrasound
ascariasis
ascending aorta (AA)
ascending aorta hypoplasia
ascending aortic aneurysm
ascending colon
ascending colon herniation
ascending contrast phlebography
ascending hypoplasia of aorta
ascending phlebography
ascending tract

ascertain, ascertained
Asch intrauterine catheter
Aschoff-Tawara node
ascites
ascitic fluid
ASCVD (arterio- or atherosclerotic
   cardiovascular disease)
ASD (atrial septal defect)
ASD transcatheter occlusion with
   button device
aseptic myocarditis of newborn
aseptic necrosis
ASFP (ascending frontoparietal) artery
ASH (asymmetric septal hypertrophy)
ASHD (arteriosclerotic heart disease)
Ashcrson syndrome
Ashhurst fracture classification system
Ashhurst sign
ASIS (anterior superior iliac spine)
Ask-Upmark kidney
ASL (arterial spin labeling)
ASO (atherosclerosis obliterans)
aspect
   anterior
   anterolateral
   anteroposterior (AP)
   apical
   axial
   dorsal
   dorsolateral
   dorsoplantar
   inferior
   infrapatellar
   lateral
   lordotic
   medial
   mediolateral
   posterior
   posteroanterior (PA)
   posterolateral
   proximal
   superior
   superolateral
   ventral

Aspect computer
Aspen ultrasound system
aspergilloma
aspergillosis
aspergillotic aneurysm
aspergillus bacterial pneumonia
aspergillus bronchiolitis
aspergillus cerebral abscess
aspergillus invasion of the nervous
   system
Aspiracath catheter
aspirated debris
aspirated foreign body
aspiration
   air
   blood
   CT-guided
   foreign body
   pulmonary
   tracheal
   transtracheal
   ultrasonic
   ultrasound-guided transthoracic
      needle
aspiration biopsy
aspiration cannula
aspiration pneumonia; pneumonitis
aspiration of ova, ultrasonic guidance
   for
aspiration-tulip device for in vitro percutaneous removal of rigid clots
aspirator, Bovie ultrasound
Aspire continuous imaging (CI)
   system
asplenia
ASPS (alveolar soft-part sarcoma)
ASPVD (atherosclerotic pulmonary
   vascular disease)
ASRT (American Society of
   Radiologic Technologists)
assay
   predictive
   radioisotope clearance

assessment
  activity
  aortoiliac inflow
  invasive
  myocardial viability
  noninvasive
  quantitative Doppler
  real-time
  regional wall motion
associated adenopathy
associated sequestrum
association cortex of parietal lobes
association, megacystis-megaureter
assumed Fick cardiac output
asthmatic airways
asthmatic bronchitis
asthmatic crisis
astragalar bone
astragalocalcanean
astragalocrural
astragaloscaphoid bone
astragalotibial
astragalus (talus)
  aviator's
  fracture of
astroblastoma
astrocytic gliosis
astrocytic tumor
astrocytoma
astroglial tumor
asymmetric appearance time
asymmetric ARDS (acute respiratory
  distress syndrome)
asymmetric breast tissue
asymmetric density
asymmetry
  amplitude
  areas of
  congestive
  facial
  hypertrophic
  interhemispheric
  limb length

asymmetry *(cont.)*
  lung volume (on x-ray)
  narrowing
  septal
  skull
  thoracic
asymptomatic
asymptomatic bacteriuria
asymptomatic hematuria
asymptomatic pseudoaneurysm
asynchronous transfer mode (ATM)
asynchronous ventricular contraction
asyndetic communication
asynergic myocardium
asynergy
  infarct-localized
  left ventricular
  regional
  segmental
asystole
  Beau
  cardiac
  complete atrial and ventricular
  ventricular
asystolic pauses
ataxia, degenerative
AT-II (angiotensin II)
atelectasis
  absorption
  acquired
  acute
  acute massive
  apical
  basilar
  bibasilar discoid
  chronic
  compression
  confluent areas of
  congenital
  congestive
  dependent
  discoid
  disklike

atelectasis *(cont.)*
  initial
  linear
  lobar
  lobular
  lower pulmonary lobe
  middle pulmonary lobe
  obstructive
  patchy
  peripheral parenchymal
  perpetuation of
  platclikc
  platter-like
  primary
  reabsorption
  relaxation
  resorption
  secondary
  segmental
  slowly developing
  streaks of
  subsegmental bibasilar
  subsegmental lower lobe
  upper pulmonary lobc
atelectatic lung
ATF (anterior talofibular ligament)
atherectomized vessel
atherectomy
  directional
  directional coronary
  percutaneous coronary rotational
    (PCRA)
  retrograde
  rotational
  rotational coronary
  transcutaneous extraction catheter
atherectomy catheter
atherectomy device
  directional
  extraction
  percutaneous
  PET balloon Simpson
  rotational

atherectomy technique
  double wire
  kissing
  AthcroCath, Simpson
atheroembolism
atherogenesis
atheroma (pl. atheromata)
  carotid bifurcation
  coral reef
  protruding
atheroma formation, exuberant
atheroma molding
atheromatous abscess
atheromatous cholesterol crystal
  embolization
atheromatous debris
atheromatous degeneration
atheromatous embolism
atheromatous material
atheromatous plaque breakup by
  balloon catheter
atheromatous stenosis
athero-occlusive disease
atherosclerosis
  accelerated
  atherosclerotic
  carotid
  coronary
  extracranial carotid artery
  fatty streak
  fibrous plaque
  intimal
  intracranial carotid artery
  juxtarenal aortic
  native
  pararenal aortic
  virulent
atherosclerosis obliterans (ASO)
atherosclerotic aortic ulcer
atherosclerotic cardiovascular disease
  (ASCVD)
atherosclerotic carotid artery disease
  (ACAD)

atherosclerotic debris
atherosclerotic fatty streaks
atherosclerotic gangrene
atherosclerotic narrowing
atherosclerotic occlusive syndrome
atherosclerotic plaque
atherosclerotic stenosis
atherostenosis
atherothrombotic brain infarction
athlete's pseudonephritis
athletic heart
Atkin epiphyseal fracture
ATL (anterior tricuspid leaflet)
   ATL duplex scanner
   ATL Mark 600 real-time sector
     scanner
   ATL Neurosector real-time scanner
   ATL ultrasound system
   ATL UM 9 HDI Colorflow ultra-
     sound system
Atlantis SR intravascular ultrasound
   imaging catheter
atlantoaxial articulation
atlantoaxial fixation
atlantoaxial instability
atlantoaxial interval
atlantoaxial joint
atlantoaxial posterior membrane
atlantoaxial separation
atlantoaxial subluxation
atlantomastoid
atlanto-odontoid
atlanto-occipital fusion
atlanto-occipital junction
atlanto-occipital membrane
atlas (C1, first cervical vertebra)
   arch of
   burst fracture of
   compression fracture of
   transverse ligaments of
Atlas LP PTCA balloon dilatation
   catheter
atlas matching

Atlas ULP balloon dilatation catheter
ATM (asynchronous transfer mode)
atm. (atmospheres)
ATN (acute tubular necrosis)
atomic mass unit (amu)
atonic bladder
atonic esophagus
atonic ureter
atonic uterus
atony (atonia)
   gastric
   intestinal
   sphincter
atony of uterus
ATP (adenosine triphosphate)-sensitive
   potassium channel openers
atraumatic occlusion of vessels
atresia
   anal
   aortic
   aortic arch
   aortic valve
   biliary
   choanal
   congenital biliary
   congenital laryngeal
   duodenal
   esophageal
   extrahepatic biliary (EBA)
   familial
   infundibular
   intestinal
   intrahepatic (IHA)
   laryngeal
   mitral
   mitral valve
   nasopharyngeal
   prepyloric
   pulmonary
   pulmonary valve
   pulmonary vein
   pulmonic
   tracheal

atresia *(cont.)*
  tricuspid
  valvular
  ventricular
atresic
atretic ovarian follicle
atretic segment (of artery)
atria (pl. of atrium)
atrial activation mapping, retrograde
atrial activation time
atrial appendage
atrial arrhythmia
atrial cuff
atrial disk
atrial ectopic automatic tachycardia
atrial ectopy
atrial-femoral bypass
atrial infarction
atrial kick
atrial myxoma
atrial pacing wire, temporary
atrial partition
atrial phasic volumetric function
atrial right to left shunting
atrial septal aneurysm
atrial septal defect (ASD)
atrial septal defect occlusion (buttoned
  device)
atrial septal defect with mitral stenosis
atrial septum
atrial single and double extrastimulation
atrial situs
atrial situs solitus
atrial standstill
atrial systole
atrial thrombosis
atrial transposition
atrialized ventricle
atriocaval junction
atriofascicular tract
atriography
  contrast left
  negative contrast left

atrio-His (atriohisian)
atrio-His bypass tract
atrio-His fiber
atrio-His pathway
atriopulmonary patch
atrioseptal defect
atrioventricular (AV)
atrioventricular anulus
atrioventricular canal
atrioventricular groove
atrioventricular nodal bypass tract
atrioventricular node mesothelioma
atrioventricular orifice
atrioventricular ostium
atrioventricular ring
atrioventricular septal defect
atrioventricular septum
atrioventricular sequential pacing
atrioventricular valves (mitral and
  tricuspid)
atrium (pl. atria)
  common
  giant left
  high right
  left (LA)
  low septal right
  nontrabeculated
  oblique vein of left
  pulmonary
  respiratory
  right (RA)
  single
  thin-walled
  trabeculated
  ventricular
atrium cordis
atrium dextrum/sinistrum cordis
atrium pulmonale
atrium sinistrum
atrophic emphysema
atrophic fracture
atrophic gastritis
atrophic kidney

atrophic lesion
atrophic nonunion
atrophic thrombosis
atrophy
    alveolar
    brachial muscular
    brain
    cerebellar
    cerebral surface
    compensatory
    compression
    cortical
    degenerative
    denervation
    disuse
    dorsum sellae
    eccentric
    frontotemporal
    gastric
    hemisphere
    infraspinatus muscle
    interstitial
    kidney
    lesser (of disuse)
    lobar
    lobular lung
    localized muscular
    mesiotemporal
    multiple system (MSA)
    muscle
    neurogenic
    olivopontocerebellar
    parenchymatous
    peroneal muscular
    physiologic
    postneuritic
    primary optic
    progressive neuropathic muscle
    progressive postpolio muscle
        (PPPMA)
    quadriceps
    scapuloperoneal muscular
    spinal muscular (SMA)

atrophy *(cont.)*
    subacute denervation
    subcortical
    Sudeck osteoporotic
    sulcal
    temporal horn
    vascular
    villous
atrophy of rostrum and splenium of
    corpus callosum
atropine flush
attachment
    capsular
    cerebellar
    commissural
    dural
    fibrous
    Hudson cerebellar
    intimate (of diseased vessel)
    ligamentous
    mesenteric
    Pearson
    peritoneal
    tendinous
    vascular
attenuate
attenuated image
attenuated lumen
attenuating
attenuation
    aortic
    breast
    decreased
    diaphragmatic
    expiratory
    gamma ray
    ground-glass
    hemidiaphragm
    increased
    linear
    liver
    lower soft tissue (of the accordion
        sign)

attenuation *(cont.)*
  periportal low
  photon
  Picker SPECT attenuation
    correction
  tendon
  theophylline
  valve
attenuation artifact
attenuation coefficient on MRI scan
attenuation correction
attenuation effect
attenuation threshold
attenuation scan
attenuation value on MRI scan
attic adhesion
attrition rupture of tendon
ATV (anterior terminal vein)
ATX-70 sonosensitizer
atypical angina
atypical aortic valve stenosis
atypical chest pain
atypical bronchial pneumonia
atypical interstitial pneumonia
atypical lobular hyperplasia
atypical subisthmic coarctation
atypical verrucous endocarditis
[198]Au (gold) brachytherapy
auditory and visual functional MR
  imaging
Auenbrugger sign
Auerbach mesenteric plexus
AU5 Harmonic ultrasound system
Auger electron emitter
augmentation, abnormal
augmented bladder
augmented filling of right ventricle
augmented stroke volume
"Aunt Minnie" sign
auricle
  left
  right
auricular fissure

Aurora MR (magnetic resonance)
  breast imaging system
Aussies-Isseis unstable scoliosis
autoecholalia
autofusion
autogenous antigen
autogeneous myocutaneous flap reconstruction
autograft, shell osteochondral
autologous clot
autologous patch graft
autologous pericardial parch
autologous pericardium
autologous vein graft
automated airway tree segmentation
  method
automated angle encoder system
automated bolus detection three-
  dimensional fast gradient-recalled-
  echo sequence
automated border detection by
  echocardiography
automated cardiac flow measurement
  (ACM) ultrasound technology
automated cerebral blood flow analyzer
automated computerized axial
  tomography (ACAT)
automated edge detection
automated nodule detection
automated quantification
automated synthesis
automated table movement
automatic extraction
automatic lumen edge segmentation
automatic motion correction
autonomic denervation
autonomic dysfunction
autonomic hyperventilation
autonomic insufficiency
autonomic nervous system
autonomous nodule
autoprescanning
autoradiograph

autoradiographic localization
autoradiography, calcium-45
autoregulation, dynamic cerebral
autoregulation of cerebral blood flow
autosomal dominant polycystic kidney
  disease
autosomal recessive polycystic kidney
  disease
AutoSonix imaging system
AutoSPECT
autostereoscopic
autotopagnosia
autotransplantation of kidney
auto-triggered elliptic centric-ordered
  sequence
AV (arteriovenous)
AV (atrioventricular)
AVA (aortic valve area)
  AVA HF introducer
  AVA 3XI introducer
Avanti angiographic catheter introducer
avascular necrosis (AVN)
avascularity
AVCO aortic balloon
AVD (aortic valvular disease)
AVDO$_2$ (cerebral arteriovenous
  oxygen content difference)
Avellis syndrome
average pixel projection (APP)
averaging
  adaptive frame
  partial volume
  spike
  volume
AVF (arteriovenous fistula)
AVG (aortic valve gradient)
aviator's astragalus
AVM (arteriovenous malformation)
AVM radiotherapy
AVN (avascular necrosis)
AVP (ambulant venous pressure)
AV-Paceport thermodilution catheter

AVR (aortic valve replacement)
AVSD (acquired ventricular septal
  defect)
avulse
avulsed fracture fragment
avulsion
  arterial
  bony
  coracoid tip
  epiphysis
  iatrogenic
  ligament
  nail plate
  spinal nerve root
  traumatic
  venous
avulsion chip fracture
avulsion fracture
avulsion fragment
AVVM (angiographically visualized
  vascular malformation)
axial calcaneal position (of the foot)
axial compression forces
axial compression fracture
axial compression injury
axial CT with timed excretory
  urography
axial dimension
axial gradient echo image
axial hiatal hernia
axial images, multiecho
axial manual traction test
axial musculature
axial neuritis
axial plane
axial plantodorsal view of calcaneus
axial proton-density-weighted image
axial scan
axial section
axial sesamoid position (of the foot)
axial skeleton
axial slice
axial spin density

axial spinal system
axial transabdominal image
axial T2-weighted image
axilla (pl. axillae)
axillary-axillary bypass graft
axillary-brachial bypass graft
axillary-femoral bypass graft
axillary-femorofemoral bypass graft
axillary lymph node staging
axillary node
axillary tail of Spence
axillary vein traumatic thrombosis
axillobifemoral bypass graft
axillofemoral approach
axillofemoral bypass graft
axiographic examination
axiolateral inferosuperior trauma view
    of hip
Axiom DG balloon angioplasty
    catheter
axis (pl. axes)
    anatomic
    ankle mortise
    basibregmatic
    basicranial
    bimalleolar foot
    bowel
    celiac
    coordinate
    cortical hinge
    craniospinal
    distal reference (DRA)
    eccentric axis of ankle rotation

axis *(cont.)*
    enteroinsular
    femoral shaft
    flexion-extension
    hypothalamic-pituitary
    hypothalamic-pituitary-adrenal
    hypothalamoneurohypophyseal
        (HNA)
    leg
    long
    longitudinal
    mechanical
    metatarsal
    proximal reference (PRA)
    rotation
    single (on knee prosthesis)
    spinal
    subtalar
    transcondylar (TCA)
    vertical
    weightbearing
    Z-
axis (C2, second cervical vertebra)
axis of heart
axoid
axonopathic neurogenic thoracic outlet
    syndrome
axoplasmic flow and papilledema
Ayerza-Arrillaga disease
azotemic osteodystrophy
azygos blood flow
azygos lobe of lung
azygos vein distension

B, b

BABE ultrasound
BabyFace 3-D surface rendering ultrasound
BabyFace ultrasound system
baby formula with ferrous sulfate contrast
Baccelli sign of pleural effusion
Bachmann, anterior internodal tract of
bacillary angiomatosis
bacillary embolism
back, arching of
back-angle anomaly
back-bleeding
back crease
backfire fracture
backflow from arterial line
backflow of blood into atria
backflux
background subtraction technique
back manipulation
backrush of blood into left ventricle
backscatter characteristics of blood
backscatter electrons
backscattering
back stroke volume
backup of blood
backward flow

backward heart failure
bacteremia, pulmonary artery catheter-related
bacterial meningitis
bacterial pneumonia or pneumonitis
bacteriuria, asymptomatic
Baffe anastomosis
baffle
    atrial
    construction of intra-atrial
    hemi-Mustard pericardial
    interatrial
    intra-atrial
    intracardiac
    Mustard
    pericardial
    Senning type of intra-atrial
baffled tunnel
baffle leak
bag (see also *pouch*)
    bile
    ostomy
    stomal
bagassosis
Baggish aspiration catheter
bagpipe sign
bailout catheter

60

Baim pacing catheter
baked brain phenomenon
baker's leg (genu valgum)
BAK Vista interbody fusion system
balanced gradient echo cardiac cine
  imaging
balanced ischemia
balance, mass
bald gastric fundus
Balint syndrome
Balkan fracture frame
Balke protocol for cardiac exercise
  stress testing
Balke-Ware treadmill exercise (stress
  testing) protocol
ball-and-seat valve
ball-and-socket joint
Ball AP method (eponym)
Ball AP pelvimetry view
ball-bearing, Steinmann pin with
ball catchers' view
Ball lateral method
Ball lateral pelvimetry view
ball-occluder valve
ball of foot
ballism
ballismus
ballistic injury
ballistocardiography
ball-on-spoon appearance
balloon
  ACS SULP II
  AVCO aortic
  Ballobes gastric
  banana-shaped
  barium enema retention
  bifoil
  Blue Max
  detachable
  esophageal
  Extractor three-lumen retrieval
  Fogarty
  Garren-Edwards

balloon *(cont.)*
  gastric
  Gau gastric
  Grüntzig (Gruentzig)
  Hartzler angioplasty
  hydrostatic
  Innovante
  intra-aortic (IAB)
  intragastric
  kissing
  Kontron intra-aortic
  LPS
  Mansfield
  mercury-containing
  nondistensible
  Outcomes by Design
  Percival gastric
  Percor DL-II (dual lumen)
    intra-aortic
  Percor-Stat intra-aortic
  PET (positron emission
    tomography)
  pulsation
  Rapid-Trak
  Raptor PTCA
  rectal
  Sci-Med Express
  Sci-Med Express Monorail
  scintigraphic
  self-positioning
  slave
  Soto USCI
  Spiegelberg epidural
  Stack autoperfusion balloon
  Taylor gastric
  trefoil
  Tru-Trac high pressure PTA
  waist in the
  Vas-Cath PTA
  Wilson-Cook gastric
balloon and coil embolization
balloon angioplasty
balloon aortoplasty

balloon brachytherapy
balloon catheter fenestration
balloon catheterization to stop
  bleeding
balloon counterpulsation
balloon decompression
ballooned floor of ventricle
balloon embolization (therapeutic)
balloon-expandable esophageal probe
balloon-expandable flexible coil stent
balloon-expandable intravascular stent
balloon-expandable metallic stent
balloon-flotation pacing catheter
balloon inflation
  sequential
  simultaneous
ballooning mitral valve prolapse
  syndrome
ballooning of leaflet
balloon occlusion
balloon occlusion arteriography
balloon occlusion pulmonary
  angiography
Balloon-on-a-Wire catheter
balloon pump
balloon sizing
balloon tamponade
balloon test occlusion
balloon-tipped catheter
balloon uterine stent
ball-valve obstruction
ball valve thrombus
ball-valve tumor
ball-wedge catheter
ball wedge-pressure catheter
Baló sclerosis
Bamberger-Marie disease
Bamberger sign
banana sign
band
  alpha
  alpha frequency
  amniotic

band *(cont.)*
  anogenital
  anterior (of colon)
  AO tension
  aponeurotic
  atrioventricular
  Broca diagonal
  calf
  Clado
  constriction
  coronary
  external
  fascial
  fibroelastic
  fibromuscular
  fibrous
  free band of colon
  Gennari
  H
  Harris
  His
  Hunter-Schreger
  iliotibial (IT)
  intercaval
  internal
  Ladd
  Lane
  lateral
  longitudinal
  lucent
  Maissiat
  Marlex
  Meckel
  mesocolic
  metaphyseal
  moderator
  omental
  parenchymal
  Parham
  Parham-Martin
  parietal
  peritoneal
  pretendinous band of hand

band *(cont.)*
  Reil
  RF saturation
  scar
  septal
  septomarginal
  septum
  silicone elastomer
  Simonart
  tendinous
  transverse
banding appearance
bandlike adhesion
bandlike shadow
band of Broca
band of colon
  anterior
  free
band of density
band of deossification
band of Gennari
band of uterus
band tenodesis
bandwidth limitations
Bannister angioedema disease
Banti disease
bar
  Bill
  bony
  cartilaginous
  congenital
  fibrous
  hyoid
  median
  Passavant
  unsegmented vertebral
bar defect
barber pole sign
barber's chair sign
Barclay niche
Bard CPS system
Bardeen disk
Bardex I.C. catheter

Bard guiding catheter
Bardic cutdown catheter
Baricon (barium sulfate) imaging
  agent
Bardinet ligament
Baricon imaging agent
barium
  double tracking of
  residual
  retained
barium artifact
barium-based fecal tagging
barium column, head of
barium enema (BE)
  air contrast
  double contrast
  full-column
  therapeutic
barium enema retention balloon
barium enema through colostomy
barium enema with air contrast
barium esophagram
barium GI series, motor meal
barium-impregnated poppet
barium injection (through colostomy)
barium meal
barium sulfate imaging agent
barium suspension
barium swallow
Barkow ligament
bar-like ventral defect on myelography
Barlow hip instability test
Barlow sign
Barobag (barium sulfate) imaging
  agent
Baro-Cat (barium sulfate) imaging
  agent
Baros Effervescent Granules (sodium
  bicarbonate and tartaric acid)
Barosperse (barium sulfate) imaging
  agent
barotrauma, pulmonary
Barré-Lieou syndrome

barrel chest
Barrett disease
Barrett esophagus
barrier
   blood-brain (BBB)
   blood-spinal cord
   blood-tumor
Barth hernia
Bartholin gland abscess
Bartholin gland inflammation
Bartholin gland obstruction
Barton fracture
Bartter syndrome
basal, basally
basal chordae
basal cistern
basal ganglia calcifications
basal ganglia of cerebellum
basal joint of thumb
basal-lateral wall myocardial infarction
basal layer
basal movements
basal neck fracture
basal short axis slice
basal skull fracture
basal tuberculosis
basal vein of Rosenthal
basal zone
base
   cranial
   dorsal spinal cord horn
   Dycal
   lung
   posterior spinal cord horn
   skull
baseball elbow
baseball finger
baseball shoulder
base deficit
baseline
   Reid
   reproducible
   return to

baseline artifact
baseline mammogram
baseline of bulb
baseline standing blood pressure
baseline standing pulse rate
baseline tenting (BLT)
base of brain
base of heart
base of lung
base of metacarpal
base of phalanx
base of skull (BOS)
base of thumb
base of toe
basibregmatic axis
basic blood pressure (BP)
basic cycle length (BCL)
basic drive cycle length (BDCL)
basic rate
basicranial axis
Basic II hookwire
basilar artery insufficiency
basilar artery syndrome
basilar atelectasis
basilar cistern
basilar ectasia
basilar fracture
basilar infiltration
basilar insufficiency
basilar intracerebral hemorrhage
basilar invagination
basilar neck fracture
basilar occlusion
basilar pneumonitis
basilar pneumothorax
basilar region
basilar skull fracture
basilar sulcus
basilar suture
basilar syndrome
basilar tip aneurysm
basilar-vertebral artery disease
basilar zone infiltration

basilic vein
basioccipital bone
basiocciput tumor
basion
basket, pericardial
basketlike calcification
basocervical fracture
BAT (B-mode acquisition and targeting) imaging
batch-reading of x-rays
Batson plexus
Batson vertebral brain system
Batten disease
bat-wing appearance
bat-wing catheter
bat-wing distribution
bat wing formation
bat-wing shadow
Baudelocque diameter
Bauman angle
bauxite fibrosis of lung
bauxite pneumoconiosis
Baxter catheter
bayesian image estimation (BIE)
Bayes theorem in exercise stress
testing
Bayliss effect
Bayne classification of radial agenesis
bayonet dislocation
bayonet leg
bayonet position of fracture
Bazin disease
BB (metallic foreign body) shot
BBB (blood-brain barrier)
BBC (biceps, brachialis, coraco-
brachialis) muscles
B bile
BCA (bell clapper anomaly)
B-cell lymphoma
BDA (bile duct adenoma)
BDCL (basic drive cycle length)
BD Insyte Autoguard shielded IV
catheter

BD Introsyte-N Autoguard shielded
introducer
BE (barium enema)
beach chair position
beaded appearance of fibromuscular
dysplasia
beaded hepatic duct
beaded thickening
beading of artery
beads
methyl methacrylate
targeting
beaked cervicomedullary junction
beaking of head of talus
beaking, talonavicular
beaklike osteophyte formation
beak sign of a cortical cyst
beam
blended
cobalt-60
fan
intensity-modulated photon
lateral opposed
Lucite
multifield
open
pencil
radiation
sound
wedge-pair
wedged
beam diffraction
beam dosimetry
adjacent field x-ray
four field x-ray
large field x-ray
single x-ray
beam energy
Beamer injection stent system
Beamer stent
beam's-eye view dosimetry
beam filtration, supplemental
beam hardening artifact

beam intensity
beam linear accelerator, high energy
bent
BEAM (brain electrical activity map)
(or mapping)
BEAMnrc
beam-restricting device
bear claw ulcer
Bear-E-Yum CT (bubble-gum flavored
barium sulfate) imaging agent
Bear-E-Yum GI (bubble-gum flavored
barium sulfate) imaging agent
bear's paw hand
beat knee syndrome
beaten silver appearance of skull
Beath view
beats per minute (BPM or bpm)
Beatson combined ankle angle
beat to beat variability
Beau disease
Beau line
Beauvais disease
beavertail appearance of balloon
profile
BEBIG iodine-125 seed implant
Beckenbaugh technique
Beck triad
Béclard amputation
Béclard hernia
Beclere method to view intercondyloid
fossa in profile
becquerel (Bq)
becquerel effect
bed
bladder
capillary
gallbladder
hepatic
liver
monitor
nail
portal vascular
primary tumor

bed *(cont.)*
pulmonary
pulmonary vascular
skeletal
stomach
tumor
ulcer
vascular
beep-o-gram
Beer-Bouguer theory
Beevor sign
Behçet disease
Behr syndrome
Bekhterev arthritis
Bekhterev layer
bell clapper anomaly (BCA)
Bell-Dally cervical dislocation
Bellini duct
Bell phenomenon
belly of muscle
bend, hand-shaped
bending fracture
Benedict-Talbot body surface area
method
benign intraductal papilloma
benign liver adenoma
benign prostatic hypertrophy
benign tumor
benediction posture (of hand)
benign asbestos related pleural disease
benignity
Benink tarsal index
Bennett basic hand dislocation
Bennett basic hand fracture
Bennett lesion
Bennett fracture
benzene scintillator
benzodiazepine (BN) receptor
benzodiazepine (GABA) receptor
Berkson-Gage breast cancer survival
calculation classification
Berman angiographic catheter
Bernard-Horner syndrome

Berndt-Hardy classification of
transchondral fracture
Berndt-Hardy talar lesion staging
Bernstein catheter
Berquist view of capitellum
berry aneurysm
Bertel position
Bertel view of orbital floors and the
infra-orbital fissure
Bertillon cephalometer
beStent balloon-expandable arterial
stent
beta decay
beta particle
beta-ray applicators
beta-spectra shape factor coefficient
Bethea sign
Bethesda bone
Bethesda classification
Bett trapezium view
Beuren syndrome
beveled anastomosis
beveled edge sign
beveled electron beam cone
beveling
Bexxar Dosimetric Package (tositumomab; iodine I 131 tositumomab)
radiotherapeutic agent
Bexxar Therapeutic Package (tositumomab; iodine I 131 tositumomab)
radiotherapeutic agent
bezoar
bezoar formation
Bezold abscess
BFV (blood flow volume)
BGO (bismuth germanate oxyortho-
silicate)
biad SPECT imaging system
Bianchi nodules
biatrial myxoma
BIB (biliointestinal bypass)
bibasally
bibasilar atelectasis

bibasilar discoid atelectasis
bibeveled
bicaval cannulation
biceps
long head of (LHB)
short head of
biceps femoris muscle
bicerebral infarction
Bichat canal
Bichat fat pad
Bichat membrane
bicipital aponeurosis
bicipital groove
bicipital rib
bicipital tuberosity
bicommissural aortic valve
biconcave
biconcavity
bicondylar fracture
biconvex
bicornuate uterus
bicoronal synostosis
bicortical screw
bicuspid aortic valve
bicuspid atrioventricular valve
bicuspid valvular aortic stenosis
bicycle exercise radionuclide
ventriculography
bidirectional cavopulmonary
anastomosis
BIE (bayesian image estimation)
Bielschowsky-Jansky disease
bifascicular heart block
bifida, spina
bifid clitoris
bifidity, pulmonary artery
bifid pelvis
bifid precordial impulse
bifid ureter
bifid uterus
bifocal manipulation with distraction
bifoil balloon
bifurcate

bifurcation
  aortic
  basilar artery
  carotid
  common bile duct
  common carotid artery
  hepatic duct
  iliac
  middle cerebral artery
  patent
  pulmonary artery
  pulmonary trunk
  tracheal
  ureteral bud
bifurcation graft
bifurcation lesion
bigeminal rhythm
  atrial
  atrioventricular nodal
  bisferious pulse
  escape-capture
  nodal
  reciprocal
  ventricular
Bigliani hip projection view
bihemispheric insult
bi-ischial diameter
bilateral carotid stenosis
bilateral consolidation
bilateral hypertrophy
bilaterality of ureteral duplication
bilaterally
bilateral mammogram
bilateral small kidney
bilateral tubo-ovarian abscess
bilateral whole breast ultrasound
Bilbao-Dotter catheter
bileaflet
bile concretion
bile duct
  common (CBD)
  infundibulum of
  interlobular

bile *(cont.)*
  lobar
  preampullary portion of
  segmental
  sphincter of
bile duct proliferation
bile duct scan
bile flow
bile lake
bile peritonitis
bile plug
bile stasis
bilharzial fibrosis
bilharziasis
  cardiopulmonary
  protopulmonary
biliary atresia
biliary duct
biliary-duodenal pressure gradient
biliary dyskinesia
biliary mud
biliary obstruction
biliary passages
biliary radicle
biliary saturation index
biliary sludge
biliary stent
biliary stone
biliary structures
biliary to bowel transit
biliary tract
biliary tract imaging
biliary tree
Biligrafin imaging agent
biliointestinal bypass (BIB)
biliopancreatic bypass (BPB)
bilious pneumonia
bilirubin pigment stones (gallstones)
Bilivist (ipodate sodium) imaging
  agent
Bill bar (bone)
billowing mitral leaflet (BML)
billowing mitral valve prolapse

Billroth I type anastomosis
Billroth II type anastomosis
bilobed mass
bilobed polypoid lesion
bilobed ureterocele
bilocular stomach
biloma
bimalleolar ankle fracture
bimanual abdominorectal palpation of
    uterus
bimanual abdominovaginal palpation
    of uterus
binarize
binary image
binding, receptor
Bing-Horton syndrome
binning, projection
binocular acuity change
biocompatibility
biodegradable magnetic microclusters
biodegradable stent
Bio divYsio stent
bioeffects algorithms
Bio-Flex CS catheter
bioimpedance
biologic age
biological half-life
biological osteosynthesis
biological tissue valve
biomagnetometer, Magnes
biomechanical analysis
biomechanical imbalance
biomechanics of limb length
    discrepancy
biometry, longitudinal ultrasonic
biomodulator
bioprosthesis
biopsy (pl. biopsies)
    core
    CT (computed tomography)-guided
    CT-guided coaxial fine-needle
        aspiration
    CT-guided Tru-Cut liver

biopsy *(cont.)*
    directional vacuum-assisted
    gamma probe-assisted
    large core needle
    mammogram-guided
    mirror image breast
    MRI-guided breast
    percutaneous endomyocardial
    percutaneous pericardial
    point-in-space stereotactic
    Sonopsy 3-D ultrasound breast
    stereotactic directional vacuum-
        assisted breast
    stereotactic vacuum-assisted breast
    stereotactic vacuum-assisted
        directional
    ultrasound-guided
    ultrasound-guided anterior
        subcostal liver
    vacuum-assisted breast
biopsy of kidney
biopsy-site marker clip
BioSorb resorbable urologic stent
Biosound AU (Advanced Ultra-
    sonography) system
Biospec imaging system
biparietal bossing
biparietal diameter (BPD)
biparietotemporal hypometabolism
bipartite patella
bipartite sesamoid
bipartition, facial
bipenniform muscles of hand
biphasic contrast-enhanced helical CT
biphasic CT
biphasic CT with mesenteric CT
    angiography
biphasic curve
biplanar aortography
biplanar cardiac blood pool
    tomography
biplanar MR imaging guidance

biplane area-length method
(echocardiography)
biplane fluoroscopy
biplane left ventricular angiogram
biplane orthogonal views
biplane pelvic arteriography
biplane pelvic oblique study
biplane sector probe
biplane transesophageal
echocardiography (TEE)
bipolar gradient
bipolar hip replacement
bipolar saline-enhanced electrode
bipolar sensing, integrated
bipolar temporary pacemaker catheter
BI-RADS (breast imaging and reporting data system) of the American
College of Radiology
bird-beak configuration or narrowing
bird-beak taper at esophagogastric
junction
bird breeder's lung
birdcage coils
birdcage splint
bird fancier's lung
bird handler's lung
bird's-eye view
bird's nest filter (or bird nest filter)
birth fracture
bisection, AP malleolar
bishop's nod
Bismuth classification of benign bile
duct stricture
bismuth germanate oxy-ortho silicate
(BGO)
Bisound AP 3000 Colorflow ultrasound system
bispinous diameter
bite-wing film
bite-wing radiograph
bit-rate allocation
bituberous diameter
bivalve

biventricular assist device (BVAD)
biventricular global systolic
dysfunction
biventricular hypertrophy
biventricular transposed aorta
biventricularly
BKA (below-knee amputation)
black blood magnetic resonance
angiography (MRA)
black blood T2-weighted inversion-
recovery MR imaging
black boundary artifact
black comets artifact
black dot heel
black echo writing
Blackett-Healy shoulder position
(for teres minor or subscapularis
insertion)
Blackfan-Diamond syndrome
black lung disease
bladder
apex of
atonic
augmented
automatic
base of
calcified
centrally uninhibited
dome of urinary
exstrophy of
formation of open ileal
hypertrophic
hypotonic
large capacity
leak point pressure in
motor paralytic
myogenic
neck of
neurogenic
papilloma of
pear-shaped
refluxing spastic neurogenic
sensory paralytic

bladder *(cont.)*
  spastic
  thickened
  thick-walled
  trigone of
  uninhibited
  urinary
  uvula of
  valve
bladder abscess
bladder calculus
bladder carcinoma classification
bladder cavity
bladder contractility study
bladder contrast
bladder diverticula
bladder emptying
  complete
  incomplete
bladder endometriosis
bladder fistula
bladder floor
bladder hypertrophy
bladder inflammation
bladder laceration
bladder malignancy
BladderManager ultrasound device
bladder neck contracture
bladder neck obstruction
bladder neck stenosis
bladder outlet obstruction
bladder perforation
bladder prolapse
bladder stasis
bladder to skin fistula
bladder to uterus fistula
bladder to vagina fistula
bladder trauma
bladder tumor
bladder wall hemorrhage
blade of grass appearance
BladderScan BVI 2500 ultrasound
  scanner

BladderScan scan
BladderScan ultrasound
blade of grass sign
blade plate
blanch
bland aortic aneurysm
bland embolism
bland infarct
blast chest
bleb
  emphysematous
  myelin
  ruptured emphysematous
  subpleural
Bleck classification of metatarsus
  adductus
bleed (noun)
  GI
  herald
bleeding into the infarct
bleeding ulcer
blended beam technique
blennorrhagic swelling
blennothorax
blind access
blind catheter
blind dimple in floor of left atrium
blind-ending rectum
blind intestine
blind loop syndrome
blind pouch
blind tibial outflow tracts
blister (vesicle)
blister, fracture
blister of bone
blistering distal dactylitis (BDD)
BLN (breast localization needle)
Bloch equation
block
  acquired symptomatic AV
  air
  alveolar-capillary
  anodal

block *(cont.)*
anterior fascicular
anterograde
arborization
AV (atrioventricular)
AV Wenckebach heart
BBB (bundle branch)
BBBB (bilateral bundle branch)
bifascicular
bifascicular bundle branch
bifascicular heart
bilateral bundle branch (BBBB)
bone
bundle branch (BBB)
bundle branch heart
CerroBend
complete AV (CAVB)
complete congenital heart
complete heart (CHB)
conduction
congenital complete heart
congenital heart
congenital symptomatic AV
custom
deceleration-dependent
divisional
donor heart-lung
entrance
exit
false bundle-branch
familial heart
fascicular
filler
first degree AV
first degree heart
fixed third degree AV
heart
high grade AV
incomplete atrioventricular (IAVB)
incomplete heart
incomplete left bundle branch
    (ILBBB)

block *(cont.)*
incomplete right bundle branch
    (IRBBB)
inflammatory heart
infra-His
intermittent third degree AV
interventricular
intra-atrial
intra-His
intra-Hisian or intrahisian
intranodal
intravenous (IV)
intraventricular conduction
intraventricular heart
inverted Y
ipsilateral bundle branch
irregular
left anterior fascicular (LAFB)
left anterior hemiblock
left bundle branch (LBBB)
left posterior fascicular (LPFB)
mantle
Mobitz I or II second degree AV
multiple
paroxysmal AV
partial heart
peri-infarction (PIB)
posterior fascicular
pseudo-AV
retrograde
right bundle branch (RBBB)
second degree AV
second degree heart
selective nerve root
simple
sinoatrial (SAB)
sinoatrial exit
sinus
sinus exit
sinus node exit
supra-Hisian *or* suprahisian
sympathetic nerve
third degree AV
third degree heart

block *(cont.)*
  transient AV
  transmission
  trifascicular
  unidirectional
  unifascicular
  VA (ventriculoatrial)
  ventricular
  vesicular
  Wenckebach AV
  Wilson
blockage
  bronchus
  pulmonary artery
blocked APC (atrial premature
  contraction)
blocked artery
blocked bronchus
blocked pleurisy
blocked urethra
blocked vertex field
blocker's exostosis
blocking, alpha
Block right coronary guiding catheter
block uniform resampling (BURS)
  algorithm
Blom-Singer tracheoesophageal fistula
Blondeau view for facial bones
blood
  arterial
  deoxygenated
  egress of
  epidural
  extravasated
  heparinized
  intraparenchymal
  intraventricular
  occult
  parenchymal
  peripheral
  shunted
  sludged
  subdural

block *(cont.)*
  upstream
  venous
blood-brain barrier (BBB)
  alteration in
  defects in
  intact
blood-brain barrier osmotic disruption
blood clearance half-time
blood clot
blood-clotting mechanism
blood flow
  altered
  antegrade
  azygos
  capillary
  cerebral
  Doppler study of
  microcirculatory
  Qp (pulmonary blood flow)
  Qs (systemic blood flow)
  regional
  regional cerebral
  supratentorial cerebral
blood flow analyzer, automated
  cerebral
blood flow extraction fraction
blood flow in heart at rest
blood flow in heart during exercise
blood flow in microcirculation with
  high frequency Doppler ultrasound
blood flow on Doppler echocardiogram
blood flow probe
blood flow reserve
blood flow response
blood flow study
blood flow to tissue beyond
  obstruction
blood flow velocity
blood flow volume (BFV)
blood flow volume measurement
blood inflow

blood leak
bloodless fluid
blood oxygen level dependent (BOLD)
   functional MR imaging
blood perfusion
blood perfusion monitor (BPM)
blood plate thrombus
blood pool
   vascular
   white-appearing
blood-pool activity
blood-pool imaging
blood-pool phase image
blood-pool radionuclide angiography
blood-pool radionuclide echocardiography
blood-pool radionuclide scan
blood pressure response
blood speckle
blood-spinal cord barrier
blood stream or bloodstream
blood substitute, oxygenated
   perfluorocarbon
blood supply
   accessory
   dual
   longitudinal
blood-tumor barrier
blood velocity distribution
blood vessel necrosis
blood vessel thermography
blood vessel tumor
blood volume
   central
   circulating
   fractional moving
blood volume per minute (vol./min.)
Bloom and Obata view
blooming artifacts in ultrasonography
blooming, signal
Blount disease
blow-in fracture
blowing pneumothorax

blowout, aortic stump
blowout fracture
BLT (baseline tenting)
blue dye "sentinel node" method
Blue FlexTip catheter
Blue Max triple lumen catheter
blue rubber-bleb nevus syndrome
Blumenbach clivus
Blumensaat line
Blumer rectal shelf
blunt abdominal trauma
blunt border of lung
blunt chest trauma
blunt duct adenosis
blunted costophrenic angle
blunting of posterior sulci
blunt injury
blunt trauma
blunt trauma to kidney
blurring of aortic knob
blurring of costophrenic angle
blurring of disk margins
blush
   tumor (on cerebral angiography)
   vascular (of tumor on carotid
     angiography)
BM (bowel movement)
BMC (bone mineral content)
BMD (bone mineral density)
BMI (body mass index)
BMIPP SPECT scan
BML (billowing mitral leaflet)
B-mode (B-scan)
   longitudinal
   pseudocolor
B-mode acquisition and targeting
   (BAT) imaging
B-mode echocardiography
B-mode echography
B-mode ultrasound
BMP (bone marrow pressure)
BNCT (boron neutron capture
   therapy)

BN receptor
BO field variation
board
  Dome Imaging RX20
  Intel PC Link2
bobby pin-like configuration
Bochdalek, foramen of
Bochdalek hernia
body (pl. bodies)
  alignment of vertebral
  carotid
  coccygeal
  esophageal
  foreign
  foreign (retained)
  Gamna-Gandy
  geniculate
  height of vertebral
  intra-articular
  juxtarestiform
  Luys
  mamillary
  navicular
  ossified
  osteocartilaginous
  osteochondritic loose
  pacchionian
  pineal
  restiform
  retained foreign
  rhinencephalic mamillary
  rice joint
  scapular
  trapezoid
body background activity
body box plethysmography
body coil
body contour orbit, body artifacts
  due to
BodyFlex port
body habitus
body mass index (BMI)
body of vertebra

body section radiography
body surface area (BSA)
body surface potential mapping
Boeck sarcoid
Boehler (Böhler) angle
boggy synovitis
boggy synovium
Bogros space
Böhler (see *Boehler*) angle
Bohr effect
BOLD (blood oxygenation level
  dependent)
  BOLD contrast enhancement
  BOLD effect
  BOLD image
  BOLD MR imaging
  BOLD response
  BOLD signal
Boltzmann distribution factor
bolus
  air
  contrast
  dynamic
  electron
  intravenous
  simple
  special
  tracer
  water
bolus challenge test
bolus chase
bolus chase imaging technique
bolus chase technique in angiography
  and MRI scan
bolus chase three-dimensional MR
  digital subtraction angiography
bolus contrast enhancement
bolus intravenous injection
bolus tracking
bolus transit
Bonanno suprapubic catheter
bombardment, alpha particle

bone
  accessory
  accessory navicular
  acetabular
  acromial
  alar
  Albers-Schönberg (Schoenberg)
    marble
  Albrecht
  alveolar
  alveolar supporting
  ankle
  anvil
  arch of
  areolae of
  articular lamella of
  articular tubercle of temporal
  astragalar
  astragalus
  astragalocalcanean
  astragalocrural
  astragaloscaphoid
  astragalotibial
  atrophy of
  autogenous
  basal
  basilar
  basioccipital
  basisphenoid
  Bertin
  Bethesda
  bicortical iliac
  blade
  bleeding
  Bonfiglio
  breast
  bregmatic
  Breschet
  brittle
  bundle
  calcaneal
  calcaneus
  Calcitite

bone *(cont.)*
  calvarial
  cancellated
  cancellous
  cannon
  capitate
  carpal
  cartilage
  cavalry
  central
  chalky
  cheek
  chevron (V-shaped)
  coccygeal
  coccyx
  coffin
  collar
  compact
  continuity of
  convoluted
  coronary
  cortical
  cortical cancellous
  costal
  coxal
  cranial
  crest of iliac
  cribriform
  cubital
  cuboid
  cuneiform
  dead
  dense
  dense structure of
  depression of nasal
  dermal
  destruction of
  devitalized portion of
  diastasis of cranial
  displaced fragment of
  dorsal talonavicular
  eburnated
  elbow

bone *(cont.)*
  endochondral
  enteral
  epactal
  epihyal
  epihyoid
  epiphysis
  epipteric
  episternal
  erosion of epiphyseal
  ethmoid
  exercise
  exoccipital
  femoral
  fibular
  first cuneiform
  flank (ilium)
  flat
  florid
  Flower
  fourth turbinated
  fracture running length of
  fragile
  fragment of
  frontal
  Goethe
  greater multangular (trapezium)
  hamate
  haunch
  heel
  heterotopic
  highest turbinated
  hip
  hollow
  hooked
  humeral
  hyoid
  hyperplastic
  iliac
  iliac cancellous
  immature
  incarial
  incisive

bone *(cont.)*
  incomplete fracture of
  incus
  infected
  inferior turbinated
  inflammation of
  innominate
  intermaxillary
  intermediate cuneiform
  interparietal
  intracartilaginous
  intrachondral
  intramembranous
  irregular
  ischial
  ivory
  ivorylike
  jaw
  knuckle
  lacrimal
  lamellar
  lenticular (of hand)
  lentiform
  lesser multangular (trapezoid)
  lingual
  long
  long axis of
  lunate
  lunocapitate
  luxated
  malar
  mallcolar
  malleolus
  marble
  mastoid
  mature
  maxillary
  maxilloturbinal
  medial cuneiform
  medullary
  membrane of
  metacarpal
  metatarsal

bone *(cont.)*
  metastasis to
  metatarsal
  middle cuneiform
  middle turbinate
  morcellized
  mortise of
  multangular
  nasal
  navicular
  necrotic
  neoplasm of
  newly woven
  Nicoll
  occipital
  odontoid
  orbicular
  orbitosphenoidal
  os calcis
  os trapezium
  os trapezoideum
  ossifying fibroma of long
  osteonal
  osteopenic
  osteoporosis of
  osteoporotic
  pagetoid
  palatine
  parietal
  pedal
  pelvic
  perichondral
  perilesional
  periosteal
  periotic
  peroneal
  petrosal
  petrous
  petrous temporal
  phalangeal
  Pirie
  pisiform
  pneumatic

bone *(cont.)*
  porous
  postsphenoid
  post-traumatic atrophy of
  preinterparietal
  premaxillary
  presphenoid
  primitive
  proliferation of
  prominence of
  pterygoid
  pubic
  pyramidal
  quadrilateral
  radial
  refractured
  replacement
  resurrection
  reticulated
  rider's
  Riolan
  rudimentary
  sacral
  scaphoid
  scapular
  sclerotic
  scroll
  second cuneiform
  semilunar
  septal
  sesamoid
  shank
  shin
  short
  sieve
  sphenoid
  sphenoidal turbinated
  sphenoturbinal
  splintered
  split thickness cranial
  spoke
  spongy
  squamo-occipital

bone *(cont.)*
squamous
squamous-type
stirrup
subchondral
superior turbinated
subperiosteal new
substitution
supernumerary
supernumerary sesamoid
supracollicular spike of cortical
suprainterparietal
supraoccipital
suprapharyngeal
suprasternal
supreme turbinate
sutural
tail
talus
tarsal
temporal
thick
thigh
thoracic
three-cornered
tibia
trabecular
trapezium (greater multangular)
trapezoid (lesser multangular)
trapezoid of Henle
trapezoid of Lyser
triangular
triangular wrist
triquetral
triquetrum
tubular
tuberculosis of
tumor-bearing
turbinate
turbinated
tympanic
tympanohyal
ulnar

bone *(cont.)*
ulnar sesamoid
unciform
upper jaw
vascular
vesalian
Vesalius
vomer
weightbearing
wing of sphenoid
wormian
woven
wrist triquetrum
xiphoid
yoke
zygomatic
bone abscess
bone absorption
bone age according to Greulich
and Pyle
bone age ratio
bone allograft
bone atrophy
bone block
bone cement, Surgical Simplex P
radiopaque
bone chip
bone core
bone debris
bone dehiscence
bone demineralization
Bone Densitometer, QDR-1500 or
QDR-2000
bone densitometry
T-score on
Z-score on
bone density, increased
bone density measurement
bone density study
bone density test
bone deposits, endochondral
bone destruction, localized
bone destructive process

bone dysplasia
bone ends
bone erosion
bone formation
  new
  sparsity of
  subperiosteal new
bone-forming sarcoma
bone-forming tumor
bone fracture
bone fragment
bone graft
bone growth stimulator
bone imaging
bone implant
bone infarct
bone infection
bone involvement
bone island
bone length study
bonelet
bone marrow edema pattern on MR
  imaging
bone marrow embolism
bone marrow involvement
bone marrow scintigraphy
bone mass, loss of
bone maturation
bone metastases, occult
bone "mets" (slang for metastases)
bone mineral content (BMC) study
bone mineral density (BMD)
bone mineralization
bone or joint pathology
bone phase image
bone pinhole
bone plate
bone plug
bone powder
bone remodeling
bone resorption
bone scan (see also *imaging*)
  isotope

bone *(cont.)*
  triple phase
  TSPP rectilinear
bone scintigraphy
bone screw
bone sequestrum
bone shaft
bone sliver
bone spicule
bone spur
bone substance
bone survey
bone-tendon exposure
bone window
bony (see also *bone*)
bony abnormality
bony ankylosis
bony apposition
bony architecture
bony avulsion
bony bridging
bony callus formation
bony change
bony decompression
bony defect (acoustic window)
bony deformity
bony deposit
bony destruction
bony disruption
bony eburnation
bony encroachment
bony enlargement
bony erosion
bony excrescence
bony exostosis
bony fracture
bony fragment
bony fusion
bony healing
bony island
bony landmark
bony lysis
bony necrosis and destruction

bony osteophyte
bony overgrowth
bony pelvis
bony proliferation
bony prominence (spur)
bony protuberance
bony rarefaction
bony reabsorption
bony resorption
bony ridge
bony sclerosis
bony skeleton
bony spicule
bony spur
bony spurring
bony stability
bony structures, demineralized
bony thorax
bony tufts of fingers
bony union, solid
"boomerang" ovoid-shaped tendon
Boorman classification of gastric
    cancer
boost
    brachytherapy
    electron
    electron beam
    interstitial
    tumor bed
boot-shaped heart
boot-top fracture
borborygmus (pl. borborygmi)
border
    alveolar
    anterior
    antimesenteric
    cardiac
    ciliated
    corticated
    crescentic
    heart
    inferior
    interosseous

border *(cont.)*
    lateral
    lower sternal (LSB)
    medial
    mid-left sternal
    posterior
    sternocleidomastoid muscle
    superior
    upper sternal
borderline
borderline ovarian tumor
borderline pelvis
border of heart
    anterior
    inferior
    left
    posterior
    right
    superior
border zone
border zone-region infarction
Borg scale of treadmill exertion
Born approximation
Bornholm disease
boron neutron capture therapy
    (BNCT)
BOS (base of skull)
Bosniak classification
Bosniak renal cystic mass classifica-
    tion
boss
bosselated
bosselation
bossing
    biparietal
    frontal
    occipital
Boston LINAC (linear accelerator)
Bosworth fracture
Botallo duct
Botallo foramen
Botallo ligament
both-bone forearm fracture

bottle sign
bottoming out of prosthetic component
Bouchard disease
Bouchard node
bouche de tapir (tapir's mouth)) in
  muscular dystrophy
Bouillaud disease
bounce point artifact
boundary
  bone marrow
  lumen
  tumor
Bourneville disease
Bourneville-Pringle disease
boutonnière deformity of finger
Bouveret disease
Bouveret-Hoffmann syndrome
Bovie ultrasound aspiration
Bowditch effect
Bowditch staircase phenomenon
bowed legs
bowel
  aganglionic
  apple-peel
  dead
  dilated loops of
  distal small
  fluid-filled loop of
  hypotensive shock
  infarcted
  intussuscepted
  irritable
  ischemic
  kinked
  kink in
  large
  multiple loops of small
  proximal small
  small
  strangulated
bowel and bladder dysfunction
bowel contents
bowel continuity

bowel fills and evacuates satisfactorily
bowel follow-through, small (SBFT)
bowel gas
  displacement of
  superimposed
bowel gas displaced by extraperitoneal
  blood and urine
bowel gas pattern
bowel involvement
bowel laceration
bowel loop
bowel lumen
bowel motion
bowel movement (BM)
bowel obstruction
bowel pattern
bowel peristalsis
bowel prep (preparation) (see *enema*)
  CoLyte
  Dulcolax
  Emulsoil
  Evac-Q-Kit
  Evac-Q-Kwik
  Fleet
  GoLytely
  HalfLytely
  inadequate
  OCL
  Tridrate
  X-Prep
bowel preparation before barium
  enema
bowel preparation before colonoscopy
bowel rest
bowel series, small
bowel shadows, superimposition of
bowel syndrome
  irritable
  spastic
bowel wall
bowel wall enhancement, abnormal
bowel wall outpouchings
Bowen disease

bowing deformity
bowing of mitral valve leaflet
bowing of tendons
bowleg (genu varum)
bowler hat sign
bowler's thumb
Bowman angle
Bowman capsule
Bowman space
bowstring sign
bowstring tear
bowstringing
bow-tie sign of cervical fracture
box
   anatomic snuffbox
   ligamentous
   snuffbox
   view
boxer's elbow
boxer's fracture of metacarpal
boxer's knuckle
boxer's punch fracture (of fifth
   metacarpal)
Boyd formula
Boyd-Griffin classification
Boyd type II fracture
Bozzolo sign
BP (arterial blood pressure)
BPB (biliopancreatic bypass)
BPD (biparietal diameter)
BPD (bronchopulmonary dysplasia)
BPM (blood perfusion monitor)
B-port implant infusion port
BPS spinal angiographic catheter
Bq (becquerel)
Braasch bulb with whistle catheter tip
Bracco system
brace, bracing (removed for imaging
   studies)
bracelet, ^{89}Sr (strontium)
braces artifact
brachial artery compression
brachial artery cuff pressure

brachial artery pulse pressure
brachial-basilar insufficiency
brachial bypass
brachial neuritis
brachial plexus compression
brachial plexus injury
brachial plexus neuritis
brachiocephalic (innominate)
brachiocephalic arterial aneurysm
brachiocephalic artery
brachiocephalic ischemia
brachiocephalic lymph nodes
brachiocephalic trunk of aorta
brachiocephalic vein
brachiocephalic vessel
brachiocubital
brachioradialis muscle
brachiosubclavian bridge graft fistula
   (BSBGF)
brachium (pl. brachia)
brachium of colliculus
brachycephalic head shape
brachycephaly
brachydactyly
brachymetatarsia
BrachySeed iodine I 125 (^{125}I) implant
   seeds
BrachySeed palladium Pd 103 (^{103}Pd)
   implant seeds
brachytherapy (radiotherapy)
   afterloading
   balloon
   BEBIG iodine I 125 (^{125}I) seed
      implant
   BrachySeed palladium Pd 103
      (^{103}Pd) seeds
   CT-guided
   endobronchial
   endovascular
   episcleral plaque
   gold ^{198}Au
   HDR (high dose rate)
   iodine ^{125}I

brachytherapy *(cont.)*
  iodine ^{192}I
  interstitial
  intracavitary
  intraluminal
  intraoperative high dose rate
    (IOHDR)
  low dose radiation (LDR) seed
  palladium 103 (^{103}Pd) implantation
  permanent
  prostate
  remote afterloading (RAB)
  Syed-Neblett
  Symmetra iodine ^{125}I seed
  volumetric interstitial
  ytterbium ^{169}Yb
brachytherapy boost
BrachyVision software for brachytherapy
Bradbury-Eggleston syndrome
Bradbury-Eggleston triad
Braden flushing reservoir
bradykinin
bradyphemic
bradyphrenia
Bragard sign
Bragg angle
Bragg curve
Bragg ionization peak
Bragg law
Bragg peak photon beam therapy
Bragg peak radiosurgery
braided diagnostic catheter
brain
  architecture of
  atrophic lesion of the
  edematous
  inflammation of
  metastasis to
  split
  unicameral
  Virchow-Robin spaces of the
  water on the
  wet

brain abscess
brain activity
brain anoxia
brain atrophy
brain contusion
brain cyst
brain-dead patient
brain death
brain disease, organic (OBD)
brain dysfunction
brain electrical activity map (or mapping) (BEAM)
brain fiber tracking
brain function
brain ischemia
brain laceration
brain lesion, atrophic
brain mantle
brain map
brain mapping
brain mass
brain parenchyma, bleeding into
brain perfusion scintigraphy
brain perfusion SPECT
brain plasticity
brain scan (see *imaging*)
brain stem compression
brain stem demyelination
brain stem disease
brain stem displacement
brain stem glioma tumor
brain stem hemorrhage
brain stem infarct
brain stem infarction
brain stem ischemia
brain stem lesion
brain stem pyramidal tract
brain stem reticular formation
brain stem signs
brain surface matching technique
brain swelling
brain syndrome, organic (OBS)
brain to background ratio

brain tumor
brain water diffusion
brain window
branch (pl. branches) (see also *artery*)
  acute marginal
  anterior cutaneous
  arterial
  AV (atrioventricular) groove
  bifid aortic
  bifurcating
  bronchial
  caudal
  circumflex
  cutaneous lateral
  diagonal
  digital
  distal
  feeding
  first diagonal
  first major diagonal
  first septal perforator
  inferior cardiac
  inferior wall
  large obtuse marginal
  left bundle
  marginal
  midmarginal
  motor
  muscular
  nonlingular
  obtuse marginal (OMB)
  paired parietal
  paired visceral
  perforating
  phalangeal
  posterior descending
  posterior intercostal
  posterior ventricular
  proper digital nerve
  pudendal
  ramus
  ramus intermedius artery
  ramus medialis
  right bundle

branch *(cont.)*
  second diagonal
  segmental
  septal
  septal perforating
  side
  subcostal
  superior phrenic
  unpaired parietal
  unpaired visceral
  ventricular
branched calculus
branches of vein
branching line
branching linear structure
branching, mirror-image brachiocephalic
branching tubular structure
branch of artery
branch point
Branham sign (arteriovenous fistula)
Brasdor method
Brattstrom method (skyline patella)
Brattstrom view
Braun tumor
bread-and-butter heart
bread-and-butter pericarditis
bread-crumbling movement
"bread-loaf" technique (for obtaining
  tomographic slices)
breakthrough vasodilatation
breakthrough visualization
breast
  accessory
  atrophic
  contralateral
  cystic
  cystic disease of
  fibroadenoma of
  fibrocystic
  heterogeneously dense
  shoemaker's
  tail of
breast abscess

breast adenoma
breast artifact
breast attenuation
breast biopsy system, Mammotome
  handheld minimally invasive
breast bone or breastbone
breast calcification
breast duct
breast fibrocystic disease stages:
  adenosis
  cystic disease
  mazoplasia
breast hypertrophy
breast imaging
breast imaging and reporting data
  system (BI-RADS) of the American College of Radiology
breast implant capsule
breast localization needle (BLN)
breast localizer
breast mass lesion with poorly defined
  margins
breast microcalcifications
breast parenchyma
breast shadow
breast skin satellite metastasis
breaststroker's knee
breast thrombophlebitis
breast tissue, attenuation by
breast ultrasound
breath-hold cine MR
breath-hold contrast-enhanced three-
  dimensional MR angiography
breath-hold fast recovery optimized
  fast spin echo imaging
breath-hold fast spin echo or multishot
  spin echo echo-planar imaging
breath-hold GRE sequences
breath-hold MR cholangiography
breath-hold MR imaging
breath-hold T1-weighted MP-GRE
  MR imaging
breath-hold ungated imaging

breath-hold velocity-encoded cine MR
  imaging
breathing
  ataxic
  labored
breathing artifact
breathing feedback
breathless when wheezing
breath pentane measurement
breath, shortness of (SOB)
breech presentation
bregma
bregmatic bone
Bremer AirFlo Vest for thoracic
  stabilization
Bremer Halo Crown system
bremsstrahlung, directional
bremsstrahlung scan
Brenner tumor
Breschet sinus
Brescia-Cimino shunt
Brett syndrome
Brevi-Kath epidural catheter
Brewerton view (metacarpals and
  phalanges), *not* Breuerton
bridegroom's palsy
bridge (bridging)
  arteriolovenular
  bone
  bony
  interthalamic
  meniscal
  mucosal
  osseous
  osteophytic
  skin
  ventral
  Wheatstone
bridge autograft
bridged loop gap resonator
bridge-graft fistula (BGF)
Bridgeman view
Bridge X3 renal stent

bridging osteophytes
bright contrast enhancement
bright highly mobile echoes
brightly increased renal parenchymal
    echogenicity
brightness-time curves
bright pixel values
bright red flush
bright signal on MRI
brim sign
brim, thickened pelvic
B ring of esophagus
Brinton disease
brisement therapy
Brissaud syndrome
Bristol-Myers system
BriteMax sheath introducer
brittle bone
brittle bones failure
broadband noise detection error
    artifact
broad band of pleural fluid
broadband transducer
broad-based
broad beam absorption
broad beam geometry
Broadbent inverted sign
broadening, dipolar
broad ligament abscess
broad ligament endometriosis
broad ligament hematoma
broad ligament laceration
broad maxillary ridge
Broca convolution
Broca diagonal band
Broca motor speech area of the brain
Broca region
Brock middle lobe syndrome
Brockenbrough catheter, modified
    bipolar
Brockenbrough mapping catheter
Brockenbrough needle

Broden subtalar joint view I and II,
    not Brodan
Brodie abscess
Brodie bursa
Brodie disease
Brodie knee
Brodie ligament
Brodie metaphyseal abscess
Brodmann cytoarchitectonic fields
bromospiperone
bromodeoxyuridine labeling index
bromophenol blue
bronchi (pl. of bronchus) (see
    bronchus)
bronchial adenoma
bronchial annular cartilage
bronchial arteriography
bronchial artery embolization
bronchial asthma
bronchial branch
bronchial bud
bronchial calculus
bronchial caliber
bronchial cartilage, absent
bronchial collapse on forced
    expiration
bronchial collateral circulation
bronchial cyst
bronchial dehiscence
bronchial diameter
bronchial distortions
bronchial erosion
bronchial kinking
bronchial lumen
bronchial mucosa
bronchial mucosal edema
bronchial obstruction
bronchial pneumonia
bronchial provocation testing
bronchial reactivity
bronchial septum
bronchial smooth muscle spasm

bronchial spasm
bronchial stenosis
bronchial stricture
bronchial tree
bronchial type B disease
bronchial vessels
bronchiectasis
  acquired
  capillary
  congenital
  cylindrical
  cystic
  dry
  follicular
  fusiform
  Polynesian
  postinfectious
  recurrent
  saccular
  tuberculous
  varicose
bronchiectasis-bronchomalacia
  syndrome
bronchiectasis-ethmoid sinusitis
bronchiectatic pattern
bronchiolar carcinoma
bronchiolar edema
bronchiolar emphysema
bronchiolar narrowing
bronchiolar obstruction
bronchiolar passages, narrowing of
bronchiole (pl. bronchioli)
  alveolar
  conducting
  lobular
  respiratory
  terminal
bronchiolitis
  aspergillus
  constrictive
  diffuse pan-
  exudative
  proliferative

bronchiolitis *(cont.)*
  respiratory
  smoker's
  vesicular
bronchiolitis obliterans with
  organizing pneumonia (BOOP)
bronchioloalveolar carcinoma
bronchiolocentric abnormalities
bronchiolus (pl. bronchioli)
bronchiospasm
bronchiostenosis
bronchitic
bronchitis
bronchitis obliterans
bronchitis with bronchospasm
bronchoadenitis
bronchoalveolar cell carcinoma
bronchoarterial bundles
bronchocavernous
bronchocele
bronchocentric granulomatosis
bronchocentric inflammatory infiltrate
bronchoconstriction
  exercise-induced
  isocapnic hyperventilation-induced
bronchoconstrictor
bronchocutaneous fistula
bronchodilatation or bronchodilation
bronchogenic carcinoma
bronchogenic cyst
bronchogram
bronchographic
bronchography
  air
  bilateral
  fiberoptic
  fluid-filled
  tantalum
  unilateral
broncholith
broncholithiasis
bronchomalacia
bronchomediastinal lymph trunk

bronchoplegia
bronchopleural fistula with empyema
bronchopleuropneumonia
bronchopneumonia
  bibasilar
  hemorrhagic
  hypostatic
  inhalation
  postoperative
  subacute
  tuberculous
  virus
bronchopneumonitis
bronchopulmonary atelectasis
bronchopulmonary dysplasia (BPD)
bronchopulmonary lymph node
bronchopulmonary segment
bronchoradiography
bronchoscope
  Jackson
  Jackson-Olympus
  Karl Storz
bronchoscopy
  preoperative
  virtual CT
bronchosinusitis
bronchospasm
  paradoxical
  uncontrolled
bronchospastic effects
bronchostaxis
bronchostenosis
bronchotracheal
bronchovascular bundles
bronchovascular markings
bronchus (pl. bronchi)
  accessory cardiac
  anterior
  anterior basal
  apical
  apicoposterior
  beaded
  branch
  cardiac

bronchus *(cont.)*
  contracted
  dilated
  edematous
  eparterial
  extrapulmonary
  granulomatous inflammation of
  hyparterial
  inferior
  inferior lobe
  inflamed
  inflammation of
  intermediate
  intrapulmonary
  lateral basal
  left main
  left main stem
  lingular
  lobar
  main stem
  major
  medial
  medial basal
  medium-sized
  middle lobe
  mucoid impaction of
  normal-appearing
  posterior
  posterior basal
  primary (right and left)
  principal
  right lobe
  right main
  right main stem
  secondary
  secretion-filled
  segmental
  stem
  subapical
  subsegmental
  superior
  superior lobe
  tracheal

Brooker classification of heterotopic
  ossification
Brostrom-Gordon arthrography
Broviac atrial catheter
brown atrophy
Brown-Dodge method for angiography
brown fat artifact
brown induration of lung
brown lung
brown pulmonary induration
brown tumor (osteoclastoma)
brow presentation
Bruce protocol (exercise stress testing)
  modified
  standard
  treadmill exercise
brucellosis, cerebral
Bruck disease
Brücke (Bruecke) muscle
Bruel-Kjaer ultrasound scanner
Bruker console
Bruker CSI MR system
Bruker NMR spectrometer
Bruker PC-10 relaxometer
Brunner gland adenoma
Brunner gland of duodenum
Brunnstrom-Fugl-Meyer (BFM) arm
  impairment assessment
BRW (Brown-Roberts-Wells) CT
  stereotaxic guide
Bryant sign
BSA (body surface area)
BSA ejection fraction
B-scan (B-mode) ultrasound
B-72.3 labeled with ^{111}In bubble
bubble
  cavitating
  collapsing
  double (sign)
  Garren-Edwards gastric (GEG)
  Garren gastric
  gastric
  gastric air

bubble *(cont.)*
  indium ^{111}In
  intragastric
  soap (appearance)
bubble-enhanced sonoporation
bubble-gum flavored barium sulfate
  (see *Bear-E-Yum*)
bubble oscillations
bubble resonance
bubble ventriculography
bubbly lung syndrome
bubbly opacity
buccal object rule
Buchbinder Omniflex catheter
Buchbinder Thruflex catheter
bucket-handle fracture
bucket-handle tear
bucket-handle tear of knee meniscus
buckle fracture
buckle, wire-fixation
buckled innominate artery syndrome
buckling of mitral valve, midsystolic
Buck modification of Cobey view
  (hindfoot coronal alignment)
Bucky imaging device
Bucky view
bud
  bronchial
  capillary
  dorsal pancreatic
  end
  vascular
  ventral pancreatic
Budd-Chiari syndrome
Budge, ciliospinal center of
Budin-Chandler anteversion
  determination
BUdR (bromodeoxyuridine, now
  broxuridine) radiosensitizer
Buerger-Gruetz disease
Buerger thromboangiitis obliterans
  disease
buffalo hump

Buford complex
Buhl desquamative pneumonia
bulb
  aortic
  arterial
  baroreceptor in the carotid
  baseline of
  carotid
  dental
  duodenal
  end
  heart
  high jugular (HJB)
  inferior jugular vein
  internal jugular
  jugular
  olfactory
  superior jugular vein
bulbar abnormality
bulbar intracerebral hemorrhage
bulbar septum
bulbar urethral stricture
bulb of occipital horn of lateral
  ventricle
bulb of posterior horn of lateral
  ventricle
bulbomembranous urethral stricture
bulbourethral gland abscess
bulbourethral gland duct
bulbosity
bulbous stump
bulbous urethra
bulb-tip catheter
bulbus (noun), bulbous (adj.)
bulge
  bilateral anterior chest
  disk
  late systolic
  palpable presystolic
  parasternal
  precordial
  suprasternal
bulging disk

bulk laxative
bulk, muscle
bulk susceptibility artifact
bulky tumor
bulla (pl. bullae)
bulla formation
bullet
  hollow-point
  stabilizing
  tri-point
bullet-shaped vertebra
bullet trajectory
bull's-eye deformity
bull's-eye images
bull's-eye map
bull's-eye mapping
bull's eye polar map
bull's-eye sign
bull neck appearance
bullous edema
bullous emphysema
bullous lung disease
bump
  hip
  inion
  runner's
bumper fracture
bundle
  aberrant
  artery-vein-nerve
  AV (atrioventricular)
  Bachmann
  bronchoarterial
  bronchovascular
  common
  fascicular
  Flechsig bundle in cerebellum
  Gierke respiratory
  Gowers bundle in cerebellum
  His
  intercostal
  intercostal neuromuscular
  James

bundle *(cont.)*
  Keith sinoatrial
  Kent
  Kent-His
  maculoneural
  Mahaim
  main
  neurovascular
  Pick
  Schultze
  sinoatrial
  Thorel
  vascular
bundle bone
bundle branch block (BBB) (on EKG)
bundle branch reentry (BBR)
bundle function
bundle of His
bundle of Kent accessory bypass fibers
bundle of Stanley Kent
bundle of Vicq d'Azyr
bunion formation
bunk bed fracture
Burdach, column of
burden, angiogenic
burden score
Bureau-Barriere syndrome
Burgess below-knee amputation
Burke syndrome
burned-out endometriosis
burned-out tabes
burning
  selective hole
  substernal
Burns space
bursa (pl. bursae)
  Achilles
  adventitious
  anserine
  bicipitoradial
  Brodie
  calcaneal

bursa *(cont.)*
  Fleischmann
  flexor
  intermediate
  intermetatarsophalangeal
  ischiogluteal
  Luschka
  Monro
  olecranon
  omental
  plantar
  popliteal
  prepatellar
  radial
  retrocalcaneal
  subacromial
  subdeltoid
  suprapatellar
  trochanteric
  ulnar
bursal adhesion
  subacromial
  subdeltoid
bursal flap
bursal fluid
bursal sac
bursitis (pl. bursitides)
  anserine
  bicipital
  calcaneal
  chronic retrocalcaneal
  infracalcaneal
  intermetatarsophalangeal
  intertubercular
  ischiogluteal
  olecranon
  patellar
  pigmented villonodular (PVB)
  postcalcaneal (posterior calcaneal
    bursitis)
  posterior calcaneal
  prepatellar

bursitis *(cont.)*
  radiohumeral
  retrocalcaneal
  septic
  subacromial
  subdeltoid
  Tornwaldt
  trochanteric
bursography, magnetic resonance
  (MR)
bursolith
burst (compression) fracture of the
  atlas
burst fracture of spiral column
bursting fracture
Burton sign
Burwell-Charnley classification of
  fracture reduction
Bush DL ureteral illuminating catheter
Busquet disease
butterfly flap
butterfly fracture fragment
butterfly pattern of infiltrates
butterfly shadow
butterfly-type glioma
butterfly view (rectosigmoid section of
    large intestine)
  AP (anterior-posterior)
  LPO (left posterior oblique)
  PA (posterior-anterior)
  RAO (right anterior oblique)
buttock sign
button
  aortic
  duodenal
  patellar
  subdural
button sequestrum
button toe amputation
buttonhole fracture
buttonhole opening
buttonhole rupture

buttonhole stenosis
buttress, frontozygomatic
buttressing
buttress plate
BVAD (biventricular assist device)
BVR (basal vein of Rosenthal)
BVS (biventricular support system)
BV2 needle
bypass
  aortoiliofemoral
  aortorenal
  aortosubclavian-carotid
  aortosubclavian-carotid-axillary-
    axillary
  aorta to first obtuse marginal
    branch
  aorta to LAD
  aorta to marginal branch
  aorta to posterior descending
  aortofemoral
  aortic-superior mesenteric
  aortobifemoral
  aortocarotid
  aortoceliac
  aortocoronary
  aortocoronary-saphenous vein
  aortofemoral
  aortofemoral-thoracic
  aortoiliac
  aortoiliac-popliteal
  aortoiliofemoral
  aortopopliteal
  aortorenal
  apico-abdominal
  atriofemoral artery
  axillary
  axillary-axillary
  axillary-brachial
  axillobifemoral
  axillofemoral
  axillopopliteal
  brachial

bypass *(cont.)*
　cardiopulmonary (CPB)
　carotid-axillary
　carotid-carotid
　carotid-subclavian
　common hepatic-common
　　iliac-renal
　coronary
　coronary artery (CAB)
　cross femorofemoral
　crossover
　distal arterial
　dorsal pedal
　DTAF-F (descending thoracic
　　aortofemoral-femoral)
　EC-IC (extracranial-intracranial)
　extended tibial in situ
　extra-anatomic
　extracranial-intracranial (EC-IC)
　fem-fem (femorofemoral)
　femoral-above-knee popliteal
　femoral crossover
　femoral distal popliteal
　femoral-tibial-peroneal
　femoral to tibial
　femoral vein-femoral artery
　femoral venoarterial
　femoroaxillary
　femorodistal
　femorofemoral
　femorofemoral crossover
　femorofemoropopliteal
　femoroperoneal
　femoropopliteal
　femoropopliteal saphenous vein
　femorotibial
　"fem-pop" (femoropopliteal)
　heart-lung
　hepatorenal saphenous vein
　hypothermic cardiopulmonary
　iliofemoral
　iliopopliteal

bypass *(cont.)*
　ilioprofunda
　iliorenal
　infracubital
　infrainguinal stenosis
　in situ
　intracranial arterial
　ipsilateral nonreversed greater
　　saphenous vein
　left atrium to distal arterial aortic
　left heart
　lesser saphenous vein in situ
　Litwak left atrial-aortic
　mammary-coronary artery
　marginal circumflex
　microscope-aided pedal
　nonreversed translocated vein
　normothermic cardiopulmonary
　obtuse marginal
　off-pump coronary artery (OPCAB)
　partial
　partial cardiopulmonary
　percutaneous femorofemoral
　　cardiopulmonary
　popliteal
　popliteal in situ
　popliteal to distal in situ
　pulsatile cardiopulmonary
　renal artery-reverse saphenous vein
　reversed
　right heart
　saphenous vein
　sequential in situ
　subclavian-carotid
　subclavian-subclavian
　superior mesenteric artery
　supraceliac aortofemoral
　temporary aortic shunt
　thoracic aortofemoral artery
　tibial in situ
　total cardiopulmonary
　upper extremity in situ

bypass circuit
bypass graft
bypass tract
   atrio-Hisian or atriohisian
   AV (atrioventricular) nodal
   concealed

bypass *(cont.)*
   fasciculoventricular bypass
   nodo-Hisian
   nodoventricular
   right ventricular
byte mode

C, c

C (carbon) (an element)
CA (coronary artery)
"cabbage" (CABG)
CABG (coronary artery bypass graft)
CABS (coronary artery bypass surgery)
Cacchione syndrome
cachexia, lymphatic
CAD (computer-aided [or assisted] design [or diagnostics])
CAD (coronary artery disease)
CADASIL (cerebral autosomal dominant arteriopathy with subcortical infarcts and leukoencephalopathy)
cadmium iodide detector
CADstream dedicated image processing system for breast MRI
caecum (cecum)
CAEP (chronotropic assessment exercise protocol)
Caffey disease
CA15-3 antigen radioimmunoassay imaging agent
cage
   bony thoracic
   osseocartilaginous thoracic
CAH (congenital adrenal hyperplasia)

Cahoon view to demonstrate styloid processes of skull
cake kidney
cake, omental
calamus scriptorius
calcaneal bone
calcaneal fracture
calcaneal inclination angle
calcaneal spur
calcaneocavus (clubfoot)
   talipes calcaneus
   talipes cavus
calcaneoclavicular ligament
calcaneocuboid joint
calcaneocuboid ligament
calcaneofibular (CF) ligament
calcaneonavicular coalition
calcaneoplantar angle
calcaneotibial fusion
calcaneovalgocavus
calcaneovalgus flatfoot
calcaneovalgus, pes
calcaneus
   pes
   sulcus
   talipes
calcar avis

calcar femorale
calcar pedis
calcar, pivot of
calcareous deposits
calcarine cortex
calcarine fissure
calcarine sulcus
calcific aortic stenosis
calcific arteriosclerosis
calcific artery
calcification
  aneurysmal wall
  annular
  aortic
  aortic valve
  arterial
  artery
  basal ganglia
  basketlike
  breast
  cartilage
  cerebral
  choroid plexus
  clustered
  coarse vascular
  conglomerate
  coronary
  coronary artery
  costal cartilage
  curvilinear
  dentate nuclei
  dural
  dystrophic
  eccentric
  eggshell
  falx
  fine
  focal
  foci of
  free body
  glial tumor
  granulomatous
  gyriform

calcification *(cont.)*
  idiopathic pleural
  intervertebral cartilage
  intervertebral disk
  intracardiac
  intracranial
  irregular
  laminated
  ligamentous
  linear
  lymph node
  malignant-type
  medial collateral ligament
  metastatic
  mitral annular
  mitral ring
  mitral valve
  Mönckeberg (Moenckeberg)
  mottled
  multiple
  myocardial
  node
  normal
  parietal pericardial
  Pellegrini-Stieda
  periarticular
  pericardial
  pericardium
  periductal
  periventricular
  pineal gland
  plaque
  plaquing
  popcorn
  premature
  questionable
  renal mass
  rice grain
  secondary
  sella turcica
  soft tissue
  stippled
  subannular

calcification *(cont.)*
  suspicious
  target
  thrombus
  thyroid adenoma
  tramline cortex
  valve
  valvular leaflet
  visceral pericardial
calcific density
calcific matrix
calcific plaque
calcific round body
calcific shoulder tendinitis
calcific spur
calcified bladder
calcified bladder mass
calcified breast implants
calcified fetus
calcified leaflet
calcified mass
calcified meconium
calcified outline of cyst
calcified phleboliths in pelvis
calcified uterine fibroid
calcifying
calcinosis circumscripta
calcinosis, tumoral
calcis, os
calcium (Ca) (an element)
  ^{45}Ca
  ^{47}Ca
calcium deposit
calcium deposition
calcium hydroxyapatite
calcium, intracardiac
calcium layering
calcium scoring
calculated clearance time
calculation
  bayesian
  Cerenkov
  gap

calculation *(cont.)*
  Monte Carlo
  multiplane dosage
  radiation dosimetry
  spectrophotometric
  volume implant
calculus (pl. calculi) (see also *stone*)
  alvine
  articular
  biliary
  bladder
  branched
  bronchial
  cat's eye (in common bile duct)
  decubitus
  dislodged
  echogenic
  encysted
  fibrin
  gallbladder
  gastric
  hard nodular urinary
  hemic
  hepatic
  impacted
  infection
  intestinal
  jackstone
  joint
  kidney
  lacteal
  lucent
  lung
  mammary
  metabolic
  mulberry
  nephritic
  nonopaque
  opaque
  oxalate
  pancreatic
  primary renal
  primary vesical

calculus *(cont.)*
  pocketed
  prostatic
  radiopaque
  radiopaque vesical
  renal
  salivary
  secondary renal
  spermatic
  staghorn
  staghorn renal
  stomach
  stonelike
  ureteral
  urethral
  urinary tract
  uterine
  vesical
Caldani ligament
Caldwell occipitofrontal view
calf muscle pump (anatomical)
calf vein thrombus
caliber
  bronchus
  internal
  luminal
  medium
  modest
  narrow
  tracheal
  vessel
  wide
calibration, absolute-peak efficiency
calibration failure artifact
calibration method
calibrator
caliceal blunting
caliceal clubbing
caliceal crescents
caliceal deformity
caliceal dilatation
caliceal diverticulum

caliceal system
caliectasis (or caliectasia)
California disease (coccidioidomycosis)
caliper
calix (pl. calices) (also calyx, calyces)
  dilated
  dilation of
  major
  minor
  renal
  obstructed
callosal agenesis
callosal dysgenesis
callosal formation
callosal gyrus
callosal lesion
callosal sulcus
callosomarginal artery
callosum, corpus
callous (adj.)
callus
  bony
  bridging
  central
  definitive
  ensheathing
  external
  florid
  fracture
  intermediate
  permanent
  provisional
callus distraction
callus formation (*not* callous)
callus weld
calvaria (pl. calvariae)
calvarial bone
calvaria, salt and pepper
Calvé-Perthes disease
calyx (see *calix*)
CAM 5.2 antibody
camelback sign

camera
 ADAC gamma
 Anger gamma
 Anger-type scintillation
 APEX 409
 APEX 415
 CeraSPECT
 CID
 Cidtech
 Digirad gamma
 DSI
 dual head gamma
 Elscint
 Elscint dual detector cardiac
 four-head
 gamma
 GE gamma
 GE single detector SPECT-
  capable
 GE Starcam
 GE Starcam single crystal
  tomographic
 Haifa
 Helix
 Israel
 MEDX gamma
 multicrystal
 multicrystal gamma
 Picker
 Pixsys FlashPoint
 R&F
 rotating gamma
 scintillation
 Siemens gamma
 slip-ring
 SP6
 Starcam
 Technicare
 three-head
 Trionix
 Vertex
 Vision
camera distortion

camera, dual head coincidence
cameral fistula
Camp-Coventry view of intercondylar
 notch
Camper chiasma
camptocormia
camptodactyly
Camurati-Engelmann disease
CAMV (congenital anomaly of mitral
 valve)
CAN (contrast-associated nephropathy)
canal
 abdominal
 accessory
 adductor
 Alcock
 alimentary
 alveolar
 alveolodental
 ampulla of semicircular
 anal
 anterior condyloid
 anterior semicircular
 arachnoid
 Arantius
 archenteric
 Arnold
 arterial
 atrial
 atrioventricular (AV)
 auditory
 basipharyngeal
 Bernard
 Bichat
 biliary
 birth
 bony semicircular
 Böttcher
 Braune
 Breschet
 calciferous
 carotid
 caroticotympanic

canal *(cont.)*
  carotid
  carpal
  caudal
  central
  central spinal
  cerebrospinal
  cervical (of uterus)
  cervical axillary
  cervicoaxillary
  ciliary
  Civinini
  Cloquet
  cochlear
  common atrioventricular
  complex atrioventricular
  condylar
  condyloid
  connecting
  Corti
  Cotunnius
  craniopharyngeal
  crural
  Cuvier
  deferent
  dental
  dental root
  dentinal
  diploic
  Dorello
  Dupuytren
  endocervical
  endodermal
  ethmoid
  ethmoidal
  eustachian
  external auditory
  facial
  facial nerve
  fallopian
  femoral
  femoral medullary
  Ferrein

canal *(cont.)*
  flexor
  Fontana
  galactophorous
  ganglionic
  Gartner
  gastric
  genital
  greater palatine
  gubernacular
  Guyon
  gynecophoric
  Hannover
  haversian
  hemal
  Henle
  Hensen
  Hering
  hernial
  Hirschfeld
  His
  Huguier
  Hunter
  Huschke
  hyaloid
  hydrops
  hypoglossal
  iliac
  incisive
  incisor
  inferior dental
  infraorbital
  inguinal
  inioendineal
  interdental
  interfacial
  intersacral
  intestinal
  intramedullary
  Jacobson
  lacrimal
  lateral
  lateral semicircular

canal *(cont.)*
lingual vascular
Löwenberg (Loewenberg)
lumbar
mandibular
marrow
mastoid
maxillary
medullary
mental
Müller (Mueller)
musculotubal
narrowing of spinal
nasal
nasolacrimal
nasopalatine
neural
neurenteric
notochordal
Nuck
nutrient
obstetric
obturator
olfactory
optic
orbital
palatine
palatomaxillary
palatovaginal
paraurethral
parturient
pelvic
pericardioperitoneal
perivascular
persistent atrioventricular
persistent common atrioventricular
petrous carotid
pharyngeal
pleural
pleuropericardial
pleuroperitoneal
portal
posterior semicircular

canal *(cont.)*
principal artery of pterygoid
pterygoid
pterygopalatine
pudendal
pulmoaortic
pulp
pyloric
recurrent
Reichert
Richet tibio-astragalocalcaneal
Rivinus
root (of tooth)
Rosenthal
sacculocochlear
sacculoutricular
sacral
Santorini
Schlemm
scleral
semicircular
sheathing
small (of chorda tympani)
Sondermann
sphenopalatine
sphenopharyngeal
spinal
spinal cord
Stensen
Stilling
subsartorial
Sucquet-Hoyer
superior semicircular
supraorbital
tarsal
temporal
Theile
tibial medullary
tibio-astragalocalcaneal of Richet
tight spinal
Tourtual
tubal
tubotympanic

canal *(cont.)*
    tympanic
    umbilical
    uniting
    urogenital
    uterine
    uterocervical
    uterovaginal
    utriculosaccular
    vaginal
    Van Hoorne
    ventricular
    Verneuil
    vertebral
    vesicourethral
    vestibular
    vidian
    Volkmann
    vomerine
    vomerorostral
    vomerovaginal
    vulvouterine
    zygomaticofacial
    zygomaticotemporal
canal decompression
Canale-Kelly classification of talar
    neck fracture
canaliculus (pl. canaliculi)
    apical
    auricular
    bile
    bone
    cochlear
    haversian
    innominate
canalization
Canavan disease
Canavan-van Bogaert-Bertrand disease
cancellated bone
cancellous bone
cancellous tissue
cancellus

cancer (see also *carcinoma, lesion,
    sarcoma, tumor*)
    aniline
    betel
    chimney sweep's
    clay pipe
    contact
    cystic
    dendritic
    dye worker's
    hereditary
    latent
    melanotic
    metachronous lung
    mule-spinner's
    oat cell
    occult
    paraffin
    pitch worker's
    swamp
    tar
    tubular
cancer embolus
cancerization
candle wax appearance of bone
C angle
Cannon-Boehm point
Cannon catheter
Cannon point
Cannon ring
Cannon segmentation
cannula (pl. cannulae, cannulas)
    aspiration
    Cohen
    Cohen/Jarcho
    Core
    DeRoyal surgical
    double lumen
    EndoTIP
    evacuating
    femoral artery
    Gyne-Flo Leventhal

cannula *(cont.)*
  Hasson
  Hasson blunt-end
  Hasson intrauterine
  Hasson laparoscopy
  Hasson SAC (stable-access
    cannula)
  high flow
  Humi inflatable uterine
  inflow
  infusion
  inlet
  internal jugular venous
  intra-arterial
  intraventricular
  Iotec flexible
  Jacobs
  Jarcho
  LaparoSac single use
  large bore inflow
  large egress
  Leventhal Gyne-Flo
  Litwak
  LV (Fleft ventricular) apex
  Margolin HSG (hysterosalpingo-
    graphy)
  metallic tip
  MultAport
  needle
  outflow
  outlet
  perfusion
  peripheral
  Reuter
  Rubin
  single bore
  small egress
  two-stage
  vena cava
  venousF
  ventricular
  washout

cannulation
  aortic
  arterial
  atrial
  bicaval
  direct caval
  left atrial
  ostial
  retrograde
  selective
  single cannula atrial
  two-stage venous
  venoarterial
  venous
  venovenous
cannulation catheter
cannulization
  selective
  subselective
Canon scanner
Cantelli sign
cap
  duodenal
  fibrous
  hilar
  knee
  phrygian
  pleural
  thin
CAP (community-acquired
  pneumonia)
capacious veins
capacitator, MOS
capacity
  absorptive
  bladder
  closing
  cranial
  functional bladder
  lung
  respiratory
  vasodilatory

capillary (pl. capillaries)
  arterial
  bile
  continuous
  lymph
  Meigs
  sinusoidal
  venous
capillary bed
capillary blood volume
capillary bud
capillary congestion
capillary density
capillary embolism
capillary filling, compensatory
capillary filling time
capillary fracture
capillary hydrostatic pressure
capillary hyperpermeability
capillary leak (or leakage)
capillary-lymphatic malformation
  (CLM)
capillary malformation (CM)
capillary permeability
capillary pneumonia
capillary pressure
capillary pulsation
capillary refill
capillary resistance test
capillary-venous malformation (CVM)
capillary walls
capillary wedge pressure, pulmonary
capital epiphysis (CE) angle
capital extension
capital flexor
capital fragment
capital mover
capitate bone
capitellum
capitellum view to demonstrate
  fracture of radial head
capitolunate joint
capitular epiphysis

capitulum costae
capitulum fibulae
capitulum humeri
capitulum mandibulae
capitulum radii
capitulum ulnae
Caplan syndrome
capsular imbrication
capsular ligament rupture
capsular plane
capsular reefing
capsular thrombosis
capsule
  adrenal
  articular
  auditory
  Bowman
  breast implant
  cartilage
  cricoarytenoid articular
  cricothyroid articular
  dorsal
  external
  facet
  fatty renal
  fibrous
  fibrous renal
  Gerota
  Glisson
  glomerular
  hepatic
  internal
  joint
  limb of anterior
  metatarsophalangeal (MTP) joint
  liver
  multicystic ovaries with thickened
  organ
  PillCam video
  plantar
  posterolateral
  prostatic
  pseudolipoma of Glisson

capsule *(cont.)*
  redundant
  renal
  rim of
  splenic
  suprasellar
  talonavicular
  thyroid
  tumor
  wrist
capsule endoscopy
capsulocaudate infarction
capsulolabral complex
capsuloperiosteal envelope
capsuloputaminal infarction
capsuloputaminocaudate infarction
captopril renal scan
captopril renography
capture, boron neutron
caput medusae
Carabello sign (rise in arterial blood
  pressure; do not confuse with
  Carabelli dental sign)
carbogen radiosensitizer imaging agent
carbon (C) (an element)
  ^{11}C acetate
  ^{11}C butanol
  ^{11}C carbon monoxide
  ^{11}C carfentanil
  ^{11}C deoxyglucose
  ^{11}C FLU
  ^{11}C flumazenil
  ^{11}C imaging agent
  ^{11}C labeled cocaine
  ^{11}C labeled fatty acids
  ^{11}C L-159
  ^{11}C L-884
  ^{11}C L-methylmethionine
  ^{11}C methionine
  ^{11}C methoxystauro-sporine
  ^{11}C N-methylspiperone
  ^{11}C N-methylspiroperidol (NMS)
  ^{11}C nomifensine

carbon *(cont.)*
  ^{11}C palmitate
  ^{11}C palmitic acid radioactive
  ^{11}C raclopride
  ^{11}C thymidine
carbon dioxide (see CO_2)
carbon dioxide laser
carbon-loaded thermoluminescent
  dosimeter
carbuncle of kidney
carcinoid syndrome
carcinoma (also *cancer, sarcoma,
  tumor*)
  acinous cell
  acinar cell
  adenocystic
  adenosquamous
  adnexal
  adrenocortical
  aldosterone-producing
  aldosterone-secreting
  alveolar
  alveolar cell
  ameloblastic
  anaplastic (of thyroid gland)
  angiosarcoma of vulva
  apocrine
  Bartholin gland
  basal cell
    alveolar
    comedo
    cystic
    multicentric
    nodulo-ulcerative
    pigmented
    sclerosing
    superficial
  basaloid
  basosquamous cell
  Bellini duct
  bile duct
  bilharzial
  bladder

carcinoma *(cont.)*
  breast
  bronchioalveolar
  bronchiolar
  bronchogenic
  cavitary squamous cell
  cavitating
  cerebriform
  cervical
  "chimney sweep's" (of skin of
    scrotum)
  cholangio-
  cholangiocellular
  chorionic
  choroid plexus
  clear cell
  colloid
  colon
  colorectal
  comedo
  corpus
  corticol
  cortisol-producing
  cribriform
  cutaneous metastatic breast
  cylindrical
  cystic
  differentiating pancreatic
  ductal
  ductal transitional cell of prostate
  duct cell
  Dukes *(not* Duke's)
  eccrine
  embryonal
  embryonal cell
  endobronchial
  endometrial
  epidermal
  epidermoid
  epithelial ovarian
  esophageal
  exophytic
  extrahepatic bile duct

carcinoma *(cont.)*
  familial breast
  fibrolamellar hepatocellular
  fibrolamellar
  FIGO stage
  follicular
  gallbladder
  gastric
  gelatinous
  genital
  giant cell (of thyroid gland)
  glandular
  glans
  granulosa cell
  hepatic
  hepatocellular (HCC)
  hereditary papillary renal
  hereditary prostate
  hormone-sensitive breast
  Hürthle cell
  hypernephroid
  hypervascular hepatocellular
  infantile embryonal
  infiltrating ductal
  infiltrating lobular
  inflammatory
  inflammatory breast
  intracystic papillary
  intraductal
  intraepidermal
  intraepithelial
  intraepithelial endometrial
  invasive
  invasive bladder
  invasive lobular
  invasive squamous cell
  juvenile embryonal
  kidney
  Kulchitzky cell
  large cell
  leiomyosarcoma vulvar
  lenticular
  leptomeningeal

carcinoma *(cont.)*
liposarcoma vulvar
lobular
lung
malignant fibrous histiocytoma
medullary
melanotic
meningeal
Merkel cell
metastatic
metatypical
microinvasive
micropapillary
moderately well-differentiated
mucinous
mucinous gastric
mucoepidermoid
mucous
nasopharyngeal
neuroendocrine
node-negative breast
noninfiltrating lobular
noninvasive
nonmucinous gastric
nonpapillary renal cell (RCC)
non-small cell
oat cell
occult cervical
osteoid
ovarian
Paget
pancreatic
pancreatic acinar cell
papillary
pelvic
penile
perforated
periampullary
polypoid
poorly differentiated
preinvasive
prickle cell
primary

carcinoma *(cont.)*
primary intraosseous
prostate
prostatic
pulmonary
rectal
rectosigmoid
renal
renal cell (RCC)
renal pelvic urothelial
residual
retinoblastoma hereditary human
rhabdomyosarcoma vulvar
scar
schistosomal bladder
schneiderian
scirrhous
sclerosing hepatic (SHC)
sebaceous
sessile nodular
sigmoid
signet-ring
small cell
small cell lung (SCLC)
small round cell
spiculated breast
spindle cell
squamous cell (SCC)
string cell
superficial bladder
superficial depressed
superficial
terminal
testicular
thyroid
tonsillar
transitional cell (TCC)
tubular
undifferentiated
undifferentiated squamous cell
urethral
urothelial
uterine cervix

carcinoma *(cont.)*
    uterine corpus
    vaginal
    verrucous
    villous
    vulvar
    well-differentiated
carcinoma de novo
carcinoma en cuirasse
carcinoma ex pleomorphic adenoma
carcinoma in situ
    ductal (DCIS)
    lobular (LCIS)
    squamous cell
    urothelial
carcinoma in situ of cervix
carcinoma in situ of penis
carcinoma-specific monoclonal
    antibody (technetium Tc 99m
    antimelanoma murine monoclonal
    antibodies)
carcinomatosis
    lymphagitic
    peritoneal
carcinomatous adenopathy
carcinomatous mastitis
carcinomatous meningitis
carcinosarcoma
carcinosis
carcinoma-specific monoclonal
    antibody (technetium Tc 99m
    antimelanoma murine monoclonal
    antibodies)
card, Intel Plink Ethernet
Cardarelli sign
cardia
    crescent of
    gastric
    patulous
cardiac antrum
cardiac apex
cardiac atrial shunt

cardiac blood pool imaging, gated
    equilibrium
cardiac border
cardiac branch
cardiac catheter
cardiac catheterization
cardiac compensation
cardiac compression
cardiac contractility
cardiac contraction
cardiac creep
cardiac cycle
cardiac death, sudden
cardiac decompensation
cardiac decompression
cardiac denervation
cardiac dilatation
cardiac dynamics
cardiac effusion
cardiac enlargement
cardiac failure
cardiac fibroma
cardiac fibrosarcoma
cardiac filling pressure
cardiac fossa
cardiac ganglion, Wrisberg
cardiac gated MRA
cardiac gated PGSE sequence
cardiac gated respiration
cardiac gating
cardiac hamartoma
cardiac hemangioma
cardiac hypertrophy
cardiac impression on liver
cardiac index (CI)
cardiac infarct
cardiac insufficiency
cardiac involvement
cardiac irritability
cardiac laminography
cardiac lipoma
cardiac long axis view

cardiac lung
cardiac lymphangioma
cardiac mapping
cardiac margins
cardiac metastases
cardiac monitor
cardiac MRI
cardiac muscle fibers
cardiac myxoma
cardiac node
cardiac notch
cardiac output (CO)
cardiac output = stroke volume x
  heart rate (vol./min.)
cardiac overload (or overloading)
cardiac perforation
cardiac positron emission tomography
  (PET)
cardiac probe
Cardiac Protect computed tomography
cardiac pumping ability
cardiac radiation syndrome
cardiac radiography
cardiac recovery
cardiac reserve
cardiac rhabdomyoma
cardiac rhabdomyosarcoma
cardiac rupture
cardiac sarcoma
cardiac scan
cardiac series
cardiac shadow
cardiac shape
cardiac short axis MR imaging
cardiac short axis view
cardiac shunt
cardiac silhouette
cardiac sling
cardiac standstill
cardiac steady state
cardiac stomach
cardiac tamponade
cardiac teratoma

cardiac thrombosis
cardiac tumor embolization
cardiac valve
cardiac valve mucoid degeneration
cardiac vasculature
cardiac vasculopathy
cardiac vein, great
cardiac waist
cardiac wall motion
cardinal sign
cardioangiography
CardioCamera imaging system
cardiochalasia
CardioCoil self-expanding coronary
  stent
cardiocutaneous syndrome
Cardio Data MK3 Holter scanner
cardiodilator
cardiodynia
cardioesophageal (CE) junction
cardiofacial syndrome
CardioFix Pericardium patch
cardiogenesis
cardiogenic embolic stroke
cardiogenic embolism
cardiogenic pulmonary edema
cardiogenic shock
Cardiografin (diatrizoate meglumine)
  imaging agent
cardiogram
cardiography
  apex (ACG)
  esophageal
  precordial
  ultrasonic (UCG)
  vector
cardiohepatic
cardiohepatomegaly
cardiointegram (CIG)
cardiokymography (CKG)
Cardiolite (technetium Tc 99m
  sestamibi) imaging agent
cardiology, invasive

cardiomegaly
 alcoholic
 borderline
 familial
 globular
 hypertensive
 iatrogenic
 idiopathic
 postoperative
cardiomotility
cardiomyopathy
 alcoholic dilated
 amyloidotic
 apical hypertrophic (AHC)
 arrhythmogenic right ventricular
 beer-drinker's
 beriberi
 concentric hypertrophic
 congenital dilated
 congestive
 constrictive
 diabetic
 diffuse symmetric hypertrophic
 dilated (DCM)
 end stage
 familial hypertrophic (FHC)
 Friedreich ataxic
 hypertrophic (HCM)
 hypertrophic obstructive (HOC or
   HOCM)
 idiopathic
 idiopathic dilated (IDC)
 idiopathic restrictive
 infantile
 infectious
 infiltrative
 ischemic
 ischemic congestive
 left ventricular
 metabolic
 mucopolysaccharidosis
 myotonia atrophica
 noncoronary

cardiomyopathy *(cont.)*
 nonischemic congestive
 nonobstructive
 obliterative
 obscure
 obstructive
 obstructive hypertrophic
 peripartum
 peripartum dilated
 postmyocarditis dilated
 postpartum
 primary
 restrictive (RCM)
 right ventricular
 right-sided
 secondary
 tachycardia-induced
 thyrotoxicotic
 toxic
cardionecrosis
cardionephric
cardioneural
cardiopathy
 hypertensive
 infarctoid
 obscure
cardiophrenic angle
cardiophrenic junction
cardioplegic needle
cardiopneumatic
cardioptosis, Wenckebach
cardiopulmonary arrest
cardiopulmonary bilharziasis
cardiopulmonary bypass (CPB)
cardiopulmonary deterioration
cardiopulmonary insufficiency
cardiopulmonary obesity
cardiopulmonary support system (CPS)
cardiopuncture
cardiopyloric
cardiorenal disease
cardiorespiratory sign
cardiorrhexis

cardiosclerosis
CardioSEAL septal occluder
cardioselective agent
cardiospasm
Cardio Tactilaze peripheral
  angioplasty laser catheter
cardiotherapy
cardiothoracic index
cardiothoracic ratio (CTR)
Cardio3DScope imaging system
cardiothyrotoxicosis
cardiotocograph
cardiotocography
cardiovalvular
cardiovascular accident (CVA)
cardiovascular anomalies
cardiovascular renal disease
cardiovascular shunt
carina of trachea
Carleton spots
C-arm digital fluoroscopy
CARMEN (cryoablation reduction of
  menstruation) procedure
C-arm fluoroscopy
C-arm portable x-ray unit
carmustine wafer
Carney syndrome
Caroli disease
caroticocavernous fistula
carotid angiography
carotid angioplasty with stenting
carotid artery
  absence of right common
  common (CCA)
  external (ECA)
  extracranial
  internal (ICA)
  intracranial
  kinking of
  petrous segment of
  redundant
  supraclinoid internal
carotid artery aneurysm

carotid artery-cavernous sinus fistula
carotid artery stenosis
carotid atherosclerotic disease
carotid atherosclerotic plaque
carotid bifurcation
carotid blowout syndrome
carotid bulb baroreceptor
carotid-carotid venous bypass graft
carotid cavernous fistula occlusion
carotid distribution TIA (transient
  ischemic attack)
carotid duplex study
carotid ejection time
carotid occlusive disease
carotid phonoangiography
carotid plexus
carotid pulse peak
carotid pulse tracing
carotid pulse upstroke
carotid shudder
carotid sinus hypersensitivity (CSH)
carotid sinus massage
carotid sinus syncope
carotid sinus syndrome
carotid siphon
carotid stenosis
carotid string sign
carotid-subclavian bypass
carotid vein
carotid wall volume
carpal arch
carpal bone
carpal boss view
carpal bridge view
carpal canal view
carpal deviation
carpal-metacarpal (see *carpometacarpal*)
carpal navicular
carpal row
carpal scaphoid bone fracture
carpal-tarsal localization
carpal tunnel release (CTR)

carpal tunnel syndrome (CTS)
carpal tunnel view
Carpenter syndrome
carpometacarpal (CMC) joint
carpophalangeal joint
carporadial articulation
carpus shortening
Carrel patch
Carrel, triangulation of
carrier
   GABA uptake
   radionuclide
carrier-free separation
Carr-Purcell-Meiboom-Gill sequence
carrying angle
Carswell grapes
Carter equation
Carter-Rowe view
Cartesian reference coordinate voxel
   array
cartilage
   accessory
   accessory nasal
   alar
   arthrodial
   articular
   annular
   arytenoid
   auditory
   auricular
   basilar
   branchial
   calcified
   cariniform
   ciliary
   circumferential
   conchal
   connecting
   corniculate
   costal
   cricoid
   cuneiform
   elastic

cartilage *(cont.)*
   ensiform
   epiglottic
   epiphyscal
   falciform
   fibroelastic
   fibrous
   floating
   hyaline
   hyaline articular
   interarticular
   loss of elasticity of
   matrix-depleted
   physeal
   pitted
   quadrangle
   roughened
   scored
   semilunar
   thinned
   thyroid
   tracheal
   triradial
   yellow
cartilage articulation
cartilage bone
cartilage joint
   primary
   secondary
   symphysis
cartilage joint space
cartilaginous ring
cartographic projection
cartwheel fracture
Carvallo sign in tricuspid regurgitation
CAS (coronary artery scan)
cascade (pl. cascades)
   abdominal
   diagnostic
cascade stomach
caseous pneumonia
Castellani disease
Castellino sign

Castillo catheter
Castleman disease
catarrhal pneumonia
CAT-CAM conversion
cat's eye calculi in common bile duct
cathartic colon
cathartic preparation
catheter
  Abramson
  Abscession fluid drainage
  Accu-Flo ventricular
  Accu-Vu sizing
  ACE
  Achiever balloon dilatation
  Ackrad balloon-bearing
  acorn-tipped
  ACS (Advanced Catheter or
    Cardiac Systems) balloon
  ACS Endura coronary dilation
  ACSJL4
  ACS mini
  ACS OTW (over the wire)
  ACS OTW Lifestream coronary
    dilatation
  ACS OTW Photon coronary
    dilatation
  ACS RX (rapid exchange)
  ACS RX Comet coronary dilatation
  ACS RX coronary dilatation
  ACS Tourguide II guiding
  AcuNav ultrasound
  AL1 or AL-1
  Alzate
  Amplatz
  Angiocath PRN flexible
  angiographic
  AngiOptic microcatheter
  angle-tip
  angiographic balloon occlusion
  Angio-Kit
  Angiomedics
  angiopigtail
  angioplasty balloon

catheter *(cont.)*
  angled balloon
  angulated
  Anthron heparinized anti-
    thrombogenic
  aortic flush pigtail
  aortic flush straight
  aortogram
  apheresis
  Arani double loop guiding
  Argyle Medicut R
  Argyle umbilical vessel
  Arrow pulmonary artery
  Arrow Twin Cath multilumen
    peripheral
  Arrow-Berman balloon
  ArrowGard Blue Line
  ArrowGard Blue Plus
  ArrowGard central venous
  Arrow-Howes multilumen
  arterial embolectomy
  AR-2 diagnostic guiding
  Asch intrauterine
  Aspiracath
  atherectomy
  AtheroCath
  Atlantis SR intravascular ultrasound
    imaging
  Atlas LP PTCA balloon dilatation
  Atlas ULP balloon dilatation
  Atri-pace I bipolar-flared pacing
  Auth atherectomy
  AV-Paceport thermodilution
  Axiom DG balloon angioplasty
  Baggish aspiration
  bail-out
  Baim pacing
  Baim-Turi monitor/pacing
  balloon
  balloon biliary
  balloon dilatation
  balloon dilating
  balloon embolectomy

catheter *(cont.)*
　balloon flotation
　balloon flotation pacing
　balloon-tipped angiographic
　balloon-tipped end hole
　balloon wedge-pressure
　ball-wedge
　Bard
　Bardex I.C.
　bat-wing
　Baxter
　BD Insyte Autoguard shielded IV
　Berman angiographic
　Bernstein
　bifoil balloon
　Bilbao-Dotter
　biliary
　Bio-Flex CS
　bipolar pacing electrode
　bipolar temporary pacemaker
　blind
　Block right coronary guiding
　Blue FlexTip
　Blue Max triple lumen
　Bonanno suprapubic
　BPS spinal angiographic
　braided diagnostic
　Brevi-Kath epidural
　Brockenbrough transseptal
　bronchial
　Bronchitrac L
　bronchospirometric
　Broviac
　Buchbinder Omniflex
　Buchbinder Thruflex
　Buerhenne steerable
　bulb-tip
　Bush DL ureteral illuminating
　Camino ICP (intracranial pressure)
　Cannon
　cannulation
　Cardio Tactilaze peripheral
　　angioplasty laser

catheter *(cont.)*
　Cardiomarker
　Castillo
　Cath-Finder
　CathLink 20 port system with
　　ChronoFlex
　Cath-Track
　Caud Λ Kath epidural
　central venous (CVC)
　Chemo-Port
　cholangiographic
　cholangiography
　ChronoFlex polyurethane
　Cloverleaf
　coaxial
　coaxial Tracker
　Cobra and Cobra 2
　cobra-shaped
　coil-tipped
　color-coded
　Comfort Cath I and II
　Conceptus fallopian tube
　Conceptus Soft Seal cervical
　Conceptus Soft Torque uterine
　Conceptus VS (variable softness)
　conductance
　ContiCath
　Cook arterial
　Cook-Cope loop suprapubic
　Cook cystotomy
　Cook hysteroscopic
　Cook pigtail
　Cook silicone balloon HSG
　Cook tissue morcellator
　Cope loop
　Cordis Brite Tip guiding
　Cordis Ducor I, II, and III
　　coronary
　Cordis Ducor pigtail
　Cordis Son-II
　coronary sinus thermodilution
　corset balloon
　coudé

catheter *(cont.)*
Councill
Cournand cardiac
CR Bard
Critikon
CVP (central venous pressure)
cystotomy
Dacron
Dale Foley
Datascope DL-II percutaneous
translucent balloon
decapolar
deflectable quadripolar
Deltec long term dual lumen
hemodialysis
DeOrio intrauterine insemination
Deseret
Dewan intrauterine insemination
diagnostic
Diasonics
dilatation balloon
DiMattina laparoscopic
directable coaxial
DLP cardioplegic
Doppler coronary
Dormia stone basket
Dorros brachial internal mammary
guiding
Dorros infusion/probing
Dotter caged balloon
double cuff dialysis
Double J
double J indwelling
double J ureteral
double lumen
double lumen femoral vein
double lumen subclavian vein
double lumen venous umbilical
double pigtail ureteral
Dow-Corning ileal pouch
drainage
Ducor balloon
Du Pen epidural

catheter *(cont.)*
Duo-Flow dual lumen
DVI Simpson AtheroCath
EAC (expandable access catheter)
E-cath tunneled epidural
EchoMark angiographic
Echosight Jansen-Anderson
intrauterine
Echosight Patton coaxial
Edwards diagnostic
eight-lumen esophageal manometry
Elecath thermodilution
electrode
El Gamal coronary bypass
Elite
embolectomy
Embryon GIFT transfer
Embryon HSG (hysterosalpingo-
graphy/hysterosonography)
end hole
Endosound endoscopic ultrasound
Endotak C lead
enhanced torque guiding
epididymal aspiration
epidural
Eppendorf
ERCP (endoscopic retrograde
cholangiopancreatography)
Erythroflex hydromer-coated
central venous
eXamine cholangiography
expandable access (EAC)
Explorer 360° rotational diagnostic
Explorer ST fixed curve diagnostic
Express PTCA
extraction
extrusion balloon
Faraday
FAST (flow-assisted, short term)
balloon
Fast-Cath introducer
female
Feth-R-Kath epidural

catheter *(cont.)*
Finesse large lumen guiding
Firlit-Sugar intermittent
Flexguard Tip
Flexi-Tip ureteral
Flexxicon Blue dialysis
Flexxicon dialysis
flotation
flow-directed microcatheter
flow oximetFry
fluid-filled
Fogarty balloon
Fogarty balloon biliary
Fogarty-Chin extrusion balloon
Fogarty embolectomy
Foley
Foley three-way
Foley ureteral
Foltz
Force balloon dilatation
French mushroom tip
F-series insemination
gadolinium-coated
gadopentetate dimeglumine-filled
Ganz-Edwards coronary infusion
Garceau tapered
Gazelle balloon dilation
Gensini coronary
Gentle-Flo suction
Gesco umbilical
Gleicher salpingography
Goldstein sonohysterography
Goodale-Lubin cardiac
Gorlin pacing
Gould PentaCath 5-lumen
    thermodilution
graft-seeking
Grollman pigtail
Groshong
Groshong double lumen
Groshong tunneled
Grüntzig (Gruentzig)
Grüntzig balloon

catheter *(cont.)*
Grüntzig Dilaca
guide
Guidezilla Softip guiding
guiding
GyneSys cervical access
GyneSys Dx diagnostic
GyneSys guidewire
GyneSys uterine cornual access
GyneSys uterine ostial access
Guidezilla guiding
Haas intrauterine insemination
Halo
Hanafee
Hartzler ACX-II and RX-014
    balloon
Hartzler LPS dilatation
Hartzler Micro II and Micro XT
headhunter
HealthShield wound drainage
heat-transmitting balloon
helical-tip Halo
helium-filled balloon
Hemocath hemodialysis
Heplock
hexapolar
Hickman indwelling
Hickman tunneled
Hidalgo
Hieshima coaxial
high fidelity microtipped
high flow
high pressure
high speed rotation dynamic
    angioplasty
HNB angiographic
H-1-H (headhunter)
hot-tip
H/S (hysterosalpingography)
HSG (hysterosalpingography)
HUMI uterine
Hurwitz dialysis
HydraCross TLC PTCA

catheter *(cont.)*
Hydrolyser microcatheter
hydrophilic-coated
hydrostatic balloon
hysterosalpingography/hystero-
sonography (H/S or HSG)
hyperthermia
IAB (intra-aortic balloon)
I-Cath
ICP (intracranial pressure)
Illumen-8 guiding
illuminating
ILUS (intraluminal ultrasound)
indwelling
indwelling urinary bladder
Infiniti
In-Flow intraurethral valved
Infuse-a-port
Innovante
Inoue balloon
Insemi-Cath
internal-external drainage
interstitial
intra-aortic balloon double lumen
intra-arterial
intra-arterial chemotherapy
Intracath
intracoronary
intrahepatic biliary drainage
Intran disposable intrauterine pressure management intrauterine
intratumoral
intrauterine injection
intravascular ultrasound
intravenous pacing
intraventricular
intrepid PTCA angioplasty
Ishida coaxial
ITC radiopaque balloon
IVUS (intravascular ultrasound)
Jackman orthogonal
Jackson-Pratt
Jansen-Anderson intrauterine

catheter *(cont.)*
JB1
JB3
JCL 3.5 guiding
Jelco intravenous
JL4 (Judkins left 4 cm curve)
Jocath coronary balloon
Jocath diagnostic
Jography angiographic
Jography balloon
Jography diagnostic
Joguide balloon
Joguide coronary guiding
Joguide diagnostic
JR5 (Judkins right 5 cm)
Judkins USCI
jugular
Katayama hysteroscopic
Kaye tamponade balloon
KDF-2.3
Kensey atherectomy
Kifa
King multipurpose coronary graft
Kinsey atherectomy
Kish urethral illuminated
KISS (kidney internal splint/stent)
Koala intrauterine pressure
Kontron balloon
Labcath
large bore
large caliber
large lumen
laser
left coronary
left heart
left ventricular sump
Lehman ventriculography
Leung coaxial
LeVeen
Lifestream coronary dilatation
Litespeed
Loc-Sure single pass
Lo-Profile balloon

catheter *(cont.)*
  Lo-Profile II balloon
  Lo-Profile steerable dilatation
  Longdwel Teflon
  low pressure
  low speed rotation angioplasty
  LPS
  Luer-Slip IAB
  Lumaguide
  Malecot
  Mallinckrodt angiographic
  MammoSite RTS (radiation therapy
    system)
  Mani
  manometer-tipped cardiac
  manometric
  Mansfield Atri-Pace 1
  Mansfield orthogonal electrode
  Mansfield Scientific dilatation
    balloon
  MapCath
  Marathon guiding
  Marrs intrauterine
  Marrs laparoscopic
  Match 35 PTA
  Maverick Monorail balloon
  Maverick over the wire balloon
  Maverick PTCA
  Maverick2 Monorail
  Maverick XL PTCA
  Max Force
  Max Force balloon
  McGoon coronary perfusion
  McIntosh double lumen
  Medicut
  Medi-Tech balloon
  medium-pressure
  Medtronic balloon
  Memory-Vu angiographic
  Metricath catheter and transducer
  Micro-Driver balloon
  Micro-Guide
  micromanometer-tip

catheter *(cont.)*
  Microvasive Rigiflex TTS balloon
  midstream aortogram
  Mikro-tip micromanometer-tipped
  Millar MPC-500
  Millenia balloon
  Mini-Profile dilatation
  Mirage over the wire balloon
  Mistique
  Mitsubishi angioscopic
  Molina needle
  Monorail balloon
  MPF
  MS Classique
  Mullins transseptal
  Multicath
  multielectrode impedance
  multifiber
  Multi-Med triple lumen infusion
  multifiber
  multilumen
  multipolar impedance
  Multipurpose-SM
  mushroom
  MVP
  MVP over the wire balloon
  Mylar
  Mystic Mongoose PTCA
  NarrowFlex intra-aortic balloon
  NarrowFlex prewrapped double
    lumen IAB
  nasobiliary
  Navi-Star diagnostic/ablation
    deflectable tip
  Navi-Star mapping
  Navius
  NBIH
  NC Raptor PTCA dilatation
  Neo PICC neonatal peripherally
    inserted central
  Neostar vascular access
  nephrostomy balloon
  nephrostomy-type

catheter *(cont.)*
  Neuhaus implantable port
  Nexus 2 linear ablation
  Niagara temporary dialysis
  NIH (National Institutes of Health)
    cardiomarker
  NIH left ventriculography
  Ninja FX PTCA dilatation
  nitrofuran delivery
  nontraumatizing
  NoProfile balloon
  Norfolk intrauterine
  NovaCath multilumen infusion
  Novy cornual cannulation
  Nycore angiography
  Nydex
  octapolar
  Olbert
  Oligon Foley
  olive-tipped
  OmniCath atherectomy
  Omniflex balloon
  Omni Flush shape Accu-Vu
  OmniMesh ablation
  OmniMesh bidirectional
  OmniMesh braided-tip
  On-Command
  one-hole angiographic
  open end ureteral
  OpenSail balloon catheter
  Opta
  Opticon
  Opti-Flow angiography
  Opti-Plast XT balloon
  Optiscope
  Optiva intravenous catheter
  Oracle Focus PTCA
  Oracle Megasonics
  Oracle Megasonics PTCA
  Oracle Micro Plus
  Oracle Micro Plus PTCA
  Orbiter PV

catheter *(cont.)*
  Oreopoulos-Zellerman peritoneal
    dialysis
  Orion balloon
  Ott intrauterine
  Outback reentry
  Outcomes by Design
  over the wire balloon
  oximetric
  Paceport
  Pacewedge dual pressure bipolar
    pacing
  pacing
  paracervical instillation
  Parodi balloon (ParCA)
  Pathfinder
  Patton laparoscopic
  PA Watch position-monitoring
  PBN hysterosalpingography
  P.D. Access over the needle
  PE Plus II balloon dilatation
  Percor DL and DL-II balloon
  Percor-Stat-DL
  Percuflex APD all-purpose with
    Fader Tip
  percutaneous
  percutaneous transhepatic biliary
    drainage (PTBD)
  percutaneous transhepatic pigtail
  Performa angiographic
  Performr (RF-Performr) electro-
    physiology catheter (*not*
    Performer)
  perfusion
  Periflow peripheral balloon
  peripheral atherectomy
  peripherally inserted central
    (PICC)
  peripherally inserted central (PICC)
  PermaCath dual lumen
  peritoneal
  peritoneal dialysis

catheter *(cont.)*
pervenous
Pezzer
Phantom V Plus
Philips
PIBC (percutaneous intra-aortic
  balloon counterpulsation)
Pico-ST II low profile balloon
pigtail
pigtail angiographic
Pipelle endometrial suction
Pollack open-end Flexi-Tip ureteral
polyethylene
PolyFlo peripherally inserted
  central
Polystan venous return
polyurethane pail-handle coiled-tip
  peritoneal dialysis
porous polyethylene dialysis
Port-A-Cath
portal
Portnoy ventricular
Positrol II
Powerline
PowerPICC
Predator angioplasty balloon
preformed
preshaped
pressure
Primopac diagnostic
Privet coaxial
probing
ProCross Rely over the wire
  balloon
Profile Plus dilatation
Proflex 5 dilatation
Pro-Flo
Pro-Flo XT
Propac diagnostic
prostatic
Pruitt-Inahara balloon-tipped
  perfusion

catheter *(cont.)*
PTBD (percutaneous transhepatic
  biliary drainage)
PTCA (percutaneous transluminal
  coronary angioplasty)
Pudenz peritoneal
pulmonary artery
pulmonary flotation
pusher
QuadraPulse radiofrequency
quadripolar
quadripolar electrode
quadripolar steerable electrode
Quanticor
Quinton Mahurkar dual lumen
  peritoneal
Quantum Maverick coronary
  balloon dilatation
Quantum PTCA
QuickFlash radial artery
Quinton
Quinton Mahurkar dual lumen
  hemodialysis
Quinton PermCath vascular access
Qwikstart
Raaf Cath vascular
Radius coronary stent delivery
RadPICC
Raimondi spring
Raimondi ventricular
Ranfac LAP-013 cholangiographic
Ranfac ORC-B cholangiographic
Ranfac XL-11 cholangiographic
Ranger PTCA
rapid-exchange PTCA balloon
  angioplasty
Rapid-Trak
RaptorRail PTCA dilatation
Rashkind septostomy balloon
recessed balloon septostomy
rectal pressure
Reddick cystic duct cholangiogram

catheter *(cont.)*
RediFurl TaperSeal IAB
RediGuard flexible IAB
red Robinson
red rubber
Release-NF (nitrofurazone Foley)
Reliance urinary control insert
Rentrop infusion
Resolve drainage
retroperfusion
Revelation microcatheter
reverse Berman angiographic
balloon
RF (radiofrequency-generated
thermal) balloon
right coronary
right heart
Rigiflex TTS balloon
Ring-McLean
Robinson
Robinson straight urethral
Rodriguez-Alvarez
Rosch
Rosch-Thurmond fallopian tube
rotatable pigtail
Royal Flush angiographic flush
Royal women's coaxial
Rsch-Uchida transjugular liver
access needle-
Rumel
Rutner percutaneous suprapubic
balloon
Samuels Micro-Scler
Sarns wire-reinforced
Schneider-Shiley
Schoonmaker multipurpose
Schwarten balloon dilatation
SciMed NC Ranger PTCA
SciMed SSC "Skinny"
Scott silicone ventricular
Seldinger
Seldinger cystic duct

catheter *(cont.)*
Select Performance balloon
dilatation
Seletz nonrigid ventricular
self-retaining
sensing
Seroma-Cath wound drainage
serrated
S.E.T. hemodialysis
Shapiro intrauterine insemination
shaver
Shaw
Sheldon
Shepard intrauterine insemination
Sherpa guiding
Sholkoff balloon hysterosalpin-
gography
Shiley-Ionescu
SHJR4s (side-hole Judkins right,
curve 4, short)
short arm Grollman
sidehole
sidewinder
Silastic
Silber aspiration
silicone Foley
silicone Malecot
silicone rubber Dacron-cuffed
Silicore
Simmons 1, 2, and 3
Simplus PE/t dilatation
Simpson peripheral AtheroCath
Simpson Ultra Lo-Profile II
balloon
single cuff dialysis
single lumen femoral vein
single lumen subclavian vein
single stage
Skinny
sliding rail
small bore
Smec balloon

catheter *(cont.)*
SMS coaxial
snare
Sof-Flex loop suprapubic
Soft-Cell
soft coaxial
Soft-Pass laparoscopic
Softip arteriography
Soft Seal Fcervical
Soft Seal transcervical balloon
soft silicone rubber dialysis
Soft Torque uterine
Softouch guiding
Soft-Vu angiographic
Soft-Vu Omni flush
Solera thrombectomy
solid-state manometry
SoloPass
Sones Cardio-Marker
Sones Hi-Flow
Sones Positrol
Soules intrauterine insemination
special steering
Spectrum silicone Foley
Speedy balloon
SPI-Argent II peritoneal dialysis
spiral-tip
Spirtos coaxial
split sheath
Spyglass angiography
Squibb
Stack perfusion coronary dilatation
Stamey-Malecot
standard Lehman
Stargate falloposcopy
steerable electrode
steering
Steerocath
Stertzer guiding
stimulating
straight flush percutaneous
subarachnoid
subclavian

catheter *(cont.)*
subcutaneous ventricular reservoir
subdural drainage
SULP II
sump
suprapubic
suprapubic urodynamic
surgically implanted hemodialysis
Swan-Ganz Guidewire TD
Swan-Ganz Pacing TD
Swan-Ganz thermodilution
swan-neck
TAC atherectomy
Talon balloon dilation
Targis
Taut cystic duct
TEC (transluminal endarterectomy)
Tefcat intrauterine
Teflon
temporary pacing
Tenacath HSG (hysterosalpingography)
Tenckhoff peritoneal dialysis
Tennis Racquet angiographic
Tesio hemodialysis access
Tesio twin
three-way
Tis-U-Trap endometrial suction
tetrapolar esophageal
thermistor
thermodilution
thrombectomy
thrombosuction
Thruflex PTCA balloon
toposcopic
Torcon NB selective angiographic
Total-Cross PTA
Tracker
transcervical
transcervical tubal access (T-TAC)
transcutaneous extraction
transducer-tipped
transluminal endarterectomy (TEC)

catheter *(cont.)*
 transluminal extraction (TEC)
 transseptal
 transvenous pacemaker
 trefoil balloon
 Triguide
 triple thermistor coronary sinus
 triple lumen
 tripolar
 T-TAC (transcervical tubal access)
 TTS (through-the-scope)
 tunneled
 tunneled hemodialysis
 Tygon
 UCAC (uterine cornual access)
 Uldall (not Udall) subclavian
  hemodialysis
 ULP (ultra-low profile)
 UltraLite flow-directed micro-
 ultrasonographic
 umbilical
 umbilical artery (UAC)
 Umbili-Cath Tecoflex umbilical
 UMI
 UOAC (uterine ostial access)
 Ureflex
 Ureflex ureteral
 ureteral
 urethral
 urodynamic loop
 UroLume flow-directed
 UroLume flow-directed micro-
 UroMax II urethral balloon
 UroQuest On-Command
 USCI Bard
 USCI Mini-Profile balloon
  dilatation
 USCI probing
 uterine cornual access (UCAC)
 uterine ostial access (UOAC)
 valvuloplasty balloon
 Van Andel
 Van Tassel pigtail

catheter *(cont.)*
 Variflex
 Vas-Cath
 Vas-Cath Flexxicon II
 Vas-Cath Opti-Flow long term
  dual lumen hemodialysis
 Vas-Cath PTA balloon
 Vas-Cath Soft-Cell permanent
  dual lumen hemodialysis
 Vector
 Vector X
 VenaSonix ultrasound
 venous
 venting
 Ventra PTA
 ventricular
 ventriculography
 VIPER PTA
 Vitalcor venous
 Voda
 Vygon Nutricath S
 Wanderer micro-
 Was-Cath
 washing
 water-infusion esophageal
  manometry
 Webster coronary sinus
 Webster orthogonal electrode
 Werlin-Ishida coaxial
 Wexler
 whistle-tip ureteral
 Williams L-R guiding
 Wilton-Webster coronary sinus
 Wishard
 Witzel enterostomy
 Xpeedior
 X-Sept
 Xtent
 Zipper balloon
 Z-Med balloon
 Zucker
catheter à demeure
catheter advanced under fluoroscopic
 guidance

catheter artifact
catheter-associated urinary tract
catheter-borne transducer
catheter damping
catheter deployment
catheter drainage
catheter exchanged over guidewire
catheter guide, Mandrin
catheter holder, Dale Foley
catheter impact artifact
catheter-induced coronary artery
    spasm
catheter introducer
    Bard Safety
    Foley
catheterization
    balloon
    cardiac
    clean intermittent (CIC)
    clean intermittent bladder
    Foley
    hysteroscopic selective
    intermittent self-catheterization
    Judkins femoral
    Mullins modification of transseptal
    Mullins sheath in transseptal
    periodic intermittent
    retrograde
    retrograde ureteral
    right heart
    self
    selective
    simultaneous right and left heart
    straight
    superselective
    suprapubic
    transnasal
    transseptal
    umbilical vein
catheterize
catheter kinking
catheter mapping
catheter migration

catheter recanalization
catheter-related upper extremity deep
    venous thrombosis
catheter sheath
catheter-skin interface
catheter tip
    acorn
    Braasch bulb with whistle
    cone
    flexible filiform
    olive
    round
    ureteral
    whistle
catheter tip hockey-stick appearance
catheter tip motion artifact
catheter-tipped manometer
catheter-tissue contact
catheter with preformed curves
catheter whip artifact
CathLink 20 port system with
    ChronoFlex catheter
Cath-Lock introducer
CathScanner ultrasound imaging
    system
CathTrack catheter locator system
CAT scan (computerized [or com-
    puted] axial tomography)
    enhanced
    nonenhanced
CAT scan cradle
CAT scan gantry
cat scratch disease
Catterall classification
cauda equina compression syndrome
caudad
Caud-A-Kath epidural catheter
caudal branch
caudal collaterals
caudal-cranial angulation
caudal regression
caudal tilt
caudal view

caudate nucleus
caudothalamic groove
cauliflower appearance
cauliflower-shaped filling defect
Causton method oblique projection to
　demonstrate sesamoids
Causton view
cava
　flat inferior vena
　juxtarenal
caval-atrial (or cavoatrial) junction
caval-pulmonary artery anastomosis
caval snare
caval tourniquet
CAVB (complete atrioventricular
　block)
cavernosography, dynamic infusion
cavernous angioma
cavernous angiosarcoma
cavernous hemangioma
cavernous sinus meningioma
cavernous transformation of the portal
　vein
cavitary lung mass
cavitary mass
cavitary squamous cell carcinoma
cavitary tuberculosis
cavitating bubbles
cavitating carcinoma
cavitating mesenteric lymph node
　syndrome
cavitating pattern
cavitation
　lobar
　multibubble
　pulmonary
　single bubble
cavitation damage
cavitation index (CI)
cavitation induced becquerel effect
cavitation induced VUV (vacuum
　ultraviolet light) effect

cavity
　abdominal
　abdominopelvic
　absorption
　air
　amniotic
　ancyroid (also ankyroid)
　axillary
　bladder
　body
　buccal
　chest
　cleavage
　coexistent
　cotyloid
　cranial
　crown
　endometrial
　epamniotic
　epidural
　funnel-shaped
　glenoid
　lung
　joint
　marrow
　Meckel
　medullary
　oral
　pelvic
　pericardial
　peritoneal
　pleural
　popliteal
　pseudoaneurysm
　pulmonary
　retroperitoneal
　saclike
　septum pellucidum
　sigmoid
　subarachnoid
　subdural
　synovial

cavity *(cont.)*
  syringomyelic
  syrinx
  thoracic
  trigeminal
  tubular
  uterine
  vaginal
  wound
cavity prostatitis
cavoatrial (caval-atrial) junction
cavogram
cavography
cavovalgus
  pes
  talipes
cavovarus
  pes
  talipes
cavovarus deformity
cavus
  global
  local
  pes
  post-traumatic
  talipes
cavus deformity
Cayler syndrome
CBF (cerebral blood flow)
CBI (convergent beam irradiation)
CBI stereotactic ring
CBT (corticobulbar tract)
CBV (cerebral blood volume)
CBV/CBF ratio
cc (cubic centimeter)
CC (conventional colonoscopy)
C-C (convexo-concave) heart valve
CCA (common carotid artery)
CCD (central collodiaphyseal) angle
CCD photodetectors
CCF (carotid cavernous fistula)
CC49 antitumor monoclonal antibody
CC49 monoclonal antibody

CCK-HIDA (HIDA-CCK scintigraphy)
CCTA (coronal computed tomographic
  arthrography)
CD (Crohn disease)
CDAI (Crohn disease activity index)
CDC (Crohn disease of colon)
CDCA (chenodeoxycholic acid)
CDE (common duct exploration)
CDH (congenital dislocation [or
  dysplasia] of hip)
CDI (color Doppler imaging)
CDP (continuous descending pressure)
CDR (computed dental radiography)
CDUS (color-flow Doppler ultra-
  sound)
CE (capital epiphysis) angle of Wiberg
CE (cardioesophageal) junction
C-E amplitude of mitral valve
CEA (carcinoembryonic antigen)
CEA scan for colorectal carcinoma
CEA-Scan (arcitumomab) (technetium
  Tc 99m arcitumomab) imaging
  agent
cecal appendage
cecal serosa
cecal sphincter
cecal volvulus
cecostomy, percutaneous
CECT (contrast enhancement of com-
  puted tomographic) head and body
  imaging
cecum (caecum)
  antimesocolic side of
  coned
  conical
  mobile
  subhepatic
Cedell fracture of talus
Cedell-Magnusson classification of
  arthritis on x-ray
Ceelen-Gellerstedt syndrome
Cegka sign
CeI scintillator

celery stalk metaphysis
C-11 or ¹¹C (carbon) acetate imaging
C-11 or ¹¹C (carbon) dihydroxyphenylalanine imaging agent for PET
scan
C-11 (¹¹C) (carbon) palmitate uptake
on PET scan
celiac and mesenteric arteriography
celiac angiography
celiac artery compression syndrome
celiac axis syndrome
celiac-bimesenteric trunk
celiac ganglia
celiac plexus
celiac trunk
celiectasia
celioma
cell-mediated immune inflammation
CEM (central extensor mechanism)
Cemax/Icon scanner
Cemax PACS platform
cement
    acrylic bone
    hydroxyapatite (HA)
    Implast bone
    methyl methacrylate
    orthopedic
    Orthoset radiopaque bone
    polymerized
    radiopaque bone
    surface
cementation
cemented Lubinus acetabular cup
cemented Reflection acetabular cup
cementifying fibroma
cement line
cement mantle
cemento-ossifying fibroma
Cencit surface scanner
center
    anechoic
    ciliospinal center of Budge
    cortical

center *(cont.)*
    diaphyseal
    emetic
    growth center of bone
    ossification
Center for Metabolic and Experi-
    mental Imaging
centigray (cGy)
centimeter (cm)
central axis depth dose
central-axis depth-dose curve
central canal
central collodiaphyseal angle (CCD)
central intraluminal saturation stripe
central laceration
central motor pathways disease
central nervous system (CNS)
central neurogenic hyperventilation
central pneumonia
central point artifact
central rays
central splanchnic venous thrombosis
    (CSVT)
central tegmental tract
central venous line placement
central venous pressure (CVP) line
centriciput
centrilobular emphysema
centrilobular region of liver
centrilobular shadow
centroparietal head region
centrum commune
centrum ovale
centrum semiovale
cephalad
cephalic angulation
cephalic index
cephalic presentation of fetus
cephalic vein
cephalization of blood flow
cephalocaudad length
cephalofacial proportionality
cephalogram

cephalohematocele
cephalohematoma, parietal
cephalometric findings
cephalometry
cephalopelvic disproportion (CPD)
cephalopelvimetry
cephalothoracopagus twins
CeraSPECT camera
cerebellar degeneration
cerebellar disease
cerebellar fiber
cerebellar hemisphere
cerebellar hemorrhage
cerebellar herniation
cerebellar infarction
cerebellar mass
cerebellar pathway
cerebellar peduncle
cerebellar syndrome
cerebellar tonsillar herniation
cerebellar tract
cerebellar vermis
cerebellopontile angle (CPA) tumor
   (also cerebellopontine)
cerebellum
   dentate nucleus of
   fetal
   midline
   petrosal
cerebra (pl. of cerebrum)
cerebral abscess
cerebral aneurysm
cerebral angiography
cerebral angioscintigraphy
cerebral aqueduct
cerebral arteries
cerebral arteriography
cerebral arteriovenous fistula
cerebral atrophy
cerebral autoregulation (CA), dynamic
cerebral autosomal dominant arteriopathy with subcortical infarcts and
   leukoencephalopathy (CADASIL)

cerebral blood flow (CBF)
cerebral blood volume (CBV)
cerebral blood volume/cerebral blood
   flow ratio
cerebral brain death
cerebral brain flow
cerebral commissure
cerebral contusion
cerebral cortex
cerebral cry
cerebral CT venography
cerebral dominance
cerebral dysfunction
cerebral dysrhythmia
cerebral edema
cerebral embolism
cerebral gigantism
cerebral glioma
cerebral hemidecortication
cerebral hemisphere
cerebral hemorrhage
cerebral hernia
cerebral herniation
cerebral hypotension
cerebral infarct (infarction)
cerebral infundibulum
cerebral ischemia
cerebral ischemic event
cerebral mantle
cerebral metabolic rate for glucose
   (CMRglu)
cerebral metabolic rate of oxygen
   (CMRO$_2$)
cerebral metabolism
cerebral mycotic aneurysm
cerebral nocardiosis
cerebral operculum
cerebral parenchyma
cerebral peduncle
cerebral perfusion pressure
cerebral perfusion SPECT scan
cerebral pneumonia
cerebral revascularization

cerebral sign
cerebral SPECT
cerebral steal syndrome
cerebral thrombophlebitis
cerebral Whipple disease
cerebral white matter
cerebri (genitive form of cerebrum)
  commotio
  contusio
  falx (hook of cerebrum)
  gliomatosis
  pseudotumor
cerebriform
cerebrohepatorenal syndrome
cerebromacular degeneration (CMD)
cerebromeningeal intracerebral
  hemorrhage
cerebropontocerebellar pathway
cerebrospinal fluid (CSF)
cerebrospinal fluid-containing lesion
cerebrospinal fluid fistula
cerebrospinal fluid flow measurement
cerebrospinal fluid leak study
cerebrospinal fluid pathway
cerebrospinal fluid rhinorrhea
cerebrovascular accident (CVA)
cerebrovascular occlusive disease
cerebrum (pl. cerebra)
  central cavity of
  cortex of
  first ventricle of
  great vein of
  lateral ventricle of
  second ventricle of
  third ventricle of
Cerenkov calculation
Cerenkov measurement
Cerenkov radiation
Cerenkov scintillation analysis
Ceretec (technetium Tc 99m
  exametazime) imaging agent
cerium (Ce) (an element)
cerium silicate imaging agent

CerroBend block
cervical aorta syndrome
cervical aortic arch
cervical CT (computed tomography)
cervical dilation
cervical disk disease
cervical dorsal outlet syndrome
cervical ectopic pregnancy locations
cervical edema
cervical endometriosis
cervical esophagus
cervical fistula
cervical fracture
cervical intervertebral foraminal MR
  phlebography (CMRP)
cervical laceration
cervical malignancy
cervical mover ligament
cervical musculature
cervical myelogram
cervical myelopathy
cervical nerve root
cervical outlet
cervical pleura
cervical rib
cervical spine (C1 to C7 vertebrae)
cervical spine dens view
cervical spine intraosseous pneumatocyst
cervical spondylosis of the spinal cord
cervical spondylosis, washboard effect
  on myelography in
cervical spondylotic myelopathy
cervical stricture
cervical triangle
cervicocerebral
cervicography
cervicomedullary junction
cervico-occipital fusion
cervicosigmoid fistula
cervicothoracolumbar
cervicotrochanteric fracture
cervicouterine junction

cervicovaginal fistula
cervicovaginal junction
cervicovesical fistula
cervigram
cervix uteri
CES (cauda equina syndrome)
cesium iodide–amorphous silicon flat-
    panel detector
Céstan-Chenais syndrome
cestodic tuberculosis
CF or CX (circumflex) artery
CFR (coronary flow reserve)
CGI (common gateway interface)
CGR biplane angiographic system
cGy (centigray)
Chaddock sign
Chagas disease
chainbead cystourethrogram
chain, obturator nodal
chain of lakes sign
chalasia
chalk (or chalky) bones
challenge
    acetazolamide
    hyperoxia
    hypotensive
chamber
    cardiac
    false aneurysmal
    infundibular
    ionization
    irradiation
    left atrial
    left ventricular
    right atrial
    right ventricular
    rudimentary outlet
    well-type ionization
    Wilson cloud
chamber compression
chamber dilatation
chamber enlargement
chamber of heart

Chamberlain line
Chamberlain-Towne view
champagne-bottle legs in Charcot-
    Marie-Tooth disease
champagne glass pelvis
Chance spinal fracture
change (pl. changes)
    cystic
    degenerative
    dystrophic
    ECMO-induced
    fibrotic
    fMRI signal
    focal degenerative
    geographic fatty
    intratumoral fatty
    lytic
    morphological
    osteoarthritic
    paroxysmal
    pre-slip
    radiation-induced
    residual limb shape
    spondylitic
    subtle
    subtle neuroanatomical
    subtle structural
    subtle white matter
    vasomotor
change-coupled device (CCD)
channel (pl. channels)
    blood
    central
    deep venous
    enlarged vascular
    gastric
    pancreaticobiliary common
    pyloric
Chaput tubercle
character cell terminal
characteristic, echo
charcoal trap
Charcot-Bouchard intracerebral
    microaneurysm

Charcot chondroma
Charcot cirrhosis
Charcot joint
Charcot-Marie-Tooth disease
Charcot triad
charge-coupled device (CCD) digitizer
charged particles
chase bolus
chase bolus imaging technique
Chassard-Lapiné ("la-pee-NAY") view
    of sigmoid colon
Chassard view (sigmoid colon)
Chausse II oblique transoral view
    of foramen jugulare
Chausse III view (temporal bone
    projection)
Chausse IV view
chauffeur's fracture
Chauffard point
Chausse view
CHD (congenital heart disease)
check-valve sheath
Chédiak-Higashi syndrome
cheekbone, cheek bone
cheese handler's (or washer's) disease
cheesy pneumonia
cheiromegaly
cheirospasm
chemically induced dynamic nuclear
    polarization
chemical pneumonia
chemical pneumonitis
chemical-selective fat saturation MR
chemical-shift artifact
chemical-shift phenomena artifact
chemical-shift ratio
chemiluminescence
chemodectoma
chemoembolization
    therapeutic
    transarterial
    transcatheter arterial
    transcatheter oily

chemonucleolysis
Chemo-Port catheter
chemoradiation therapy
chemotherapy
    adjuvant
    CT-guided intra-arterial
    induction
    intra-arterial
    multiagent
    neoadjuvant
    superselective intra-arterial
Chen-Smith image coder
Cherry keyboard
CHESS method
chest
    alar (flat)
    barrel
    blast
    cobbler's
    cylindrical
    flail
    foveated
    funnel
    globular
    hollow
    keeled
    lateral upright
    paralytic
    PA upright
    phthinoid (flat)
    pigeon
    pounding
    pterygoid (flat)
    symmetrical
    tetrahedron
chest tube
    apically directed
    atelectasis following removal of
chest wall invasion
chest wall paradoxical motion
chest x-ray (CXR), baseline
Chester disease
chevron bone

CHF (congenital hepatic fibrosis)
CHF (congestive heart failure)
Chiari-Budd syndrome
Chiari-Foix-Nicolesco syndrome
Chiari II malformation
chiasmal compression
chiasm of digits of hand
Chiba percutaneous cholangiogram
  chickenpox
chicken breast
chicken-fat clot
chickenpox pneumonia
Chilaiditi sign
Child classification of esophageal
  varices
Child-Pugh cirrhosis
chip
  cancellous bone
  corticocancellous bone
chip fracture
chiropractic x-ray films
chisel fracture
choana cerebri
choanal
cholangiocarcinoma, peripheral (PCC)
Cholangiocath
cholangiocatheter
cholangiofibromatosis
cholangiogram
cholangiography
  balloon
  breath hold MR
  catheter
  Chiba percutaneous
  common duct
  contrast selective
  cystic duct
  drip infusion (DIC)
  endoscopic retrograde (ERC)
  fine-needle percutaneous
    transhepatic (PTHC)
  fine-needle transhepatic (FNTC)
  HASTE MR

cholangiography *(cont.)*
  intraoperative (IOC)
  intraoperative MR-
  intravenous (IVC)
  magnetic resonance (MRC)
  operative
  Oriental
  percutaneous transhepatic (PTC)
  transhepatic (THC)
  recurrent pyogenic (RPC)
  serial
  single shot MR
  thin needle percutaneous
  three-dimensional portocholangi-
    ography
  transhepatic (THC)
  T-tube (TTC)
  transjugular
cholangiohepatitis
cholangiopancreatography
  endoscopic
  magnetic resonance (MR)
  retrograde (ERCP)
cholangiopathy, eosinophilic
cholangiovenous communication
cholangitis
  acute obstructive
  ascending
  chronic nonsuppurative destructive
  fibrous obliterative
  intrahepatic sclerosing
  nonsuppurative
  primary sclerosing (PSC)
  progressive suppurative
  pyogenic
  recurrent pyogenic
  sclerosing
  septic
  suppurative
cholecystectasia
cholecystitis
  acalculous
  acute

cholecystitis *(cont.)*
  calculous
  chronic
  emphysematous
  gaseous
  perforated
cholecystitis with cholelithiasis
cholecystocholangiogram
cholecystocholangiography
cholecystoduodenal ligament
cholecystogram, oral (OCG)
cholecystography
cholecystokinetic food
cholecystokinin (CCK)
cholecystokinin-pancreozymin
  (CCK-PZ)
cholecystolithiasis
cholecystopathy
cholecystoptosis
cholecystostomy
  percutaneous transhepatic
  ultrasound-guided percutaneous
choledochal cyst
choledochocele
choledocholithiasis
cholelith
cholelithiasis
cholelithoptysis
cholescintigram
cholescintigraphy
  morphine augmented
  sincalide
cholestatic liver disease
cholesteatoma
cholestasis
  intrahepatic
  neonatal
cholesterol embolization
  diffuse
  disseminated
cholesterol pleurisy
cholesterol pneumonitis
cholesterolosis of gallbladder

Choletec (technetium ^{99m}Tc mebrofenin) hepatobiliary imaging agent
Cholografin Meglumine (iodipamide
  meglumine) imaging agent
Cholografin Meglumine chondrosarcoma
  dedifferentiated
  synovial
chololith (cholelith)
chondral fragment
chondrification
chondroblastoma
chondrodiastasis
chondrodystrophia calcificans
chondrodystrophia fetalis
chondrofibroma
chondrogenic tumor
chondroid matrix
chondroitin sulfate iron colloid (CSIS)
  enhanced MRI
chondrolipoma
chondrolysis
chondroma
  Charcot
  juxtacortical
chondromalacia patellae
chondromatosis
  Henderson-Jones
  synovial
chondromatous hamartoma
chondromyofibroma
chondromyxoid fibroma (CMF)
chondromyxoma
chondromyxosarcoma
chondronecrosis
chondro-osteodystrophy
chondrophyte
chondroporosis
chondrosarcoma (see also *carcinoma,*
  sarcoma)
  differentiated
  osteo-
  osteofibro-

chondrosarcoma (cont.)
  parosteal
  synovial
chondrosarcomatosis
chondrosteoma
chondrosternal junction
Chopart ankle dislocation
Chopart joint
Choquet fuzzy integral
chorda (pl. chordae)
  basal
  cleft
  commissural
  first order
  second order
  strut
  third order
chorda magna
chorda tympani
chordae tendineae cordis
chordae Willisii
chordal rupture
chordocarcinoma
chordoepithelioma
chordosarcoma
choriocarcinoma
choriocarcinoma testicular tumor
chorionic villus sampling
choroid glomera
choroid plexus papilloma (CPP)
choroidal fissure
choroidal pericallosal artery
Christmas tree appearance on MR
Christmas tree appearance of pancreas
chromatographic separations
chromic phosphate P 32 radiotherapy
  agent
chromium (Cr) (an element)
  ^{51}Cr-labeled red blood cells
chromium-labeled red blood cells
chronic eosinophilic pneumonia
chronic fatigue syndrome
chronic focal pancreatitis

chronic inflammation
chronic lithium nephropathy
chronic obstructive hydronephrosis
chronic pneumonitis
chronic pseudoaneurysm
ChronoFlex polyurethane catheter
chronologic age
Churg-Strauss syndrome
chyliform pleurisy
chyloid pleurisy
chylous pleurisy
CI (cavitation index)
CI (continuous imaging)
Ciaglia percutaneous tracheostomy
  introducer
CID camera
Cidtech camera
CIG (cardiointegram)
cigarette smoking, pack-years of
CIIP (chronic idiopathic intestinal
  pseudo-obstruction)
ciliary ganglion
ciliated border
ciliospinal center of Budge
Cimino shunt
Cincinnati view (supine chest)
cineangiocardiography
cineangiogram
cineangiography
  aortic root
  biplane
  coronary
  left anterior oblique (LAO)
  left posterior oblique (LPO)
  left ventricular (LV)
  radionuclide
  right anterior oblique (RAO)
  right posterior oblique (RPO)
  selective coronary
  Sones technique for
  ventricular
cine-based viewing

cinecardioangiography
cine coronary angiography
cine CT (computed tomography)
  scanner
cinedefecogram
cine-esophagogram
cine-esophagram
cinefluorography
cinefluoroscopy
cine gradient-echo MR imaging
cine (high frame-rate) mode
cine-loop
cine magnetic resonance tagging
Cine Memory with color flow
  Doppler imaging
cine mode MR imaging
cine PC imaging
cine projector, Tagarno 3SD (for
  angiography)
cineradiography
cineradiology, digital
cine view in MUGA (multiple gated
  acquisition) scan
cineventriculogram
cineventriculography
cingulate gyrus
cingulate herniation
cingulate sulcus
cipher
  product
  transposition
circadian event recorder
circadian periodicity
circle
  arterial
  articular vascular
circle of Vieussens
circle of Weber
circle of Willis
Circon stent
Circon video camera

circuit
  anticoincidence
  application-specific integrated
    (ASIC)
  arrhythmia
  ASIC
  bypass
  coincidence
  doubly broadband triple resonance
    NMR probe
  macroreentrant
  magnetoresistive sensor
  microreentrant
  reentry
  shunting
circular cherry-red lesion
circular muscles
circular plane
circular syncytium
circular tomosynthesis
circulation
  allantoic
  arrested
  assisted
  balanced
  cerebrospinal fluid
  codominant
  collateral
  compensatory
  cutaneous collateral
  derivative
  extracorporeal
  fetal
  greater
  intervillous
  peripheral
  placental
  sluggish enterohepatic
  spiderweb
  systemic
  thebesian
circulation time

circulatory collapse
circulatory compromise
circulatory disturbance
circulatory embarrassment
circulatory failure
circulatory hyperkinetic syndrome
circulatory impairment
circulatory shock
circulatory stasis
circumference (of anatomical structure)
circumferential echodense layer
circumferential fracture
circumferentially
circumferential perilesional enhance-
    ment
circumflex (circ., CF, CX)
circumflex artery
circumflex branches
circumflex coronary artery
circumflex groove artery
circumflex vessels
circumscribed edema
circumscribed infiltrate
circumscribed pleurisy
circumscript aneurysm
cirrhosis
    acholangic biliary
    acute juvenile
    alcoholic
    atrophic
    biliary
    Budd
    calculus
    cardiac
    Charcot
    Child-Pugh
    cholangitic biliary
    congestive
    Cruveilhier-Baumgarten
    cryptogenic
    decompensated alcoholic
    diffuse septal
    end stage

cirrhosis (cont.)
    fatty
    focal biliary
    frank
    glabrous
    Hanot
    hepatic
    hypertrophic
    Indian childhood
    juvenile
    Laënnec
    liver
    lung
    macrolobular
    macronodular
    medionodular
    metabolic
    microlobular
    micronodular
    multilobular
    nutritional
    obstructive biliary
    periportal
    pipe-stem
    portal
    posthepatic
    postnecrotic
    primary biliary (PBC)
    progressive familial
    pulmonary
    secondary biliary
    septal
    stasis
    Todd
    toxic
    unilobular
    vascular
cirrhotic
cirsoid aneurysm
CISS (constructive interference in
    steady state) MR imaging
CISS scheme

cistern
  ambient
  basal
  basal arachnoid
  basilar
  carotid
  cerebellomedullary
  cerebellopontine
  chiasmatic
  chyle
  crural
  great
  increased basilar
  interpeduncular
  mesencephalic
  opticochiasmatic
  parasellar
  posterior
  prepontine
  quadrigeminal
  subarachnoidal
  trigeminal
cistern of chiasma
cistern of fossa of Sylvius
cistern of lamina terminalis
cistern of lateral fossa of cerebrum
cistern of Pecquet
cistern of Sylvius
cisternogram
cisternography
  air
  indium
  intrathecal gadolinium-enhanced
    MR
  isotope
  isotopic
  metrizamide CT (MCTC)
  oxygen
  radioisotope
  radionuclide
CJD (Creutzfeldt-Jakob disease)
CKG (cardiokymography)
c-Ki-ras mutation

Clado point
Clamshell occluder
Clarke-Hadfield syndrome
Clarke rule (buccal object rule)
Clark vulvar melanoma classification
classic interstitial pneumonia
classification
  AAOS acetabular abnormalities
  acromioclavicular injury
  Aitken epiphyseal fracture
  Allman acromioclavicular injury
  American Spinal Cord Injury
    Association
  Anderson-D'Alonzo odontoid
    fracture
  Antoni-A neurinoma
  AO ankle fracture
  AO-Danis-Weber ankle fracture
  Arcq
  Arthritis Impact Measurement
    Scales
  Bayne radial agenesis
  Berndt-Harty talar lesion staging
  Berkson-Gage breast cancer
    survival calculation
  Bethesda
  bladder carcinoma
  Bleck metatarsus adductus
  Bosniak
  Bosniak renal cystic mass
  Boyd-Griffin trochanteric fracture
  Brewlow malignant melanoma
  Broders tumor index
  Brooker periarticular heterotopic
    ossification (PHO)
  Burwell-Charnley fracture
    reduction
  Butcher staging
  Caldwell-Moloy
  Canale-Kelly talar neck fracture
  Carnesale-Stewart-Barnes hip
    dislocation
  Catterall

classification *(cont.)*
  Cedell-Magnusson arthritis
  Clark malignant melanoma
  Clark vulvar melanoma
  Colonna hip fracture
  Copeland-Kavat metatarso-
    phalangeal dislocation
  Danis-Weber ankle fracture
  D'Antonio acetabular
  David-Chausse (I-IV)
  DeBakey aortic
  Delbet hip fracture
  Denis
  Dickhaut-DeLee discoid meniscus
  Dubin and Amelar varicocele
  Dukes carcinoma
  Essex-Lopresti calcaneal fracture
  Evans intertrochanteric fracture
  Ficat stage of avascular necrosis
  Fielding-Magliato subtrochanteric
    fracture
  FIGO staging of adenocarcinoma
    of endometrium
  Fränkel spinal cord injury
  Freeman calcaneal fracture
  Fries score for rheumatoid arthritis
  Frykman hand fracture
  Garden femoral neck fracture
  Gartland supracondylar fracture
  Gertzbein seat belt injury
  Grantham femur fracture
  Gumley seat belt injury
  Gustilo-Anderson tibial plafond
    fracture
  Hahn-Steinthal capitellum fracture
  Hansen fracture
  Hawkins talar neck fracture
  Herbert-Fisher fracture system
  Hohl tibial condylar fracture
  Holdsworth spinal fracture
  Hughston Clinic injury
  Hunt-Hess aneurysm
  Hunt-Kosnik

classification *(cont.)*
  Hyams grading of esthesioneuro-
    blastoma
  Ingram-Bachynski hip fracture
  Jackson and Parker (of Hodgkin
    lymphoma)
  Jahss dislocation
  Jeffery radial fracture
  Jewett bladder carcinoma
  Jones
  Judet epiphyseal fracture
  Kalamchi-Dawe congenital tibial
    deficiency
  Kernohan brain tumor
  Kiel non-Hodgkin lymphoma
  Kilfoyle condylar fracture
  King classification of thoracic
    scoliosis
  Kistler subarachnoid hemorrhage
  Klatskin tumor
  Kocher-Lorenz capitellum fracture
  Kostuik-Errico spinal stability
  Kyle fracture
  Lauge-Hansen ankle fracture
  Letournel and Judet (acetabular
    fractures)
  Lukes-Butler non-Hodgkin
    lymphoma
  Mason radial fracture
  Mazur ankle evaluation
  McLain-Weinstein spinal tumor
  Merland perimedullary
    arteriovenous fistula
  Meyers-McKeever tibial fracture
  Milch elbow fracture
  Modic
  MSTS (Musculoskeletal Tumor
    Society) staging system
  Mueller humerus fracture
  multiaxial
  Neer shoulder fractures I, II,
    and III
  Neer-Horowitz humerus fracture

classification *(cont.)*
Nevaiser frozen shoulder
Newman radial fracture
Nurick spondylosis
NYHA (New York Heart Association) congestive heart failure
O'Brien radial fracture
Ogden epiphyseal fracture
Olerud and Molander fracture
Ovadia-Beals tibial plafond fracture
osteoarthritis grading
Pauwels femoral neck fracture
Pennal
Pennal and Tile pelvic girdle injury
Pipkin femoral fracture
Poland epiphyseal fracture
Rappaport lymphoma
Ratliff avascular necrosis
Riordan club hand
Riseborough-Radin intercondylar
fracture
Rockwood acromioclavicular injury
Rowe calcaneal fracture
Rowe-Lowell fracture-dislocation
Ruedi-Allgower tibial plafond
fracture
Russell-Rubinstein cerebrovascular
malformation
Rye Hodgkin disease
Sage-Salvatore acromioclavicular
joint injury
Sakellarides calcaneal fracture
Salter-Harris fracture
Salter-Harris-Rang epiphyseal
fracture
Schatzker fracture
Seinsheimer femoral fracture
Shelton femur fracture
Smith sesamoid position
Sorbie calcaneal fracture
Steinbrocker rheumatoid arthritis
Steinert epiphyseal fracture
Steward-Milford fracture

classification *(cont.)*
talocalcaneal index
Thompson-Epstein femoral fracture
Tile
Tile-Pennal
TNM (tumor size, nodal involvement, metastatic progress)
Tönnis (Toennis) hip dysplasia
Tronzo intertrochanteric fracture
Trunkey fracture
Vostal radial fracture
Watanabe discoid meniscus
Watson-Jones
Weinstein-Boriani-Biagini spinal
tumor
Wiberg patellar types
Wilkins radial fracture
Winquist-Hansen femoral fracture
Wolfe breast carcinoma
Young-Burgess
Zickel fracture
Claude syndrome
clavicle
clavicular head of sternocleidomastoid
clavicular notch
clavipectoral fascia
clawfoot deformity
pes arcuatus
pes cavus
claw hand (or clawhand)
clawtoe deformity
Claybrook sign
clay shoveler's fracture
CLC (Clerc-Levy-Cristesco) syndrome
clean intermittent bladder catheterization (CIC)
clean intermittent catheterization
clean shadow
cleansing, digital subtraction bowel
clearance, aerosol
clearance curve
clearance half-time
clear cell of kidney

clear zone
cleavage fracture
cleavage plane, subintimal
Cleaves axial hip projection
Cleaves axial shoulder projection
Cleaves method (hip)
Cleaves method (shoulder)
cleaving, plaque
Cleeman sign
cleft
    anal
    branchial
    first visceral
    gill
    interinnominoabdominal
    meniscal
    olfactory
    pudendal
    retrosomatic
    synaptic
    ventricular
cleft chordae
cleft leaflet
cleidocranial dysostosis
Cleland ligament in the hand
Clements-Nakayama method (to view
    acetabulum and femoral head)
clenched fist view
Clerc-Levy-Cristesco (CLC) syndrome
clicking pneumothorax
clinical correlation
clinical sequelae
clinical target volume
Clinical Ultrasonic Bone Sonometry
    (CUBA)
clinicopathological analysis
clinodactyly
clinoid ligament
clip
    aneurysm
    biopsy-site marker
    marking
    metallic
    surgical

clip deployment
clip migration
clipping, ureteral
clitoral hypertrophy
clitoris, bifid
clivus, Blumenbach
clivus meningioma tumor
CLO (congenital lobar overinflation)
cloacal anomaly
clockwise whirlpool sign
clonogen number
clonogenicity
C-loop of duodenum
closed-break fracture
closed dislocation
closed fracture
closed spinal dysraphism
close-up view
closure
    growth center
    native aortic valve
    percutaneous transcatheter ductal
        (PTDC)
    physeal
    threatened vessel
    tricuspid valve
    valve
clot
    agonal (or agony)
    autologous
    blood
    chicken-fat
    marantic
    passive
    preformed
    sentinel
    subarachnoid
    subdural
    subtle
clot-filled lumen
clot lysis
clouding, alveolar
cloudy swelling of heart

Cloverleaf catheter
cloverleaf deformity
cloverleaf-shaped lumen
cloverleaf skull
clubfoot deformity
clubhand deformity
club-shaped (anatomical structure)
clumsy-hand syndrome
cluneal nerve
clustered calcification
clustered calcifications on mammo-
    gram
clustered microcalcifications
clustering algorithm
cluster plots
clusters, K-means
cm (centimeter)
CMD (cerebromacular degeneration)
CMF (chondromyxoid fibroma)
CMJ (corticomedullary junction)
    phase imaging on CT scan
CMR (congenital mitral regurgitation)
CMRglu (cerebral metabolic rate for
    glucose)
$CMRO_2$ (cerebral metabolic rate of
    oxygen glucose metabolite)
CMRP (cervical intervertebral
    foraminal MR phlebography)
CMT (Charcot-Marie-Tooth) disease
CMV (cytomegalovirus)
C/N (contrast to noise) ratio (CNR)
CNS (central nervous system)
CO_2 (carbon dioxide)
    CO_2 angiography
    CO_2 cylinder
    CO_2 generator
    CO_2 insufflation
    CO_2 laser
    CO_2 negative contrast media
    CO_2 retention
CO (cardiac output) (L/min)
coagulation
    disseminated intravascular
    microwave

coagulation defect
coagulative interstitial laser
coal miner's (also coal worker's) lung
coalesce
coalescence
coalescent multiple intrarenal abscess
coalition
    bony
    calcaneonavicular
    carpal
    fibrous
    intercarpal
    lunate-triquetral
    Minaar classification of
    osseous
    subtalar
    talocalcaneal
    tarsal
coalition view (calcaneotalar coalition)
coaptation of leaflet
coaptation point
coapted leaflets
coarctation
    aortic
    atypical
    atypical subisthmic
    congenital isthmic
    isthmic
    juxtaductal
coarctation of aorta
    adult-type
    infantile-type
    juxtaductal
    postductal
    preductal
    reversed
coarctation, reversed
coarse nodular ultrasound pattern
coarse thickening of interstitial struc-
    tures
Coats disease
coaxial catheter, Hieshima
coaxial steering

coaxial Tracker catheter
cobalt-chromium alloy
cobalt radioactive source
cobalt-60 beam
cobalt-60 gamma knife radiosurgical
    treatment
cobbler chest syndrome
cobblestone appearance
cobblestone appearance of mucosa on
    small bowel follow-through
cobblestone pattern
Cobb scoliosis angle
Cobb syndrome
Cobey-Saltzman view
Cobey view of hindfoot
Cobra (and Cobra 2) catheter
cobra head appearance
cobra head effect
cobra head sign
Cobra over the wire balloon catheter
cobweb appearance
cobweb pattern
coccidioidal granuloma
coccidioidoma
coccidioidomycosis
    desert
    disseminated
    latent
    Posadas-Wernicke
    primary
    progressive
    San Joaquin Valley
    secondary
    valley
coccidioidomycosis arthritis
coccygeal body
coccygeal bone
coccygeal spine
coccygeopubic diameter
coccyx
cochlear implant
cockade image (for intraosseous
    lipoma of the calcaneus)

Cockayne syndrome
cocking injury
cockscomb deformity
cock-up deformity of toe
Co-Cr-Mo (cobalt-chromium-
    molybdenum) alloy implant metal
Co-Cr-W-Ni (cobalt-chromium-
    tungsten-nickel) alloy implant metal
COD (computerized optical
    densitometry)
coded-aperture imaging
coder
    Chen-Smith
    ICS (improved Chen-Smith)
codfish vertebrae
codivilla extension
Codman angle
Codman Hakim programmable valve
Codman sign
Codman triangle
codominant circulation
codominant system
codominant vessel
Codonics color printer
coefficient
    absorption
    attenuation
    beta-spectra shape factor
    curve fit
    diffusion
    linear absorption
    linear attenuation
    mass attenuation
    partition
    stiffness
CO_2 enema
coeur en cuirasse
coeur en sabot
coffee bean sign
coffee worker's lung
Cohen cannula
Cohen/Jarcho cannula
coherent scattering

coil
  aneurysmal
  birdcage
  birdcage-type head
  body
  collagen-filled interlocking
    detachable
  crossed
  dedicated phased-array
  defibrillation
  detachable
  double breast
  electrolytically detachable
  endoanal
  endoesophageal MRI
  endorectal
  endoscopic quadrature RF
  endovaginal
  endovascular
  flexible surface
  Flex-S
  GDC (Guglielmi detachable)
  Gianturco occlusion
  Gianturco wool-tufted wire
  Golay
  Gore 1.5T Torso Array surface
  gradient
  gradient sheet
  Guglielmi detachable (GDC)
  head
  Helmholtz
  High Performance Detach
    embolization
  immediately detachable
  Intercept prostate microcoil
  Intercept urethra microcoil
  Intercept Vascular 0.030" internal
    MR
  interlocking detachable
  intraurethral
  liver
  Medrad MRInnervu endorectal
    colon probe

coil *(cont.)*
  modified birdcage
  opposed loop-pair quadrature
    NMR
  optimized transmit-receive
  orthogonal RF
  platinum
  quadrature RF receiver
  radiofrequency (RF)
  receiver
  RF (radiofrequency)
  right ventricular
  saddle
  sensing
  shim
  solenoid surface
  surface
  Surgi-Vision Intercept urethral
  Surgi-Vision urethral MRI
    microcoil
  three-axis gradient
  torso phased-array (TPAC)
coiled spring appearance of intussuscepted bowel
coil embolization (therapeutic)
coiling of stent
coil-occluded
coil occlusion
coil-tipped catheter
coil to vessel diameter
coincidence circuit
coincidence-summing correction
coin lesion
CO labeled with O-15 imaging agent
Colapinto transjugular liver biopsy
  needle
Colcher-Sussman AP projection
  (pelvimetry view)
Colcher-Sussman lateral projection
  (pelvimetry view)
COLD (chronic obstructive lung
  disease)
cold nodule

cold spot myocardial imaging
colic impression on the liver
Colinet-Caplan syndrome
colitis
    chronic ulcerative (CUC)
    Crohn
    familial ulcerative
    focal
    fulminant
    fulminating ulcerative
    granulomatous transmural
    ischemic
    mucous
    myxomembranous
    pseudomembranous (PMC)
    radiation
    radiation-induced
    regional
    single stripe (SSC)
    transmural
    ulcerative (UC)
colitis polyposa
colitis ulcerosa gravis
collagen-filled interlocking detachable
    coils
collagen tissue proliferation
collagen vascular disease
collapse
    left lower lobe
    postoperative acute massive
    subtle
collapse of anatomical structure
collapse of jugular venous pressure
collapsing bubbles
collar
    implant
    periosteal bone
collar bone
collar-button abscess
collar-button appearance in colon
collateral
    bridging
    porto-azygos

collateral *(cont.)*
    retrograde
    septal
collateral blood flow
collateral blood supply
collateral branch
collateral channel
collateral circulation
collateral eminence
collateralization
collateral ligament
collateral sulcus
collateral system
collateral vessel
collecting duct
collecting system
collection, juxtacaval fat
collection of contrast material
Colles fracture
Colles ligament
Collet-Sicard syndrome
collicular fracture
colliculus (pl. colliculi)
    facial
    seminal
collimated
collimation
    detector
    dynamic multileaf
    tertiary
collimation CT
collimation scanning
collimation width
collimator
    APC-3
    APC-4
    converging
    diverging
    Eureka
    fan-beam
    Lehr-par
    long bore
    Machlett

collimator *(cont.)*
  Micro-CAST
  multileaf
  multirod
  parallel-hole
  pinhole
  slant hole
  Summit LoDose
collimator exchange effect
collimator helmet
collimator plugging pattern
collimator scatter
collision, inelastic
colloid cystic tumor
colloid oncotic pressure (COP)
colloid shift on liver-spleen scan
colloid shift on scan
colocolic anastomosis
colocolic intussusception
colocutaneous fistula
colography, CT
Colombo count
colon
  anterior band of
  ascending
  descending
  distal
  free band of
  giant
  iliac
  inflammation of
  lateral reflection of
  lead-pipe
  left
  malposition of
  mega-
  mesosigmoid
  midsigmoid
  pelvic
  perisigmoid
  redundant sigmoid
  right
  sigmoid

colon *(cont.)*
  spastic
  transverse
colon cutoff sign
colonic diverticulum
colonic haustra
colonic motility
colonic pit
colonic polyp
colonic tuberculosis
colonography
  CT
  multidetector row CT
  thin section multidetector row CT
colonoscope, Olympus CF-1T100L
  forward-viewing video colonoscope
colonoscopy, virtual
coloptosis
color amplitude imaging
color-coded catheter
color-coded duplex sonography
color-coded pulmonary blood flow
  image
color-coded real-time sonography
color correction, multi-illuminant
color Doppler imaging (CDI)
color Doppler ultrasound
color duplex interrogation
color duplex sonography
color duplex ultrasound
color duplex ultrasound-guided percutaneous transluminal angioplasty
color flow Doppler sonographic guidance
color flow Doppler ultrasound
  (CDUS)
color-flow duplex imaging of vein
  graft
colorectal (CR)
colorectal adenoma
colorectal mucosa
color flow Doppler

color flow Doppler real-time 2-D
   blood flow imaging
color flow duplex imaging
color flow mapping
colorimetric color reproduction
color power transcranial Doppler
   sonography
color reproduction, colorimetric
color space conversion
color space, C-Y
color space interpolator
color ultrasound
colosigmoid resection
colostomy, diverting
colovaginal fistula
colovesical fistula
colpocele
colpoptosis
column
   anal
   anterior gray (of spinal cord)
   Bertin
   branchial efferent
   Clarke
   contrast medium
   Lissauer
   renal
   variceal
   vertebral
column extraction method
columning of dye
columnization of imaging agent
column mode sinogram images
column of Burdach
column of dye
column of Morgagni
column theory, Letournel and Judet
   classification and (of acetabular
   fractures)
CoLyte bowel prep
Combidex (ferumoxtran-10) imaging
   agent

Combidex multifunctional MR
   imaging agent
combination flow and pressure loads
combined cystogram-nephrostogram
combined flexion phenomenon
combined modality radiation therapy
combined leukocyte-marrow imaging
combined multisection diffuse-
   weighted and hemodynamically
   weighted echo planar MR imaging
combined Myoscint/thallium imaging
combined thallium-Tc-HOMPAO
   imaging
comb sign on CT scan
comet tail sign
comma sign in truncus arteriosus
comminuted bursting fracture
comminuted fracture
commissural attachments
commissural chordae
commissural leaflet
commissural point
commissure
   anterior (AC)
   anteroseptal
   cerebral
   fused
   gray commissure of spinal cord
   posterior (PC)
   scalloped
   tectum
   valve
   vestigial
   white commissure of spinal cord
common bile duct (CBD)
common carotid artery (CCA)
common cavity phenomenon
common duct cholangiogram
common duct stone
common femoral artery
common gateway interface (CGI)
common iliac artery

common sheath reimplant
communicating hydrocephalus
communicating vein
communication
  asyndetic
  interatrial
communis, extensor digitorum
community-acquired (bacterial)
  pneumonia (CAP)
Comolli sign
compact bone
comparison
  histopathologic
  yield
comparison view
compartment
  anterior
  anterior mediastinal
  deep posterior
  extensor
  extradural
  infracolic
  infratentorial
  lateral
  medial
  patellofemoral
  plantar
  posterior
  posterolateral
  posteromedial
  superficial posterior
  supracolic
compartment lesion, posterior
compartment syndrome
Compass stereotactic frame
compatible
compensated composite spin lock
  pulse
compensated congestive heart failure
compensation
  cardiac
  cardiac gating
  lens-distortion

compensation *(cont.)*
  respiratory
  scatter
  section-select flow
compensator
  scattering foil
  tissue deficit
compensatory emphysema
compensatory enlargement
compensatory hypertrophy
compensatory renal hypertrophy
competent valve
competitive adsorption
complete atrioventricular block
complete atrioventricular dissociation
complete bladder emptying
complete dislocation
complete fracture
complete heart block
complex
  AIDS dementia (ADC)
  amygdala-hippocampal
  amygdaloid nuclear
  ankle joint (AJC)
  anterior communicating artery
  antibody-antigen
  apical
  arcuate
  atrial
  auricular
  Buford
  capsulolabral
  caudal pharyngeal
  dentomaxillofacial
  diisocyanide-triisocyanide ^{99m}Tc
  discoligamentous
  echo
  Eisenmenger
  fabellofibular
  foot–ankle
  gadolinium
  gastrocnemius–soleus
  gastroduodenal artery

complex *(cont.)*
 Ghon
 Ghon-Sachs
 hallux valgus–metatarsus primus
  varus
 hindfoot joint
 hippocampal-amygdaloid
 inverted Y
 ligamentous
 Lutembacher
 mantle
 MION-gene
 multiform ventricular
 nipple-areola
 oxidized
 post-transplantation
 primary
 Ranke
 salvo of premature ventricular
 sesamoid
 sling ring
 subluxation
 superior olivary
 symptom
 syndesmotic ligament
 tibiocalcaneal joint
 triangular fibrocartilaginous
  (TFCC)
 transluminal coronary artery
  angioplasty
 ventricular premature
 vertebrobasilar
 von Meyenburg complex
 zygomatic-malar (ZMC)
complex blocking
complex dynamic pharyngeal and
 speech evaluation by cine recording
complex electron arc therapy
compound dislocation
compound fracture
compression
 aqueduct
 axial

compression *(cont.)*
 brachial artery
 brachial plexus
 brain stem
 cardiac
 celiac artery
 chamber
 chiasmal
 contoured tilting
 cord
 dynamic
 extrinsic
 fingerprint image
 iliocaval
 image
 interfragmental
 irreversible
 JPEG
 limited
 local
 lossy wavelet
 magnification and spot
 manual
 multiplanar
 nerve root
 neurovascular
 optic nerve
 orbital mass
 plaque
 pulmonary
 pulmonary artery
 radicular
 rapid thoracic
 root
 sequential
 spinal cord
 spot
 thermal
 ultrasound-guided pseudoaneurysm
 ureteral
 wavelet
 wedge
compression atelectasis

compression fracture (burst)
compression paddle
compression plate and screws
compression ratio
compression syndrome
compression ultrasonography
compromise
 circulatory
 renal
 respiratory
 umbilical cord
 ureteral vascular
compromised flow
Compton scattering cross-section
Compton suppression spectrometer
Compuscan Hittman computerized
 electrocardioscanner
computed axial tomography (CAT)
 scan
computed CT scanned projection
 radiography
computed CT SPR (computed tomographic scanned projection radiography)
computed dental radiography (CDR)
computed ejection fraction
computed radiograph
computed rotational osteography
computed sonography, Acuson
computed tomographic angiography
 (CTA)
computed tomographic colonography
 (CTC)
computed tomographic scanned
 projection radiography
computed tomography (see *CT*)
computed tomography angiographic
 portography (CTAP)
computed tomography dose index
 (CTDI)
computed tomography during arterial
 portography (CTAP)
computed tomography enteroclysis

computed tomography laser mammography (CTLM)
computed tomography pulmonary
 embolus (CT PE) protocol
computed tomography scan (see *CT*)
computed transmission tomography
computer-aided design (CAD)
computer-aided diagnosis scheme
computer, Aspect
computer-assisted intracranial navigation
computer-assisted retrograde drilling
computer-assisted stereotactic resection
 of deep-seated and superficial
 lesions
computer-assisted volumetric stereotactic resection
computer-generated images
computerized (or computed)
 tomography (CT)
computerized axial tomography (CAT)
 with contrast
computerized axial tomography (CAT)
 without contrast
computerized cranial tomography
 (CCT)
computerized optical densitometry
 (COD)
computerized phonoenterography
computerized texture analysis of lung
 nodules and lung parenchyma
Computerized Thermal Imaging
 system
computerized tomographic hepatic
 angiography (CTHA)
computerized tomographic hepatic
 angiography (CTHA)
computerized tomographic scan
computerized tomography guidance
 for placement of radiation therapy
 fields
computerized tomography guidance
 for stereotactic localization

computerized tomography-guided
ncedlc biopsy
computerized transverse axial
tomography (CTAT)
computer subtraction techniques
conal papillary muscle
concatenation
Concato disease
concave
concavity
concealed hemorrhage
concentrating defect
concentration, abnormal
concentric hourglass stenosis
concentric hypertrophy
Concentric retriever system (CRS)
concept, gooseneck
Conceptus fallopian tube catheter
Conceptus Robust guidewire
Conceptus Soft Seal cervical catheter
Conceptus Soft Torque uterine catheter
Conceptus VS (variable softness)
    catheter
concha (pl. conchae)
concomitant boost radiotherapy
concordant results
concretion
    bile
    fecal
concurrent radiation therapy and
    chemotherapy
conducting loop, closed
conductive development
conductivity, vascular hydraulic
conduit
    detour
    ileal
conduit valve
condylar fracture
condylar lift-off, fluoroscopy-guided
condyle
    external
    femoral

condyle *(cont.)*
    lateral
    medial
    occipital
    tibial
condyloid joint
C1-C5 segments of internal carotid
    artery
C1-C7 cervical vertebrae
cone
    arterial
    bevelled electron beam
cone and socket bone
cone-beam image
cone-beam projection
cone-beam reconstruction algorithm
cone catheter tip
cone disk
cone-down (coned-down) view
coned-down appearance of colon
coned-down view
cone of extraocular muscles (on MRI
    scan)
cone view
configuration
    back to back
    biventricular
    dome and dart (on cardiac
        catheterization)
    horizontal dipole
    stellate
    winged
confirmatory needle localization
confocal microscopy
conformal neutron and photon
    radiotherapy
conformal radiation therapy
congenital absence
congenital anomaly
congenital cardiac malformation
congenital diaphragmatic hernia
congenital esophageal stenosis
congenital hernia

congenital pyriform aperture stenosis
congenital renal lymphangiectasia
congenital rubella pneumonitis
congenital stricture
congenital vascular malformation
congestion
  active
  asymmetric pulmonary
  capillary
  cardiac
  centrilobular
  cerebral
  chronic passive
  hepatic
  hypostatic
  intravascular
  passive vascular
  pulmonary vascular
  splenic
  symmetric
  vascular
  venous
congestive asymmetry
congestive atelectasis
congestive cardiomyopathy
congestive cirrhosis
congestive heart failure (CHF)
conglomerate calcification
congruity, joint
conical cecum on radiography
conical heart
conjoined
conjoined leaflet
conjoined twins
conjugate diameter
conjugate gradients
conjugate overshooting
conjugate, true
Conn syndrome
connection, ISDN (teleradiology)
connective tissue
  areolar
  dense

connective *(cont.)*
  peribronchial
  regular
  reticular
  subcutaneous
connective tissue proliferation
connective tissue septa
conoid ligament
conotruncal anomaly, congenital
conotruncal malformation
conoventricular defect
Conrad-Bugg trapping of soft tissue in
  ankle fracture
Conradi-Hünermann syndrome
Conray-30 imaging agent
Conray-43 imaging agent
Conray-280 imaging agent
consecutive dislocation
console
  Bruker
  SMIS
consolidated infiltrate
consolidation
  air-space
  alveolar
  bilateral
  confluent
  dense
  exudative
  ill-defined
  lobar
  lung parenchyma
  nonhomogeneous
  parenchymal
  patchy air-space
  peripheral
  pulmonary
  segmental
  unilateral
consolidative change
consolidative pneumonia
consolidative process
conspicuity

constant, Planck
constant tilt wave
constellation of findings; symptoms
constitutional symptoms
constriction
   airway
   hourglass
   occult pericardial
   postglomerular arteriolar
   tangential
constriction band syndrome
constriction of hip capsule, hourglass
constrictive bronchiolitis
constrictive pericarditis
construction artifact
construction of intestinal ureter
constructive interference in steady
   state (CISS) magnetic resonance
   imaging
contact B-scan ultrasound
contents
   abdominal
   bone mineral (BMC)
   bowel
   brain water
   digestive tract
   gastric
   intestinal
ContiCath catheter
contiguous images (in CT scan)
contiguous slices
continuity, gastrointestinal
continuity of bone
continuous arterial spin-labeling perfusion MR imaging
continuous descending pressure (CDP)
continuous wave (CW) high intensity
   ultrasound energy (HIUE)
continuous imaging (CI), Aspire
continuously rolling platform table
continuous wave (CW)
continuous wave Doppler
   echocardiography

continuous wave Doppler ultrasonography
continuous wave laser system
continuous wave high frequency
   Doppler ultrasound system
Continuum MR-compatible infusion
   system
contour
   irregular hazy luminal
   isodose
   S
   scalloping
   undulating
contoured tilting compression
   mammography
contour extraction
contour following algorithm
contour mapping
contracted bladder
contracted gallbladder
contracted pelvis
contractile function
contraction
   cicatricial
   concentric
   left atrial
   peristaltic
   tertiary
contraction stress test (CST)
contracture
   Dupuytren
   elbow
   fixed flexion
   flexion-adduction
   gastroc/soleus (gastrocnemius/
     soleus)
   hip flexion
   ischemic
   joint
   knee flexion
   muscle
   myocardial
   myostatic

contracture *(cont.)*
  scar
  secondary
  soft tissue
  Volkmann ischemic
  web
contralateral
contralateral breast
contralateral subtraction technique
contralesional
contrast
  area of enhanced
  bladder
  extravasated
  extravasation of
  intravascular
  iodinated
  nondiluted
  short scale
contrast agent-induced nephropathy
contrast ascending up the vertebral
  column
contrast-associated nephropathy (CAN)
contrast echocardiography
contrast-enhanced coded phase-
  inversion harmonic ultrasound
contrast-enhanced color Doppler
contrast-enhanced CT scan
contrast-enhanced dynamic snapshot
contrast-enhanced hepatic CT
contrast-enhanced in vivo proton MR
  spectroscopy
contrast-enhanced MR
contrast-enhanced power Doppler
contrast-enhanced radiographic
  examination
contrast-enhanced scan
contrast-enhanced thoracic CT
contrast-enhanced ultrasound
contrast enhancement, blood oxygenation level dependent (BOLD)
contrast enhancement of computed
  tomographic (CECT)

contrast epididymogram
contrast esophagography
contrast extravasation
contrast-filled stomach
contrast-limited adaptive histogram
  equalization
contrast material-enhanced MRI scan
contrast medium (pl. media) (see
  imaging agent)
contrast reaction
contrast reaction with anaphylaxis
contrast resolution
contrast selective cholangiogram
contrast to noise (C/N) ratio (CNR)
contrast vasogram
contrast venography
contrast ventriculography
contrecoup fracture
control
  fluoroscopic
  image
  radiographic
  roentgenographic
controlled bladder filling
controlled lung volume
contusion pneumonia
conus arteriosus
conus artery
conus branch ostia
conus, club-shaped
conus ligament
conus medullaris
conus septum
conventional colonoscopy (CC)
conventionally fractionated stereotactic
  radiation therapy
conventional spin echo MR imaging
  vs. breath-hold fast spin echo or
  multishot spin echo echo-planar
  imaging
conventional study
convergence zone
convergent beam irradiation

converging collimator
convergent color Doppler imaging
conversion
  color space
  spontaneous
converter
  analog to digital (A to D)
  digital to analog (D to A)
  motion-compensating format
  real-time format
  reusable flange
convex linear array
convexity
convexobasia
convolution
  Arnold
  ascending frontal
  ascending parietal
  Broca
  cerebral
  Gratiolet
  Heschl
  occipitotemporal
  Zuckerkandl
convolution mask
Cook arterial catheter
Cook-Cope loop suprapubic catheter
Cook cystotomy catheter
Cook hysteroscopic catheter
Cook silicone balloon HSG catheter
Cook tissue morcellator catheter
Cooley-Tukey fast Fourier transform
  alignment algorithm
Cooper hernia
Coopernail sign
coordinate axis (pl. axes)
coordinate, Cartesian
coordinates (X, Y, and Z) for target
  lesion
COPD (chronic obstructive pulmonary
  disease)
Cope point
coplanar contour points

copper (Cu) (an element)
  ^{64}Cu
  ^{62}Cu PTSM imaging agent
  ^{62}Cu pyruvaldehyde-bis-(4N-thio-
    semicarbazone) imaging agent
  Cu/Zn (copper-zinc)-SOD
copper filtration
co-precipitation
coprolith
coprostasis
coracoacromial arch
coracoacromial ligament
coracoacromial process
coracohumeral ligament
coracoid notch
coracoid process
coracoid tuberosity
cor (heart)
cor adiposum
cor arteriosum
cor biloculare
cor bovinum
cord
  condyle
  fibrous
  hepatic
  Lissauer tracts of spinal
  medullary
  pretendinous
  rostral spinal
  sacral spinal
  spermatic
  spinal
  tethered
  triangular
  vocal
  Weitbrecht
cordate pelvis
cord compression
cord embarrassment
cor dextrum
cord hematoma
Cordis Brite Tip guiding catheter

Cordis Ducor brachial I, II, and III
coronary catheter
Cordis-Ducor-Judkins catheter
Cordis multipurpose access port
(MPAP)
Cordis Son-II catheter
Cordis tantalum stent
cordlike filling defect
cordlike mass
Cordonnier ureteroileal loop
cord prolapse
corduroy arteries
corduroy artifact
corduroy cloth pattern on myelogram
bore biopsy
core biopsy needle
core, bone
Core cannula system
coregistration, morphological and
physiological image
coregistration of CT
cor mobile
cor pendulum
cor pulmonale (c. pulmonale)
cork handler's lung disease
corkscrew appearance
corkscrew esophagus
Cornelia de Lange syndrome
Cornell protocol (exercise stress
testing)
corner fracture
cornflake esophageal motility study
corn oil and ferric ammonium citrate
contrast imaging agent
cornu (pl. cornua)
cornual ectopic pregnancy locations
cornual obstruction
coronal computed tomographic
arthrography (CCTA)
coronal CT reformation
coronal CT scan of sinuses
coronal image, multiecho

coronal maximum-intensity projection
(MIPcor)
coronal oblique plane
coronal orientation
coronal plane
coronal projection
coronal reoriented slices, segmentation
in
coronal section
coronal slab
coronal slice
coronal SPIR image
coronal suture
coronal synostosis
coronal T1-weighted MR image (spin
echo)
coronal view
coronary angiography
left (LCA)
right (RCA)
coronary artery (see *artery*)
coronary artery disease (CAD)
coronary artery ostia
coronary artery scan (CAS) by
Ultrafast CT
coronary artery scoring
coronary artery steal syndrome
coronary artery tree
coronary atherosclerosis
coronary balloon angioplasty
coronary branch ostial lesion
coronary bypass graft patency
coronary calcification
coronary-cameral fistula
coronary cineangiography
coronary cusp
coronary fistula
coronary flow reserve (CFR)
coronary groove
coronary heart disease (CHD)
coronary microvascular functional
reserve

coronary (artery) perfusion pressure
(CPP)
coronary reserve
coronary sinus (CS)
coronary sinus of Valsalva
coronary spasm
coronary steal phenomenon
coronary steal syndrome
coronary-subclavian steal syndrome
coronary sulcus
coronoid fossa
coronoid process
Coroskop C cardiac imaging
system
corpora cavernosography
corpora fornicis
corpora restiformia
corpus callosum, splenium of
corpus cavernosum abscess
corpus cavernosum fibrosis
corpus cavernosum hematoma
corpus cavernosum hypertrophy
corpus luteum hemorrhage
corpus Luysii
corpus sterni
corpus striatum
corpus uteri
corrected for distortion
correction
    accidental
    attenuation
    automatic motion
    coincidence-summing
    fuzzy logic contrast
    inhomogeneity
    multi-illuminant color
    Picker SPECT attenuation
    summing
    surface variable attenuation
    trend
correction filter
correlation
    clinical
    explant pathologic

correlation *(cont.)*
    functional
    histologic
    histopathologic-CT
    imaging-anatomic
    imaging-pathologic
    in vivo
    mammographic histopathologic
    morphological
    radiologic-anatomic
    radiologic-pathologic
correlation analysis
correlation algorithm (CR)
Correra line
Corrigan pneumonia
Corrigan sign
corrugated air column
corset balloon catheter
corset, Rissser plaster
cortex (pl. cortices)
    adrenal
    articular
    auditory
    bilateral orbital frontal
    bone
    calcarine
    cerebellar
    cerebral
    entorhinal
    femoral
    frontal
    lymphatic
    mesial-frontal
    motor
    nonolfactory
    opercular
    orbitofrontal
    ovarian
    parastriate
    parietal
    perirolandic parietal
    peristriate
    perisylvian
    premotor

cortex *(cont.)*
   primary auditory
   primary visual
   pyriform
   renal
   rolandic
   sensorimotor
   somatosensory
   striate
   visual
cortical activity
cortical adenoma
cortical atrophy
cortical bone
cortical branch
cortical carcinoma
cortical defect
cortical deficit
cortical dysfunction
cortical fetal maturation
cortical gray matter
cortical hinge axis
cortical hyperintensity
cortical hyperostosis
cortical infarcts
cortical intracerebral hemorrhage
cortical ischemia
cortical motor area
cortical necrosis
cortical ring sign
cortical scintigraphy
cortical sign
cortical signet ring shadow
cortical spoking
cortical sulci
cortical thumb
cortical tuber
cortical versus cancellous bone
cortical white matter
corticated border
corticocallosal dysgenesis
corticocancellous strut
corticocerebellar connection

corticogram
corticography
corticomedullary junction (CMJ)
corticomedullary junction (CMJ)
   phase imaging on CT scan
corticomedullary phase (CP)
corticospinal motor pathway
corticospinal tract
Corti organ
corundum smelter's lung
Corvisart syndrome
cosine transform
costa fluctuans decima
costae spuriae
costae verae
costal angle
costal bone
costal cartilage
costal groove
costal interarticular cartilage
costal margin
costal margin syndrome
costal notch
costal pleura
costal pleural reflection
costal process
costal sulcus
costal surface
costal tubercle
costocervical artery
costocervical trunk
costochondral joint
costochondral junction
costochondritis
costoclavicular syndrome
costoclavicular test
costodiaphragmatic recess
costolateral
costomediastinal recess
costophrenic (CP) angle blunting
costophrenic recess
costophrenic septal lines
costophrenic sulcus

costosternal angle
costosternal malformation
costotransverse joint
costovertebral angle (CVA)
costovertebral articulation
costovertebral joint
costoxiphoid ligament
COSY H-1 MR spectroscopy
cottage loaf appearance
cottage loaf deformity
cottage loaf sign
Cotton ankle fracture
Cotton-Berg syndrome
cotyloid cavity
cotyloid notch
couch view
cough fracture of rib
coulomb (C)
Councill catheter
count
   Cerenkov
   direct liquid scintillation
counter
   Geiger
   proportional
counter-current aortography
counter-occluder
counterpulsation
counterstaining technique in intraoperative ultrasonography of liver
counting, double label
coup
Cournand cardiac catheter
course
   postinfarction
   serpiginous
course of anatomical structure
coursing of gas
Courvoisier gallbladder
Courvoisier sign of malignancy
covered Gianturco stent
covered retrievable, expandable nitinol
   stent

Cowden disease
cowl-shaped obstruction
Cowper duct
Cowper gland abscess
Cowper ligament
coxa adducta
coxa brevis
coxa flexa
coxa magna
coxa plana
coxa saltans
coxa senilis
coxa valga
coxa vara luxans
Coyle trauma method (to view radial
   head and/or coronoid process)
CP (costophrenic) angle
CPA (cerebellopontile or cerebellopontine angle)
CPAD (chronic peripheral arterial
   disease)
CPB (cardiopulmonary bypass)
CPD (cephalopelvic disproportion)
CPI (conventional planar imaging)
CPMG sequence
c. pulmonale (cor pulmonale)
Cr (chromium) (an element)
CR (colorectal)
CR (computed radiology)
CR Bard catheter
CR-39 nuclear tract detector
crablike lesion on mammogram
crabmeat-like appearance
craniad
cranial and caudal angulations
cranial angled view
cranial nerves (12)
   I (olfactory)
   II (optic)
   III (oculomotor)
   IV (trochlear)
   V (trigeminal)
   VI (abducens)

cranial *(cont.)*
   VII (facial)
   VIII (vestibulocochlear)
   IX (glossopharyngeal)
   X (vagus)
   XI (spinal accessory)
   XII (hypoglossal)
cranial nerve involvement
cranial suture
cranial vessel
cranial view
craniocaudad projection
craniocaudal displacement
craniocaudal view
craniocervical junction
craniodorsal head view (for hip)
craniofacial duplication
craniofacial dysjunction fracture
craniomandibular syndrome
cranio-orbital deformity
craniopharyngioma, adamantinomatous
craniopharyngioma tumor
craniosclerosis
craniospinal axis
craniospinal hemangioblastoma
craniosynostosis
cranioventral head view (for hip)
craniovertebral junction
cranium
cranium bifidum occultum
crater, ulcer
crazy-paving appearance
crazy-paving pattern of the lungs
crazy-paving sign
creation and reformation
creep, periosteal
cremasteric artery
crenulation
crescent artifact
crescent, caliceal
crescentic lumen
crescent-in-doughnut sign (for
   intussusception)

crescent-shaped fibrocartilaginous disk
crescent sign on x-ray
crest
   acoustic
   acousticofacial
   alveolar
   ampullary
   arched
   arcuate
   articular
   basilar
   buccinator
   conchal
   deltoid
   dental
   ethmoidal
   falciform
   frontal
   ganglionic
   gingival
   gyral
   iliac
   infundibuloventricular
   pubic
   sacral
   supraventricular
   terminal (of right atrium)
   tibial
   urethral
Creutzfeldt-Jakob disease (CJD)
cribriform bone
cribriform plate
cribriform process
cricoarytenoid
cricoid cartilage
cricopharyngeal diverticulum
cricopharyngeal sphincter
cricopharyngeus muscle
cricothyroid cartilage
cricothyroid membrane
crinkle artifact
crinkling, mucosal
crisscross heart

criteria (pl. of criterion)
AAST (American Association for
the Surgery of Trauma)
American Association for the
Surgery of Trauma (AAST)
NINDS-AIREN
error sum
CRL (crown-rump length)
Crohn disease (CD)
Crohn ileocolitis
Crohn regional enteritis
Cronkhite-Canada syndrome
cross-aortic
crossbridge cycle (cycling)
cross-collateralization
cross-correlation technique
crossed cerebellar diaschisis
crossed-coil design
crossed ectopic kidney
crossed embolism
crossed-fused renal ectopia
crossed renal ectopia
crossed sciatica sign
crossed signs
crossed testicular ectopia
cross-filling
cross-fused ectopic kidney
crossing vasculature
crossing vessels
cross ligament
cross-linked polystyrene (PET scan)
crossover of activity
cross-pelvic collateral vessel
cross-section, Compton scattering
cross-sectional image
cross-sectional imaging technique
cross-sectional slice images of the
    breast
cross-sectional zone
cross-table lateral film
cross-talk effect artifact
cross-trigonal tunnel
cross-union

Crouzon disease
crowded carpal sign
crowding of bronchovascular markings
Crowe pilot point
crown artifact
crown, halo
crown-rump length (CRL)
CRS (Concentric retriever system)
CRT (cathode ray tube)
cruciate ligament
crucipage twins
crura of diaphragm (left and right)
crus (leg) (pl. crura)
    diaphragmatic
    lateral
    left
    medial
    right
crushing of ureter
crushing-type injury
Cruveilhier ulcer
crux cordis (crux of heart)
cry, cerebral
cryoablation
    Endocare renal
    endometrial
    transperineal prostatic
cryoablation for prostate cancer
cryoablation reduction of menstruation
    (CARMEN) procedure
CRYOCare cryosurgical system
CRYOCare endometrial cryoablation
    system
CRYOCare laser treatment for prostate
    carcinoma
cryocauterization
cryoconization of cervix
cryogel, polyvinyl alcohol (PVA)
CRYOguide ultrasound system
cryolesion
cryomagnet
cryoreductive surgery
cryosurgical lesion

cryosurgery, map-guided
crypt
  anal
  enamel
  epithelium
  ileal
  Lieberkühn (Lieberkuehn)
  Luschka
  Morgagni
cryptococcoma
cryptogenic organizing bacterial
  pneumonia
cryptogenic organizing pneumonia
CrystalEyes shutter glasses
crystallography
Cs (cesium) (an element)
CS (coronary sinus)
CSA (cross-sectional area)
CSDH (chronic subdural hematoma)
CSF (cerebrospinal fluid)
CSF-suppressed T2-weighted 3D
  MP-RAGE MR imaging
CSI (coronary stenosis index)
  CSI-enhanced MRI
  CSI spectroscopy
C sign
C-60 teletherapy
CSL (central sacral line)
Cs131 (Cesium-131) Seed isotope
C-spine (cervical spine)
CSS (carotid sinus syndrome)
CST (contraction stress test)
CST (corticospinal tract)
CT (cardiothoracic) ratio
CT (computed tomography)
  biphasic
  cine
  collimation
  contrast-enhanced
  coregistration of
  dental
  dual energy
  dual isotope single photon

CT *(cont.)*
  electron beam
  enhanced
  expiratory
  gated cardiac
  helical
  helical thin section
  high resolution
  high spatial resolution cine
    (HSRCCT)
  high temporal resolution cine
    (HTRCCT)
  indirect
  lipiodol
  multidetector (MDCT)
  multidetector row spiral
  multiphasic
  nonenhanced
  peripheral quantitative (pQCT)
  quantitative spirometrically
    controlled CT angiography with
    volume rendering
  renal helical CT (RHCT)
  single photon emission (SPECT)
  single energy spectrum quantitative
  16-detector row
  sliding-thin-slab maximum intensity
    projection
  slip-ring
  SPECT (single photon emission)
  spiral
  superselective angio-
  thallium-201 single photon emission
  thermoacoustic
  thin collimation multidetector row
    spiral
  thin section
  thin section excretory phase
  thin slice
  thoracic
  three-dimensional processed
    ultrafast
  three-phase helical

CT *(cont.)*
 transmissionx
 triphasic spiral
 triple phase helical
 two phase
 two phase helical
 ultrafast
 ultrafast CT electron beam
  tomography
 unenhanced helical
 water-contrast
 Z-dependent
CTA (computed tomographic
 angiography)
CTA dosimetry
CT angiogram sign
CT angiographic portography (CTAP)
CTAP (computed tomography during
 arterial portography)
CTAP (CT angiographic portography)
CTAP-1 (first scan CT arterial
 portography)
CT arrowhead sign
CT arterial portography (CTAP)
CT arteriography
CT arthrography
CTAT (computerized transverse axial
 tomography)
CT attenuation value
CTA-2 (second scan CT arterial
 portography)
CT bone window photography
CTC (computed tomographic colonog-
 raphy)
CT cisternogram, metrizamide
 (MCTC)
CT colonography
CT colonography with teleradiology
CT densitometry
CT-directed hookwire localization
CT enteroclysis
CT fluoroscopy
 half scan cone-beam
 real-time

CT gantry
CT-guided aspiration
CT-guided brachytherapy
CT-guided coaxial fine-needle aspira-
 tion biopsy
CT-guided intra-arterial chemotherapy
CT-guided needle biopsy
CT-guided percutaneous biopsy
CT-guided PEG (percutaneous endo-
 scopic gastrostomy)
CT-guided stereotactic surgery
CT-guided transthoracic percutaneous
 ethanol injection
CT-guided transsternal core biopsy
CT-guided Tru-Cut liver biopsy
CT-guided ultrasound
CTHA (computerized tomographic
 hepatic angiography)
CT holography (CTH)
CT imaging error
CT laser mammography (CTLM)
CT-LINAC or CT-Linac (computed
 tomography with linear accelerator)
 imaging
CTLM (computed tomography laser
 mammography)
CT Max 640 scanner
CT myelography
CT9000 scanner
CT9800 scanner
CT PE (computed tomography
 pulmonary embolus) protocol
CT PEG (CT-guided percutaneous
 endoscopic gastrostomy)
CT peritoneography
CT pulmonary angiography
CT reconstruction image
C-TRAK hand-held gamma detector
CT scan directed needle biopsy
CT scan, field-guided
CT scanned projection radiography
CT scan with contrast
CT scanner (see *scanner*)

CT sialography
CT/SPECT fusion
CT SPR (computed tomographic
scanned projection radiography)
CT stereotaxic guide
CT urography
CT with MR, single photon emission
CTDI (computed tomography dose
index)
CTH (computerized tomographic
holography)
CTHA (computerized tomographic
hepatic angiography)
CTI 933/04 ECAT scanner
CTI PET scanner
CTLM (computerized tomographic
laser mammography)
CTLV (cross-table lateral view)
CT/MRI-compatible stereotactic
headframe
CT/MRI-defined tumor slice image
CT/MRI-defined tumor volume image
CTR (cardiothoracic ratio)
CTS (carpal tunnel syndrome)
CTT (central tegmental tract)
Cu (copper) (an element)
CUBA (Clinical Ultrasonic Bone
Sonometry)
cube vertices
cubic centimeter (cc)
cubic convolution interpolation
cubic packing
cubic voxels
cubital fossa
cubital tunnel syndrome
cubitocarpal
cubitoradial
cubitus valgus
cubitus varus
cuboid bone
cubonavicular joint
cue
  biopsy
  exclusionary

cue (cont.)
  inclusionary
  preclusionary
cue-based image analysis
cuff
  aortic
  atrial
  inflow
  musculotendinous
  rectal muscle
  right atrial
  rotator
  suprahepatic caval
cuff abscess
cuffing, peribronchial
cuff rupture
cul-de-sac
  Douglas
  dural
cul-de-sac hernia
Cullen sign
culprit lesion
culprit vessel
cumulative effect
cuneiform bone of carpus
cuneiform fracture-dislocation
cuneiform joint
cuneiform mortise
cuneus
cup
  acetabular
  hip replacement
  migration of acetabular
  prosthesis
  retroversion of acetabular
cup-and-spill stomach
CUP (cancer of unknown primary)
cup-shaped acetabulum
cupula
  diaphragmatic
  pleural
Curix Capacity Plus film processing
  system

curled-up position
curlicue ureter
Curling ulcer
Curracino-Silverman syndrome
Currarino triad
current
　gradient drive
　pulsing
　tube
curvature (see also *curve*)
　angular
　anterior
　backward
　cervical
　dorsal kyphotic
　flattening of normal lordotic
　gingival
　greater
　humpbacked spinal
　kyphotic
　lesser
　lumbar
　normal cervical
　radius of
　stomach
curvature anisotropy
curvature of stomach
　greater
　lesser
curve (pl. curves)
　biphasic
　Bragg
　brightness-time
　central-axis depth-dose
　cervical spine
　clearance
　depth-dose
　dilution
　dye dilution
　flattening of normal
　flow time
　free induction delay
　gaussian

curve *(cont.)*
　glow
　isoclosed
　lumbar lordotic
　lung count
　nonstructural
　normal lordotic
　pulmonary time activity
　renal flow
　renogram
　sigmoid
　signal intensity time
　spline
　superincumbent spinal
　thoracic spine
　time-attenuation
　time-density
　time-intensity
　videodensity
　washout
curved-array transducer
curved planar reformations
curved-slab maximum intensity
　projections (MIPs)
curved vessels
curve fit coefficient
curvilinear calcification
curvilinear defect
curvilinear subpleural lines
Cushing syndrome
Cushing ulcer
cushion defect
cushion, endocardial
cushion sign
Cu (copper)
cusp
　accessory
　anterior
　aortic
　asymmetric closure of
　conjoined
　coronary
　dysplastic

cusp *(cont.)*
  fibrocalcific
  fishmouth
  fusion of
  intact valve
  left coronary
  left pulmonary
  mitral valve
  noncoronary
  perforated aortic
  posterior
  pulmonary valve
  right coronary
  ruptured aortic
  semilunar valve
  septal
  tricuspid valve
  valve
cusp degenerator
cusp motion
cusp shots (films)
custom block
custom shielding blocks
cut (pl. cuts)
  off-center
  tangential
  tomographic
cut and cine film
cutaneous hemorrhage
cutaneous myiasis of the breast
cutaneous tumor
cut-film technique
cutis laxa
cutting balloon percutaneous transluminal angioplasty
Cuvier, canal of
CVA (cerebrovascular accident)
CVA (costovertebral angle)
CVBS (congenital vascular–bone
  syndrome)
C-VEST ambulatory radionuclide
  monitoring system
CVIS imaging device

CVM (congenital vascular malformation)
CVM (cryptic vascular malformation)
CVP (central venous pressure)
  catheter
CV Peri-Guard patch
CW HIUE (continuous wave high
  intensity ultrasound energy)
CX or CF (circumflex) artery
CX-1 metastases
CXR (chest x-ray), baseline
C wave pressure on right atrial
  catheterization
CyberKnife radiosurgery
cyberradiology
Cyberware system
cycle
  aberrant
  cardiac
  forced
  gastric
cycling, phase
cyclohexane scintillator
cyclops lesion
cyclosporin A-induced fibroadenoma
  of the breast
cyclotron (see also *scanner*)
  medical
  multiparticle
C-Y color space
cylinder, CO_2
cylindrical projection map
cylindroma
cyllosis
Cyriax syndrome
cyst
  acoustic
  adenocarcinoma
  adenomyotic
  Bartholin
  Blessig
  bone
  branchial

cyst *(cont.)*
  branchial cleft
  bronchogenic
  calcification of
  cerebral
  corpus luteum
  cortical
  dentigerous
  dermoid
  endometrial
  epidermal
  epidermal inclusion
  epidermoid
  epithelial
  fluid-filled
  follicular
  functional ovarian
  ganglion
  hemorrhagic
  hydatid
  inclusion
  joint
  lumbar facet joint synovial
  mammary
  meibomian
  mesenteric
  mesothelial
  morgagnian
  mucinous
  mucous
  müllerian
  multilocular
  multiloculated
  myxoid
  nabothian
  neoplastic
  non-neoplastic
  ovarian
  ovarian follicular
  pancreatic
  paratubal
  parovarian
  pericardial

cyst *(cont.)*
  pineal
  pituitary
  primordial
  prostatic
  renal
  retention
  serous
  solitary bone
  tailgut
  tarsal
  testicular
  thin-walled
  thyroglossal duct
  umbilical
  unilocular
  wolffian
cystadenoma
  mucinous
  unilocular macrocystic serous
cystic angiomatosis
cystic artery
cystic change
cystic duct angiogram
cystic duct cholangiogram
cystic duct remnant
cystic duct stump
cystic echinococcosis
cystic emphysema
cystic fibrosis
cystic hydroma
cystic hygroma
cystic lysis
cystic mazoplasia
cystic medionecrosis
cystic neoplasm
cystic nephroma
cystic osteofibromatosis
cystic pulmonary emphysema
cystic renal lesion
cystic sac
cystic teratoma
cystic tumor

cystic wall
cystitis
  eosinophilic
  hemorrhagic
cysto-atrial shunt
cystocele, protrusion of
cystocolpoproctography fluoroscopic
  imaging
Cysto-Conray (now Conray-43)
  (iothalamate meglumine injection
  43%)
Cysto-Conray II (iothalamate meglumine injection 17.2%) imaging
  agent
Cystografin (diatrizoate meglumine)
  imaging agent
cystogram
cystography
  AP 10-15° caudad
  delayed
  double voiding
  excretory
  postdrainage
  postvoiding
  radionuclide (RNC)

cystography *(cont.)*
  retrograde
  RPO 30° voiding
  stress
  triple voiding
  voiding
cystometry, magnetic resonance
cystoproctogram, dynamic
cystoscopic urography
cystoscopy, virtual
cystosonography, echo-enhanced
cystotomy
cystotomy catheter
cystourethrogram, voiding (VCUG)
cystourethroscopy
cytoarchitectonic abnormality
cytoarchitectonic field, Brodmann
cytokine cascades
cytomegalic inclusion disease
cytomegalovirus pneumonitis
Cytomel suppression test
cytometry
  flow
  multicolor flow

D, d

D (diaphragmatic)
dacryocystography
Dacron catheter
Dacron-covered stent-graft
Dacron onlay patch graft
Dacron Sauvage patch
Dacron stent
dacryocystography
dacryocystoplasty, fluoroscopically
    guided
DAF (dynamic axial fixator)
DAVF (dural AV fistula, spinal)
dagger sign
Dagradi classification of esophageal
    varices
DAH (diffuse alveolar hemorrrhage)
DAI (diffuse axonal injury)
Dale Foley catheter
DALM (dysplasia with associated
    lesion or mass)
damage
    cavitation
    iatrogenic
D'Amato sign in pleural effusion
dammed-up CSF (cerebrospinal fluid)
dampened obstructive pulse
dampened pulsatile flow

dampened waveform
damping of catheter tip pressure
dancer's fracture
Dance sign
Dandy-Walker cyst
Dandy-Walker deformity
Dandy-Walker syndrome
Danelius-Miller method (for viewing
    hip and pelvis)
Danelius-Miller modification of
    Lorenz method (for viewing hip
    and pelvis)
Dane particle
Danis-Weber classification of ankle
    fractures
D'Antonio classification of acetabular
    abnormalities
DANTE sequence
DANTE-selective pulses
Dardik Biograft
dark pixel values
dark region
darkroom error
Darrach-Hughston-Milch fracture
DASA (distal articular set angle)
Daseler-Anson classification of
    plantaris muscle anatomy

169

data
  radiology outcomes
  volumetric image
data acquisition time
data-clipping detection error artifact
data log, ICD
data sets
data spike detection error artifact
Datascope DL-II percutaneous
  translucent balloon catheter
Datascope System 90 balloon pump
daughter abscess
daughter product
David-Chausse classification (I-IV)
Davies-Colley syndrome
Davies endomyocardial fibrosis
Dawbarn sign
DBM (demineralized bone matrix)
DBP (diastolic blood pressure)
DBS (directional bremsstrahlung
  splitting)
DC (direct current) offset artifact
DC (dynamic compression) plate
DCA (directional color angiography)
DCA (directional coronary angioplasty)
DCA (directional coronary atherec-
  tomy)
DCBE (double contrast barium
  enema)
DCIS (ductal carcinoma in situ)
DCP (dynamic compression plate)
DCS (distal coronary sinus)
dD/dt (derived value on apex
  cardiogram)
DDD (double dose delay)
DDH (developmental dysplasia of hip)
DDT (fluorescein dye disappearance
  test)
dead space, anatomical
dead time
death
  brain
  cerebral

debilitation
debris
  aspiration of
  atheromatous
  atherosclerotic
  bone
  calcium
  cholesterol
  extra-articular
  foreign
  gelatinous
  grumous
  intimal
  intra-articular
  joint
  necrotic
  particle
  particulate
  thallium
De Broglie wavelength
Debye-Scherrer photographic
  technique
decalcification
decalcified dorsum sellae
decannulated
decannulation
decapolar catheter
decapsulation of kidney
decay
  alpha
  beta
  exponential
  free induction
decay rate
decay series
decay time
deceleration time
decelerative injury
dechondrification
decidua
decidual cyst
decidual reaction
decidual sac

deciduous
decimalized variance map
declamping
decoding
 document image (DID)
 Viterbi
decompensated congestive heart
 failure
decompensation
 cardiac
 chronic respiratory
 end stage adult cardiac
 end stage fetal cardiac
 hemodynamic
 respiratory
 ventricular
decompress
decompression
 balloon
 canal
 cardiac
 endoscopic
 gastric
 hydrostatic
 intestinal
 laser-assisted disk (LDD)
 long tube
 microvascular (MVD)
 percutaneous transhepatic (PTD)
 peripheral nerve
 portal
 surgical
 transduodenal endoscopic
 tube
 variceal
decompression tube
deconditioning
deconvolutional analysis
deconvolution, statistical
decortication
 cardiac
 chemical

decortication *(cont.)*
 heart
 lung
decoupling
decreased attenuation
decreased uptake
decreased uptake with patchy distribution
decryption algorithms
DecThreads software
decubitus film
decubitus position
 dorsal
 lateral
 ventral
decubitus ulcer
decubitus view
decussation
dedicated phased-array coil
deep arch
deep artery
deep cardiac plexus
deep diverticulum
deep Doppler velocity interrogation
deep hyperthermia treatment
deep inspiration CT angiography
deep interloop abscess
deep lateral femoral notch sign
deep lesion
deep pelvic abscess
deep respirations
deep-seated lesion
deep-seated tumor
deep-shelled acetabulum
deep sulcus sign
deep veins
deep vein thrombosis
deep venous aplasia
deep venous channel
deep venous incompetence
deep venous insufficiency (DVI)
deep venous thrombosis (DVT)

deep white matter track
defecation
defecogram
defecographic study
defography
defect (see also *deformity*)
  acquired ventricular septal (AVSD)
  anastomotic
  anteroapical
  aortic septal
  aorticopulmonary
  ASD (atrioseptal defect)
  atrial ostium primum
  atrioseptal (or atrial septal) (ASD)
  atrioventricular canal
  atrioventricular septal
  bar
  bar-like ventral (in myelography)
  birth
  bony
  bridging of
  cardiofacial
  cauliflower-shaped
  chain of lakes filling
  chiasmatic
  chondral
  coagulation
  cold
  concentrating
  concomitant
  congenital
  conoventricular
  contiguous ventricular septal
  cordlike filling
  cortical
  craniotomy
  crista supraventricularis septal
  curvilinear
  cushion
  developmental
  discoid filling
  endocardial cushion
  extradural

defect *(cont.)*
  fibrous cortical
  field
  filling
  fixed
  fixed intracavitary filling
  fixed perfusion
  focal plaquelike
  frondlike filling
  frontal
  fusiform
  global cortical
  hernia
  hot
  inferoapical
  infracristal septal
  infracristal ventricular septal
  infundibular ventricular septal
  interatrial septal (septum)
  intercalary
  interventricular conduction
  interventricular septal (IVSD)
  intra-atrial conduction
  intra-atrial filling
  intraluminal
  intraluminal filling
  intraventricular conduction
  ischemic
  junctional
  juxta-arterial ventricular septal
  juxtatricuspid ventricular septal
  linear
  lobulated filling
  lucent
  luminal
  luteal phase
  mapping of
  matched V/Q (ventilation-perfusion)
  membranous ventricular septal
  muscular ventricular septal
  myocardial perfusion
  neural tube
  nonsubperiosteal cortical

defect *(cont.)*
nonuniform rotational (NURD)
open neural tube
optic nerve
osseous
osteochondral (of the glenoid fossa)
ostium primum
ostium secundum
partial AV (atrioventricular) canal
pear-shaped
perfusion
peri-infarction conduction (PICD)
perimembranous ventricular septal
PG-related
photopenic
plication
polypoid filling
posteroapical
postinfarction ventriculoseptal
postoperative skull
pouching
radial ray
radiolucent filling
Rastelli type A, B, or C
    atrioventricular canal
restrictive ventilatory
reversible
reversible ischemic
reversible perfusion
scan
scintigraphic perfusion
secundum atrial septal
segmental
segmental bone
septal
sinus venosus
soft tissue
spontaneous closure of
stellar
subcortical
subperiosteal cortical
supracristal septal

defect *(cont.)*
supracristal ventricular
supracristal ventriculoseptal
Swiss cheese ventricular septal
transient perfusion
trochlear
type I (supracristal) ventricular
    septal
type II (infracristal) ventricular
    septal
type III (canal type) ventricular
    septal
type IV (muscular) ventricular
    septal
V-Q, VQ (ventilation-perfusion)
valvular
ventilation
ventilation-perfusion (V-Q, VQ)
ventral hernia
ventricular septal or
    ventriculoseptal (VSD)
wedge-shaped
wire-related
defective communication between
    cardiac chambers
defects in blood-brain barrier
deferential artery
deferens, ductus
defervesce
defervesced
deficit
    focal
    lateralizing
    perfusion
    posterior column
    pulse
    residual
    reversible (or resolving) ischemic
        neurologic (RIND)
    significant residual deficit
    space
    subtle

deficiency
  Aitken femoral
  alpha-1-antitrypsin
  molybdenum cofactor
  pyruvate dehydrogenase complex
deficiency disease
Definity (perflutren) imaging agent
deflectable quadripolar catheter
deflectable-tip catheter
deformans
  osteitis
  osteochondrodystrophia
  Paget osteitis
deformity (also see *defect*)
  Akerlund
  angular
  aortic valve
  Arnold-Chiari
  back-knee
  bell clapper
  biconcave
  bifid thumb
  bone
  bony
  boutonnière (of finger)
  bowing
  bull's-eye
  buttonhole
  calcaneus
  caliceal
  cavovarus
  cavus
  chain of lakes
  Charcot
  checkrein
  clawfoot
  clawhand
  clawtoe
  cloverleaf
  clubhand
  cockscomb
  cock-up
  codfish

deformity *(cont.)*
  compensatory
  congenital
  contracture
  cottage loaf
  coxa vara
  cranio-orbital
  cubitus valgus
  cubitus varus
  curly toe
  Dandy-Walker
  digital
  digitus flexus
  dinner-fork
  DISI (dorsal intercalary segment
    instability)
  duodenal bulb
  equinovalgus
  equinovarus
  equinovarus hindfoot
  equinus
  Erlenmeyer flask-like
  eversion-external rotation
  femoral head
  flatfoot
  flexible spastic equinovarus
  flexion
  forefoot abduction
  funnel-like
  genu valgum
  genu varum
  gibbous
  gooseneck outflow tract
  gunstock
  Haglund
  hallux abductovalgus
  hallux flexus
  hallux malleus
  hallux rigidus
  hallux valgus
  hallux varus
  hammertoe
  hatchet-head

deformity *(cont.)*
Hill-Sachs
hindbrain
hindfoot
hockey-stick tricuspid valve
hourglass
Ilfeld-Holder
internal rotation
intrinsic minus
intrinsic plus
J-hook
J-sella
joint
keyhole
Kirner
lobster-claw
Madelung
mallet
mallet finger
mermaid
metatarsus adductocavus
metatarsus adductovarus
metatarsus adductus
metatarsus atavicus
metatarsus latus
metatarsus primus varus
metatarsus varus
Michel
mitral valve
nasal tip
neuropathic midfoot
pannus
parachute mitral valve
pectus excavatum
pencil-in-cup
perigastric
pes cavus
pes planus
phrygian cap
pigeon breast
planovalgus
plantar flexion-inversion
procurvature

deformity *(cont.)*
pseudo-Hurler
pulmonary valve
recurvatum
reduction
rockerbottom foot
rolled edge
rotational
round shoulder
sabre shin
scimitar
seal-fin
shepherd's crook
silver-fork
snowman
spastic equinovarus
spastic hindfoot valgus
splay foot
split foot
Sprengel
static foot
stepdown shoulder
supination
supratip nasal tip
swan-neck
swan-neck finger
talus foot
testicular
thumb-in-palm
torsional
trefoil
tricuspid valve
trigger finger
triphalangeal thumb
turned-up pulp
ulnar drift (motor)
uterine myoma
valgus
valgus heel
varus
Velpeau
vertical talus foot
VISI

deformity *(cont.)*
  Volkmann
  wasp-tail (in Duchenne dystrophy)
  wedging
  whistling
  Whitehead
  windblown
  windswept
defunctionalization
defuzzification algorithm
degassed tap water
degenerated leaflet
degeneration
  angiolithic
  anterior pillar
  articular cartilage
  atheromatous
  atrophic
  ballooning
  bone
  bony
  brain
  breast
  calcareous
  cardiac
  cardiac valve mucoid
  cardiomyopathic
  cartilaginous
  cerebellar
  cerebromacular (CMD)
  cobblestone
  collagen
  colloid
  cortical cerebellar
  corticobasal ganglionic
  corticostriatospinal
  cusp
  cystic
  Doyne familial colloid
  Doyne honeycomb
  dystrophic
  esophageal
  fatty

degeneration *(cont.)*
  fibrinoid
  fibrinous
  fibroid
  gray matter
  heart
  hepatic
  hepatocerebral
  hepatolenticular
  Holmes cerebellar
  Holmes cortical cerebellar
  honeycomb
  hyaline
  hydropic
  hypertensive vascular
  intimal
  lipoid
  lipoidal
  liquefaction
  malignant
  Menzel olivopontocerebellar
  mitral valve
  Mönckeberg
  mucoid
  mucous
  mural
  muscular
  myocardial
  myocardial cellular
  myocardial fibers
  myxomatous
  olivopontocerebellar
  pancreas
  pancreatic
  paraneoplastic cerebellar
  parenchymatous cerebellar
  paving stone
  primary progressive cerebellar
  progressive
  Regnauld-type great toe
  renal tubular
  retinal
  retrograde

degeneration *(cont.)*
  rim
  sclerotic
  secondary
  senile
  spinal
  spinocerebellar
  spongy
  spongy white matter
  subacute combined spinal cord
  testicular
  thyroid
  trabecular
  traumatic
  wear and tear
  Zenker
degenerative ataxia
degenerative atrioventricular node
  disease
degenerative change
degenerative disease
degenerative disk disease
degenerative joint disease (DJD)
degenerative spurring
DeGimard syndrome
deglutition
deglutition mechanism
deglutition paralysis
deglutition pneumonia
deglutition syncope
Degos disease
degradation, image quality
degree, noncircularity
degree of correction
degree of distortion
degrees of supination
Dehio test
dehiscence
  aortic homograft anastomotic
  bone
  bronchial
  perivalvular
  prosthesis

DEI (diffraction-enhanced imaging)
de la Camp sign
de Lange syndrome
Delarnette scanner
delay
  developmental
  regrowth
  temporal phase
  time (echo)
  trigger
delayed excretion of contrast media
delayed films
delayed images
delayed phase
delayed gastric emptying
delayed resolution of pneumonia
delayed transport of tracer
delayed traumatic intracerebral
  hematoma (DTICH)
delayed union
delayed visualization
delay time, echo
Delbet fracture classification
Delbet sign
deleterious effect
delicate crepitation
delineation
delineation of margins
delivery, timed bolus
Delmege sign of tuberculosis
DELTAmanager MedImage system
Delta 32 TACT three-dimensional
  breast imaging system
Deltec long term dual lumen hemodialysis catheter
deltoid branch of posterior tibial
  artery
deltoid ligament
deltopectoral groove
demagnetization field effect
demand (standby)
demarcate
demarcated

demarcation line
De Martini-Balestra syndrome
dementia
Demianoff sign
demifacets
demilune
demineralization, bone
demineralization from disuse
demineralized bone matrix (DBM)
demodulator
demographic data
Demons-Meigs syndrome
de Musset sign (aortic aneurysm)
de Mussey point or sign (pleurisy)
demyelinating disease
demyelination
    brain stem
    large fiber
    posterior column
    postinfectious
    segmentFal
demyelinative disorder
denatured technetium Tc 99m RBCs
dendritic lesion
Deneer method (to view acetabulum)
denervated area
denervation atrophy
Denis classification of spinal injury
    (A to E)
de novo
de novo lesion
dens (odontoid process of axis)
dense breasts, heterogeneously
dense metaphyseal band sign
dens fracture
dens view of cervical spine
densitometer
    Achilles+
    bone
    CT
    DEXA (dual energy x-ray
        absorptiometry)
    Discovery bone

densitometer *(cont.)*
    Discovery QDR
    DPX-IQ
    dual photon
    Expert-XL
    Hologic 2000
    Norland bone
    photon
    Prodigy bone
    single photon
densitometry
    accuDEXA bone
    DEXAscan bone
    dynamic spiral CT lung
    fan-beam
    Norland bone
    Prodigy bone
    QDR-1500 bone
    QDR-2000 bone
    Sahara
    three-dimensional CT
density (pl. densities)
    air
    area of increased
    asymmetric
    bands of
    bone mineral (BMD)
    calcific
    calcified
    capillary
    diffuse reticular
    discrete perihilar
    double
    echo
    fluid
    gas
    ground glass
    hazy
    homogeneous soft tissue
    hydrogen
    ill-defined
    increased
    linear

density *(cont.)*
  masslike
  metallic
  mottled
  nodular
  nuclear
  ovoid-shaped calcific
  patchy
  perihilar
  pleural
  proton
  pulmonary
  radiographic
  radiolucent
  radiopaque
  retroareolar
  retrocardiac
  ropy
  soft tissue
  spicular
  spin
  teardrop-shaped
  tissue
  trabecular bone equivalent (TBED)
  variations in
  water
  wedge-shaped
density matrix theory
dental CT
dental cyst
dental scan
dental vertical root fracture
DentaScan
dentate fracture
dentate ligament
dentate line
dentate nucleus
dentate suture of skull
dentato-olivary pathway
dentatorubral-pallidoluysian atrophy
dentinogenesis imperfecta
dentomaxillofacial complex
dentoskeletal relationship

denudation, areas of
denude
denuded
denuding
DeOrio intrauterine insemination
  catheter
deossification
dependent atelectasis
dependent extracellular fluid
  accumulation
dependent lung
dephasing
  intravoxel
  signal
dephasing gradient
depiction, magnetic resonance
depiction of vasculature
deployment, clip
deposit
  calcium
  metastatic
deposition
  calcium
  callus
  iron
  spontaneous
  submucosal fat
deposition rate
depreotide (technetium Tc 99m
  depreotide) imaging agent
depressed and compound fracture
depressed fracture
depressed skull fracture
depression
  fragment
  hemidiaphragm
  reciprocal
  sinus node
  spinal cord
  subtle
depth
  lesion
  photon interaction

depth-dose curves
depth-dose distribution
depth of invasion
depth of wall invasion
depth perception
de Quervain fracture
derangement, internal
derby hat fracture
Dercum disease
dermatofibrosarcoma protuberans
dermoid cyst
dermoid tumor
derotate
derotated
derotation
DeRoyal surgical cannula
Derrick intrauterine insemination
   catheter
DES (diffuse esophageal spasm)
Desault dislocation
Desault fracture
descending aorta
descending aorta–pulmonary artery
   shunt
descending colon
descending duodenum
Deseret angiocatheter
de Seze angle (see *angle of Lequesne*
   and *angle de Seze*)
desmalgia
desmectasis
desmocytoma
desmodynia
desmoid
desmoma
desmoplasia
desmoplastic
desmoplastic metastases
desmoplastic small round cell tumor
   of the abdomen
desmosis
desquamative interstitial pneumonia
   (DIP)

D'Espine sign
detachable balloon
destruction, bone (or bony)
destructive lesion
destructive process
destructive tumor
detachable coils
detail
   exquisite
   suboptimal
detecting, collision
detecting module
detection
   automated nodule
   magnetic resonance (MR)
   occult
   quadrature
   radioactivity
   radwaste radioactivity
detection and quantification
detection zone
detector
   adaptive array
   amorphous silicon flat-panel
   annular
   cadmium iodide
   cesium iodide-amorphous silicon
     flat-panel
   CR-39 nuclear tract
   diode
   Doppler blood flow
   GE (General Electric)
   glass track
   HPGe
   passive track
   selenium
   Si (Li)
   sodium detector
   solid state nuclear track
   Wang-Binford edge
detector array
detector collimation

deterioration
  progressive
  uniform
Determann syndrome
determination
  particle size
  void
detour conduit
detritus
Deutschländer disease
devascularization, paraesophagogastric
developer artifact
development
  conductive
  delayed
  insulative
  interval
  torpid
developmental delay
Deventer diameter
deviated septum
deviation
  angular
  aortic
  carpal
  fracture
  left axis (LAD)
  mediastinal
  radial
  right axis (RAD)
  rotary
  septal
  tracheal
  ulnar
device
  accuDEXA bone mineral density
    assessment
  ACMI ulcer measuring
  ACS anchor exchange
  Add-On Bucky imaging
  Aestiva/5 MRI anesthesia machine
  Angio-Seal hemostatic puncture
    closure

device *(cont.)*
  Apogee ultrasound
  Arrow PICC radiology
  artificial left ventricular assist
    (LVAD)
  ASD transcatheter occlusion with
    button
  aspiration-tulip
  atherectomy
  atrial septal defect occlusion
    buttoned
  beam-restricting
  biventricular assist (BVAD)
  BladderManager ultrasound
  Bovie ultrasound aspirator
  BRW (Brown-Roberts-Wells) CT
    stereotaxic guide
  Bucky imaging
  change-coupled (CCD)
  charge-coupled (CCD)
  CVIS imaging
  diffracting Doppler transducer
  Doppler Intra-Dop intraoperative
  dynamic multileaf collimator
    (DMLC)
  DynaWell medical compression
  Eclipse ST cyclotron used with
    PET scan imagers
  electronic portal imaging (EPID)
  Elscint Planar
  Escort balloon stone extractor
  FlashPoint image-guided surgical
    instruments
  Fujinon Sonoprobe
  GE 0.5 tesla double doughnut
    magnet MRI machine
  HeartMate LVAD (left ventricular
    assist device)
  hemostatic puncture closure
    (HPCD)
  IMED intravenous infusion
  intraoperative x-ray visualization
    of fixation

device *(cont.)*
  Innovante dilator
  Innovante retrieval
  left ventricular assist (LVAD)
  Leksell stereotaxic
  Mammotome handheld minimally
    invasive breast biopsy
  Mark II Kodros radiolucent awl
  MediPort implanted vascular access
  Micro-Imager high resolution
    digital camera
  Mini C-arm
  Miser tube
  MOS capacitor
  Navarre interventional radiology
  NB200 vascular access
  neck-bridge
  Olympus EU-M30S endoscopic
    ultrasonography receiver
  Optistat power contrast injector
  OsteoAnalyzer
  PercuGuide
  PerDUCER pericardial access
  PGK (Panos G. Koutrouvelis,
    M.D.) stereotactic
  Probe cardiac
  Rashkind double umbrella
  right ventricular assist (RVAD)
  SAVANT (Surgical Anatomy
    Visualization and Navigation
    Tools)
  Sceratti goniometer
  sequential compression
  Signa SP/i 0.5T MR imaging unit
  Simpson atherectomy
  stereotactic add-on
  SurgiScope
  suture-ligated embolization
    microcoils
  synchronization
  Telos radiographic stress
  unbuttoning of

device *(cont.)*
  ventricular assist (VAD)
  Versalab ultrasonic medical
  device-independent (DVI)
  DeVilbiss ultrasound nebulizer
  devitalized tissue
  devoid of circulation
  Dewan intrauterine insemination
    catheter
  DEXA (dual energy x-ray absorptiom-
    etry)
  DEXA densitometer
  DEXA scan
  DEXA scan for bone density determi-
    nation
  Dexter-Grossman classification of
    mitral regurgitation
  dextrocardia
  dextrocardiac
  dextrogastria
  dextrogastric
  dextroposed
  dextroposition
  dextrorotatory
  dextrorotoscoliosis
  dextroscoliosis
  dextrotransposition (D-transposition) of
    great vessels
  dextrotropic
  dextroversion of heart
  DFA (hallux dorsiflexion angle)
  DFP (diastolic filling pressure)
  DGR (duodenogastric reflux)
  diabetic gastroparesis
  diabetic mastopathy
  diacondylar fracture
  diadochokinesia
  diadochokinesis
  diagnosis
    clinical
    differential
    empirical

diagnosis *(cont.)*
  noninvasive
  pathologic
  postoperative
  preoperative
  presumptive
  radiologic
  remote
  roentgenographic
  sonographic
  tentative
  ultrasound
  working
diagnostic efficacy analysis
diagnostic procedure
diagnostic radiology
diagnostic radiopharmaceutical
diagnostic range ultrasound
diagonal branch of artery
diagonal conjugate diameter
dialysis kidney
diamagnetic shift
diamagnetic susceptibility
diametaphyseal
diametaphysis
diameter (or dimension)
  anteroposterior (AP)
  aortic (AD)
  aortic root
  artery
  Baudelocque
  bi ischial
  biparietal (BPD)
  bronchial
  cardiac
  coccygeopubic
  coil to vessel
  conjugate
  Deventer
  diagonal conjugate
  gestational sac (GS)
  increased AP (anteroposterior)
  intercristal

diameter *(cont.)*
  internal conjugate
  intertuberal
  left anterior internal (LAID)
  left atrial
  left ventricular internal (LVID)
  Lohlein
  luminal
  maximum AP (anteroposterior)
  midsagittal (MSD)
  minimal luminal
  narrow anteroposterior
  orthonormal
  pelvic
  pulmonary vein
  right ventricular internal (RVID)
  sacropubic
  spinal cord
  stenosis
  transverse
  valve
  vessel
diamond-shaped anastomosis
diaphanography
diaphragm
  aponeurotic portion of
  arcuate ligaments of
  Bucky
  central tendon
  crus (pl. crura) of
  depressed
  dome of
  duodenal
  elevated
  eventration of
  free air under the
  leaf (or leaves) of
  muscular crus of
  pelvic
  polyarcuate
  Potter-Bucky
  respiratory
  sella turcica

diaphragm *(cont.)*
  tenting of
  thoracoabdominal
  twigs to pelvic
  urogenital
diaphragmatic attenuation
diaphragmatic contour
diaphragmatic creep
diaphragmatic crus (pl. crura)
diaphragmatic cupula
diaphragmatic dome
diaphragmatic elevation
diaphragmatic eventration
diaphragmatic hernia
diaphragmatic hiatus
diaphragmatic pericardium
diaphragmatic pleura
diaphragmatic wall myocardial
  infarction
diaphyseal cortical mortise
diaphyseal dysplasia
diaphyseal fracture
diaphysis (pl. diaphyses)
diaplasis
diarthrodial joint
diaschisis, crossed cerebellar
Diasonics ultrasound scanner
diastasis
  fracture
  sutural
  syndesmotic
  tibiofibular
diastolic blood pressure (DBP)
diastolic counterpulsation
diastolic depolarization phase
diastolic filling period
diastolic gating
diastolic overload
diastolic perfusion pressure
diastolic pressure-time index (DPTI)
diastolic velocity (cm/sec)
diastrophic dwarfism
diathermy, ultrasound

diatrizoate meglumine imaging agent
diatrizoate sodium imaging agent
DIC (drip infusion cholangiography)
DICC (dynamic infusion cavernosometry and cavernosography)
dichromate dosimeter
Dickhaut-DeLee classification of
  discoid meniscus
DICOM (Digital Imaging and Communications in Medicine) interface
DID (document image decoding)
didactylism
didelphia
Didiee shoulder view (glenoid fossa)
diencephalic herniation
diencephalon
DIET fast SE imaging
DIET method of fat suppression
DIF (digital image fusion) procedure
differences
  not-so-subtle
  subtle
differencing filter
differential diagnosis
differential lesion pattern
differential loading
differential renal function (DRF) on
  MR urography
differentiated
differentiated chondrosarcoma
differentiating pancreatic carcinoma
differentiation
diffracting Doppler transducer device
diffraction
  beam
  high resolution
  high temperature
  x-ray
diffraction-enhanced imaging (DEI)
diffraction peak
diffuse alveolar hemorrhage (DAH)
diffuse axonal injury (DAI)
diffuse esophageal spasm (DES)

diffuse idiopathic skeletal hyperostosis
  (DISH)
diffuse infiltrating tumor
diffuse near-infrared spectroscopy
diffuse nodularity
diffuse opacity (opacities)
diffuse panbronchiolitis
diffuse pattern
diffuse pneumonia
diffuse thickening
diffuse uptake
diffusion
  anisotropic
  brain water
  spectral
  thermal
diffusion and perfusion magnetic
  resonance imaging
diffusion anisotropy
diffusion coefficient
diffusion coefficient reversal
diffusion magnetic resonance imaging
diffusion pulse sequence
diffusion tensor imaging (DTI)
diffusion tensor magnetic resonance
  imaging (MRI)
diffusion tensor MR imaging
diffusion-weighted echo-planar
  imaging
diffusion-weighted imaging
diffusion-weighted pulse sequence
DiGeorge syndrome
digestion
digestive system
digestive tract
Digirad gamma camera
digit (pl. digits)
  accessory
  arthrodesed
  flail
  replanted
  sausage
  supernumerary
  syndactylization of

digital Add-On Bucky x ray image
  acquisition system
digital branches
digital cineradiology
digital circular tomosynthesis
digital equipment system
digital fluoroscopy, FluoroPlus
  Roadmapper
digital frequency analysis
digital fundus imager
digital holography system
digital ICG (indocyanine green)
  fluorescein dye) videoangiography
digital image fusion (DIF) procedure
digital imaging
Digital Imaging and Communications
  in Medicine (DICOM) protocol
digital imaging processing (DIP)
digitally fused CT and radiolabeled
  monoclonal antibody SPECT
  images
digital mammography
digital parabola
digital pelvic examination
digital radiography
digital rectal examination
digital rotational angiography (DRA)
digital runoff
digital storage (in cineangiography)
digital subtraction angiogram
digital subtraction angiography (DSA)
digital subtraction bowel cleansing
  with mucosal reconstruction
digital subtraction imaging technique
digital subtraction macrodacryocystography
digital subtraction pulmonary
  angiogram
digital subtraction rotational
  angiography
digital to analog converter
digital tomosynthesis (breast imaging
  technique)

digital unraveling
digital vascular imaging (DVI)
digital videoangiography
digital x-ray tomosynthesis
digitized slices
digitized spinography
digitizer (see *scanner)*
Digitizer Director imaging
digitorum
Digitron digital subtraction imaging
  system
Digitron DVI/DSA computer
digiti manus (fingers)
digiti pedis (toes)
digitus annularis (ring finger)
digitus medius (middle finger)
digitus minimus (little finger)
digiti primus (thumb)
digitus secundus (index finger)
digitus valgus
digitus varus
dihydroxyphenylalanine (DOPA),
  C-11-labeled, for PET scans
diisocyanide-triisocyanide ^{99m}Tc
  complexes
dilatation (also dilation)
  alveolar
  anal
  aneurysmal
  annular
  aortic root
  appreciable
  arrested
  arterial
  artery by balloon catheter
  ascending aorta
  balloon
  bile duct
  biliary
  bowel
  bowel loop
  bronchial
  bronchiolar

dilatation *(cont.)*
  caliceal
  cardiac
  cavitary
  cervical
  chamber
  colonic
  common duct
  diffuse aortic
  distal ureteral
  ductal
  Eder-Puestow
  endoscopic
  esophageal
  extrahepatic biliary cystic
  fluoroscopically guided balloon
    (FGBD)
  fusiform
  gastric
  hepatic web
  idiopathic pulmonary artery
  idiopathic right atrial
  intestinal
  intrahepatic bile duct
  intrahepatic biliary cystic
  intraluminal
  left ventricular
  megacolon
  multiple mural
  myocardial
  pancreatic ductal
  percutaneous balloon
  percutaneous transluminal balloon
    (PTBD)
  periportal sinusoidal
  pneumatic bag esophageal
  pneumatic balloon catheter
  poststenotic
  probe
  prognathous (or prognathic)
  pulmonary artery
  pulmonary trunk idiopathic
  pulmonary valve stenosis

dilatation *(cont.)*
  rectal
  respiratory bronchiolar
  right ventricular
  sequential
  sulcus
  terminal bronchiolar
  tortuous vein
  transient left ventricular
  transvaginal uterine cervical dila-
    tion with fluoroscopic guidance
  tubular
  ureteral
  ureteric
  urethral
  vein
  ventral
  ventricular wall
dilatation and hypertrophy
dilate
dilated calices
dilated veins due to obstruction of the
  hepatic portal circulation
dilation (see *dilatation*)
dilation of calices
dilution curve
dilution, isotopic
DIMAQ integrated ultrasound workstation
DiMattina laparoscopic catheter
dimension
  absolute artery
  aortic root
  arterial
  axial
  end systolic
  intraluminal
  intrathoracic
  left atrial
  left ventricular end diastolic
    (LVEDD)
  left ventricular end systolic
    (LVESD)

dimension *(cont.)*
  left ventricular internal (LVID)
  left ventricular internal diastolic
    (LVIDD)
  left ventricular internal end diastole
    (LVIDd)
  left ventricular internal end systole
    (LVIDs)
  left ventricular systolic (LVs)
  luminal
  right ventricular (RVD)
diminished systemic perfusion
diminutive vessel
dimple of bone
dinner-fork deformity
diode detector
diode, infrared light-emitting
diode laser
DIP (desquamative interstitial
  pneumonia)
DIP (digital imaging processing)
  algorithms
DIP (distal interphalangeal) joint
diplegia spinalis brachialis traumatica
diploic
dipolar broadening
dipolar interaction
dipole antenna, loopless
diprosopus
dipyridamole echocardiography test
dipyridamole handgrip test
dipyridamole infusion test
dipyridamole thallium stress test
dipyridamole thallium-201
  scintigraphy
dipyridamole thallium
  ventriculography
dipyridamole tomographic thallium
  stress test
directable coaxial catheter
direct caval cannulation
direct current ablation (DCA)
direct current (DC) energy

direct fracture
direct hernia
direction, aboral
directional bremsstrahlung splitting
  (DBS)
directional color angiography (DCA)
directional coronary angioplasty
  (DCA)
directional coronary atherectomy
  (DCA)
directional vacuum-assisted biopsy
direct liquid scintillation count
directly coupled sample changer
  system
direct MR arthrography
director, grooved
direct puncture phlebography
direct radioiodination
DirectRay imaging device
DirectView CR 900 imaging system
direct visualization
dirofilariasis
dirty fat sign
dirty mass
dirty shadowing
disarticulate
disarticulation
disc (see *disk)*
discernible findings
discogenic
discogram
discography
diskogram
diskography
discoid atelectasis
discoid lateral meniscus
discoid shadow
discoligamentous complex
discontinuity
discordant nodule
Discovery bone densitometer
Discovery LS imaging system
Discovery QDR densitometer

discrepancy
  leg length
  limb length
discreta, porokeratosis plantaris
discrete (separate) (not *discreet)*
discrete absorbance
discrete bleeding source
discrete lesion
discrete mass
discrete perihilar density
discrete subvalvular aortic stenosis
  (DSAS)
discrete tumor
discriminant analysis
discriminate
discrimination
discriminator
discus (disci)
disease, disorder, or condition
  acquired
  adiposis dolorosa
  advanced cortical
  air-space
  airways
  Albers-Schönberg (Schoenberg)
  alcoholic liver (ALD)
  Alexander
  Alpers
  Alzheimer (AD)
  amyloid
  antiphospholipid syndrome
  aortic valvular disease (AVD)
  aortoiliac
  Apert
  arterial degenerative
  arteriosclerotic cardiovascular
    (ASCVD)
  arteriosclerotic heart (ASHD)
  arteriosclerotic peripheral vascular
  ascariasis
  athero-occlusive
  atherosclerotic cardiovascular
    (ASCVD)

disease *(cont.)*
  atherosclerotic carotid artery
    (ACAD)
  atherosclerotic heart
  atherosclerotic pulmonary vascular
    (ASPVD)
  autosomal dominant polycystic
    kidney
  avascular necrosis
  Ayerza-Arrillaga
  Bamberger-Marie
  Bannister angioedema
  Banti
  Barrett esophageal
  basilar-vertebral artery
  Batten
  Bazin
  B-cell lymphoma
  Beau
  Beauvais
  Behçet
  benign asbestos related pleural
  Bielschowsky-Jansky
  black lung
  Blount
  Bornholm
  Bouchard
  Bouillaud
  Bourneville
  Bourneville-Pringle
  Bouveret
  Bowen
  brain stem
  breast cystic
  breast fibrocystic
  Brinton
  Brodie
  bronchial type B
  Bruck
  Buerger thromboangiitis obliterans
  Buerger-Gruetz
  bullous lung
  Busquet

disease *(cont.)*
  Caffey
  California coccidioidomycosis
  Calvé-Perthes
  Camurati-Engelmann
  Canavan
  Canavan-van Bogaert-Bertrand
  cardiorenal
  cardiovascular renal
  Caroli
  carotid atherosclerotic
  carotid occlusive
  Castellani
  Castleman
  cat scratch
  central motor pathways
  cerebellar
  cerebral Whipple
  cerebrovascular occlusive
  cervical disk
  Chagas
  champagne-bottle legs in Charcot-
    Marie-Tooth
  Charcot-Marie-Tooth (CMT)
  cheese handler's (or washer's)
  Chester
  cholangiohepatitis
  cholestatic liver
  chondrosarcoma
  choriocarcinoma
  chronic obstructive lung (COLD)
  chronic obstructive pulmonary
    (COPD)
  chronic peripheral arterial (CPAD)
  Coats
  coccidioidomycosis
  collagen vascular
  Concato
  congenital heart disease (CHD)
  constrictive bronchiolitis
  cork handler's lung
  coronary artery (CAD)
  coronary heart (CHD)

disease *(cont.)*
  Cowden
  Creutzfeldt-Jakob (CJD)
  Crohn (CD)
  Crouzon
  cryptogenic organizing pneumonia
  cytomegalic inclusion
  deficiency
  degenerative
  degenerative atrioventricular node
  degenerative disk
  degenerative joint (DJD)
  Degos
  demyelinating
  demyelinative disorder
  Dercum
  Deutschländer
  dirofilariasis
  disk
  disseminated
  Dubin-Sprinz
  Duroziez mitral stenosis
  eccentric plaque
  emphysematous type A
  Engelmann
  Engel-Recklinghausen
  Erb disease
  Erdheim-Chester
  esophageal motility disorder
  EtOH-associated liver
  evacuation disorder
  Ewing sarcoma
  exanthematous
  exogenous lipoid pneumonia
  extracranial carotid occlusive
  Fabry
  Fahr-Volhard
  Farber
  Favre
  Fenwick
  Flatau-Schilder
  flax-dresser's
  Fleischer

disease *(cont.)*
  fluffy rarefaction of Paget
  Forestier
  Fraley syndrome
  Freiberg
  Freiberg-Kohler
  fulminant course of
  fulminant herpes hepatitis
  functional bowel
  functional disorder
  Gairdner
  Gandy-Nanta
  Garré
  gastric motor disorder
  gastroesophageal reflux (GERD)
  Gaucher
  Gee-Herter
  gestational trophoblastic
  Glénard
  glial
  global cardiac
  Gorham
  graft-versus-host (GVHD)
  Graves
  Gull
  Hagner
  Hand-Schüller (Schueller)-
    Christian
  hard metal
  Hartnup
  Heath-Edwards classification of
    pulmonary vascular
  Heberden
  Heckathorn
  Heerfordt syndrome
  hemorrhagic (of newborn)
  Henderson-Jones
  hepatic veno-occlusive
  hepatic venous web
  hepatobiliary
  heterogeneous system
  Hodgkin
  Hoffa

disease *(cont.)*
Horton
Huchard
Huppert
hyaline membrane
hypertensive heart
hypertensive renal
hypertensive vascular
idiopathic
idiopathic calcium pyrophosphate
  dihydrate (iCPPD) deposition
idiopathic inflammatory bowel
  (IBD)
idiopathic mural endomyocardial
ileocolic
iliac artery
iliac atherosclerotic occlusive
infectious
inflammatory
inflammatory bowel (IBD)
inflammatory paranasal sinus
inherently unstable condition
inoperable
interstitial lung disease (ILD)
intimal atherosclerotic
intractable bleeding disorder
intrapulmonary
intrathoracic lymphoproliferative
  disorder
intrauterine cytomegalic inclusion
intrinsic
intrinsic pulmonary
iron storage
ischemic
ischemic heart (IHD)
Jaffe-Lichtenstein
Jansen
Joubert syndrome
juvenile Paget
Kahler
Kashin-Bek
Kawasaki
Keshan

disease *(cont.)*
Kienböck
Kikuchi-Fujimoto
Kimura
kinky-hair syndrome
Kinnier-Wilson
knee knob of Osgood-Schlatter
Köhler
Köhler-Pellegrini-Stieda
Krabbe
Kümmell
Kussmaul-Maier
kyphoscoliotic heart
Lane
large vessel
Larsen-Johansson
Legg-Calvé-Perthes (LCP)
Legg-Calvé-Waldenström
LeinerF
leptomeningeal
Letterer-Siwe
Lhermitte-Duclos
Libman-Sacks endocarditis
Lichtman radiographic classifica-
  tion of Kienböck
littoral cell angioma
liver hydatid
Löfgren syndrome
Lyme
MacLean-Maxwell
Majocchi
malaria
malignant peripheral nerve sheath
  tumor (MPNST)
malignant pleural mesothelioma
  (MPM)
mammary tuberculosis
maple syrup urine
Marie-Bamberger
Marie-Strümpell
Marie-Tooth
Martin
Meigs

disease *(cont.)*
　Ménétrier
　Menkes kinky-hair syndrome
　metastatic
　miliary lung
　Miller
　Milroy
　Milton angioedema
　mixed connective tissue
　mixed restrictive-obstructive lung
　Moschcowitz
　motility disorder
　moyamoya
　MPM (malignant pleural meso-
　　thelioma)
　MPNST (malignant peripheral
　　nerve sheath tumor)
　multicystic mesothelioma
　multiple hamartoma syndrome
　Münchmeyer
　mushroom picker's
　myelodysplastic syndrome
　myocardial granulomatous
　necrobiotic xanthogranulomatosis
　necrotizing fasciitis
　neurofibromatosis
　Niemann-Pick
　nonspecific esophageal motility
　　disorder (NEMD)
　obstructive airway
　obstructive pulmonary (OPD)
　occult distant metastatic
　Ollier
　orbital pseudotumor
　organic brain (OBD)
　Osgood-Schlatter
　Osler
　osteochondromatosis
　Paas
　Paget
　paragonimiasis
　parenchymal lung
　Payr

disease *(cont.)*
　Pel-Ebstein
　Pellegrini-Stieda
　pelvic inflammatory (PID)
　peptic ulcer (PUD)
　peripheral air-space
　peripheral arterial occlusive
　peripheral lung
　peripheral vascular (PVD)
　Perthes
　Petit
　Pick
　pigmented villonodular synovitis
　plexiform neurofibromatosis
　Plummer
　pneumonia, cryptogenic organizing
　polycystic kidney
　polycystic ovary (or ovarian)
　　syndrome
　Pompe
　popliteal artery occlusive
　post-transplant coronary artery
　post-transplant lymphoproliferative
　　disorder (PTLD)
　Preiser
　primary diffuse large B-cell
　　lymphoma
　Proteus syndrome
　PTLD (post-transplant lympho-
　　proliferative disorder)
　pulmonary collagen vascular
　　(PCVD)
　pulmonary veno-occlusive
　Quincke angioedema
　radiation pericardial
　radiation-induced lung (RILD)
　ragpicker's
　RCC (renal cell carcinoma)
　reactive airways (RAD)
　Recklinghausen
　Reiter
　renal cell carcinoma (RCC)
　renal parenchymal

disease *(cont.)*
  Rendu-Osler-Weber
  restrictive lung
  restrictive-obstructive lung
  reversible airways (RAD)
  reversible obstructive airway
    (ROAD)
  rhabdomyosarcoma
  rheumatic heart (RHD)
  rheumatic valvular
  rheumatoid arthritis-associated
    interstitial lung
  rhythm disorder
  Riedel thyroiditis
  right-left disorder
  RILD (radiation-induced lung)
  Roger (maladie de Roger)
  Ruysch
  Rye Hodgkin
  sacroiliac
  Sandhoff
  sarcoma botryoides
  schistosomiasis
  Schlatter-Osgood
  Schmitt
  Schmorl
  sclerosing mesenteritis
  Sertoli-Leydig cell tumor
  sickle cell
  Sinding-Larsen-Johansson (SLJD)
  single vessel
  sinistral portal hypertension
  skip lesions of Crohn disease
  small volume
  snufftaker's pituitary
  steno-occlusive
  Still (juvenile rheumatoid arthritis)
  strongyloidiasis
  Strümpell-Lorrain
  Strümpell-Marie
  subarachnoid metastatic
  Swediaur

disease *(cont.)*
  systemic disorder affecting heart
    function
  systemic lupus erythematosus
  Thiemann
  three-vessel coronary
  thromboembolic disease (TED)
  thyrocardiac
  tibial artery
  tibioperoneal occlusive
  Trevor
  trypanosomiasis
  upper respiratory tract
  valvular (VD)
  valvular heart
  vanishing bile duct syndrome
  Vaquez
  vascular occlusive
  veno-occlusive (VOD)
  venous thromboembolic (VTED)
  vertebrobasilar
  VOD (veno-occlusive)
  von Gierke
  Waldenström
  Weber-Osler-Rendu
  Weil (named for Adolf Weil)
  Westphal-Strümpell
  Whipple
  Williams syndrome
  Wilms tumor
  Wilson
  Winiwarter-Buerger
  Winiwarter-Manteuffel-Buerger
  woolsorter's inhalation
disease-free vessel wall
DISH (diffuse idiopathic skeletal hyperostosis)
dishpan fracture
dish-shaped acetabulum
DISI (dorsal intercalary segment
  instability)
DISIDA (diisopropyliminodiacetic
  acid) scan

disimpaction
disintegration of plaque by laser
  pulses
disjointing
disk (also disc)
  acromioclavicular joint
  anal
  articular
  atrial
  Bardeen primitive
  Bowman
  bulge (or bulging)
  cartilaginous (of epiphysis)
  cervical vertebral
  chorionic
  contained
  crescent-shaped fibrocartilaginous
  distal radioulnar joint
  embryonic
  epiphyseal
  extruded
  fibrocartilaginous
  fibrous ring of
  fixation
  frayed
  growth
  H
  hard
  Hensen
  herniated
  herniated cervical
  herniated intervertebral (HID)
  herniated lumbar
  herniated lumbosacral intervertebral
  herniated sacral
  herniated thoracic intervertebral
  I
  interarticular
  intervertebral
  intra-articular
  isotropic
  locking
  lumbar vertebral

disk *(cont.)*
  lumbosacral vertebral
  mandibular
  massive herniated
  Merkel tactile
  midline herniation of
  noncontained
  placental
  protruded (or protruding)
  ruptured
  sequestered
  slipped intervertebral
  soft
  sternoclavicular joint
  tactile
  temporomandibular joint
  thoracic vertebral
  thoracolumbar vertebral
  triangular
  vacuum
  vertebral
disk bulge
disk bulging
disk disease
disk displacement
diskectomy, fluoroscopic
disk extrusion
disk fragment
disk herniation
disk interspace
diskitis, infectious
disklike atelectasis
disk margin
disk maturation
diskogram
diskography (discography)
  intranuclear
  intervertebral
diskovertebral infection
disk plication
disk poppet
disk protrusion
disk space height

disk space, linear radiolucency in the
disk space narrowing
disk to magnetic field orientation
disk water signal
dislocate, dislocated
dislocation
 anterior
 anterior-inferior
 Bankart
 bayonet
 Bell-Dally
 Bennett
 boutonnière
 bursting
 central
 Chopart
 chronic recurrent
 closed
 complete
 complicated
 compound
 consecutive
 Desault
 divergent
 facet
 fracture
 frank
 gamekeeper's
 habitual
 Hill-Sachs
 incomplete
 irreducible
 isolated
 Jahss
 Kienböck (Kienboeck)
 Lisfranc
 lunate
 milkmaid's
 Monteggia
 Nélaton
 nonreducible
 nontraumatic
 open
 Otto

dislocation *(cont.)*
 partial
 pathologic
 perilunate
 posterior
 primitive
 recent
 recurrent
 simple
 Smith
 subtle mobile atlantoaxial
 swivel
 traumatic
 ulnar nerve
 volar perilunate
dislocation fracture
dislodged calculus
dismembered pyeloplasty
disobliteration, carotid
disorder (see *disease*)
disparate
disparity of maturation
disphenoid extraction
dispersion, intravoxel phase (IVPD)
displaced fat pad sign
displacement
 craniocaudal
 disk
 Ellis Jones peroneal
 lateral
 trabecular
 volar
displacement field-fitting MR imaging
displacement maneuver
displacement of kidney
display
 multiparametric color composite
 pseudocolor B-mode
 real-time
 shaded-surface
disproportion
 cephalopelvic (CPD)
 fiber-type
 ureterocele

disrupted plaque
disruption
  perivalvular
  traumatic
dissecans
  osteochondritis (OD)
  osteochondrosis
dissect
dissecting aneurysm
dissecting hematoma
dissection
  aneurysmal
  aortic
  arterial
  descending aorta
  spontaneous
  Stanford type B aortic
  type A aortic
  type B aortic
dissection propagation
disseminated atheromatous
  embolization
disseminated cholesterol embolization
disseminated disease
disseminated intravascular coagulation
  (DIC)
disseminated sclerosis
disseminated tuberculosis
distal articular set angle (DASA)
distal coronary sinus (CS)
distal interphalangeal (DIP) joint
distally
distal part of prostatic urethra
distal right ureter
distal splenorenal shunt (DSRS)
distal ureteral dilation
distal urethra
distal urethral stenosis
distalward
distance
  focal
  interarch
  intercaudate

distance *(cont.)*
  interlaminar
  internuclear
  interopercular
  interorbital
  interpediculate
  interridge
  interslice
  interspinous
  metatarsal protrusion
  minimum interbone (MID)
  object-film (OFD)
  source-image (SID)
  source-skin (SSD)
  surface
distance-based block classification
distance transform-based skeletonization
distant metastases
distant metastatic disease, occult
distend
distended
distensible
distensibility
distention
  abdominal
  bladder
  colonic
  gaseous
  gastric
  intestinal
  neck vein
  pelvicaliceal
  postprandial
  rectal
  ureteral
  vesical
disto-occlusal
distortion
  additive white gaussian noise
  architectural
  bronchial
  camera

distortion *(cont.)*
  degree of
  elliptical
  esophageal
  focal
  geometric
  head frame
  image
  lens
  lung architecture
  minimal radiographic
  pincushion
  pituitary stalk (PSD)
  pressure-induced
  radiographic pincushion
  residual
  S
  severe
  shape
  significant
  tracheal
  Y-shaped
distortion-corrected image
distortion-free image
distortion of limitations of image
  reconstruction algorithm artifact
distraction
  callus
  fracture fragment
  hyperflexion injury
  joint
  physeal
  segment
  small step
  soft tissue
distraction gap
distraction osteogenesis
distribution
  anatomic
  anomalous
  binomial
  blood velocity
  Boltzmann

distribution *(cont.)*
  catecholamineF
  centrilobular
  depth dose
  diffuse
  gaussian
  geometric
  inhomogeneous
  inhomogeneous tracer
  mottled
  peribronchial
  perivascular
  reverse
  rimlike calcium
  spectral noise
  trace element
  uniform
distributive shock
disturbance, functional
disuse
  demineralization from
  lesser atrophy of
disuse atrophy
disuse osteoporosis
diurnal variation
diuretic renal imaging
diuretic renal scan
dive-bomber discharges
divergent dislocation
diverging collimator
diversion, biliopancreatic
diverticulitis
  acute
  chronic
  colonic
  Meckel
  sigmoid
diverticulosis
diverticulum (pl. diverticula)
  acquired
  bladder
  caliceal or calyceal
  colonic

diverticulum *(cont.)*
  cricopharyngeal
  deep
  epiphrenic
  esophageal
  fallopian tube
  false
  functional
  Ganser
  Graser
  hepatic
  hypopharyngeal
  IDD (intraluminal duodenal)
  intestinal
  intraluminal duodenal (IDD)
  intramural
  inverted Meckel
  juxtapapillary
  Kirchner
  Kommerall
  left-sided bladder
  Meckel
  metanephric
  midesophageal
  Nuck
  perforated
  periampullary
  pharyngoesophageal
  pulsion
  Rokitansky
  traction
  urethral
  Vater
  vesical
  widemouthed mucosal
  Zenker
diverting colostomy
divisional block
divisionary line (in bipartite sesamoid)
divisum, pancreas
divot
Dixon method of fat suppression
Dixon method of phase unwrapping

Dixon quantitative chemical shift
  magnetic resonance imaging
DJD (degenerative joint disease)
DJJ (duodenojejunal junction)
DKS (Damus-Kaye-Stansel)
  anastomosis
D-loop, ventricular
D-loop ventricular situs
DMA (distal metatarsal angle)
D-malposition of aorta
DMI (Diagnostic Medical
  Instruments) analyzer
DMI (diaphragmatic myocardial
  infarction)
DMLC (dynamic multileaf collimator)
DMPE (^{99m}Tc-bis-dimethylphosphono-
  ethane)
DMVA (direct mechanical ventricular
  actuation)
DNA, plasmid
DNA ploidy pattern
DNA-MION
DOBI (dynamic optical breast imaging
  system)
dobutamine echocardiography
dobutamine stress echocardiography
dobutamine stress echocardiography
  (DSE) imaging
dobutamine thallium angiography
DOBV (double outlet both ventricles)
document image decoding (DID)
document-recognition algorithm
Dodd perforating vein group
Dodge method for ejection fraction
dog artifact
dog-leg sign
dolichocephaly
dolichocolon
dolichoectasia
dolichoesophagus
dolichosigmoid
dolichostenomelia
DOLV (double outlet left ventricle)

domain, Fourier
dome
  anterior talar
  atrial
  diaphragmatic
  bladder
  liver
  shoulder
  talar
  weightbearing acetabular
dome and dart configuration on
  cardiac catheterization
Dome Imaging RX20 board
dome of urinary bladder
dome-shaped heart
dome-shaped roof of pleural cavity
dome sign
dominance
  coronary artery
  hemispheric
  mixed
  right ventricular
  shared coronary artery
dominant
  anatomically
  autosomal
dominant hemisphere
dominant left coronary artery
dominant mass
dominant right coronary artery
doming, diastolic
doming of leaflet
doming of valve
D1 (diagonal branch #1)
donor kidney
donut sign (also doughnut)
dopamine D1 agonist
dopamine D2 receptor
dopamine transporter
Doplette monitor
Doppler
  color flow
  continuous wave

Doppler *(cont.)*
  contrast-enhanced color
  contrast-enhanced power
  duplex
  duplex B-mode
  gray-scale
  intraoperative
  pocket
  power
  pulsed wave
  range-gated pulsed
  real-time
  spectral
Doppler blood flow detector
Doppler blood flow monitor
Doppler blood flow velocity signal
Doppler blood pressure
Doppler color flow mapping
Doppler color spectral analysis
Doppler coronary catheter
Doppler-derived stroke distance
Doppler echocardiography
  continuous wave (CW)
  pulsed wave
Doppler flow probe study
Doppler flow signal
Doppler flow-imaging system, real-
  time two-dimensional
Doppler flowmetry
Doppler frequency shift
Doppler imaging
Doppler insonation
Doppler Intra-Dop intraoperative
  device
Doppler phenomenon
Doppler pulse
Doppler Resistive Index (DRI)
Doppler shift
Doppler shift principle
Doppler signal
Doppler signal enhancers
Doppler spectral analysis
Doppler spectral waveforms

Doppler tissue imaging (DTI)
Doppler ultrasonic blood flow detector
Doppler ultrasonic fetal heart monitor
Doppler ultrasonic velocity detector
Doppler ultrasonography
Doppler ultrasound, high frequency
  (HFD)
Doppler ultrasound intestinal blood
  flow measurement
Doppler ultrasound segmental blood
  pressure testing
Doppler venous examination
Doppler waveform analysis
Dorendorf sign of aortic arch
  aneurysm
Dormia basket catheter
Dornier scanner
Dorros brachial internal mammary
  guiding catheter
dorsal branch
dorsal capsule
dorsal decubitus position
dorsalis pedis pulse
dorsal lithotomy position
dorsal metacarpal ligament
dorsal pedal bypass
dorsal pedal pulse
dorsal position
dorsal ramus of spinal nerve
dorsal recumbent position
dorsal root entry zone (DREZ) lesion
dorsal root ganglia (DRG)
dorsal spine (D1 to D12)
dorsal spinocerebellar tracts
dorsal subaponeurotic space
dorsal subcutaneous space
dorsal supine position
dorsal union twins
dorsalward
dorsal wing fracture
dorsal wrist ligament
dorsiflexion
dorsiflexor

dorsoanterior
dorsocephalad
dorsolateral
dorsolaterally organized sequestration
dorsoplantar talonavicular angle
dorsoplantar view
dorsoposterior
dorsoradial
dorsorostral
dorsum pedis
dorsum sellae
DORV (double outlet right ventricle)
Dos Santos needle for aortography
dose (pl. doses)
  absorbed
  bolus
  divided
  fraction
  fractionated
  incremental
  integral
  iodine
  lethal
  loading
  maintenance
  median lethal
  multiple scan average (MSAD)
  normalized average glandular
  reduced radiation
  tapering
  titrated
  tracer
dose index, computed tomography
  (CTDI)
dose response relationship
dose volume histogram
dose volume relationship
dosimeter
dosimetric penumbra
dosimetry
  beam's-eye view
  carbon-load thermoluminescent
  CTA

dosimetry *(cont.)*
dichromate
electron
EPR
free-radical
high dose film
LiF thermoluminescence
thermoluminescent
transmission
dosing, titrated
dots, subpleural
Dotter caged balloon catheter
Dotter-Judkins PTA (percutaneous
    transluminal angioplasty)
double-acting actuator
double aortic arch
double barrel aorta
double barrel lumen
double breast coil
double bubble sign
double bubble ultrasound appearance
    of fetus
double camelback sign of knee
double clamping
double contour
double contrast arthrography
double contrast barium enema
    (DCBE)
double cuff dialysis catheter
double density
double dose delay (DDD)
double dose gadolinium imaging
double doughnut magnet (GE Signa
    0.5 T)
double echo chemical shift in-phase
    and opposed-phase FLASH MR
    images
double echo three-point Dixon method
    fat suppression
double exposure artifact
double exposure drift artifact
double fracture
double halo sign on CT scan

double helical CT scan
double helix acquisition on CT scan
double inlet left ventricle/double outlet
    both ventricles
double inlet ventricles
double J indwelling catheter
double J indwelling stent
double J ureteral catheter
double J ureteral stent
double label
double label counting
double line sign
double lumen femoral vein catheter
double lumen subclavian vein catheter
double lumen venous umbilical
    catheter
double outflow
double outlet both ventricles (DOBV)
double outlet left ventricle (DOLV)
double outlet right ventricle (DORV)
double outlet right ventricle (I–IV)
    syndrome
double outline
double PCL (posterior cruciate
    ligament) sign on MRI
double phase technetium-99m
    sestamibi imaging
double photon absorptiometry (DPA)
double pigtail ureteral catheter
double pneumonia
double-populated detector ring
double spin echo proton spectroscopy
double spiral CT arterial portography
double strand, intracellular DNA
double stripe sign
double systolic apical impulse
double tracking of barium
double-walled fibroserous sac
double wall sign
double wire atherectomy technique
doubly broadband triple resonance
    NMR probe circuit
doughnut (also donut)

doughnut configuration on thallium
imaging
doughnut, double (MRI magnet)
doughnut magnet
doughnut-shaped prolapsing leaflet
doughnut sign
Douglas abscess
Douglas bag method for determining
cardiac output
Douglas
cul-de-sac of
pouch of
Dow-Corning ileal pouch catheter
dowager's hump
dowel
Dow method for measuring cardiac
output
down-folding epiglottis
downscatter
downstream sampling method
Down syndrome
downward displacement of apical
impulse
downward sloping
doxorubicin, liposomal
dP/dt (upstroke pattern on apex
cardiogram), peak
DPA (double [or dual] photon absorptiometry)
D point
DPTI (diastolic pressure-time index)
DPX-IQ densitometer
DRA (digital rotational angiography)
DRA (distal reference axis)
drainage
aberrant venous
anomalous
percutaneous antegrade biliary
percutaneous transhepatic (PTD)
transvaginal ultrasound-guided
drainage stent
draining vein pressure (DVP)
draped aorta

DRC (dynamic range control) algorithm used in digital radiography
Drennan metaphyseal-epiphyseal angle
Dressler post-myocardial infarction
syndrome
DREZ (dorsal root entry zone) lesion
DRF (differential renal function) on
MR urography
DRG (dorsal root ganglia)
DRI (Doppler Resistive Index)
drifting wedge pressure
drilling, computer-assisted retrograde
drip infusion cholangiography (DIC)
driven equilibrium pulse
dromedary kidney
drooping lily appearance
drooping lily sign
drop finger
drop foot
drop metastases
dropsy (hydrops)
drop test for pneumoperitoneum
drowned lung
Drummond marginal artery
Drummond sign of aortic aneurysm
dry pleurisy
dry swallow on esophageal manometry
Drystar dry imager
DS (duplex sonography)
DSA (digital subtraction angiography)
frameless stereotaxic
intra-arterial
intravenous
DSAS (discrete subvalvular aortic
stenosis)
DSC (dynamic susceptibility contrast)
MR imaging
D-shaped vessel lumen
DSI camera
D signal
DTAF-F (descending thoracic
aortofemoral-femoral) bypass
DTI (diffusion-tensor imaging)

DTI (Doppler tissue imaging)
DTICH (delayed traumatic intracere-
    bral hemorrhage [or hematoma])
DTI-FT (diffusion-tensor imaging/
    fiber tractography)
D to E slope on echocardiography
DTPA (technetium Tc-99m pentetate
    kit) imaging agent
DTPA renography
DTPA, technetium bound to
D-transposition (dextrotransposition) of
    great arteries
D2 dopamine receptors
DU (duplex ultrasound)
dual atrioventricular node pathway
dual balloon method
dual blood supply
dual contrast study
dual display mode
dual echo DIET fast SE imaging
dual echo sequence
dual energy contrast-enhanced digital
    subtraction mammography
dual energy x-ray absorptiometry
    (DEXA)
dual GRE pulse sequences
dual head coincidence camera
dual head gamma camera system
dual head SPECT
dual isotope scanning
dual isotope single photon emission
    CT
dual lookup table algorithm
dual modality PET/CT
dual phase protocol
dual phase scan
dual phase spiral CT scan
dual phase ^{99m}Tc-sestamibi imaging
dual photon absorptiometry (DPA)
dual photon densitometry
dual x-ray absorptiometry (DXA)
Dubin and Amelar varicocele classifi-
    cation

Dubin Johnson syndrome
Dubin-Sprinz disease
Ducor-Cordis pigtail catheter
Ducor HF (high flow) catheter
Ducor tip
duct
    aberrant
    aberrant bile
    accessory hepatic
    accessory pancreatic
    alveolar
    amniotic
    arterial
    Bartholin
    beaded hepatic
    bile
    biliary
    Botallo
    branchial
    breast
    bucconeural
    bulbourethral gland
    canalicular
    carotid
    choledochous
    cochlear
    collecting
    common
    common bile (CBD)
    common gall
    common hepatic
    Cowper
    craniopharyngeal
    cystic
    cystic gall
    deferent
    distal bile
    efferent
    ejaculatory
    endolymphatic
    excretory
    extrahepatic bile
    frontonasal

duct *(cont.)*
  fusiform widening of
  galactophorous
  gall
  Gartner
  gasserian
  genital
  Guérin
  Haller aberrant
  hepatic
  Hering
  His
  hypophyseal Rathke
  interlobular bile
  intrahepatic biliary
  involution of
  lacrimal
  lactiferous
  Leydig
  lobal bile
  lymph
  lymphatic
  main pancreatic (MPD)
  mammary
  mesonephric
  metanephric
  middle extrahepatic bile
  milk
  Müller (Mueller)
  mullerian
  normal caliber
  obstruction of
  occlusion of breast
  omphalomesenteric
  ovarian
  pancreatic
  paramesonephric
  paraurethral
  perilobular
  preampullary portion of bile
  prepapillary bile
  primordial
  pronephric

duct *(cont.)*
  prostatic
  Rathke
  renal
  right hepatic
  Santorini
  Schüller (Schueller)
  secretory
  segmental bile
  seminal
  Skene
  spermatic
  stenosis of breast
  Stensen
  subvesical
  terminal bile
  testicular
  thoracic
  thyroglossal
  umbilical
  urogenital
  vitellointestinal (VID)
  wolffian
  Vater
  vitelline
  Wirsung
  wolffian
ductal arch
ductal architecture
ductal carcinoma in situ (DCIS)
ductal constriction
ductal dilatation
ductal ectasia
ductal epithelial hyperplasia
ductal hyperplasia
ductal pattern
ductal remnant
duct ectasia
duct obstruction
duct of Bellini
duct-penetrating sign
ductule
ductular proliferation

ductus arteriosus
  patent (PDA)
  persistent
  persistent patency of
  reversed
ductus arteriosus patency
ductus deferens artery
ductus venosus patency
Dulcolax bowel prep
dumb terminal
dumbbell-shaped shadow
dumbbell tumor
dumbbell-type neuroblastoma
dumping syndrome
Duncan Howe (no hyphen; first and
  last name) flexion and extension
  views of lumbar spine
Dunlap, Swanson, and Penner acetabular projection
Dunlap-Rippstein method
Dunn and Rippstein technique to view
  femoral neck
duodenal adenoma
duodenal atresia
duodenal bulb
duodenal cap
duodenal C-loop
duodenal duplication
duodenal erosion
duodenal impression on liver
duodenal loop
duodenal papilla
duodenal seromyectomy
duodenal sweep
duodenal switch
duodenal terminus
duodenal tumor, periampullary
duodenal ulcer
duodenal ulcer perforation (DUP)
duodenal wind sock sign
duodenitis
  chronic atrophic
  erosive

duodenobiliary pressure gradient
duodenogastric reflux
duodenography, hypotonic
duodenojejunal angle
duodenojejunal junction (DJJ)
duodenopancreatic reflux
duodenum
  C-loop of
  curve of
  descending
  distal
  first portion of
  scarified
  second portion of
  suspensory muscle of
  third portion of
duodenum deformed by scarring
Duo-Flow dual lumen catheter
DUP (duodenal ulcer perforation)
Du Pen epidural catheter
duplex Doppler scan
duplex Doppler sonography (DS)
duplex Doppler ultrasound
duplex imaging, color-flow
duplex kidney
duplex pulsed-Doppler sonography
duplex scan
  color flow
  renal
duplex screening test
duplex sonography (DS)
duplex ultrasound (DU)
duplex ultrasound
duplicated renal collecting system
duplication
  craniofacial
  esophageal
DuPont CRONEX x-ray film
DuPont Rare Earth Imaging System
DuPont scanner
Dupuytren contracture
Dupuytren fracture

dura
  attenuated
  bulging
Dura-Guard patch
dural arteriovenous malformation
dural attachment(s)
dural AV fistula (DAVF), spinal
dural ectasia
dural fold
dural impingement
dural sac
dural scar
dural sheath
dural sinus thrombosis (DST)
dural tail sign
dural tear
dural venous sinus thrombosis
dura mater of brain
dura mater of spinal cord
Duret lesion
Durham flatfoot
Duroziez mitral stenosis disease
DUS (dynamic ultrasound of
  shoulder)
Dusart syndrome
Dutt view (PA oblique of cribriform
  plate)
Duverney fracture
dV/dt (contractility)
DVI (deep venous insufficiency)
DVI (device-independent)
DVI (digital vascular imaging)
DVI Simpson AtheroCath
DVP (draining vein pressure)
DVT (deep venous thrombosis)
dwarfism
  achondroplastic
  deprivation
  Lorain-Lévi
  pituitary
  renal
  Russell-Silver
  Walt Disney

dwarf pelvis
dwell time
DWI (diffusion weighted imaging)
DXA (dual x-ray absorptiometry)
^{166}Dy (dysprosium) ^{166}Ho
  holmium in vivo generator
dye (see *imaging agent)*
dye extravasation
dye fluorescence index (DFI)
dye punch fracture
dynamic absorptivity
dynamic beat filtration
dynamic bolus
dynamic cerebral autoregulation (CA)
dynamic computerized tomography
  (CT)
dynamic conformal therapy
  (irradiation)
dynamic contrast-enhanced subtraction
  study
dynamic cystoproctogram
dynamic filtering
dynamic helical scan imaging
dynamic hyperpolarized 3He (helium)
  magnetic resonance imaging
dynamic infusion cavernosography
dynamic infusion cavernosometry and
  cavernosography (DICC)
dynamic lineshape effects
dynamic multileaf collimator (DMLC)
dynamic optical breast imaging system
  (DOBI)
Dynamic PACSPlus imaging system
dynamic pedobarography
dynamic radiotherapy
dynamic range control (DRC) algorithm used in digital radiography
dynamic single photon emission
  tomography
dynamic snapshot
Dynamic Spatial Reconstructor (DSR)
  scanner
dynamic spiral CT lung densitometry

dynamic susceptibility contrast (DSC)
magnetic resonance imaging
dynamic susceptibility-weighted contrast-enhanced MR imaging
dynamic tagging magnetic resonance
angiography
dynamic three-dimensional ultrasound
imaging
dynamic ultrasound of shoulder (DUS)
dynamic volume-rendered display
dynamic volumetric SPECT
dynamic wedge
Dynarad portable imaging system
DynaWell medical compression device
dynode
dynograph
dysbaric osteonecrosis
dyschezia
dyschondroplasia
dyscollagenosis
dyscrasic fracture
dysfunction
    hemodialysis graft
    positional
    swallowing
dysfunctional uterine hemorrhage
dysgenesis
    alar
    anorectal
    callosal
    corticocallosal
    epiphyseal
    gonadal
dysgerminoma tumor
dyshormonogenesis
dyskinesia
    bile duct
    biliary
    regional
    tardive
    anterior wall
    anteroapical
    left ventricular

dyskinesia *(cont.)*
    segmental wall motion
    wall motion
dysmaturity, pulmonary
dysmotility, esophageal
dysosteogenesis
dysostosis
    cleidocranial
    craniofacial
    metaphyseal
dysostosis multiplex
dysostosis, Nager acrofacial
dyspepsia
dyspeptic
dysphagia
    contractile ring
    esophageal
    liquid food
    oropharyngeal
    postvagotomy
    pre-esophageal
    progressive
    sideropenic
    soft food
    solid food
    vallecular
dysphagia inflammatoria
dysphagia lusoria
dysphagia nervosa
dysphagia paralytica
dysphagia spastica
dysphagia valsalviana
dysplasia
    acetabular
    acromelic
    acromesomelic
    acropectorovertebral
    arteriohepatic
    bone
    bronchopulmonary
    cleidocranial
    congenital (of hip) (CDH)
    congenital polyvalvular

dysplasia *(cont.)*
  cranioskeletal
  developmental
  diaphyseal
  endocardial
  epiarticular osteochondromatous
  familial arterial fibromuscular
  fibromuscular (FMD)
  fibrous
  foot
  mesomelic
  microscopic cortical
  mandibuloacral
  mammary
  metaphyseal
  Mondini
  monostotic fibrous
  multicystic
  multiple epiphyseal
  Namaqualand hip
  oculoauriculovertebral (OAV)
  odontoid
  osseous
  perimedial
  polyostotic fibrous
  polypoid
  progressive diaphyseal
  pulmonary valve (PVD)
  retroareolar
  right ventricular
  sheetlike
  Sponastrime

dysplasia *(cont.)*
  spondyloepiphyseal
  Streeter
  tricuspid valve
  thymic
  ventricular
  ventriculo-radial
dysplasia with associated lesion or
  mass (DALM)
dysplastic white matter
dyspnea on exertion
dysprosium (^{166}Dy) ^{166}Ho holmium
  in vivo generator
dysraphism
  closed spinal
  occult spinal
  spinal
dyssynergia
  biliary
  detrusor-sphincter
  regional
  segmental
dyssynergy
dystocia
  fetal
  shoulder
dystopia
dystopic
dystrophic change
dystrophic degeneration
dystrophy, Jeune asphyxiating thoracic
dysuria

E, e

EAC (expandable access catheter)
E:A ratio on echocardiogram
early arterial phase
early-phase termination
early pneumonitis
early venous filling
Eastman Kodak scanner
Eaton agent pneumonia
EBA (extrahepatic biliary atresia)
EBCT (electron-beam computed
  tomography)
EBDA (effective balloon dilated area)
Eberth line
EBIORT (electron beam intraoperative
  radiotherapy)
EBRT (external beam radiation
  therapy)
Ebstein sign
eburnation, bony
ECA (external carotid artery)
E-CABG (endarterectomy and
  coronary artery bypass graft)
E.CAM dual head emission imaging
E.CAM+ coincidence-imaging
E-cath tunneled epidural catheter
eccentrically placed lumen
eccentric atherosclerotic plaque

eccentric atrial activation
eccentric axis of rotation of the ankle
eccentric calcification
eccentric coronary artery
eccentric ectopic pregnancy locations
eccentric hypertrophy
eccentricity index
eccentric ledge
eccentric lesion
eccentric plaque disease
eccentric position (of structure)
eccentric stenosis
eccentric vessel
ecchondroma
Eccocee compact ultrasound
  diagnostic system
eccrine angiomatous hamartoma
ECG (electrocardiogram)
  ECG-gated reconstructed multi-
    detector row CT coronary
    angiography
  ECG-gated reconstruction
  ECG gating
  ECG-synchronized digital
    subtraction angiography
  ECG-triggered multidetector
echinococcosis, alveolar

echo (slang for echocardiogram)
echo (pl. echoes)
  amphoric
  atrial
  bright
  dense
  highly mobile
  internal
  solid
  homogeneous
  inhomogeneous
  linear
  median level
  metallic
  navigator
  shower of
  sonographic
  specular
  spin
  swirling smokelike
  thick
  ultrasonographic
  ultrasound
  ventricular
echocardiogram (see *echocardiography*)
echocardiogram adenosine
echocardiographic automated border
echocardiography (echocardiogram)
  akinesis on
  ambulatory Holter
  A-mode
  anterior left ventricular wall
    motion
  apical
  apical five-chamber view
  apical left ventricular wall motion
    on
  apical two-chamber view
  B bump on anterior mitral valve
    leaflet
  B-mode
  biplane transesophageal

echocardiography *(cont.)*
  blood pool radionuclide
  cardiac output
  color flow imaging Doppler
  continuous loop exercise
  continuous wave (CW) Doppler
  contrast
  contrast-enhanced
  cross-sectional two-dimensional
  CW (continuous wave) Doppler
  D to E slope on
  detection
  dipyridamole
  dobutamine stress
  Doppler
  dyskinesis on
  echo-free space on
  endometrial
  epicardial Doppler
  E point on
  exercise
  Feigenbaum
  fetal (in utero)
  four-chamber
  hypokinesis on
  inferior left ventricular wall
    motion on
  intracardiac (ICE)
  intracoronary contrast
  intraoperative cardioplegic contrast
  in utero
  late systolic posterior displacement
    on
  lateral left ventricular wall motion
    on
  left ventricular long axis
  long axis parasternal view
  loss of an "a" dip on
  MCE (myocardial contrast
    echocardiography)
  M-mode Doppler
  multiplanar transesophageal
  myocardial contrast (MCE)

echocardiography *(cont.)*
  myocardial perfusion
  parasternal long axis view
  parasternal short axis view
  pharmacologic stress
  postcontrast
  posterior left ventricular wall
    motion on
  postexercise
  postinjection
  postmyocardial infarction
  precontrast
  preinjection
  premyocardial infarction
  pulsed Doppler
  pulsed-wave (PW) Doppler
  real-time
  renal sinus
  resting
  right ventricular short axis
  sector scan
  SEE IT substernal epicardial
  septal wall motion on
  short axis view
  signal averaged
  single shot fast spin (SSFSE)
  stress
  subcostal short axis view
  subxiphoid view of
  three-dimensional (3D or 3-D)
  transesophageal (TEE)
  transthoracic (TTE)
  transthoracic three-dimensional
  two-dimensional (2D or 2-D)
  two-chamber
  ventricular wall motion
echo characteristics on ultrasound
Echo-Coat biopsy needle
Echo-Coat localization needle
Echo-Coat ultrasound biopsy needles
echocolonoscope
echo complex
echo contrast

echo contrast variability imaging
echo delay time (TE)
echo dense (or echodense)
echo density
echoencephalography
echo-enhanced cystosonography
echo-enhanced transcranial color-
  coded ultrasound
EchoEye 3-D ultrasound imaging
  system
EchoEye ultrasound imaging system
echo FLASH MR
EchoFlow blood velocity meter system
  (BVM-1)
echo-free area
echo-free central zone
echo-free space
echogastroscope
echogenic
echogenicity
echogenic immunoliposomes (ELIPs)
echogram, echography
  B-mode
  ophthalmic biometry by ultrasound
  transrectal
  transvaginal
echography for placement of radiation
  therapy fields
echoic
echoicity
echolucent plaque
EchoMark angiographic catheter
echo pattern
  homogeneous
  inhomogeneous
echophonocardiography
echo planar (or echo-planar) imaging
  (EPI)
  FLAIR
  multishot
  one-shot
  MR (magnetic resonance)
  pulse sequence
  sequence

echo reflectivity
echo reverberation
EchoSeed (iodine-125) brachytherapy
Echosight Jansen-Anderson intrauterine catheter
Echosight Patton coaxial catheter
echo signature
echo-tagging technique
echo texture (also echotexture)
echo time (TE)
echo train length (ETL)
Echovar Doppler system
ECI (Ensemble contrast imaging)
ECIC (extracranial-intracranial)
  arterial bypass
ECHO therapy
Eclipse ST cyclotron used with PET
  scan imagers
ECRB (extensor carpi radialis brevis)
  muscle
ECRL (extensor carpi radialis longus)
  muscle
ECT acquisition
ectasia
  alveolar
  annuloaortic
  basilar artery
  coronary artery
  diffuse arterial
  duct
  ductal
  dural
  mammary
  mammary duct
  mammary ductal
  renal tubular
  tubular
  ureteral
  vascular
ectatic emphysema
ectatic ureter
ectocardia

ectopia
  crossed kidney
  crossed renal
  crossed testicular
  renal
  renal cross-fused
  testis
  ureteral
ectopic beat
ectopic bone growth in joint
ectopic decidua
ectopic endometrium
ectopic focus (pl. foci)
ectopic impulse
ectopic kidney
ectopic papilla
ectopic pregnancy (EP)
  aborted
  hemorrhage in
  persistent
  ruptured
  tubal ring in
ectopic pregnancy locations
  abdominal
  ampullar tube
  cervical
  cornual (interstitial)
  eccentric
  extrauterine
  fallopian tube
  heterotopic
  infundibular tubal
  interstitial
  intraligamentous
  intramural
  isthmic tubal
  ovarian
  peritoneal
ectopic test
ectopic testis
ectopic thyroid tissue
ectopic ureter

ectopic ureterocele
ectopic urethral orifices
ectopic wall motion abnormality
ectopy
ectrodactyly
ECU (extensor carpi ulnaris) muscle
EDA (extravasation detection accessory)
EDAMS (encephaloduroarteriomyosynangiosis)
EDAS (encephaloduroarteriosynangiosis)
EDB (extensor digitorum brevis) muscle
EDC (extensor digitorum communis) muscle
eddy (pl. eddies)
eddy current artifact
eddy formation
edema
    acute pulmonary
    acute urethral
    alveolar
    alveolar pulmonary
    angioneurotic
    antral
    brain
    bronchiolar
    brown
    bullous
    bullous-like
    capillary permeability
    cardiac
    cardiogenic pulmonary
    cardiopulmonary
    cerebral
    bullous
    cervical
    chemical pulmonary
    chronic
    circumscribed
    collateral
    compressive

edema *(cont.)*
    cyclical
    cyclic idiopathic
    diffuse
    fingerprint
    focal
    frank pulmonary
    fulminant pulmonary
    generalized pulmonary
    gestational
    high altitude pulmonary (HAPE)
    hypervolemic pulmonary
    idiopathic
    ileocecal
    inflammatory
    interstitial
    interstitial pulmonary
    intracompartmental
    laryngeal
    leg
    liver
    local
    localized
    lymphatic
    lymph-
    malignant brain
    massive pulmonary hemorrhagic
    mediastinal
    mild
    negative image of pulmonary
    nephrotic
    nerve root
    neurogenic pulmonary
    noncardiac pulmonary
    noncardiogenic pulmonary
    osmotic
    paroxysmal pulmonary
    passive
    patchy
    pericholecystic
    pericystic
    perihilar
    perineoplastic

edema *(cont.)*
  periorbital
  peripheral
  peritumoral
  perivascular
  postoperative pulmonary
  pulmonary
  reexpansion pulmonary
  renal
  reperfusion (after lung transplanta-
    tion)
  solid (of lungs)
  stasis
  subglottic
  submucosal
  supraglottic
  terminal
  thalamic
  trace
  vasogenic
  venous
  vernal (of lung)
  visceral
edema fluid
edema neonatorum
edematous tissues
edentulous
edge
  boundary
  leading
  ligament reflecting
  ligament shelving
  liver
  Poupart ligament shelving
  sawtooth
  shelving
  sternal
  tentorial
  trailing
edge boundary artifact
edge detection angiography
edge effect

edge-enhanced error diffusion
  algorithm
edge misalignment artifact
edge profile acutance
edge-region pixel
edge ringing artifact
EDH (epidural hematoma)
EDL (extensor digitorum longus)
  muscle
Edmondson Grading System for
  hepatocellular carcinoma
EDQ (extensor digiti quinti) muscle
EDRT (endothelium-derived relaxant
  factor)
EDTMP (ethylenediaminetetramethy-
  lenephosphonate) (radiotherapy
  agent samarium Sm 153 lexidronam)
EDV (end diastolic volume)
EDVG (epididymography plus vasography)
Edwards diagnostic catheter
EDXRF (energy dispersive x-ray
  fluorescence) spectrometer
EF (ejection fraction)
EFF (electromagnetic focusing field)
  probe
efface
effaced gastric folds
effaced trabeculations
effacement
  cistern
  cisterna magna
  dural sac
  nerve root sheath
  sulcus
  ventricle
effect
  adverse
  anisotropic
  Anrep
  artifact
  attenuation

effect *(cont.)*
  Bayliss
  becquerel
  BOLD (blood oxygenation level
    dependent)
  Bohr
  BOLD
  Bowditch
  bronchodilator
  bronchomotor
  cavitation induced becquerel
  cavitation induced VUV (vacuum
    ultraviolet light)
  cobra head
  collimator exchange
  Compton
  copper wire
  cumulative
  deleterious
  demagnetization field
  Dotter
  dottering
  dynamic lineshape
  edge
  effect, fisheye
  flow-related enhancement
  halo
  hemispheric mass
  hemodynamic
  lag
  magic angle
  magnetization transfer
  masquerading
  mass
  neurotoxic
  purse-stringing
  reservoir
  silver wire
  snowplow
  stalk-section
  subtle
  vasodilatory
  Venturi

effect *(cont.)*
  washboard
  water relaxation
  Wolff-Chaikoff
effective refractory period (ERP)
effective renal blood flow (ERBF)
effective renal plasma flow (ERPF)
efferent arteriolar resistance
efferent digital nerve
efferent duct obstruction
efferent view
effervescent agent
efficacious
efficacy
  clinical
  drug therapy
  treatment
efficiency
  absolute-peak
  full energy peak
  valvular
effluent
effort
  inspiratory
  respiratory
  suboptimal
effort-dependent
effort thrombosis
effuse
effused chyle
effusion
  cardiac
  exudative
  free pleural
  hemorrhagic
  inflammatory joint
  ipsilateral pleural
  joint
  layering
  liquid pleural
  loculated
  loculated pleural
  malignant

effusion *(cont.)*
  noninflammatory joint
  parapneumonic
  pericardial (PE)
  pleural
  pleurisy with
  pleuropericardial
  pseudochylous
  serofibrinous pericardial
  subdural
  subpleural
  taut pericardial
  tuberculous
effusion artifact
effusion of blood in pleural cavity
eFlexTrial Probe2000
EG (esophagogastric) junction
Egan mammography
Egawa sign
egg-shaped congruous acetabulum
eggshell border of aneurysm
eggshell-like calcification
eggshell nodal calcification
egress of blood
EHL (extensor hallucis longus)
  muscle
EHM (extrahepatic metastasis)
EHT (electrohydrothermo-electrode
  or electrohydrothermal electrode)
eigenvector analysis
eigenvector, principal
8 x 8 pixel-block
eighth nerve tumor
Einthoven triangle
EIP (extensor indicis proprius) muscle
Eisenmenger complex
Eisenmenger syndrome
ejection, accelerated
ejection fraction (EF)
  area-length method for
  basilar half
  blunted
  BSA (body surface area)

ejection *(cont.)*
  cardiac
  computed
  depressed
  digital
  Dodge method for
  gallbladder
  global
  globally depressed
  interval
  Kennedy method for calculating
  left ventricular (LVEF)
  one-third
  regional
  resting left ventricular
  right ventricular (RVEF)
  systolic
  thermodilution
  well-preserved
ejection fraction acoustic
  quantification, left ventricular
ejection fraction by first pass
  technique
ejection phase index
ejection sound
  palpable aortic
  palpable pulmonic
ejection time
  increased left ventricular
  prolonged
EJV (external jugular vein)
EKG or ECG (electrocardiogram)
EKG-gated multislice
EKG-gated reconstruction
EKG-gated spin echo
EKG-synchronized digital subtraction
  angiography
EKG-triggered, flow-compensated,
  gradient echo image
Ektascan laser printer
El Gamal coronary bypass catheter
elaborate
elastic cross-section

elastic recoil of artery
elastic stable intramedullary nailing
    (ESIN)
elastic subtraction algorithms
elastic subtraction spiral CT
    angiography
elasticity
elasticity imaging
elastography
    intravascular ultrasound
    magnetic resonance (MRE)
    one-dimensional transient
    phase contrast magnetic resonance
    steady state
    transient
    ultrasonic
elastomyofibrosis
elbow
    baseball pitcher's
    boxer's
    floating
    golfer's
    javelin thrower's
    Little Leaguer's
    milkmaid's
    pulled
    reverse tennis
    tennis
    thrower's
    wrestler's
elbow fat pad sign
ELCA (excimer laser coronary angio-
    plasty)
Elecath thermodilution catheter
elective cardiac arrest and subsequent
    reperfusion
electric joint fluoroscopy
electrocardiogram (ECG or EKG)
electrocardiography
electrocardiogram-gated MRI
electrocardiogram-gated SPECT
electrocardiogram tracing
electrocardiographic gating

electrocardiographic gating with
    electron beam CT technology
electrocardiographic variant
electrocardiography, electrocardiogram
    (ECG or EKG)
electrocardiography-gated echo-planar
    imaging
electrocardiography-triggered navigator
    cardiac motion prescanning
electrocardiophonogram
electrocardioscanner, Compuscan
    Hittman computerized
electrocautery, radiofrequency
electrocorticographic evaluation
electrode
    bipolar saline-enhanced
    electrohydrothermal
    electrohydrothermo-electrode
    Medelec DMG 50 Teflon-coated
    monopolar
electrode monitoring
electrogastrogram
electrogastrography
electrolytes
electrolytic
electrolytically detachable coil
electromagnet, structured coil
electromagnetic blood flow study
electromagnetic heating of tumor
electromagnetic interference (EMI)
electromechanical dissociation (EMD)
    of heart
electrometer
electromyogram
electromyography
electron and x-ray diffraction patterns
electron arc therapy
electron(s), backscatter
electron beam angiography of
    coronary arteries
electron beam boost
electron beam computed tomography
    (EBCT)

electron beam CT scanner
electron beam dynamic CT
electron beam intraoperative radiotherapy (EBIORT)
electron boost
electron bolus
electron dosimetry
electron equilibrium loss
electronic portal imaging
electronic portal imaging device
(EPID)
electron linear accelerator
electron microscopy
electron photon field matching
electron production, secondary
electron spin resonance (ESR)
electron volt (eV)
electrophilic radioiodination
electrophoresis
electroplethysmography
electrostatic potential
electrovectorcardiogram
electrovectorcardiography
electrovibratography (EVG)
elements
 antimony
 calcium (Ca)
 carbon (C)
 cerium (Ce)
 cesium (Cs)
 chromium (Cr)
 copper (Cu)
 fluorine (F)
 gadolinium (Gd)
 gallium (Ga)
 holmium (Ho)
 indium (In)
 iodine (I)
 iridium (Ir)
 krypton (Kr)
 manganese (Mn)
 nitrogen (N)
 oxygen (O)

elements *(cont.)*
 palladium (Pd)
 phosphorus (P)
 potassium (K)
 rhenium (Re)
 rubidium (Rb)
 samarium (Sm)
 selenium (Se)
 strontium (Sr)
 tantalum (Ta)
 technetium (Tc)
 thallium (Tl)
 uranium (U)
 xenon (Xe)
elephant pelvis
elevated diaphragms
elevated hemidiaphragms
elimination kinetics
Elite double loop catheter
Ellestad protocol for treadmill stress
test
elimination, matched mask bone
ELIPs (echogenic immunoliposomes)
ellipsoid joint
elliptical
elliptic centric contrast-enhanced
magnetic resonance angiography
elliptic centric-ordered sequence
elliptic centric view ordering
elliptical distortion
ellipticity index
Ellis fracture of zygomaticomaxillary
complex (ZMC)
Ellis-Garland line
Ellis line
Ellis sign
elongated heart
elongation and tortuosity
eloquent areas of brain
ELPIDA architecture
Elscint camera
Elscint CT scanner
Elscint dual detector cardiac camera

Elscint Gyrex Prestige 2.0T MR
   imaging system
Elscint Privilege 0.5 T MR imaging
   system
Elscint Planar device
Elscint Twin CT scanner
Elsner syndrome
eluted
elution
elutriation
embarrassment
   circulatory
   cord
   midbrain function
   nerve root
   respiratory
embedding of stent coils
embolectomy, percutaneous balloon
emboli (pl. of embolus), "shower" of
embolic agent, Embol-78 liquid
embolic cerebral infarction
embolic event
embolic gangrene
embolic infarct
embolic material, nidus of
embolic obstruction
embolic occlusion
embolic phenomenon
embolic pneumonia
embolic shower
embolic stroke
embolism (also embolus)
   air
   amniotic fluid
   arterial
   arterial stenosis
   atheromatous
   bacillary
   bile pulmonary
   bland
   bone marrow
   cancer
   capillary

embolism *(cont.)*
   cardiogenic
   catheter-induced
   cellular
   cerebral
   cerebral fat
   cholesterol
   coronary artery
   cotton fiber
   crossed
   direct
   fat
   fibrin platelet
   foam
   gas
   gas nitrogen
   hematogenous
   infective
   intracranial
   intraluminal
   lymphogenous
   massive
   miliary
   multilobar pulmonary
   multiple
   obturating
   occluding spring
   oil
   pantaloon
   paradoxical
   peripheral
   plasmodium
   polyurethane foam
   prosthetic valve
   pulmonary (PE)
   pulmonary venous-systemic air
   pyemic
   recurrent
   renal cholesterol
   retinal
   retrograde
   riding
   septic

embolism *(cont.)*
  septic pulmonary
  silent cerebral
  straddling
  submassive pulmonary
  thrombus
  trichinous
  tumor
  venous
  visceral
embolization
  alcohol
  angiographic (AE)
  angiographic variceal
  atheromatous cholesterol crystal
  balloon therapeutic
  balloon and coil
  bronchial artery
  cardiac tumor
  cholesterol
  chronic lung
  coil (of unwanted vessel)
  coil (therapeutic)
  diffuse cholesterol
  disseminated atheromatous
  disseminated cholesterol
  embryonal cell testicular tumor
  Embryon GIFT transfer catheter
  Embryon HSG (hysterosalpingog-
    raphy/hysterosonography)
    catheter
  embryoscopy
  endovascular
  fibroid
  flow-directed
  Gelfoam powder
  Ivalon
  massive
  microvascular
  percutaneous transvenous
  selective percutaneous transhepatic
  selective renal artery
  septic

embolization *(cont.)*
  Silastic bead
  stent
  subsegmental transcatheter arterial
    (STAE)
  super selective
  super selective adrenal arterial
  super selective transcatheter
  therapeutic
  tract
  transarterial
  transcatheter oily chemo-
    embolization
  transcatheter variceal
  transhepatic (THE)
  uterine arterial (UAE)
embolization of vascular malformation
embolization transcatheter therapy
embolotherapy, catheter
Embol-78 liquid embolic agent
embolus (pl. emboli) (see *embolism)*
embolus trap, Mobin-Uddin
embryonal cell carcinoma
embryonal tumor
embryonal vein
embryonic anastomosis
embryonic aortic arch
embryonic branchial arch
EMED scanner
emergent
emergently
emesis
EMF (endomyocardial fibrosis)
EMI CT scanner
eminence
  arcuate
  articular
  collateral
  cruciate
  cruciform
  deltoid
  facial
  frontal

eminence *(cont.)*
  genital
  hypothenar
  iliopubic
  iliopectineal
  intercondylar
  intercondyloid
  medial
  median
  occipital
  pyramidal
  thenar
  thyroid
  tibial
emission and transmission data
emission filter
emission probability
emit, emitted
emitter
  alpha particle
  Auger electron
emphysema
  alveolar
  alveolar duct
  atrophic
  bronchiolar
  bullous
  centriacinar
  centrilobular
  chronic
  chronic hypertrophic
  chronic obstructive
  chronic tuberculous
  compensating
  compensatory
  congenital lobar
  cystic
  cystic pulmonary
  diffuse
  distal acinar
  distal lobular
  ectatic
  false

emphysema *(cont.)*
  focal dust
  gangrenous
  generalized
  giant bullous
  glass blower's
  hypoplastic
  idiopathic unilobar
  infantile lobar
  interlobular
  interstitial
  intestinal
  liquefactive
  lobar
  localized obstructive
  lung
  mediastinal
  neck
  necrotizing
  neonatal cystic pulmonary
  obstructive
  oxygen dependent
  panlobular
  paracicatricial
  paraseptal
  pericicatricial
  postoperative
  postsurgical
  pulmonary
  pulmonary interstitial (PIE)
  pulmonary subcutaneous
    encephalitis
  senile
  skeletal
  small-lunged
  subcutaneous
  substantial
  surgical
  traumatic
  unilateral
  unilateral pulmonary
  vesicular

emphysematous bleb
emphysematous bulla
emphysematous cholecystitis
emphysematous COPD (chronic
    obstructive pulmonary disease)
emphysematous epididymitis
emphysematous gastritis
emphysematous lungs
emphysematous pyelitis
emphysematous pyelonephritis
emphysematous type A disease
empirical therapy
emplaced (verb)
empty collapsed lung
empty delta sign
empty lumen
emptying time
emptying, tortuous
empty sella syndrome
empyema
    chest
    gallbladder
    interlobar
    latent
    left-sided
    loculated
    metapneumonic
    pericardial
    pleural
    pulsating
    right-sided
    spinal
    subdural
    synpneumonic
    thoracic
    tuberculous
empyema pericardium
empyema with pachypleuritis
emulsion
en bloc
encapsulated abscess
encapsulated brain abscess
encapsulated radioactive "seeds"

encasement, vascular
encephalitic
encephalitis, Nipah virus
encephalocele with cranium bifidum
encephaloclastic lesion
encephalocystocele
encephalodysplasia
encephalography
    air
    A-mode
encephaloid
encephalolith
encephaloma
encephalomalacia
encephalopathy, sporadic subcortical
    arteriosclerotic
enchondral ossification
enchondroma
enchondromatosis
encircle
encircled
encircling
encirclement
encoded-Fourier
encoded, wavelet-
encoding gradient
encoding, sensitivity
Encompass cardiac network
encroachment
    bony
    foraminal
    luminal
encryption algorithms
encryption, scheme
en cuirasse, cor
encysted calculus
encysted hernia
encysted pleurisy
endarterectomy and coronary artery
    bypass graft (E-CABG)
end diastole
end diastolic flow
end diastolic polar map

end diastolic pressure
end diastolic pressure-volume relation
end diastolic velocity (EDV)
end diastolic volume (EDV)
end expiratory lung volume (FRC)
end expiratory pressure
end inspiratory pressure
endoanal coil
endoanal MR imaging
endoanal sonography
endobrachyesophagus
endobronchial brachytherapy
endobronchial carcinoma
endobronchial neoplasm
endocardial activation mapping
endocardial catheter mapping
endocardial cushion defect
endocardial fibroelastosis
endocardial fibrosis, Davies
endocardial mapping
endocardial pocket
endocarditis
    aortic valve
    atypical verrucous
    Libman-Sacks
    Loeffler
    pulmonary artery catheter-
      associated
endocardium
    disc of
    wafer of
Endocare Horizon prostatic stent
ENDOcare nitinol urinary stent
Endocare renal cryoablation
endocavitary applicator system
endochondral bone
endochondral ossification
EndoCoil biliary stent
endocranium
endocrine fracture
endodermal cyst
endoergic reaction
endoesophageal MRI coil

end of atrial systole
endogenous arteriovenous fistula
endogenous callus formation
endoleak
endoluminal stent
endolymphatic duct
endolymphatic sac
endometrial ablation
    laser
    Microsulis
    NovaSure
    PEARL
    rollerbar *or* roller bar electrode
endometrial ablator
endometrial cryoablation
endometrial echo
endometrial echocardiogram
endometrial malignancy
endometrial polyp
endometrial stromal sarcoma
endometrioid tumor
endometriosis
    abdominal
    adhesive
    appendiceal
    bladder
    broad ligament
    burned-out
    cervical
    colonic involvement of
    fallopian tube
    implantation theory of
    intestinal
    intra-abdominal
    lung
    myometrial
    ovarian
    patchy
    peritoneal
    rectal
    rectovaginal nodules of
    sciatic
    studding of

endometriosis *(cont.)*
  stromal
  ureteral
  uterine
  vaginal
  vulvar
endometriosis in skin of scar
endometriosis of cul-de-sac of
  Douglas
endometriosis of rectovaginal septum
  and vagina
endometriosis uterus
endometrium, ectopic
endomyocardial biopsy, ultrasonic
  guidance for
endomyocardial fibrosis, mural
end-on vessel
endophlebitis
Endo-P-Probe
endoprosthesis
  biliary
  double lumen
  double pigtail
  large bore bile duct
  polytetrafluoroethylene-covered
    nitinol
  self-expanding metallic
endorectal coil
endorectal ileal pouch
endorectal ileal pull-through
endorectal magnetic resonance
  imaging
endorectal ultrasonography
end organ
endoscope
  echocolonoscope
  echogastroscope
  Jackson bronchoscope
  Jackson-Olympus bronchoscope
  Karl Storz bronchoscope
  Littmann stethoscope
  Olympus angioscope

endoscope *(cont.)*
  Olympus CF-1T100L forward-
    viewing video colonoscope
  Olympus EVIS Q-200V video
    endoscope
  Olympus GF-UM130 ultrasound
    gastroscope
  Pentax EUP-EC124 ultrasound
    gastroscope
  Reichert flexible sigmoidoscope
  Sonde enteroscope
  SurgiScope
  ultrasound stethoscope
  Valle hysteroscope
endoscopic bougienage
endoscopic catheterization
endoscopic optical coherence tomography (EOCT)
endoscopic quadrature RF coil
endoscopic retrograde cholangiography
  (ERC)
endoscopic retrograde cholangiopancreatography (ERCP)
endoscopic retrograde pancreatic duct
  cannulation
endoscopic retrograde parenchymography (ERP)
endoscopic sclerosing therapy
endoscopic ultrasonography
endoscopic ultrasound (EUS)
endoscopic ultrasound-assisted band
  ligation
endoscopic ultrasound-guided fine
  needle aspiration (EUS-FNA)
endoscopic washing pipe
endoscopic water pick
endoscopically
endoscopist
endoscopy
  capsule
  virtual
  VIVENDI virtual

endoskeleton
EndoSonics IVUS/balloon dilatation
   catheter
endosonogram
endosonography
Endosound endoscopic ultrasound
   catheter
endosteal callus
endosteal revascularization
endosteal surface
endosteum
endosystolic volume (ESV)
endotenon
endothelialization of stent
endothelialized vascular grafts
endotheliomatous meningioma
endothelium
   arterial
   pulmonary capillary
   squamous
endothelium-derived contracting factor
endothelium-derived relaxant factor
   (EDRF)
EndoTIP cannula
Endotrac carpal tunnel release system
endotracheal (ET) tube intubation
endovaginal coil
endovaginal sonography
endovaginal transducer
endovaginal ultrasonography (EVUS)
endovaginal ultrasound (EVUS)
endovaginal sonography
endovascular aortic graft
endovascular brachytherapy
endovascular coil
endovascular coil embolization
   procedure
endovascular embolization
endovascular flow wire study
endovascular stent-graft
endovascular therapy
endovascular ultrasonography

endplate
   hyaline-cartilage (of intervertebral
      disk)
   vertebral body
endpoint, measurable
end pressure artifact
end stage rejection
end stage renal failure
end systolic polar map
end systolic pressure-volume relation
end systolic reversal
end systolic volume (ESV) index
end to end anastomosis
end to side anastomosis
Enecat CT (barium sulfate) imaging
   agent
enema (see also *bowel prep*)
   air
   air contrast barium
   analeptic
   barium (BE)
   blind
   CO_2
   contrast
   Cortenema retention
   double contrast barium (DCBE)
   flatus
   Fleet
   full column barium
   Gastrografin
   HalfLytely and bisacodyl tablets
      bowel prep kit
   Harris flush
   hydrocortisone
   hydrogen peroxide
   Kayexalate
   lactulose
   mesalamine
   methylene blue
   nuclear
   phosphate
   Phospho-Soda (Fleet)
   prednisolone
   retention

enema *(cont.)*
  Rowasa
  saline cleansing
  single contrast barium
  small bowel
  soapsuds (SSE)
  steroid foam
  sulfasalazine
  tap water
  theophylline olamine
  water soluble contrast
enemas administered until clear
energy
  beam
  kinetic
  low photon
  treatment
  variable
energy decays
energy dispersive x-ray fluorescence
  (EDXRF) spectrometer
energy transfer process
en face view
Engelmann disease
Engel-Recklinghausen disease
engorged collecting system
engorged tissues
engorged veins
engorgement
  circumferential perilesional
  mucosal
  parenchymal
  pulmonary artery
  vascular
  venous
  wedge-shaped perilesional
Enhance deblurring method
enhanced imaging
Enhancer (barium sulfate) imaging
  agent
enhancement
  contrast
  Doppler flow signal

enhancement *(cont.)*
  heterogeneous isodense
  isodense
  nodule
  nonhomogeneous
  PALA
  peak
  signal
  vascular MR contrast
enhancement morphology
enhancement pattern
enhancement rate, instantaneous
enhancing lesion
enlargement
  cardiac silhouette
  chamber
  compensatory
  hilar lymph node
  mediastinal lymph node
enophthalmic
en plaque, meningioma
Ensemble contrast imaging (ECI)
ensiform appendix
ensiform process
EnSite 3000 imaging system
ensued
ensuing
enteral alimentation
enteral bone
enteral nutrition (EN)
enterobiliary
enterocele sac
enteroclysis, computed tomography
enterococcus
enterocutaneous fistula
enterocystoma
enteroenteral fistula
enteroinsular axis
enterolith
enteropathy, protein-losing
enteroperitoneal abscess
enteroptosis
enterourethral fistula

enterovaginal fistula
enterovesical fistula
Entero Vu (barium sulfate for suspension) imaging agent
enthesophytes, subacromial
entrapment
artery
gas
guide-wire
nerve
soft tissue
entrapment syndrome
Entristar skin-level gastrostomy tube
Entrobar (barium sulfate [methyl-
cellulose diluent]) imaging agent
entry slice phenomenon (artifact MRI)
entry zone
enucleated
envelope, soft tissue
environment, fibroblastic
environmental implication
environmental plutonium
enzymes, fluid
EOL (end of life)
EORTC (European Organization for
Research and Treatment of Cancer)
eosinophilic cholangiopathy
eosinophilic cystitis
eosinophilic granuloma
eosinophilic pneumonia
EP (ectopic pregnancy)
eparterial bronchus
EPB (extensor pollicis brevis) muscle
EPBF (effective pulmonary blood
flow)
ependymoma
malignant
myxopapillary
spinal cord
ephemeral pneumonia
EPI (echo planar imaging)
Epi-C (barium sulfate) imaging agent
epicardial attachment

epicardial Doppler echocardiography
epicardial Doppler flow transducer
epicardial fat pad
epicardial imaging
epicardial implantation
epicardial reflection
epicardial space
epicardial surface
epicardial tension
epicardial vessels, vasorelaxation of
epicardium
epicondylar fracture
epicondyle
epicortical lesion
epicranial aponeurosis
epicranial subaponeurotic hemorrhage
EPID (electronic portal imaging
device)
epidermal growth factor
epidermoid cyst
epidermoid tumor
epididymal adenomatoid tumor
epididymal aspiration catheter
epididymal ligament
epididymis
appendix of
body of
edema of
inflammation of
interstitial congestion of
ligament of
lobule of
sinus of
tail of
epididymitis, emphysematous
epididymogram, contrast
epididymography
epididymography plus vasography
(EDVG)
epididymo-orchitis
epidural abscess
epidural blood
epidural catheter

epidural cavity
epidural hematoma
epidural hemorrhage
epidural mass
epidural space
epidural venography
epidurogram
epidurography
epigastric discomfort
epigastric distress
epigastric hernia
epigastrium
epiglottic disruption
epiglottis, down-folding
epilepsy-causing brain tumors
epilepsy, temporal lobe
epileptic focus
epileptogenic foci
epileptogenic zone
epiphrenic diverticulum
epiphyseal arrest
epiphyseal chondroblastic growth
epiphyseal coxa vara
epiphyseal disk
epiphyseal fracture
epiphyseal growth
epiphyseal hyperplasia
epiphyseal plate
epiphyseal (or epiphysial)
epiphysis (pl. epiphyses)
   annular
   atavistic
   capital
   capital femoral
   capitular
   hypertrophy of
   ischemic
   Perthes
   pressure
   slipped
   slipped capital femoral (SCFE)
   slipped upper femoral (SUFE)
   stippled

epiphysis *(cont.)*
   tibial
   traction
epiploic appendagitis
episcleral plaque brachytherapy
episode, silent ischemic
episodic colic
epispadias
Epistar subtraction angiography
epistaxis, spontaneous
epitendineum
epithalamus
epithelial malignancy
epithelial membrane antigen (EMA)
   antibody
epithelial-myoepithelial carcinoma
epithelialization, creeping
epithelioid hemangioendothelioma
epithelioid sarcoma
epithelium of urinary bladder
epitrochlear
EPL (extensor pollicis longus) muscle
E point on apex cardiogram
E point of cardiac apex pulse
E point to septal separation (EPSS)
eponychium
Eppendorf catheter
EPR dosimetry
EPSS (E point to septal separation)
EQP (extensor quinti proprius)
equalization
   contrast-limited adaptive histogram
   histogram
   multiscale adaptive histogram
   peripheral
   x-ray beam
equalization of pressure
equalized diastolic pressures
equation
   Bloch
   Kety
   Larmor
   Stewart-Hamilton

equilibrium angiocardiography
equilibrium factor
equilibrium MUGA scan
equilibrium phase
equilibrium point
equilibrium radionuclide angiocardiography
equilibrium radionuclide angiogram
equilibrium view
equinus deformity
equipment artifact
equipment
   interventional
   real-time
equipment artifact
equivocal findings
equivocal lesion
Eraso projection of jugular foramina
Erb disease
Erb-Duchenne-Klumpke injury to
   brachial plexus
ERBF (effective renal blood flow)
Erb point (of heart)
ERC (endoscopic retrograde
   cholangiography)
ERCP (endoscopic retrograde
   cholangiopancreatography)
ERCP manometry
Erdheim-Chester disease
Erdheim cystic medionecrosis
Erdheim I syndrome
ERE (external rotation in extension)
erect position
erect view
erectile dysfunction
erector spinae
ERF (external rotation in flexion)
ergonovine test
erosion
   articular
   bony
   bronchial
   duodenal

erosion *(cont.)*
   epiphyseal
   gastric
   gastric antral
   graft-enteric
   joint
   linear
   osteoclastic
   pedicle
   plaque
   salt and pepper duodenal
   tumor
erosion of articular surface
erosive gastritis
ERP (effective refractory period)
ERP (endoscopic retrograde parenchymography)
   atrial
   ventricular
ERPF (effective renal plasma flow)
error
   darkroom
   Hausdorff
   interpretive
   isocenter placement
   magnification
   mean-square
   operator-dependent
   photoreceptor fractional velocity
   positioning
   raster spacing
   sensing
   size estimation
error diffusion method
error sum criterion
erythema of joint
erythematosus
   lupus
   systemic lupus
escape beat
escape interval
escape mechanism, ventricular

escape of air into lung connective
    tissue
escape-peak ratio
Escherichia coli bacterial pneumonia
Escort balloon stone extractor
E sign on x-ray
ESIN (elastic stable intramedullary
    nailing)
ESOLAN program
EsophaCoil biliary stent
esophageal achalasia
esophageal adenoma
esophageal A ring
esophageal B ring
esophageal distortion
esophageal duplication
esophageal dysmotility
esophageal fold
esophageal hiatus
esophageal inlet
esophageal motility disorder,
    nonspecific (NEMD)
esophageal obturator airway
esophageal plexus
esophageal reflux
esophageal spasm
esophageal spasm mimicking
    myocardial infarction
esophageal varices
esophageal web
esophageal window
esophagitis
esophagogastric fat pad
esophagogastric junction
esophagogram
esophagography
esophagorespiratory fistula (ERF)
esophagospasm
esophagram
    barium swallow
    contrast

esophagus
    achalasia of
    aperistaltic
    A ring of
    Barrett
    B ring of
    cervical
    columnar-lined
    corkscrew (diffuse esophageal
        spasm)
    distal
    dysmotile
    nutcracker
    spastic
    thoracic
    tortuous
    upper thoracic
ESP (end systolic pressure)
ESP/ESV ratio
ESR (electron spin resonance)
ESR measurement
Essex-Lopresti calcaneal fracture
esthesioneuroblastoma
estimated blood loss (EBL)
estimation
    bayesian image (BIE)
    fractional moving blood volume
    MR volume
    volume
estrogen-producing ovarian tumor
estrogen-receptor positive (ER+)
    tumor
estrogen-receptor-negative (ER-) tumor
estrogen receptor status
estrogen-secreting testicular tumor
ESV (end systolic volume)
ESVI (end systolic volume index)
ESWI/ESVI (end systolic wall stress
    index/end systolic volume index)
ESWL (extracorporeal shock wave
    lithotripsy)
ET (ejection time)

ET (endotracheal)
ctching, track
ethanol, ethanolism
ethanol injection, percutaneous
ethanol therapy
ethiodized oil
Ethiodol (ethiodized oil) imaging agent
ethmoid bone
ethmoid sinus
cthmoidal canal
ethmoidal foramen
ethmoidal meningoencephalocele
ethylene vinyl alcohol copolymer
   thrombotic agent
etiology undetermined
etiology unknown
ETL (echo train length)
ETL 3D FSE imaging
E to A changes
E-TOF (time of flight) detecting
   module
E to F slope of valve on echocardiogram
EtOH (ethanol; ethyl alcohol)
EtOH-associated liver disease
e-Touch technology
ETT (exercise tolerance test)
ET (endotracheal) tube
EU (excretory urography)
eukinesis
EU-M30S endoscopic ultrasonography
   receiver from Olympus
Eureka collimator
European Organization for Research
   and Treatment of Cancer (EORTC)
"euro radiology" (phonetic for
   uroradiology)
eurysternum
EUS (endoscopic ultrasound)
EUS (endoscopic ultrasonography)
EUS-FNA (endoscopic ultrasound-
   guided fine needle aspiration)
euthyroid sick syndrome

eV (electron volt)
Evac-Q-Kit
Evac-Q-Kwik bowel prep
evacuating cannula
evacuation
   colonic
   digital rectal
   precipitate
evacuation proctography
evaluation
   biological
   electrocorticographic
   functional
   in vitro
   initial staging
   noninvasive
evacuation disorder
evaluation of deep veins for patency
   and valvular reflux
evaluation of glucose metabolism
evanescent
Evans blue imaging agent
Evans fracture classification system
Evans syndrome
EVD (external ventricular drain)
even distribution of echoes in
   ultrasonography
event
   adverse
   atrial sensed (As)
   cardinal
   embolic
   inciting
   ischemic
   morbid
   precipitating
   untoward
   ventricular sensed
event counter
event marker
event recorder
eventration (peaking)
eventration of diaphragms

eversion sprain
evert, everted
EVG (electrovibratography)
evolution, stroke in
Evolution XP ultrafast CT scanner
evolving stroke
EVUS (endovaginal ultrasonography,
  ultrasound)
EVUS (endovaginal ultrasound)
Ewald test meal
Ewart sign
Ewing sarcoma
Ewing tumor
ExAblate 2000 system
exacerbate, exacerbated
exacerbation, acute
exaggeration of pelvic venous plexuses
exam (examination)
eXamine cholangiography catheter
exametazime imaging agent
exanthematous disease
excavatum, pectus
Excelart Planissimo scanner
Excelart short bore MRI
excellent prognosis
excessive joint play
exchange
  air
  catheter
  coupling
  guidewire
  narrowing
excimer (from "excited dimer")
excimer laser
excimer laser coronary angioplasty
  (ELCA)
excitation
  TCR rebound
  variable flip angle
  wave of
excitation filter
excitation function measurement
excitation profile

excitation-spoiled fat-suppressed T1-
  weighted SE images
exclusionary cue
exclusion-HPLC technique
exclusion, subtotal gastric
excrescence, bony
excrete
excretory function
excretory intravenous pyelography
excretory phase
excretory urogram
excretory urography (EU)
excursion
exenteration
  anterior pelvic
  total pelvic
exercise echocardiography
exercise first pass LVEF
exercise images
exercise-induced ischemia
exercise intolerance
exercise load (kpm/min)
exercise, modified stage
exercise oximetry
exercise strain gauge venous
  plethysmography
exercise stress-redistribution
  scintigraphy
exercise thallium-201 stress test
exercise thallium-201 tomography
exhalation
exit site of catheter
exit wound
Exner plexus
exocardia
exoccipital bone
exoergic reaction
Exogen SAFHS (sonic accelerated
  fracture healing system)
exogenous invasion
exogenous lipoid pneumonia
exogenous obesity
exogenous pneumonia

exophytic adenocarcinoma
Exorcist respiratory compensation
  technique
exostosis (pl. exostoses)
  blocker's
  bony
  epiphyseal
  hereditary multiple
  hypertrophic
  impingement
  marginal
  retrocalcaneal
  tackler's
  traction
  turret
expandable access catheter (EAC)
expanded lung
expanding intracranial mass
expansile lesion
expansile lytic lesion
expansion
  complete stent
  emphysematous
  fluid
  fusiform
  lung
  rapid fluid
  stent
Expert-XL densitometer
expiration, quantitative CT during
expiratory chest
expiratory computed tomography
expiratory flow
explant pathologic correlation
exploration, common bile duct
  (CBDE)
exploration of pseudoaneurysm
Explorer ST fixed curve diagnostic
  catheters
Explorer 360° rotational diagnostic
  catheter
Explorer X 70 intraoral radiography
  system

exponential decay
exponential shape
exponential simultaneous waveforms
exposure
  asbestos
  bone-tendon
  double
  intraperitoneal
exposure variation
Express over the wire balloon catheter
expression
  acute phase gene
  HER-2 neu oncoprotein
expression vector
exquisite detail
exsanguinate, exsanguinated
exstrophy
extended pattern
extended tibial in situ bypass
extension
  basal
  Buck
  Codivilla
  extraaxial
  hilar
  intracavitary
  medial
  parenchymal
  parietal
  suprasellar
  tumor
extension injury of spine
extensive dissection
extensor
  apparatus
  mechanism
extensor carpi radialis brevis (ECRB)
  muscle
extensor carpi radialis longus (ECRL)
  muscle
extensor digitorum communis (EDC)
  muscle

extensor digitorum longus (EDL)
  muscle
extensor hallucis longus (EHL) muscle
extensor hood mechanism
extensor indicis proprius (EIP) muscle
extensor pollicis brevis (EPB) muscle
extensor pollicis longus (EPL) muscle
extensor quinti proprius (EQP) muscle
extensus, hallux
exteriorization
external beam radiation therapy
  (EBRT)
external blow over a full bladder
external carotid artery (ECA)
external carotid steal syndrome
external fixation
external heat generating source
external hemorrhage
external hernia
external hyperthermia treatment
external iliac artery
external inguinal ring
external jugular vein
external oblique aponeurosis
external os of uterus
external ring
external ventricular drain (EVD)
external wire fixation
extirpation of saphenous vein
extra-articular fracture
extra-adrenal chromaffin tissue
extra-adrenal sites
extra-articular resection
extra-axial fluid collection, crescent-
  shaped
extracapillary lesion
extracapsular dissection
extracapsular fracture
extracardiac anomalies
extracardiac collateral circulation
extracardiac malformation
extracardiac right to left shunt
extracavitary-infected graft

extracavitary prosthetic arterial graft
extracerebral intracranial glioneural
  hamartoma
extracorporeal membrane oxygenation
  (ECMO) therapy
extracorporeal photochemotherapy
extracorporeal shock wave lithotripsy
  (ESWL)
extracranial carotid artery atherosclerosis
extracranial carotid occlusive disease
extracranial cerebral circulation
extracranial-intracranial bypass (ECIC)
extracranial neoplasm
extracranial vessel
extraction
  automatic
  contour
  disphenoid
  first pass
  fringe skeleton
  stone
  vascular segmentation and
extraction catheter
  transcutaneous
  transluminal
extraction catheter atherectomy
extraction column
extraction method
extracutaneous intrathoracic involvement
extradural abscess
extradural artery
extradural compartment
extradural defect
extradural space
extradural tumor
extradural vertebral plexus of veins
extragonadal
extrahepatic bile ducts, dilated
extrahepatic biliary atresia (EBA)
extraintestinal
extraluminal air

extraluminal imaging agent
extraluminal endarterectomy
extraluminal fluid
extramedullary hemangioma
extramedullary hematopoiesis
extraneous material
extraovarian mass
extraparenchymal cyst
extrapericardial dissection
extraperitoneal excision of lower
  one-third of ureter
extraperitoneal rupture
extraperitoneal space
extrapleural drainage
extrapleural hemorrhage
extrapleural space
extrapolate
extrapolation
extrapulmonary injury
extrapulmonary tuberculosis
extrapyramidal tract
extrarenal pelvis
extraskeletal osteosarcoma
extrathecal injection
extrathecal nerve roots
extrathoracic obstruction
extrauterine ectopic pregnancy
  locations
extrauterine gestation
extrauterine pregnancy
extravasated blood
extravasated contrast
extravasated imaging agent
extravasation
  bile
  blood
  contrast
  dye
  fluid
  intravascular content
  joint fluid
  radiopaque fluid
  urinary

extravasation detection accessory
  (EDA)
extravasation of contrast
extravascular fluid
extravascular mass
extravascular pressure
extraventricular obstruction
extravesical opacification
extremity (pl. extremities)
  lower (LEs)
  upper (UEs)
extrinsic carpal ligaments
extrinsic compression of trachea
extrinsic foot muscles
extrinsic lesion
extrinsic sick sinus syndrome
extrude
extruding
extrusion, disk
extubate
extubation
exuberant atheroma formation
exuberant granulation tissue
exudate
exudation
exudation of fibrin-rich fluid
exudative bronchiolitis
exudative consolidation
exudative effusion
exudative pericardial fluid
exudative pleurisy
exudative tuberculosis
ex vacuo, hydrocephalus
ex vivo magnetic resonance imaging
eyelet, rod
eye-of-the-tiger sign
eye shield
  lead
  tungsten
eye-view 3D-CRT

F, f

F (fluorine) (an element)
FAB (French/American/British)
    classification
Fab (fragment antigen binding)
    fragment
fabella
fabellofibular complex
Fabry disease
FAC (ferric ammonium citrate)
    imaging agent
face, en
facet (also facette)
    articular
    atlas
    capitate
    clavicular
    corneal
    costal
    flat
    hamate
    inferior
    inferior costal
    inferior medial
    Lenoir
    locked
    lunate

facet (cont.)
    scaphoid
    squatting
    superior
    superior articular
    superior costal
    transverse costal
facet capsule disruption
facet dislocation
facet jamming and hypomobility
facet joint
facet joint vacuum
facet surface of vertebra
facet syndrome
facet tropism
faceted gallstone
facial asymmetry
facial bipartition
facial fracture
facial nerve (seventh cranial nerve)
facial nerve canal
facies ossea
facile synthesis
facing of metacarpal heads
facioauriculovertebral (FAV)
    syndrome

faciostenosis
FACScan (fluorescence-activated cell
  sorter) flow cytometer
FACSVantage cell sorter
FACT (focused appendix computed
  tomography)
factitial
factor (pl. factors)
  Boltzmann
  EDRT
  endothelium-derived relaxant
    (EDRT)
  epidermal growth
  equilibrium
  geometry
  NOMOS correction
  overrelaxation
  prognostic
  recurrent human granulocyte
    colony stimulating (r-met
    HuG-CSF)
  technical
  wedge
Fader Tip ureteral stent
Fahr-Volhard disease
FAI (functional aerobic impairment)
failed back surgery syndrome (FBSS)
failure
  adrenal
  cardiac
  congestive heart (CHF)
  hepatic
  liver
  heart
  multiple organ
  multisystem
  pituitary
  postinfarction
  pulmonary
  renal
  respiratory
  vein graft
  ventricular

Fairbanks changes on x-ray
falciform ligament
falcine region
falcotentorial meningioma
falcula
falcular
fallen fragment
fallopian tube abscess
fallopian tube, accessory
fallopian tube diverticula
fallopian tube ectopic pregnancy
  locations
fallopian tube endometriosis
fallopian tube occlusion
falloposcopy (with imaging)
Fallot, tetralogy of
fallout, signal
false aneurysm
false channel
false color scale
false diverticulum
false emphysema
false lumen
false profile view
false sac
falx
  calcification of
  cerebral
falx cerebelli
falx cerebri
falx meningioma
familial adenomatous polyposis (FAP)
familial aortic dissection
familial avascular necrosis of
  phalangeal epiphysis
familial cardiomegaly
familial cavernous malformation
familial goiter
familial hypophosphatemic rickets
fan angle
fan beam
fan-beam collimator
fan-beam densitometry

fan-beam dual energy x-ray absorptiometry (DEXA) scan
fan-beam formula
fan-beam projection
fan-beam reconstruction
Fanconi-Hegglin syndrome
fan-shaped view
FAP (femoral artery pressure)
Faraday catheter
faradic (electrical) stimulation
Farber disease
Farber syndrome
far field
farmer's lung
fascia
  anal
  antebrachial
  anterior rectus
  axillary
  bicipital
  brachial
  broad
  buccopharyngeal
  Camper
  cervical
  clavipectoral
  Cloquet
  Colles
  cremasteric
  crural
  cribriform
  Cruveilhier
  deep
  deltoid
  dentate
  diaphragmatic
  endopelvic
  endothoracic
  extraperitoneal
  Gerota
  iliac
  infraspinous
  investing

fascia *(cont.)*
  lateral oblique
  lateroconal
  lumbar
  medial geniculate
  obturator
  obturator internus
  palmar
  parietal pelvic
  pelvic
  perineal
  psoas
  quadratus femoris
  renal
  rim of
  Scarpa
  Sibson
  subcutaneous
  superficial
  superficial temporalis
  superficial temporoparietal
  thoracolumbar
  visceral pelvic
fascia lata (but *tensor fasciae latae*)
fascial plane
fascial rent
fascial sling
fascial thickening
fascial tract
fasciculus (pl. fasciculi)
  arcuate
  lenticular
  longitudinal
  longitudinalis medialis
  medial longitudinal (MLF)
fasciitis, necrotizing
fasciogram
FAST (flow-assisted, short term)
FAST balloon catheter
Fastcard
fast cardiac phase contrast cine
  imaging
Fast-Cath introducer catheter

fast dynamic volumetric x-ray CT
fast-FLAIR technique
fast flow lesions
fast flow malformation
fast flow vascular anomaly
fast Fourier spectral analysis
fast Fourier transform (FFT)
fast fractionation
fast GE (Fastcard) sequences
fast low-angle shot (FLASH)
fast multiplanar spoiled gradient-
  recalled (FMPSPGR) imaging
fast-neutron therapy
fast PC cine MR sequence with
  echo-planar gradient
fast phase-contrast MRI
fast routine production
fast SE (FSE) imaging
fast SE and fast IR (FMPIR) imaging
fast SE train
fast short tau inversion recovery (fast
  STIR)
fast spin echo acquisition
fast spin echo MR imaging
fast spin echo T2-weighted image
fast spoiled gradient-recalled (FSPGR)
  MR imaging
fast STIR (short tau inversion
  recovery)
fat
  abdominal
  dietary
  digital process of
  extraperitoneal
  ischiorectal pad of
  pericolonic
  perihilar
  perinephric
  perirectal
  perirenal
  preperitoneal
  properitoneal
  protruding

fat *(cont.)*
  renal
  subcutaneous
fatal dose of radiation
fatal exsanguination
fatal herniation
fat- and water-suppressed T2-weighted
  images
fat-blood interface (FBI) sign
fat C2 sign
fat embolism syndrome (FES)
fat embolus, cerebral
fatigability
fatigue damage
fatigue fracture
fatigue, progressively severe
fat line, subcutaneous
fat metabolism
fat pad
  abdominal
  antimesenteric
  foveal
  heel
  Hoffa
  infrapatellar
  ischiorectal
  pericardial
  scalene
fat pad sign
fat plane
FAT SAT (fat saturation) technique
fat, scattered
fat selective presaturation
fat signal intensity
fat-suppressed three-dimensional
  spoiled gradient-echo FLASH MR
  imaging
fat suppression, double echo three-
  point Dixon method
fat suppression pulse
fat suppression technique
fatty acid metabolism
fatty degeneration

fatty filum terminale
fatty infiltration of liver
fatty liver
fatty meal sonogram (FMS)
fatty replacement of the pancreas
fatty streak atherosclerosis
fatty tumor
fat-water interface
fauces (pl. of faux)
    anterior pillar of
    arch of
fault, sagittal plane
faulty colloid preparation with excess
    aluminum
faulty RF (radiofrequency) shielding in
    MRI scanner room artifact
faux (see *fauces)*
faux profil ("foh pro-feel") (FP) view
    (oblique view of hip in standing
    position)
faveolate
Favre disease
FB (foreign body)
FBI (fat-blood interface) sign
FBP (filtered back-projection) method
FBS (failed back syndrome)
FBSS (failed back surgery syndrome)
FCLA (fluoresceinyl Cypridina
    luminescent analogue)
FCR (flexor carpi radialis) muscle
FCS (full cervical spine) series of
    x-rays
FCU (flexor carpi ulnaris) muscle
FDC (flexor digitorum communis)
    muscle
FDDNP-PET scan
FDG ([18]fluorodeoxyglucose; fludeoxy-
    glucose F-18) imaging agent
FDG-blood flow mismatch
FDG-labeled positron imaging
FDG myocardial imaging
[18]FDG-PET scan
FDG SPECT

FDI (first digital interosseous) muscle
FDI (frequency domain imaging)
    (in ultrasound)
FDL (flexor digitorum longus) muscle
FDP (fibrin degradation products)
    on MRI
FDP (flexor digitorum profundus)
    muscle
FDQ (flexor digiti quinti) muscle
FDQB (flexor digiti quinti brevis)
    muscle
FDS (flexor digitorum sublimis)
    muscle
FDS (flexor digitorum superficialis)
    muscle
Fe-Ex orogastric tube magnet
feasible alternatives
feathery appearance
fecal impaction
fecal incontinence
fecal mass
fecal material, retained
fecal residue
fecalith
fecalogram (slang)
fecaloid
fecaloma
fecal tagging
fecaluria
feces
    impacted
    inspissation of
feculence
feculent
Federici sign
feedback
    breathing
    real-time respiratory
feeder arteries
feeder veins
feeding artery to aneurysm
feeding branch of artery
feeding mean arterial pressure
    (FMAP)

feeding vessel
feet-first position
Feigenbaum echocardiogram
F-18 fluoromisonidazole (FMISO)
Feiss line
Feist-Mankin position (recumbent
    oblique projection)
Feldaker syndrome
Feldkamp algorithm
felon
Felty syndrome
female catheter
female urethra
femoral artery pseudoaneurysm
fem-pop (slang for femoral-popliteal)
    bypass
feminine aorta, small
feminizing tumor
femoral above-knee popliteal bypass
femoral anteversion
femoral aortic flush catheter
femoral approach for cardiac
    catheterization
femoral artery
femoral artery pressure
femoral bone
femoral capital epiphysis
femoral condyle
femoral head and neck
femoral head deformity
femoral head vascularity
femoral hernia
femoral neck
femoral pulse
femoral tuberosity
femoral vein
femoral vein percutaneous insertion
femoral venoarterial bypass
femoral venous approach
femoral view
femoroaxillary bypass
femorocrural graft
femorodistal bypass

femorodistal popliteal bypass graft
femorofemoral approach
femorofemoral bypass
femorofemoral bypass graft
femorofemoral crossover
femoroperoneal bypass graft
femoroperoneal in situ vein bypass
    graft
femoropopliteal angioplasty
femoropopliteal artery
femoropopliteal atheromatous stenosis
femoropopliteal bypass
femoropopliteal bypass surgery
femoropopliteal Gore-Tex graft
femoropopliteal thrombosis
femorotibial angle (FTA)
femorotibial bypass graft
femtoliter (fL)
femur (pl. femora)
    apex of
    body of
    greater trochanter of
    head and neck of
    head of
    lesser trochanter of
    neck of
    nutrient artery of
femur length (FL)
fender fracture
fenestra (pl. fenestrae)
fenestration
    aortic
    aortopulmonary
    apical
    cusp
    interchordal space
fenestration occlusion
fenestration of dissecting aneurysm
Fenwick disease
Ferguson view of sacroiliac joints
Feridex (ferumoxides) imaging agent
Fermi-Eyges-Hogstrom (FEH) algo-
    rithm to calculate dose distribution

ferric ammonium citrate (FAC)
  imaging agent
ferric ammonium citrate-cellulose
  paste
ferric chloride imaging agent
FerriSeltz (ferric ammonium citrate)
  [FAC] imaging agent
ferrocalcinosis, familial cerebral
ferromagnetic objects creating artifacts
    on imaging studies
  bra underwire
  button
  cigarette lighter
  clothing with metal object
  earring
  hair coloring
  hairpin
  make-up
  metal mesh in toupee or wig
  necklace
  paper clip
  pen
  political button
  probe
  ring
  shunt
  tooth filling
  watch
  zipper
ferromagnetic properties
ferromagnetic relaxation
ferruginous bodies
ferumoxides-enhanced MR imaging
ferumoxsil imaging agent
ferumoxtran-10 imaging agent
FES (fat embolism syndrome)
fetal biophysical profile
fetal bradycardia
fetal cardiac anomalies
fetal cerebellum
fetal cerebral ventricular morphology
fetal chromosome abnormality

fetal death
  early
  intermediate
  late
fetal echocardiogram
fetal echocardiography in utero
fetal gallbladder
fetal heart
fetal heart failure
fetal hydrops
fetal imaging in utero
fetal lobe
fetal lobulation
fetal lung volume
fetal magnetic resonance imaging
fetal magnetocardiography
fetal malformation
fetal-maternal hemorrhage
fetal midface
fetal motion or movement
fetal-pelvic disproportion
fetal-pelvic index
fetal placenta
fetal pole
fetal position
fetal small parts
fetal sonography
fetal tumor
fetal ultrasonography
fetal umbilical vein injection under
  sonographic guidance
Feth-R-Kath epidural catheter
fetomaternal hemorrhage
fetometry
fetus (pl. fetuses)
  amorphous
  anomalous
  calcified
  growth-retarded
  impacted
  intrauterine
  maturity of

fetus *(cont.)*
  nonviable
  paper-doll
  parasitic
  placenta of
  presentation of
  previable
  retained dead
  small parts of
  stunted
  tissue of
  umbilical artery in
  viable
fetus in fetus
fetus papyraceus
FFA (free fatty acid) scintigraphy,
  labeled
FFE sequences
F-4500 Fluorescence Spectrophotometer
FFP (fresh frozen plasma)
FFT (fast Fourier transform) image
FGBD (fluoroscopically guided
  balloon dilatation)
FHB (flexor hallucis brevis) muscle
FHC (familial hypertrophic cardiomyopathy)
FHL (flexor hallucis longus) muscle
FI (full-scan with interpolation)
  method/projection
fiber (pl. fibers)
  cardiac muscle
  muscle
  myocardial
  skeletal muscle
  sling muscle
fiberoptic angioscopy
fiberoptic bronchography
fiberoptic light source
fiberoptic tapers
fiberoptic video glasses
fiber tractography (FT)
fibrillate

Fibrimage technetium Tc 99m imaging
  agent
fibrin calculus
fibrin clot
fibrin degradation products (FDP) on
  MRI
fibrin glue, percutaneous
fibrin mass
fibrinogen
  radiolabeled
  technetium ^{99m}Tc-labeled
fibrinogen degradation
fibrinolysis
  intrapleural
  ophthalmic arterial
fibrinolytic treatment
fibrinopurulent pleurisy
fibrinous pneumonia
fibrin sleeve stripping
fibrin split products
fibroadenoma
fibroadipose tissue
fibroblast radiosensitivity
fibroblastic meningioma
fibroblastic proliferation
fibroblastoma, perineural
fibrocalcific cusps
fibrocalcification
fibrocartilage
  circumferential
  intra-articular plates of
  triangular
fibrocartilaginous disk
fibrocartilaginous plate
fibrocollagenous connective tissue
fibrocystic breast syndrome
fibrocystic residual
fibrodysplasia ossificans progressiva
fibroelastoma of heart valve
fibroelastoma, papillary
fibroepithelial polyp
fibrofatty mesenteric proliferation
fibrofatty pulvinar hypertrophy

fibroglandular tissue
fibrohistiocytic tumor
fibroid
  calcified
  intramural
  pedunculated
  uterine
fibroid adenoma
fibroid embolization
fibroid lung
fibroid myocarditis
fibroid uterus
fibrolamellar hepatocarcinoma
fibrolamellar hepatocellular carcinoma
fibrolipoma
fibroma
  aponeurotic
  cementifying
  cemento-ossifying
  chondromyxoid (CMF)
  desmoplastic
  heart
  juvenile ossifying
  meningeal
  nonossifying
  nonosteogenic
  ossifying
  osteogenic
  periosteal
  subcutaneous
fibroma-thecoma tumor of ovary
fibromatosis
fibromuscular dysplasia (FMD)
fibromuscular lesion
fibromuscular ridge
fibromyoma
fibromyxoma, odontogenic
fibronodular
fibro-osseous lesion
fibro-osseous tunnel
fibrosarcoma
fibrosclerosis of breast
fibrosclerotic

fibrosed muscles
fibroserous pericardial sac
fibrosing inflammatory pseudotumor
fibrosis (pl. fibroses)
  alcoholic
  arachnoid
  basilar
  bilharzial
  confluent
  congenital hepatic (CHF)
  corpus cavernosum
  cystic
  diffuse interstitial pulmonary
    (DIPF)
  endocardial
  endomyocardial (EMF)
  idiopathic interstitial
  idiopathic pulmonary (IPF)
  idiopathic retroperitoneal
  interstitial
  interstitial pulmonary
  leptomeningeal
  mediastinal
  meningeal
  myocardial
  nodal
  nodular subepidermal
  noncirrhotic portal (NCPF)
  panmural
  penile
  pericentral
  periductal
  perimuscular
  perineal
  periportal
  periureteral
  periureteric
  pipestem
  portal
  portal to portal
  postradiation
  progressive perivenular alcoholic
    (PPAF)

fibrosis *(cont.)*
 pulmonary
 radiation-induced
 renal
 replacement
 retroperitoneal
 subadventitial
 subintimal
 subserosal
 Symmers
FibroSpect study
fibrotic cavitating pattern
fibrotic kidney
fibrotic tissue
fibrous ankylosis of multiple joints
fibrous capsule of kidney
fibrous dysplasia ossificans
 progressiva
fibrous goiter
fibrous nonunion
fibrous plaques
fibrous pleural adhesions
fibrous pneumonia
fibrous tissue proliferation
fibrous pneumonia
fibrous tumor
fibrous union
fibroxanthoma
fibroxanthosarcoma
fibula
 apex of
 nutrient artery of
fibular bone
fibular notch
fibulotalocalcaneal (FTC) ligament
Ficat classification of femoral head
 osteonecrosis
Ficat-Marcus grading system
Ficat stage of avascular necrosis
Fick equation
Fick method for calculating cardiac
 output
FID (free induction delay)

fiducial movement
field
 collapsed lung
 disk to magnetic
 fringe
 Gibbs random
 high power
 insonifying wave
 large hinge angle electron
 low power
 lower lung
 lung
 mantle
 Markov random
 midlung
 near
 oscillating magnetic
 rf or RF (radiofrequency)
 stray neutron
 tangential breast
 tesla (T)
 upper lung
field alignment
field-dependent
field-fitting technique
field gradient
field-guided CT scan
field H of Forel
Fielding-Magliato classification of
 subtrochanteric fracture
field lock
field of view (FOV) imaging
field variation, BO
Fiessinger-Rendu syndrome
fifth compartment
fifth cranial nerve (trigeminal nerve)
fifth intercostal space
fifth left interspace
fifth rib
fighter's fracture
FIGO stage of carcinoma
figure, acetabular teardrop
figure of 8 modeling

figure of 8 wire
figure-3 sign
filariasis
filar lipoma
file transfer protocol, FTP
filiform appendix
filigree pattern
fill and spill of dye (in fallopian tubes)
filling
  atrial
  augmented
  capillary
  controlled bladder
  decreased left ventricular
  incomplete
  left atrial
  left ventricular
  passive
  peak
  rapid
  reduced
  retrograde
  ureteral
  venous
  ventricular
  vessel
filling defect
  air-bubble
  cordlike
  radiolucent
  ureteral
filling factor
filling phase, rapid
filling pressure
filling rate, peak
film (see also *position, projection, view*)
  Accu-Flo dura
  AP (anteroposterior)
  bite-wing
  chest
  chiropractic
  comparison

film *(cont.)*
  cross-table lateral
  decubitus
  digital subtraction
  DuPont Cronex x-ray
  expiratory
  flat plate
  GLP7
  high contrast
  lateral
  lateral decubitus
  limited
  low contrast
  low dose
  manual subtraction
  oblique
  outside
  overhead
  PA (posteroanterior)
  photo-plotter
  plain
  port
  portable
  postevacuation
  postvoid
  postvoiding
  preliminary
  prone
  radiochromic
  scout
  sequential
  serial
  skull
  spot
  stress
  suboptimal
  subtraction
  supine
  UP7
  upright
  working
film alternator
film-based viewing

film changer, Sanchez-Perez automatic
filmless imaging
film slippage
filter
    bird's nest percutaneous IVC
        (inferior vena cava)
    caval
    correction
    differencing
    emission
    excitation
    Gianturco-Roehm bird's nest vena
        caval
    Greenfield vena caval
    inferior vena caval
    Innovante
    IVC (inferior vena cava)
    Kalman
    Kimray-Greenfield caval
    Mobin-Uddin umbrella
    Mobin-Uddin vena caval
    noise-reduction
    percutaneous inferior vena cava
        (IVC)
    prophylactic IVC
    Simon nitinol percutaneous IVC
    Simon nitinol vena cava filter
    translation-invariant
    umbrella
    Venatech percutaneous IVC
    wall
    Wiener
filtered-back projection
filtering, dynamic
filtration
    copper
    dynamic beat
    glomerular
    post beat
filum, fatty
filum terminale, fatty
fimbriated end of fallopian tube

finding (pl. findings)
    angiographic
    auscultatory
    cardinal
    cephalometric
    characteristic
    concomitant
    equivocal
    focal
    indeterminate
    lateralizing
    no discernible
    ominous
    pathognomonic
    salient physical
    scanty
    specious
    spurious
    voxel-based morphometric
fine calcification
fine needle
fine-needle biopsy, ultrasound-guided
fine reticular pattern
fine-speckled appearance
Finesse large lumen guiding catheter
finger
    angle
    baseball
    base of
    bolster
    clubbed
    drop
    fingers
    football
    hippocratic
    index
    jammed
    jersey
    little
    long
    mallet
    middle

finger *(cont.)*
  pedicle
  pulley of
  pulp of
  replantation of
  replanted
  ring
  sausage
  spade
  speck
  spider
  stoved
  trigger
  webbed
finger fracture
finger fracture dissection
fingerlike projection
finger of tumor
finger opposition
finger pad
fingerprint image compression
finger pulley
fingertip amputation
fingertip pad
firing of ectopic atrial focus
firing temperature
Firlit-Sugar intermittent catheter
firm uterus
first pass effect
first pass extraction
first pass imaging
first pass MUGA
first pass myocardial perfusion MR
first pass radionuclide exercise
  angiocardiography
first pass study
first pass view
first portion of duodenum
first trimester nuchal translucency
fish-eye effect
fish flesh appearance
fishhook appearance of ureter
fishhooking of ureters

fish meal worker's lung
fishmouth configuration of mitral
  valve
fishmouth stenosis
fishmouth vertebra
fish scale gallbladder
Fisk projection of bicipital groove
FISP (gradient echo sequence)
FISP sequence
fission track analysis of urine
fissula
fissuration
fissure
  abdominal
  anal
  anterior median (of cord)
  antitragohelicine
  auricular
  brain
  calcarine
  callosomarginal
  central
  cerebellar
  cerebellopontine or cerebellopontile
  cerebral
  choroidal
  chronic
  collateral
  cutaneous
  decidual
  dentate
  displacement of interhemispheric
  glaserian
  hippocampal
  horizontal
  interhemispheric
  lateral
  longitudinal
  lung
  main
  oblique (of lung)
  occipital
  oral

fissure *(cont.)*
  palpebral
  portal
  rolandic
  studded
  superior orbital
  supraorbital
  sylvian
  umbilical
fissure fracture
fissure in ano
fissure of Rolando
fissure of Sylvius
fissure sign
fistula
  abdominal
  anal
  anorectal
  aorta-left ventricular
  aorta-right ventricular
  aortic sinus
  aortic sinus to right ventricle
  aortocaval
  aortoduodenal
  aortoenteric
  aortoesophageal
  aortopulmonary
  aortosigmoid
  arteriovenous (AV, AVF)
  AV (arteriovenous)
  biliary
  biliary-cutaneous
  biliary-duodenal
  biliary-enteric
  bilioenteric
  bladder
  bladder to skin
  bladder to uterus
  bladder to vagina
  Blom-Singer tracheoesophageal
  branchial
  Brescia-Cimino AV
  brachiosubclavian bridge graft
    (BSBGF)

fistula *(cont.)*
  bridge-graft (BGF)
  bronchobiliary
  bronchocavitary
  bronchocutaneous
  bronchoesophageal
  bronchopleural
  cameral
  carotid artery-cavernous sinus
  carotid cavernous
  carotid-cavernous sinus
  cerebral arteriovenous
  cerebrospinal fluid
  cervical
  cervicosigmoid
  cervicovaginal
  cervicovesical
  cholecystenteric
  cholecystocholedochal
  cholecystocolonic
  cholecystoduodenal
  cholecystoduodenocolic
  choledochal-colonic
  choledochoduodenal
  chylous
  coil closure of coronary artery
  colocutaneous
  colonic
  colovaginal
  colovesical
  complex anorectal
  congenital
  congenital pulmonary arteriovenous
  coronary
  coronary arteriosystemic
  coronary arteriovenous
  coronary artery cameral
  coronary artery-pulmonary artery
  coronary artery to right ventricular
  coronary-cameral
  coronary-pulmonary
  CSF (cerebrospinal fluid)
  cystic

fistula *(cont.)*
  duodenocolic
  dural arteriovenous (AVF)
  durocutaneous
  Eck
  endogenous arteriovenous
  enterocutaneous
  enteroenteral
  enteroenteric
  enterourethral
  enterovaginal
  enterovesical
  esophagorespiratory
  external biliary
  extrasphincteric anal
  fecal
  gastric
  gastrocolic
  gastroduodenal
  gastrojejunal-colic
  gastrojejunocolic
  genitourinary
  graft-enteric
  hepatic
  hepatic arteriovenous
  hepatopleural
  horseshoe
  H-type
  iatrogenic
  ileosigmoid
  intersphincteric anal
  intestinoureteral
  intestinouterine
  intestinovaginal
  intestinovesical
  intradural arteriovenous
  intradural retromedullary arterio-
    venous
  intrahepatic AV
  intrapulmonary arteriovenous
  jejunocolic
  kidney arteriovenous
  lacteal

fistula *(cont.)*
  lower ureter and vagina
  mammary
  Mann-Bollman
  mediastinal
  mesenteric
  microvenoarteriolar
  mucous
  orofacial
  pancreatic
  pancreatic cutaneous
  pancreaticopleural
  paraprosthetic-enteric
  parietal
  perineovaginal
  persistent bronchopleural
  pilonidal
  pleural
  pleurocutaneous
  premedullary arteriovenous
  pseudoaneurysm of arteriovenous
  pulmonary arteriovenous
  radial artery to cephalic vein
  radiation
  rectal
  rectolabial
  rectourethral
  rectovaginal
  rectovesical
  rectovesicovaginal
  rectovestibular
  rectovulvar
  respiratory-esophageal
  retroperitoneal
  saphenous vein
  seminal vesicle
  sigmoidovaginal
  sigmoidovesical
  spermatic
  spinal dural arteriovenous
  splanchnic AV
  splenic AV
  suprasphincteric

fistula *(cont.)*
  thoracic
  thrombosed dialysis
  tracheobronchial
  tracheoesophageal (TE or TEF)
  transdural
  transsphincteric anal
  trigeminal cavernous
  umbilical
  ureteral
  ureter and skin
  urethral
  urethra and penile skin
  urethra and vagina
  ureterocutaneous
  ureterocervical
  ureterovaginal
  urethroperineal
  urethroperineovesical
  urethrorectal
  urethroscrotal
  urethrovaginal
  urethrovesical
  urethrovesicovaginal
  urinary
  urinary tract
  urogenital
  uterine
  uteroperitoneal
  uterorectal
  uteroureteric
  uterovaginal
  uterovesical
  uterus to abdominal wall
  vaginal
  vaginoperineal
  vaginovesical
  vesical
  vesicocervicovaginal
  vesicocolic
  vesicocutaneous
  vesicoenteric
  vesicointestinal

fistula *(cont.)*
  vesicoperineal
  vesicorectal
  vesicosigmoidovaginal
  vesicoureteral
  vesicoureterovaginal
  vesicouterine
  vesicovaginal
  vesicovaginorectal
  vitelline
fistula formation
fistula in ano
fistula tract study
fistulogram
fistulography
fistulous tract
511-keV high energy imaging
5-iodoacetamidofluorescein imaging
  agent
5-iodo-2-deoxyuridine imaging agent
5 MHz sonography
5 MHz transducer (ultrasound)
5 mm collimation
five-view chest x-ray
fixed airway obstruction
fixed area of narrowing in large
  airway
fixed defect
fixed grid stereologic method
fixed intracavitary filling defect
fixed mass
fixed perfusion defect
fixed pulmonary valvular resistance
fixed segment of bowel
fixed shaped coplanar or nonplanar
  radiation beam bouquet
fL (femtoliter)
FL (femur length)
FL/AC ratio (femur length to
  abdominal circumference)
flabby heart
flaccid
Flack sinoatrial node

flail chest
flail digit
flail foot
flail joint
flail mitral leaflet
flail mitral valve
flail shoulder
FLAIR (fluid-attenuated inversion
   recovery) sequences
FLAIR-FLASH imaging (see *FLASH*)
flake fracture of the hamate
flaking of cartilage in osteoarthritis
flame appearance
flamingo views (stress views of
   symphysis pubis)
flank bone (ilium)
flank pain
flank position
flap
   bone
   entry
   intimal
   liver
   muscle
   necrotic
   osteoplastic
   pedicle
   pericardial
   pleural
   scimitar-shaped
   subclavian
flaplike valves
flap valve ventricular septal defect
flare
   condylar
   metaphyseal
   tibial
   trochanteric
flare phenomenon
FLASH (fast low-angle shot)
   FLASH images
   FLASH 3D sequence
flashlamp-pulsed dye laser

FlashPoint image-guided surgical
   instruments
flask, vascular
Flatau-Schilder disease
flat bone
flatfoot deformity
flat-hand test
flat inferior vena cava
flat lined (verb)
flat-panel megavoltage imager
flat pelvis
flat plate of abdomen
flattened longitudinal arch of foot
flattening of normal lumbar curve
flat time-intensity profile
flaval ligament
flawed image
flax-dresser's disease
flea-bitten kidney
Flechsig tract
Fleet bowel prep
Fleischer disease
Fleischmann bursa
Fleischner lines
Fleischner sign
fleur de lis pattern
Flexguard tip catheter
flexibility
flexible cardiac valve
flexible filiform catheter tip
flexible suction cannula
flexible surface coil
flexible surface-coil-type resonator
   (FSCR)
flexible-tip guidewire
flexion deformity
flexion-distraction injury of spine
flexion, extension, and oblique
   positions
flexion maneuver on cervical spine
   x-ray
flexion-rotation injury of spine
Flexi-Tip ureteral catheter

flexor carpi ulnaris (FCU) muscle
flexor digitorum profundus (FDP)
   muscle
flexor digitorum superficialis (FDS)
   muscle
flexor hallucis longus (FHL) muscle
flexor pollicis longus (FPL) muscle
flexor tendon
Flex-S coil
FlexStrand cable
flexure
   caudal
   cephalic
   cerebral
   cervical
   colonic
   cranial
   duodenojejunal
   hepatic
   left colic
   left colonic
   right colic
   right colonic
   sigmoid
   splenic
Flexxicon Blue dialysis catheter
Flexxicon dialysis catheter
FlimFax teleradiology system
flip angle
flip-flop phenomenon
flipper hand
flips, value
Flo-Coat (barium sulfate) imaging
   agent
Flo-Rester vessel occluder
floating head
floating kidney
floating leaflets
floating table
flocculation on barium enema
flocculent foci of calcification
flocculonodular lobe of cerebellum
flocculonodular tumors

flock worker's lung
Flo-Coat (barium sulfate) imaging
   agent
flood section
floor
   bladder
   fibromuscular pelvic
   inguinal
   pelvic
   sellar
floppy aortic valve
floppy mitral valve
Flo-Rester vessel occluder
florid adenosis
florid new bone
flotation catheter
flow
   antegrade
   antegrade bile
   antegrade blood
   antegrade diastolic
   aortic (AF)
   axoplasmic
   azygos
   azygos blood
   backward
   blood
   cerebral blood (CBF)
   cerebral brain
   cerebrospinal fluid (CSF)
   chronic reserve
   collateral
   collateral blood
   compromised
   coronary blood
   coronary reserve (CRF)
   dampened pulsatile
   decreased cerebral blood
   effective pulmonary blood (EPBF)
   effective pulmonic
   effective renal blood (ERBF)
   effective renal plasma (ERPF)
   expiratory

flow *(cont.)*
    forward
    Ganz method for coronary sinus
    great cardiac vein (GCVF)
    hepatofugal
    hepatofugal portal venous
    hepatopetal
    high velocity
    inspiratory
    insufficient pulmonary arterial
    intercoronary collateral
    laminar
    left to right
    maximum midexpiratory
    midexpiratory tidal
    mitral valve
    myocardial blood (MBF)
    peak
    peak expiratory (PEF)
    peak tidal expiratory flow
    physiologic
    pulmonary blood (PBF)
    pulmonic output
    pulmonic versus systemic
    Qp (pulmonary blood flow)
    Qs (systemic blood flow)
    redistribution of pulmonary
        vascular
    regional cerebral blood (rCBF)
    regional myocardial blood
    regurgitant
    regurgitant systolic
    restoration of
    retrograde
    retrograde systolic
    reversed vertebral blood (RVBF)
    sluggish
    systemic blood (SBF)
    systemic output
    time-averaged
    tissue
    total cerebral blood (TCBF)
    transmitral

flow *(cont.)*
    tricuspid valve
    turbulent blood
    turbulent intraluminal
flow arrest
flow-compensated gradient-echo
    sequence
flow-compromising lesion
flow cytometry
flow cytometry DNA analysis
flow cytometry Tpot (potential
    doubling time)
flow dependent obstruction
flow-directed balloon catheter
flow-directed microcatheter
flow effect artifact
flow-guided Inoue balloon
flow images
flow-induced artifact
flowing spin
FloWire Doppler ultrasound
flow-limited expiration
flow mapping technique
flowmeter
flowmetry
    blood
    Doppler
    laser-Doppler (LDF)
    Narcomatic
    Parks 800 bidirectional Doppler
    pulsed Doppler
    Statham electromagnetic
flow quantification
flow redistribution
flow-related enhancement effects
flow scan, radionuclide
flow signal
flow study
flow-time curve
flow velocity profile
flow velocity signals
flow velocity waveforms
flow void

flow void artifact
flow void sign
flow volume
flow volume curve
flow volume loop (in spirometry
    reports)
fluctuant abscess
fluctuant lesion
fluctuant mass
fludeoxyglucose (^{18}F)
fluffy infiltrate
fluffy rarefaction of Paget disease
fluid
    amniotic
    articular
    ascitic
    bursal
    cavitary
    cerebrospinal (CSF)
    cystic
    extraluminal
    extravascular
    free
    free abdominal
    free pelvic
    high signal (on MRI) intratendinous
        collection of
    interstitial
    joint
    leakage of cerebrospinal
    localized mediastinal
    loculated
    pelvic
    pericardial
    pericholecystic
    peritoneal
    pleural
    prostatic
    serosanguineous
    spinal
    subgaleal cerebrospinal
    synovial
fluid accumulation in tissues

fluid-attenuated inversion recovery
    (FLAIR) imaging
fluid collection, loculated
fluid density
fluid enzymes
fluid expansion, rapid
fluid extravasation
fluid-filled bronchograms
fluid-filled mass in uterus
fluid flow between capillaries and
    interstitial tissue
fluid-fluid level
fluidification
fluid level
fluid mass
fluid overload
fluid resorption
fluid retention
fluid volume
fluid wave
fluke
    liver
    lung
Fluoratec technetium-based imaging
    agent
fluorescein angiography
fluorescein dye disappearance test
    (DDT)
fluorescein uptake
fluorescence spectroscopy
fluoresceinyl Cypridina luminescent
    analogue (FCLA)
fluorine (F) (an element)
    ^{18}F (fluorine-18, F-18)
    ^{18}FDG (fluorine-18 2-deoxy-D-
        glucose) PET scan
    ^{18}F estradiol (FES)
    ^{18}F fluoro-DOPA
    ^{18}F fluorodeoxyglucose
    ^{18}F fluorodeoxyglucose PET scan
    ^{18}F fluoromisonidazole
    ^{18}F labeled derivatives of
        m-tyrosine

fluorine *(cont.)*
   ^{18}F labeled HFA-134a
   ^{18}F labeled polyfluorinated ethyl
   ^{18}F methyl tyrosine
   ^{18}F N-methylspiperone
   ^{18}F spiperone
   ^{18}F 2-deoxyglucose (^{18}FDG)
      uptake on PET scan
   ^{18}F uptake
fluorocarbon-based ultrasound contrast
   agent
FluoroCatcher digital last-image hold
fluorodeoxyglucose (FDG) radioactive
   tracer
fluorography, spot-film
fluoroimmunoassay
fluorometer
fluorometry
   image intensification
   portable C-arm intensifier
   two-plane
FluoroNav virtual fluoroscopy system
Fluoropassiv thin-wall carotid patch
FluoroPlus angiography
FluoroPlus Cardiac real-time digital
   imaging
FluoroPlus Roadmapper digital
   fluoroscopy system
FluoroScan mini C-arm imaging
   system
fluoroscope (see *fluoroscopy*)
fluoroscopically guided balloon dilatation (FGBD)
fluoroscopically guided dacryocystoplasty
fluoroscopic assistance
fluoroscopic control, advanced under
fluoroscopic cystocolpoproctography
fluoroscopic diskectomy
fluoroscopic guidance
fluoroscopic localization
fluoroscopic road-mapping technique
   in angioplastic vascular procedures

fluoroscopic view
fluoroscopy
   airway
   biplane
   C-arm
   C-arm digital
   chest
   digital
   electric joint
   FluoroPlus Roadmapper digital
   half scan cone-beam CT
   mobile
   Orca C-arm
   real-time CT
   region of interest
FluoroPlus angiography
FluoroPlus Roadmapper digital
   fluoroscopy system
fluoroscopy-guided condylar lift-off
fluoroscopy-guided subarachnoid
   phenol block (SAPB)
Fluoro Tip cannula
FluoroTrak surgical navigation system
flush aortogram
flush aortography
flushed
flushing of catheter
flush, pituitary
flutamide-associated liver toxicity
fluttering of valvular leaflet
fluximetry
fluxionary hyperemia
fluttering of valvular leaflet
flying angel view (lateral thoracic
   inlet)
fly-through, stereoscopic
fly-through viewing, PVR
FMA cephalometric measurement
FMAP (feeding mean arterial
   pressure)
FMD (fibromuscular dysplasia)
FMH (first metatarsal head)
FMISO (F-18 fluoromisonidazole)

FMPIR (fast SE and fast IR) imaging
FMPSPGR (fast multiplanar spoiled
gradient-recalled) imaging
FMPSPGR sequence
FMR (functional MR) imaging
fMRI or FMRI (functional magnetic
resonance imaging)
fMRI signal change
FMS (fatty meal sonogram)
FNH (focal nodular hyperplasia)
FNTC (fine-needle transhepatic
cholangiogram)
foam cell
foam embolus
foamy exudate in air spaces
focal abnormality
focal and diffuse lung texture analysis
focal area of hemorrhage
focal area of hypometabolism
focal calcification
focal changes
focal damage
focal deficit
focal degenerative change
focal dilatations of air spaces
focal distance
focal distortion
focal eccentric stenosis
focal edema
focal endocardial hemorrhage
focal epileptiform activity
focal hepatic hot spot
focal hyperinflation
focal infiltrating tumor
focal inflammation in febrile
granulocytopenia
focal interstitial infiltrate
focal intimal thickening
focal lesion
focal mass
focal nodular hyperplasia (FNH)
focal perivascular infiltrate
focal plaquelike defect

focal pooling of tracer
focal stenosis
focal uptake
focal wall motion abnormality
focal white matter signal abnormalities
foci of calcification
foci of tumor
focus (pl. foci)
   Assmann
   atrial
   ectopic
   epileptogenic
   hemorrhagic
   hypermetabolic activity
   hypoechoic
   junctional
   mesial frontal
   midline parasagittal
   multiple
   occipital
   radiolucent
   shadowing
   Simon
   tumor
focused extracorporeal ultrasound
focused-heat tumor ablation
Fogarty adherent clot catheter
Fogarty arterial embolectomy catheter
Fogarty balloon biliary catheter
Fogarty-Chin extrusion balloon
   catheter
fog (or fogging) effect on CT
Foix-Alajouanine syndrome
fold (pl. folds)
   adipose
   alar
   amniotic
   aryepiglottic
   caval
   cecal
   cholecystoduodenocolic
   circular
   circulator

fold *(cont.)*
  costocolic
  Douglas
  duodenojejunal
  duodenomesocolic
  effaced gastric
  epigastric
  esophageal
  falciform
  flattened duodenal
  gastric
  gastropancreatic
  genital
  giant gastric
  glossopalatine
  gluteal
  Guérin
  haustral
  Hensing
  hepatopancreatic
  ileocecal
  ileocolic
  Kerckring
  Kohlrausch
  mucosal
  Nélaton
  palatopharyngeal
  paraduodenal
  peritoneal
  prepyloric
  rectal
  rectouterine
  rugal
  sacrogenital
  semilunar
  sentinel
  sigmoid
  spiral
  superior duodenal
  superior transverse rectal
  thickened
  vestigial
folded fundus of gallbladder

folded step ramp
folding-potential analysis
Foley catheter
Foley catheterization
Foley three-way catheter
Foley ureteral catheter
folinic acid, low dose
follicle (pl. follicles)
  aggregated
  aggregated lymphatic
  anovular ovarian
  atretic ovarian
  gastric
  gastric lymphatic
  graafian
  intestinal
  malpighian
  nabothian
  ovarian
  primordial
  ruptured
  thyroid
  unruptured
follicular lymphoma
follow-through, small bowel
follow-up or followup (n., adj.)
  examination
follow up (v.)
Fonar Stand-Up FMRI scanner
Fonar-360 MRI scanner
Fontan anastomosis of atrial
  appendage to pulmonary artery
fontanel (fontanelle)
fontanelle
  anterior
  anterolateral
  bregmatic
  bulging
  closed
  cranial
  frontal
  fused
  Gerdy

fontanelle *(cont.)*
  mastoid
  occipital
  open
  overriding sutures of
  posterior
  posterolateral
  sagittal
  sphenoid
  tense
  triangular
foot (pl. feet)
  arch of
  arcuate artery of
  articulations of
  calcaneocavus
  Charcot
  digital artery of
  flail
  Friedreich
  Madura
  perforating artery of
  phalanges of
  rockerbottom
football finger
footballer's ankle
football sign
footling presentation
foramen (pl. foramina)
  alveolar
  anterior condyloid
  aortic
  apical
  arachnoidal
  blind
  Bochdalek
  Botallo
  carotid
  cecal
  conjugate
  costotransverse
  cranial

foramen *(cont.)*
  emissary sphenoidal
  epiploic
  ethmoidal
  frontal
  greater palatine
  great sacrosciatic
  greater sciatic
  intertransverse
  interventricular
  intervertebral
  Luschka
  Magendie
  Monro
  Morgagni
  sacrosciatic
  spinous
  stylomastoid
  sublabral
  superior maxillary
  vertebral
  Winslow
foramen magnum of skull
foramen ovale, patent
foramina (pl. of foramen)
foraminal encroachment
foraminal space
force (pl. forces)
  axial compression
  pascals of (SI units)
  reserve
  rotational
  shearing
  stroke
  torsional impaction
  transverse plane
Force balloon dilatation catheter
forcefully wedged
forearm
forefoot
  mid- and
  narrowing of

foreign body (FB)
  metallic
  retained
  tracheobronchial
foreign body aspiration
foreign body in respiratory passages
foreign body reaction
foreign body upper airway obstruction
foreign material artifact
Forestier disease
forking of sylvian aqueduct
format
  cylindrical
  hemodynamic
  slice
  three-dimensional
  two-dimensional
formation
  anomalous
  bat-wing
  bezoar
  brain stem reticular
  bunion
  callosal
  callus
  eddy
  exuberant atheroma
  fistula
  gas
  giant cell
  glomeruloid
  Gothic arch
  gray reticular
  hernia
  hippocampal
  hippocampus-amygdala (HAF)
  honeycomb
  lateral reticular
  marginal osteophyte
  mesencephalic reticular
  midbrain reticular (MRF)
  neointimal
  new bone

formation *(cont.)*
  osteophyte
  palisade
  paramedian pontine reticular
  periosteal bone
  paramedian pontine reticular
    (PPRF)
  pseudoaneurysm
  reticular
  rouleaux
  saccular
  secondary stricture
  spur
  subsequent hernia
  thrombus
formation of open ileal bladder
forme fruste (pl. formes frustes)
forme tardive
formication
formidable risk
formula
  Bayesian
  fan-beam
Forney syndrome
forniceal rupture
fornix (pl. fornices), flattening of
fornix cerebri
Forrester syndrome
forward failure
forward flow
forward flow of velocity
forward heart failure
forward subluxation
forward transport
forward triangle method
forward velocity (on Doppler)
fossa (pl. fossae)
  acetabular
  adipose
  amygdaloid
  anconeal (also anconal)
  antecubital
  anterior recess of ischiorectal

fossa *(cont.)*
  articular
  axillary
  bony
  condylar
  coronoid
  cranial
  crural
  cubital
  digastric
  digital
  duodenal
  duodenojcjunal
  epigastric
  femoral
  floccular
  gallbladder
  glenoid
  Gruber
  hyaloid
  iliac
  infraspinous
  infrasternal
  infratemporal
  intercondylar
  intercondyloid
  interpeduncular
  intrauterine
  ipsilateral iliac
  ischiorectal
  Jobert
  navicular
  obturator
  olecranon
  ovarian
  pararectal
  paravesical
  patellar
  pituitary
  popliteal
  posterior
  prostatic
  pterygopalatine

fossa *(cont.)*
  radial
  renal
  retroappendiceal
  rhomboid
  Rosenmüller (Rosenmueller)
  sphenoidal
  supravesical
  Sylvius
  temporal
  Treitz
  valve of navicular
  Waldeyer
fossa ovalis
fossa ovalis cordis
Foster-Kennedy syndrome
four-chamber apical view
four-chamber plane on echocardiography
4D Cardio-View scanner
four-dimensional (4D) image
four-head camera
four-hour delayed thallium imaging
Fourier analysis of electrocardiogram
Fourier coefficients
Fourier domain
Fourier-encoded
Fourier transform (or transformation)
  imaging
Fourier transform infrared spectroscopy
Fourier transform Raman spectroscopy
Fourier transformation zeugmatography
Fourier two-dimensional (2D) imaging
Fourier two-dimensional (2D)
  projection reconstruction
four-part fracture
4-row scanner
four-slice coronal CT scan of sinuses
fourth branchial cleft pouch
fourth compartment
fourth cranial nerve (trochlear nerve)

fourth intercostal space
fourth left interspace
fourth ventricle tumor
four-vessel cerebral angiography
four-view chest x-ray:
    PA, lateral, both oblique
FOV (field of view) imaging
fovea
fovea centralis
fovea inferior
foveal fat pad
foveated chest
foveola, gastric
Fowler position
FP (frontopolar) artery
FPB (flexor pollicis brevis) muscle
FPL (flexor pollicis longus) muscle
F point of cardiac apex pulse
FP (faux profil ["foh pro-feel"]) view
FR4 guiding catheter
fractal analysis
fractal-based method
fraction
    absorbed
    blood flow extraction
    ejection (EF)
    necrotic
    pulmonary regurgitant
    regional brain parenchymal (RBPF)
    S-phase
    Teichholz ejection
    unattached
    ventricular ejection
fractional area
fractional moving blood volume
    estimation
fractional myocardial shortening
fractional shortening of left ventricle
fractional volumetric analysis
fractionated radiation therapy
fractionated stereotaxic radiation
    therapy
fractionation, spatial dose

fraction dose
fracture
    abduction
    acute
    acute avulsion
    adduction
    agenetic
    Aitken classification of epiphyseal
    alveolar bone
    anatomic
    angulated
    ankle mortise
    annular
    anterior column acetabular
    anterior column with posterior
        hemitransverse acetabular
    anterior wall acetabular
    AO classification of ankle
    apophyseal
    articular
    artificial
    Atkin epiphyseal
    atrophic
    avulsion
    avulsion chip
    axial compression
    backfire
    Barton
    basal neck
    basal skull
    baseball finger
    basilar femoral neck
    basilar skull
    basocervical
    bending
    Bennett
    Berndt-Harty classification of
        transchondral
    bicondylar
    bimalleolar ankle
    bipartite
    birth
    blow-in

fracture *(cont.)*
blowout
boot-top
Bosworth
both bone
both column acetabular
boxer's
Boyd type II
bucket-handle
buckle
bumper
bunk bed
burst (compression) (of atlas)
bursting
butterfly
buttonhole
Canale-Kelly talar neck
capillary
carpal navicular
carpal scaphoid bone
cartwheel
Cedell (of talus)
cemental
cementum
cervical
cervicotrochanteric
Chance spinal
chauffeur's
chevron (V-shaped)
chip
chisel
circumferential
clay shoveler's
cleavage
closed
closed break
Colles
collicular
comminuted
comminuted bursting
comminuted intra-articular
comminuted teardrop
complete

fracture *(cont.)*
complex
complicated
composite
compound
compound skull
compression (burst) (of atlas)
condylar
condylar compression
condylar split
congenital
contrecoup
corner
cortical
Cotton ankle
cough (of a rib)
crack
craniofacial dysjunction
crush
cuboid
cuneiform
dancer's
Danis-Weber classification of ankle
Darrach-Hughston-Milch
dashboard
decompression of
Denis (A,B,C,D, or E) spinal
dens
dental vertical root
dentate
depressed
depressed and compound skull
depressed skull
de Quervain
derby hat
diacondylar
diaphyseal
diastatic
direct
dishpan
dislocation
displaced
dogleg

fracture *(cont.)*
 dome
 dorsal wing
 double
 Dupuytren
 Duverney
 dye punch
 dyscrasic
 Ellis
 endocrine
 epicondylar
 epiphyseal slip
 Essex-Lopresti calcaneal
 extra-articular
 extracapsular
 facial
 fatigue
 femoral neck
 fender
 fighter's
 finger
 fissure
 flake (of the hamate)
 flexion-burst
 flexion-compression
 flexion distraction
 floating arch
 four-part
 Freiberg
 Frykman radial
 fulcrum
 Galeazzi (of radius)
 Garden femoral neck
 Gosselin
 greenstick
 grenade-thrower's
 gross
 growth plate
 Guérin
 gutter
 Hahn-Steinthal capitellum
 hairline
 hamate tail

fracture *(cont.)*
 hangman's (C2)
 Hansen
 Hawkins talar neck
 healed
 heat
 hemicondylar
 Herbert scaphoid bone
 Hermodsson
 hockey-stick
 horizontal
 horizontal maxillary
 humeral head-splitting
 hyperextension teardrop
 hyperflexion
 hyperflexion teardrop
 idiopathic
 impacted
 impacted subcapital
 impacted valgus
 incomplete
 indented (of skull)
 indirect
 inflammatory
 infraction
 insufficiency
 intercondylar
 internally fixed
 interperiosteal
 intertrochanteric
 intra-articular
 intracapsular
 intraperiosteal
 intrauterine (of fetus)
 irreducible
 ischioacetabular
 Jefferson burst
 joint
 joint depression
 Jones
 juvenile Tillaux
 juxta-articular
 kidney

fracture *(cont.)*
  Kocher
  Kocher-Lorenz classification of
    capitellum
  laryngeal
  lateral column calcaneal
  lateral wedge (of vertebral body)
  laterally displaced
  Lauge-Hansen classification of
    ankle
  Le Fort I, II, and III
  lead-pipe
  linear
  linear and depressed skull
  Lisfranc
  local compression
  local decompression
  long bone
  longitudinal
  loose
  lorry driver's
  low T humerus
  lunate
  Maisonneuve fibular
  malar
  Malgaigne pelvic
  mallet
  malunited
  mandibular
  march
  maxillary
  medial column calcaneal
  medial epicondyle
  medial malleolar
  midfacial
  midshaft
  minimally displaced
  monomalleolar ankle
  Monteggia
  Monteggia fracture-dislocation
  Montercaux
  Moore
  Mueller classification of humerus

fracture *(cont.)*
  multangular ridge
  multipartite
  multiple
  nasal
  navicular
  navicular body
  naviculocapitate
  neck
  Neer classification of shoulder
  neoplastic
  neurogenic
  neuropathic
  neurotrophic
  nightstick
  nonarticular radial head
  nondisplaced
  oblique
  occipital
  occult
  odontoid
  Ogden classification of epiphyseal
  old
  olecranon
  olecranon tip
  one-part
  open
  open-break
  osteochondral
  osteoporotic vertebral body
    compression
  Pais
  panfacial
  paratrooper
  parry
  patellar
  pathologic
  Pauwels
  pedicle
  pelvic rim
  pelvic ring
  perforating
  periarticular

fracture *(cont.)*
  peripheral
  peritrochanteric
  phalangeal
  physeal plate
  Piedmont
  pillar
  pillion
  pillow
  ping-pong
  plafond
  plaque
  plateau
  pond
  posterior column acetabular
  posterior column with posterior
    wall acetabular
  posterior element
  posterior wall acetabular
  postmortem
  Pott ankle
  pressure
  puncture
  pyramidal
  Quervain (de Quervain)
  radial head
  radial styloid process
  resecting
  retrodisplaced
  reverse Barton
  reverse Colles
  rib
  ring
  ring-sparing
  Rolando
  rotation burst
  Ruedi-Allgower tibial plafond
  sacral insufficiency
  Salter
  Salter-Harris (1 through 5)
  Salter-Harris-Rang classification of
    epiphyseal
  sandbagging (of long bones)

fracture *(cont.)*
  scaphoid
  seat belt
  secondary
  segmental
  Segond
  senile subcapital
  SER-IV (supination, external
    rotation-type IV)
  shaft
  shear
  Shepherd
  sideswipe elbow
  silver-fork (Colles)
  simple
  simple skull
  skier's
  Skillern
  sleeve
  slice
  Smith
  spiral
  splintered
  split compression
  spontaneous
  sprain
  sprinter's
  stable
  stairstep
  Steinert classification of epiphyseal
  stellate
  stellate skull
  stepoff of
  Stieda
  straddle
  strain
  stress
  stress-type
  subcapital
  subcutaneous
  subperiosteal
  subtrochanteric
  supination (see *SER-IV*)

fracture *(cont.)*
  supination-adduction
  supination-eversion
  supracondylar
  supracondylar femoral
  surgical neck
  T
  talar osteochondral
  T condylar
  T-shaped
  teardrop
  teardrop-shaped flexion-
    compression
  temporal bone
  thalamic (of calcaneal)
  three-part
  through-and-through
  tibial plafond
  tibial plateau
  tibiofibular
  Tillaux
  Tillaux-Kleiger
  tongue-type
  torsion
  torus
  total condylar depression
  transcapitate
  transcervical femoral
  transchondral talar
  transcondylar
  transepiphyseal
  transhamate
  transscaphoid
  transtriquetral
  transverse
  transverse acetabular
  transverse with posterior wall
    acetabular
  trimalleolar ankle
  triplane
  triquetral
  trophic
  T-shaped acetabular

fracture *(cont.)*
  tuft
  two-part
  ulnar styloid
  undepressed stellate
  undisplaced
  unilateral
  unstable
  ununited
  V-shaped (chevron)
  vertebra plana
  vertebral wedge compression
  vertical
  vertical shear
  wagon wheel
  Wagstaffe
  Watson-Jones navicular
  Watson-Jones spinal
  Weber C
  wedge
  wedge-compression
  wedged
  wedge flexion-compression
  willow
  Y
  Y-T
  Zickel
  zygomatic-malar complex (ZMC)
fracture classification
fracture deformity
fracture-dislocation, perilunate (PLFD)
fracture en rave
fracture fragment
fracture in close apposition
fracture line
fracture nonunion
fracture threshold
fracture zone
fragility, hereditary (of bone)
fragment
  alignment of fracture
  articular
  avulsed fracture

fragment *(cont.)*
  avulsion
  bone
  bony
  butterfly fracture
  capital
  chondral
  cortical
  disk
  displaced
  displacement of fracture
  Fab (fragment antigen binding)
  fallen
  fracture
  free
  free-floating cartilaginous
  loose
  major fracture
  osteochondral
  overriding of fracture
  retrolisthesed
  retropulsed bony
  smear
fragmentation myocarditis
fragmentation of apophysis
fragmentation therapy
Fraley syndrome
frame
  robotics-controlled stereotactic
  stereotactic head
frameless stereotaxic DSA
frameless stereotaxic guidance tools
Francisella tularensis bacterial
  pneumonia
frank dislocation
frank hemorrhage
frank pulmonary edema
frank pus
Frank sign
Frank vectorcardiogram (VCG)
Frankel classification of spinal cord
  injury (Fraenkel)
Frankel white line

Frankfort horizontal plane
Frankfort mandibular incisor angle
fraught with error
fray
fraying of edges
fraying of meniscus
FRC (functional residual capacity)
free air
free air in body cavity
free air in diaphragm
free air passage
free air under diaphragm
free body in peritoneal cavity
free-breathing black-blood coronary
  MR angiography
free-breathing cardiac MR imaging
free-breathing three-dimensional
  coronary MR angiography
free flap of cartilage
free-floating cartilaginous fragment
free fluid
free fragment
freehand interventional sonography
freehand ultrasound
free hepatic venography
free induction decay (FID)
free induction delay curve
free induction decay imaging
free induction signal
free intraperitoneal air
free intraperitoneal gas
freely movable mass
free pelvic fluid
free pericardial space
free pleural effusion
free radical
free-radical dosimeter
free wall, ventricular
free wall tract
Freiberg disease
Freiberg-Kohler disease
French 5 angiographic catheter
French MBIH catheter

French pigtail catheter
French scale for caliber of catheter
French shaft balloon
French T-tube
frequency
  halftone
  Larmor
  microbubble resonance
  precisional
  raster
  vibration
frequency analysis of Doppler signal
frequency domain imaging (FDI) in
  ultrasound
frequency offset
frequency-related peak
friability
friable lesion
friable mass
friable mucosa
friable tumor
friable vegetation
friable wall
friction-reducing polymer
Friedel Pick syndrome
Friedländer pneumonia
Friedman view of hip
Friedreich foot
fringe field
fringe skeleton extraction
fringe, synovial
fringe thinning algorithms
frogleg position
frogleg view
froglike appearance
Frohse ligamentous arcade
frondlike appearance
frondlike papillary projection
frontal abscess
frontal bone
frontal defect
frontal foramina
frontal gyrus

frontal horn of lateral ventricle
frontal lobe
frontal lobe contusion
frontal lobe dysfunction
frontal lobe lesion
frontal lobe tumor
frontal oblique view
frontal plane
frontal plane loop
frontal pole
frontal sinus
frontal suture
frontal view
frontoanterior position
frontocentral convexity
frontocentral head region
frontoethmoidal encephalocele
fronto-orbital advancement
frontoparietal
frontoparietal suture
frontopolar region
frontoposterior position
frontosphenoid suture
frontosphenoidal encephalocele
frontotemporal (FT)
frontotemporal atrophy
frontotemporal muscle
frontotemporal region
frontotransverse position
frontozygomatic buttress
frontozygomatic region
frothy colonic mucosa
Frykman classification of hand and
  wrist
FS (full scan) method/projection
FS-BURST MR imaging
F-scan
FSCR, flexible surface-coil-type
FSE (fast SE) imaging
F-series insemination catheter
FSPGR (fast spoiled gradient-recalled)
  MR imaging
FSV (forward stroke volume)

FT (fiber tractography)
FTA (femorotibial angle)
FTC (fibulotalocalcaneal) ligament
FTP (file transfer protocol)
F-1200 (and F-2000) Fluorescence
Spectrophotometer
Fuchs projection of temporal styloid
process
FUdR (5-fluorouracil deoxyribo-
nucleoside)
Fuji AC2 storage phosphor computed
radiology system
Fuji FCR9000 computed radiology
system
Fujinon Sonoprobe
Fukuyama congenital muscular
dystrophy
fulcrum fracture
fulguration of valves
full bladder ultrasound technique
full body echo planar system imager
full-blown cardiac tamponade
full column barium enema
full energy peak efficiency
full field digital mammography system
full field digital mammogram
full scan (FS) method/projection
full scan with interpolation (FI)
method/projection
full thickness button of aortic wall
full thickness Carrel button
full thickness infarction of ventricular
septum
full volume loop spirometry
full width at half maximum (FWHM)
fulminant cerebral lymphoma (in
AIDS)
fulminant course of disease
fulminant hepatic failure (FHF)
fulminant herpes hepatitis
fulminant hydrocephalus
fulminant pulmonary edema
fulminant tuberculosis

fulminating ulcerative colitis
function
abnormal tubular
atrial phasic volumetric
commissural
compromised ventricular
depressed right ventricular
contractile
excitation
excretory
exercise LV
global ventricular
inadequate ovarian
function, Kupffer cell
leaflet
left atrial (LA)
left ventricular (LV)
left ventricular systolic/diastolic
myocardial contractile
ovarian
point spread
regional left ventricular
regional ventricular
renal
renal tubular
reserve cardiac
residual renal
rest LV (left ventricular)
rest RV (right ventricular)
right and left atrial phasic
volumetric
right atrial (RA)
right ventricular (RV)
right ventricular systolic/diastolic
sinusoid reference
split
swallowing
ventricular contractility (VCF)
volumetric
functional abnormality
functional aerobic impairment (FAI)
functional bladder capacity
functional bowel disease

functional brain imaging
functional classification of congestive
  heart failure
functional correlation
functional cyst
functional disorder
functional disturbance
functional evaluation
functional impairment
functional interstitial cell testicular
  tumor
functional magnetic resonance
  imaging (FMRI)
functional MRI (fMRI)
functional nephrosis
functional ovarian cyst
functional reentry
functional refractory period (FRP)
functional residual capacity (FRC)
functional tubular impairment
functional ureteral obstruction
functional urethral length
functional uterine hemorrhage
fundal
fundoplication
fundoplication wrap
fundus (pl. fundi)
  aneurysmal
  bladder
  bald gastric
  eye
  gallbladder
  gastric
  globular
  incompetence of pelvic
  normal
  regular in outline
  stomach
  urinary bladder
  uterine
  vaginal
fundus of aneurysm
fundus of urinary bladder

fundus of uterus
fundus uteri
fungal plaque
fungal pneumonia
fungating lesion
fungoides, mycosis
fungus ball
funic souffle
funicular souffle
funiculus (pl. funiculi)
funiculus cuneatus
funiculus dorsalis
funiculus gracilis
funiculus medullae spinalis
funiculus ventralis
funnel chest
funnel deformity
funnel pelvis
funnel-shaped pelvis
FUO (fever of undetermined origin)
Fürbringer (Fuerbringer) sign
Furmaier method (skyline patella)
furosemide medication
furrier's lung
fused ankle
fused commissures
fused kidney
fused leaflet
fused papillary muscle
fused PET-CT scanner
fused physis
fusiform aneurysm
fusiform bronchiectasis
fusiform dilatation
fusiform expansion
fusiform narrowing of arteries
fusiform shadow
fusiform swelling
fusiform widening of duct
fusion
  ankle
  atlanto-occipital
  bone (bony)

fusion *(cont.)*
   calcaneotibial
   carpal-metacarpal (CMC) (also
      carpometacarpal)
   cervical
   cervical interbody
   chevron
   CT/SPECT
   diaphyseal-epiphyseal
   extra-articular hip
   facet
   image
   interbody
   interphalangeal
   interspinous process
   intra-articular knee
   joint
   metatarsocuneiform joint
   metatarsophalangeal joint
   multilevel

fusion *(cont.)*
   occipitocervical
   pantalar
   spinal
   splenogonadal
   talar body
   talocrural
   tibiocalcaneal
   tibiotalar
   transfibular
   two-stage
fusion defect
fusion of two or more vertebral
   segments
fuzzy echo
fuzzy logic contrast correction
fuzzy rules
fuzzy set theory
FWHM (full width at half maximum)
fx (fracture)

G, g

g (gram)
Ga (gallium) (an element)
GABA-BN complex
gadobenate dimeglumine imaging
  agent
gadobutrol (neutral gadolinium
  chelate) imaging agent
gadodiamide imaging agent
gadofosveset trisodium
gadolinium (Gd) (an element)
gadolinium-coated catheter
gadolinium-coated guidewire
gadolinium complex
gadolinium-enhanced spin echo MR
  imaging
gadolinium-enhanced subtracted MR
  angiography, 3-D
gadolinium-enhanced T1-weighted
  images
gadolinium, motexafin
gadolinium neutron capture therapy
  (GdNCT)
gadolinium texaphyrin (Gd-Tex)
gadolinium zeolite
Gadolite oral suspension (gadolinium
  zeolite) imaging agent

gadopentetate dimeglumine-filled
  catheter
gadopentetate dimeglumine imaging
  agent
gadoteridol imaging agent
gadoversetamide imaging agent
Gaeltec catheter-tip pressure
  transducer
Gage sign
Gairdner disease
Gaisböck syndrome
galactogram
galactography
galactose imaging agent
galactose-based ultrasound imaging
  agent
galactose imaging agent
galea aponeurotica
galeal extension of tumor
Galeazzi fracture-dislocation
Galeazzi fracture of radius
Galeazzi sign
Galen, great cerebral vein of
Galen Scan scanner
Galen teleradiology system
Gallannaugh bone plate

Gallavardin phenomenon
gallbladder
  bilobed
  body of
  chronically inflamed
  contracted
  Courvoisier
  dilated
  distended
  double
  edematous
  fetal
  fish scale
  floating
  folded fundus
  fundal portion of
  fundus of
  hourglass
  mobile
  multiseptate
  neck of
  nonvisualization of
  robin's egg blue
  stasis
  thick-walled
  thin-walled
  wandering
gallbladder bed
gallbladder calculus
gallbladder ejection fraction
gallbladder hydrops
gallbladder lift
gallbladder polyp
gallbladder stasis
gallbladder study (oral cholecystogram)
gallbladder torsion
gallbladder ultrasound
gallbladder wall abscess
Gallie H-graft
gallium (Ga) (an element)
  ^{67}Ga bone scan
  ^{67}Ga citrate radioactive imaging

gallium *(cont.)*
  ^{67}Ga-EDTA
  ^{67}Ga exam
  ^{68}Ga GABA uptake carrier
  ^{67}Ga imaging agent
gallium scan (scanning)
gallium scintigraphy
gallstone (see also *stone*)
  asymptomatic
  dissolution of
  faceted
  floating
  innocent
  radiolucent
  retained
  silent
  symptomatic
gallstone migration
GALT (gut-associated lymphoid
  tissue)
Gambro Lundia Minor artificial
  kidney
gamekeeper's thumb
gamma camera (see *camera*)
gamma counter
gamma irradiation
gamma probe
gamma probe-assisted biopsy
gamma ray attenuation
gamma spectrometric analysis
gamma unit
gamma knife for radiosurgery
Gammex RMI DAP (dose area
  product) meter
Gammex RMI scanner
Gamna-Gandy nodule
Gandy-Nanta disease
ganglia (pl. of ganglion)
ganglioglioma
gangliolysis, radiofrequency
ganglion (pl. ganglia)
  aberrant
  acousticofacial

ganglion *(cont.)*
  aorticorenal
  Acrel
  auditory
  auricular
  basal
  calcification of basal
  cardiac
  carotid
  celiac
  cervical
  cervicothoracic
  ciliary
  coccygeal
  diffuse
  dorsal root (DRG)
  ganglia
  gasserian
  geniculate
  intraosseous
  otic
  palmar
  paravertebral
  prevertebral
  petrosal
  posterior root
  radiocapitellar joint
  Scarpa
  sensory
  sphenopalatine
  submandibular
  spinal
  superior mesenteric
  sympathetic
  trigeminal
  uterine cervical
  vestibular
  Wrisberg
ganglioneuroma
ganglionic cyst in synovial tendon
  sheath
gangliosidosis, GM1 and GM2
gangrenous cholecystitis

gangrenous pneumonia
Ganser diverticulum
gantry angulation in CT-guided
  percutaneous biopsy
gantry of CT scanner
gantry of lithotripsy machine
gantry room
gantry tilt
Ganz-Edwards coronary infusion
  catheter
Ganz formula for coronary sinus flow
gap
  Bochdalek
  intersection
  interslice
gap calculation
Garceau tapered catheter
Garcin syndrome
Garden angle
Garden femoral neck fracture
Gardner-Diamond syndrome
Garland triangle
Garré disease
Garren-Edwards gastric (GEG) bubble
Garren gastric bubble
Garth apical axial oblique view of the
  shoulder
Gartland classification of supracondylar fracture
Gärtner (Gaertner) duct
gas
  abdominal
  aneurysmal wall
  bowel
  coursing of
  free subphrenic
  intravascular
  natural neon
  overlying bowel
  pulmonary
  small bowel
  soft tissue
  subcutaneous tissue
  superimposed bowel

gas accumulation under serous tunic
  of intestine
gas-bloat syndrome
gas CT cisternography
gas cupula
gas density
gas density line
gaseous distention
gaseous drainage
gaseous oxygen artifact
gas-fluid level
gas formation
gas-forming liver abscess
gas-forming organism in bowel wall
gas nitrogen embolism
gas pattern
gasserian duct
gasserian ganglion tumor
gassy
gas target
gastric adenoma
gastric air bubble
gastric antral erosion
gastric antrum
gastric balloon (see *balloon*)
gastric bubble
gastric capacity
gastric catarrh
gastric channel
gastric contents
gastric distention
gastric erosion
gastric fistula
gastric foveola
gastric fundus
gastric impression on liver
gastric lymphatic follicle
gastric mucosa imaging
gastric mucosal pattern
gastric outline
gastric partition
gastric pits
gastric pool

gastric pull-through segment
gastric reflux of bile
gastric remnant
gastric secretion
gastric ulcer
gastric window
gastrinoma, duodenal
gastritis
  acute
  antral
  atrophic
  chronic
  cirrhotic
  hemorrhagic
  hypertrophic
  necrotizing
  pseudomembranous radiation
gastroc (gastrocnemius muscle)
gastrocardiac syndrome
gastrocnemius muscle
gastrocnemius-soleus complex
gastrocnemius-soleus muscle group
gastrocolic ligament
gastrocolic omentum
gastrocystoplasty
gastroduodenal artery complex
gastroduodenitis
gastroduodenal intussusception due to
  Peutz-Jeghers syndrome in infancy
gastroduodenal stent
gastroduodenoscopy
gastroenteritis
gastroenterocolitis
gastroenteroptosis
gastroepiploic arcade
gastroepiploic artery
gastroepiploic vessel
gastroesophageal hernia
gastroesophageal incompetence
gastroesophageal junction (GEJ)
gastroesophageal reflux (GER)
gastroesophageal reflux disease
  (GERD)

Gastrografin (diatrizoate meglumine;
    diatrizoate sodium) imaging agent
Gastrografin enema
gastrohepatic bare area
gastrohepatic omentum
gastrointestinal (GI)
    GI endoscopic ultrasound
    GI tract
gastrointestinal continuity
gastrointestinal hemorrhage
gastrointestinal leiomyosarcoma
gastrointestinal plaque
gastrointestinal stromal tumor
gastrojejunocolic fistula
gastrolienal ligament
GastroMark or GastroMARK
    (ferumoxsil) imaging agent
gastroparesis
gastroptosis
gastroscopy, virtual
gastrosphincteric pressure gradient
gastrostomy, percutaneous (PG)
gas ventilation study
gas volumes
gate arrays
gated blood (pool) cardiac wall motion
    study
gated blood pool ventriculogram
gated cardiac blood pool imaging
gated cardiac CT
gated equilibrium blood pool scanning
gated exercise examination
gated imaging studies
gated inflow technique
gated magnetic resonance imaging
gated planar studies
gated radionuclide ventriculography
gated SPECT (GSPECT)
gated view (in MUGA, multiple gated
    acquisition scan)
gating (timing of images)
    cardiac
    diastolic

gating *(cont.)*
    ECG
    echocardiographic
    electrocardiographic gating with
       electron beam CT technology
    electrocardiogram
    heartbeat
    MUGA
    respiratory
    spirometric (in helical CT
       technology)
    systolic
Gaucher disease
gauge
gauss
gaussian curve
gaussian dose-volume histogram
gaussian distribution
gaussian line saturation
gaussian mode profile laser beam
gaussian noise distortion
Gaynor-Hart inferosuperior carpal
    tunnel projection
Gaynor-Hart position
Gazelle balloon dilation catheter
GBM (glioblastoma multiforme)
GBP (gastric bypass)
GBS (Guillain-Barré syndrome)
GCSF (granulocyte colony stimulating
    factor)
GCT (germ-cell tumor)
GCTSPS (germ-cell tumor with
    synchronous lesions in pineal and
    suprasellar regions)
GCVF (great cardiac vein flow)
Gd (gadolinium) (an element)
GDC (gradient distortion correction)
GE (gastroesophageal)
    GE junction
    GE reflux
GE (General Electric)
    GE CT Advantage scanner
    GE Advance PET scanner

GE (General Electric) *(cont.)*
  GE CT Hi-Speed Advantage
    system
  GE CT 8800 scanner
  GE CT Max scanner
  GE CT Pace scanner
  GE detector
  GE Discovery LS CT/PET scanner
  GE gamma camera
  GE GN300 7.05T/89 mm bore
    multinuclear spectrometer
  GE GN 500 MHz
  GE HiSpeed Advantage helical CT
    scanner
  GE HiSpeed CT scanner
GEJ (gastroesophageal junction)
gelatin sponge
GE Medical Systems
  GE 9800 high resolution CT
    scanner
  GE MR Max scanner
  GE MR Signa scanner
  GE MR Vectra scanner
  GE NMR spectrometer
  GE Omega 500 MHz
  GE QE 300 MHz GE PET
    scanner
  GE RT 3200 ADV II ultrasound
    system
  GE scanner
  GE Senographe 2000D fully digital
    mammography system
  GE Signa 5.4 Genesis MR imager
  GE Signa 5.5 Horizon EchoSpeed
    MR imager
  GE Signa MR system
  GE 0.5 tesla double doughnut
    magnet MRI machine
  GE Signa 1.5 tesla scanner
  GE Signa 1.5 T magnet
  GE Signa 4.7 MRI scanner
  GE Signa 5.2 scanner

GE (General Electric) *(cont.)*
  GE Signa 5.2 scanner with SR-230
    3-axis EPI gradient upgrade
  GE single axis SR-230 echo-planar
    system
  GE single detector SPECT-capable
    camera
  GE single photon emission com-
    puterized tomography
  GE SPECT (single photon
    emission computerized
    tomography)
  GE Spiral CT scanner
  GE Starcam single crystal tomo-
    graphic scintillation camera
Gee-Herter disease
GEG (Garren-Edwards gastric) bubble
Geiger counter
gelatinous debris
gelatinous hematoma
Gelfoam powder embolization
gemellary pregnancy
gemellus (pl. gemelli) muscle
gene delivery imaging
generalized nephrographic (GNG)
  phase imaging (CT scan)
general pattern matching
General Electric (see *GE*)
generalized
generator
  carbon dioxide
  ^{166}Dy (dysprosium)
  extraction
  ^{166}Ho (holmium in vivo)
  172Hf-172Lu (not superscripts)
  molybdenum-99
  Van de Graaff
generator-produced ^{188}Re (rhenium)
GeneSys guidewire catheter
genial tubercle of mandible
geniculate body
geniculate ganglion
geniculocalcarine region

geniculocalvarium
geniculum
genital lesion
genital prolapse
genital tract
genitourinary fistula
genitourinary tuberculosis
Gennari
  band of
  line of
  stripe of (in brain)
Gensini catheter
Gentle-Flo suction catheter
genupectoral position (knee-chest
  position)
genu valgum (knock-knee) deformity
genu varum (bowleg) deformity
geographic fatty change
geographic lesion
geometric distortion
geometry
  broad beam
  coronary vessel
  narrow beam
geometry factor
geophagia artifact
GER (gastroesophageal reflux)
GERD (gastroesophageal reflux
  disease)
Gerdy ligament
Gerdy tubercle in knee
Gerhardt sign
Gerhardt triangle
geriatric features on chest x-ray
germ-cell tumor (GCT)
germinal matrix
germinoma
  intracranial
  intramedullary spinal cord
  primary central nervous system
Gertzbein classification of seat belt
  injury
Gesco umbilical catheter

gestation
  extrauterine
  intrauterine
gestational age
gestational edema
gestational sac diameter (GS)
gestational trophoblastic disease
gestational trophoblastic neoplasia
  (GTN)
GeV (gigaelectron volt)
GF cassette
GFR (glomerular filtration rate)
Ghon complex
Ghon primary lesion
Ghon-Sachs complex
Ghon tubercle
ghosting artifact
GI (gastrointestinal)
giant aneurysm
giant aortic pseudoaneurysm
  giant cell
giant bullous emphysema
giant cell carcinoma
giant cell formation
giant cell interstitial (GIP)
giant cell interstitial pneumonia (GIP)
giant gastric folds
giant hydronephrosis
Gianturco-Roehm bird's nest vena
  caval filter
Gianturco-Rösch Z-stent esophageal
  stent
Gianturco-Roubin flexible coil stent
Gianturco-Wallace venous stent
Gianturco wool-tufted wire coil stent
giardiasis
gibbous deformity
Gibbs artifact
Gibbs phenomenon
Gibbs random field
gibbus (n.)
GIF (graphics interchange format)
gigaelectron volt (GeV)

gigantism, cerebral
Gilliam suspension of uterus
GIP (giant cell interstitial pneumonia)
girdle
  limb
  pelvic
  shoulder
girth, abdominal
Given diagnostic imaging system
gland
  absorbent
  accessory
  admaxillary
  adrenal
  Albarran
  alveolar
  anteprostatic
  aortic
  apical
  aporic
  arterial
  arteriococcygeal
  axillary sweat
  Bartholin
  bulbocavernous
  bulbourethral
  calcification of pineal
  carotid
  coccygeal
  Cowper
  Duverney
  endocrine
  globate
  glomiform
  haversian
  hilar
  interscapular
  lacrimal
  lymph
  mammary
  ovaries
  pancreas
  parathyroid

gland *(cont.)*
  parotid
  pineal
  pituitary
  prostate
  salivary
  Skene
  sublingual
  submandibular
  suprarenal
  testes
  urethral
  thymus
  thyroid
gland volume
glandular proliferation
glandular tissue
Glasgow sign
glass blower's emphysema
glasses
  CrystalEyes shutter
  red/blue anaglyph
glass eye artifact
glass track detector
Gleason grade
Gleicher salpingography catheter
Glénard disease
glenohumeral joint
glenohumeral ligament
glenoid cavity
glenoid fossa
glenoid labrum
glenoid process
GLF lymphography method
glial disease
glial nodule
glial scarring
glial tumor
GlideCath sheath
Glidewire
  long taper/stiff shaft
  Radiofocus
glioblast

glioblastoma
glioblastoma multiforme (GBM)
glioma
   anaplastic cerebral
   brain stem
   butterfly-type
   cerebral
   high grade
   intracranial
   low grade
   malignant
   nonanaplastic
   optic nerve
   pontine
   rolandoparietal
   supratentorial
glioma tumor
gliomatosis cerebri
glioneural hamartoma
gliosarcoma
gliosis
   astrocytic
   progressive subcortical
   reactive
gliosis of sylvian aqueduct
Glisson capsule
global cardiac disease
global cerebral hypoperfusion
global cerebral ischemia
global cortical defect
global ejection fraction
global hypokinesis
global hypometabolism
global left ventricular dysfunction
global left ventricular perfusion
global systolic left ventricular
   dysfunction
global tissue loss
global ventricular dysfunction
global wall motion abnormality
globally depressed ejection fraction
globe, optic
globe-orbit relationship

globoid heart
globular chest
globular fundus
globular sputum
globus hystericus
globus pallidus
globus pallidus internal (GPi) segment
Glofil-125 (iothalamate sodium I 125)
   imaging agent
glomeriform arteriovenous
   anastomosis
glomeriform arteriovenular
   anastomosis
glomerular arteriole
glomerular basement membrane
glomerular capsule
glomerular filtration agent
glomerular filtration rate (GFR)
glomerular hypertrophy
glomerular tip lesion
glomeruloid formation
glomerulonephritis
   acute
   malignant
   membranous
   necrotizing
   proliferative
   segmental necrotizing
glomus (subungual) tumor
glomus tumor of fingertip
glomus-type arteriovenous
   malformation (AVM)
glossopharyngeal nerve (ninth cranial
   nerve)
glottic larynx
glottis
glove phenomenon (artifact)
gloves, radiation-attenuating surgical
glow curve
GLP7 film
glucagon imaging agent
glucarate, radiolabeled
glucarate ^{99m}Tc hot spot imaging agent

glucarate tracer
glucose metabolism within the
    myocardium
glue, percutaneous fibrin
glutamate spectroscopy
glutathione
gluteal bonnet
gluteal lines
gluteus maximus muscle
gluteus medius muscle
gluteus minimus muscle
GNG (generalized nephrographic)
    phase imaging (CT scan)
goblet sign
goiter
    Basedow
    colloid
    cystic
    diffuse
    diving
    exophthalmic
    familial
    fibrous
    intrathoracic
    iodide
    iodine deficiency
    lingual
    multinodular
    nodular
    parenchymous
    retrovascular
    simple
    substernal
    suffocative
    thyroid
    toxic
    toxic nodular
    vascular
    wandering
Golay coil
gold Au 198 (^{198}Au) imaging agent
gold marker seeds
gold-195m imaging agent

gold-195m radionuclide
gold radioactive source
gold standard of diagnosis
Goldblatt phenomenon
Goldenhar syndrome
Goldstein sonohysterography catheter
golfer's elbow
GoLytely bowel prep
gonial angle (of mandible)
goniometer, Rippstein
gonion-gnathion plane
Goodale-Lubin cardiac catheter
Goodpasture syndrome
gooseneck concept
gooseneck deformity of outflow tract
gooseneck shape of ventricular
    outflow
Gore 1.5T Torso Array surface coil
Gore-Tex cardiovascular patch
Gore-Tex catheter
Gore-Tex soft tissue patch
gorge
gorging
Gorham disease
Gorlin catheter
Gorlin formula for aortic valve area
Gorlin hydraulic formula for mitral
    valve area
Gorlin method for cardiac output
Gorlin syndrome
Gosling pulsatility index
Gosselin fracture
Gosset, spiral band of
gossypiboma
Gothic arch formation
Gottschalk staging
Gould PentaCath 5-lumen
    thermodilution catheter
Gould Statham pressure transducer
Gouley syndrome
gout, tophaceous
gouty tophus
Gowers bundle

Gowers column
Gowers fasciculus
Gowers syndrome
GP (gastroplasty)
GPi (globus pallidus internal) segment
graafian follicle
graafian vesicle
Grace method of ratio of metatarsal
   length
grade (also grading)
   Gleason
   histologic
   Hyams
   osteoarthritis
   osteoarthritis radiographic (I-V)
   placental
   Severin
graded compression sonography
graded compression ultrasonography
graded infusion
grade 1 tear
grade 2 tear
grade 3 tear
gradient
   aortic outflow
   aortic valve (AVG)
   aortic valve peak instantaneous
   arteriovenous pressure
   atrioventricular
   biliary-duodenal pressure
   brain-core
   conjugate
   coronary perfusion
   dephasing
   diastolic
   duodenobiliary pressure
   elevated
   encoding
   end diastolic aortic–left ventricular
      pressure
   Ficoll
   gastrosphincteric pressure
   hepatic venous pressure

gradient *(cont.)*
   holosystolic
   instantaneous
   left ventricular outflow pressure
   maximal estimated
   mean mitral valve
   mean systolic
   mitral valve
   negligible pressure
   outflow tract
   peak diastolic
   peak instantaneous
   peak pressure
   peak right ventricular–right atrial
      systolic
   peak systolic (PSG)
   peak to peak pressure
   perfusion
   pressure
   pressure-flow
   pulmonary artery diastolic and
      wedge pressure (PADP-PAWP)
   pulmonary artery to right ventricle
      diastolic
   pulmonary outflow
   pulmonic valve
   rephasing
   residual
   right ventricular to main pulmonary
      artery pressure
   stenotic
   subvalvular
   systolic
   transaortic systolic
   translesional
   transmitral diastolic
   transpulmonic
   transstenotic pressure
   transtricuspid valve diastolic
   transvalvar
   transvalvular pressure
   tricuspid valve
   ventricular

gradient across valve
gradient amplifier
gradient coil
gradient distortion correction (GDC)
gradient drive current
gradient echo cine technique
gradient echo image
gradient echo imaging sequence
gradient echo MR with magnetization
  transfer
gradient echo pulse sequence
gradient echo sequence
gradient echo phase image
gradient echo pulse sequence
gradient echo sequence imaging
gradient magnetic field
gradient-recalled acquisition in a
  steady state (GRASS)
gradient-recalled echo (GRE)
gradient sheet coils
gradient waveforms
grading (see *grade*)
Graf alpha angle
Graf beta angle
graft
  AFBG (aortofemoral bypass graft)
  coronary artery bypass (CABG)
  Dacron-covered stent
  endovascular aortic
  Ochsner
  off-pump coronary artery bypass
    (OPCABG)
  OmniFlow vascular
  synthetic interposition
  transrenal arteriovenous dialysis
graft copolymer
graft-enteric erosion
grafting
Graftpatch
graft patency
graft-versus-host disease (GVHD)
Graham-Burford-Mayer syndrome
Graham-Cole cholecystography

grain-handler's lung
grainy appearance
gram (g)
gram-negative bacilli pneumonia
Grancher sign
Grancher triad
grand mal seizure
Grandy lateral cervical spine view
Granger view
Grantham classification of femur
  fracture
granularity
granular kidney
granular sparkling appearance of the
  myocardium
granulated
granulation stenosis
granulation tissue
granulocyte colony stimulating factor
  (GCSF)
granulocytic leukemia
granuloma (pl. granulomata)
  amebic
  apical
  beryllium
  calcified
  cholesterol
  coccidioidal
  coli
  eosinophilic
  epithelioid
  extravascular
  fishtank
  foreign body
  frontoethmoidal giant cell
    reparative
  Hodgkin
  inguinal
  laryngeal
  lethal midline
  lipoid
  Majocchi
  malarial

granuloma *(cont.)*
  midline
  Mignon
  miliary
  noncaseating
  paracoccidioidal
  periapical
  pseudopyogenic
  reticulohistiocytic
  rheumatic
  silicotic
  stellate
  swimming pool
  trichophytic
  tuberculous
  umbilical
  xanthomatous
granuloma annulare
granulomatosis
  allergic
  Wegener
granulomatous enterocolitis
granulomatous gastritis
granulomatous inflammation of
  bronchi
granulomatous pneumonia
granulomatous pneumonitis
granulosa cell tumor
granulosa-theca cell tumor
granulovacuolar degeneration
graphics interchange format (GIF)
graphite fibrosis of lung
Graser diverticulum
Grashey method (skull)
Grashey method (to view glenohumeral joint space)
Grashey oblique plantodorsal projection of the foot
GRASS (gradient-recalled acquisition
  in a steady state)
  GRASS MR imaging
  GRASS pulse sequence
Gratiolet convolutions

grave prognosis
Graves disease
gravid uterus
gravid uterus prolapse
gravida
gravis, myasthenia
gravitational edema
gravity drainage
gray commissure (of spinal cord)
gray hepatization stage of pneumonia
gray horns in spinal canal
gray matter
gray reticular formation
gray scale Doppler
gray scale images (imaging)
gray scale range
gray scale ultrasound
Grayson ligament in hand
gray to white matter activity ratio
gray to white matter utilization ratio
gray-white differentiation on CT scan
gray-white matter contrast ratio
gray-white matter junction
GRE (gradient-recalled echo)
  GRE breath-hold hepatic imaging
  GRE-in images
  GRE-out images
  GRE magnetic resonance imaging
greater curvature of stomach
greater multangular bone
greater saphenous vein
greater sciatic notch
greater superficial petrosal nerve
greater tarsal angle
greater trochanter
greater tuberosity
great vessels, transposition of
Greene renal implant stent
Greene sign
Greenfield IVC (inferior vena cava)
  filter
greenstick fracture
Greer EZ Access drainage pouch

grenade thrower's fracture
grenz ray
Greulich and Pyle Atlas
Greulich and Pyle, bone age
  according to
grey (see *gray*)
grid
  mammography
  megavoltage
grid and slot scan scatter reduction
grid therapy
Griesinger sign
groin adenopathy
groin mass
Grollman pigtail catheter
groove
  alveolingual
  alveolobuccal
  alveololabial
  anal intersphincteric
  anterolateral
  anteromedian
  arterial
  atrioventricular (AV)
  auriculoventricular
  basilar
  bicipital
  bronchial
  buccal
  carotid
  carpal
  cavernous
  central
  coronary
  costal
  dental
  developmental
  digastric
  esophageal
  ethmoidal
  gastric
  genital
  gingivobuccal

groove *(cont.)*
  gingivolabial
  Harrison
  infraorbital
  interatrial
  intertubercular
  interventricular
  labial
  lacrimal
  Liebermeister
  neural
  paravertebral
  radial
  radial neck
  sagittal
  Sibson
  spindle colonic
  ulnar
  urethral
  venous
  Verga lacrimal
  vertebral
Groshong catheter
Groshong double lumen catheter
Groshong tunneled catheter
Grossman scale for regurgitation
Grossman sign
ground-glass appearance of lungs
ground-glass attenuation
ground-glass density
ground-glass infiltrates in lungs
ground-glass matrix
ground-glass opacity
ground plate
ground state
Group A hemolytic streptococci
  pneumonia
group viewing
growth arrest line
growth center of bone
growth plate arrest
growth plate fracture
growth plate injury

growth plate, premature closure of
growth plate widening
Gruber fossa
Gruentzig (Grüntzig)
grumous debris
grumous tissue
Grüntzig (Gruentzig)
Grüntzig balloon catheter angioplasty
Grüntzig Dilaca catheter
Grüntzig technique for PTCA
GS (gestational sac)
GSA imaging agent for liver
   scintigraphy
Gsell-Erdheim syndrome
GSPECT (gated SPECT)
GSW (gunshot wound)
GSWH (gunshot wound to head)
GTN (gestational trophoblastic
   neoplasia)
guanylate cyclase (enzyme)
Guérin fracture
Guglielmi detachable coil (GDC)
guidance
   active biplanar MR imaging
   biplanar MR imaging
   catheter advanced under fluoro-
      scopic
   color-flow Doppler sonographic
   computerized tomography (CT)
   fetal umbilical vein injection under
      sonographic
   fluoroscopic
   frameless stereotaxic
   radiologic
   transvaginal uterine cervical
      dilation with fluoroscopic
   ultrasonic
   under fluoroscopic
Guidant introducer
Guidant sheath
guidewire
   ACS Hi-Torque Balance middle-
      weight

guidewire *(cont.)*
   Amplatz Teflon-coated
   Conceptus Robust
   flexible-tip
   gadolinium-coated
   High Performance Detach
   Innovante
   Intercept Vascular
   intravascular loopless antenna
   Jocath
   Jography
   Joguide
   J-tipped exchange
   J-tipped spring
   long taper/stiff shaft Glidewire
   Lumina
   Lunderquist
   Lunderquist-Ring torque
   Microvasive Glidewire
   Microvasive stiff piano wire
   Mustang steerable
   Navius
   Outcomes by Design steerable
   PercuSurge GuardWire system
   Phantom cardiac
   Prima laser
   Radiofocus Glidewire
   Rapid-Trak
   Redifocus
   Reflex steerable
   Shinobi Plus
   Shinobi steerable
   SilverSpeed
   Teflon-coated
   WaveWire high performance
      angioplasty
guidewire entrapment
guidewire for needle localization
Guidezilla Softip guiding catheter
guiding catheter
guiding shots
Guillain-Barré syndrome
guilt screen

Gull disease
gumma (pl. gummas or gummata)
gummas of rib
gummatous lesion
gun stock deformity
Gunn crossing sign
gunshot wound (GSW)
gunshot wound to head (GSWH)
gusset-type patch
Gustilo-Anderson classification of
    tibial plafond fracture
Gustilo classification of tibial fractures
gut (intestine)
    blind
    large
    mid-
    small
gutter
    lateral
    left
    paracolic
    parapelvic
    peritoneal
    right
    sacral
gutter fracture
Guyon canal
GVHD (graft-versus-host disease)
Gy (gray)
gymnast's wrist
gynecoid pelvis
Gyne-Flo Leventhal cannula
GyneSys cervical access
GyneSys uterine cornual access
    catheter
GyneSys uterine ostial access catheter
gyral crest
gyration
Gyrex Prestige 2.0T MR imaging
    system
gyri cerebri
gyriform calcification
gyromagnetic ratio

Gyroscan ACS NT MRI scanner
Gyroscan Intera scanner
Gyroscan, Philips
Gyroscan S15 scanner
gyrus (pl. gyri)
    angular (AG)
    annectant
    ascending parietal
    Broca
    callosal
    central
    cingulate
    contiguous supramarginal
    dentate
    fasciolar
    first temporal
    flattening of
    frontal
    fusiform
    Heschl transverse
    hippocampal
    inferior frontal
    inferior temporal
    infracalcarine
    insular
    lamination of
    lateral occipitotemporal
    lingual
    marginal
    medial occipitotemporal
    middle frontal
    middle temporal
    occipital
    occipitotemporal
    olfactory
    orbital
    paracentral
    parahippocampal
    paraterminal
    parietal
    postcentral
    posterior central
    precentral

gyrus *(cont.)*
   preinsular
   quadrate
   short insular
   subcallosal
   subcollateral
   superior frontal
   superior parietal lobule
   superior temporal
   supracallosal
   supramarginal
   temporal

gyrus *(cont.)*
   transverse temporal
   Turner marginal
   uncal
   uncinate
gyrus cerebelli
gyrus cingulatus
gyrus cinguli
gyrus fornicatus
gyrus hippocampi
gyrus isthmus fornicatus
gyrus rectus

H, h

Haas intrauterine insemination catheter
Haas view (head)
habenula
habitus
  body
  gracile
  large
Haemophilus influenzae pneumonia
HAF (hippocampus-amygdala
  formation)
Hagar probe
Haglund deformity
Hagner disease
Hahn-Steinthal classification of
  capitellum fracture
Haid Universal bone plate system
Haifa camera
Haim-Munk syndrome
hairline crack in bone cortex
hairline fracture
hair-on-end sign
Hajdu-Cheney syndrome
HAL (hip axis length)
Hale syndrome
half axial projection
half dose enhanced MRI with MT
  (magnetization transfer)

half-filtered imaging agent
half-Fourier acquisition single shot
  turbo spin echo (HASTE)
half-Fourier imaging (HFI)
half-Fourier three-dimensional
  technique
half-life
  antibody
  biological
  effective
  radioactive
  short
HalfLytely and bisacodyl tablets bowel
  prep kit
half-moon artifact
half-moon mark artifact
half-moon shape
half scan (HS)
half scan cone-beam CT fluoroscopy
half scan fan-beam weighting
half scan method/projection
half scan with extrapolation (HE)
  method/projection
half scan with interpolation (HI)
  method/projection
half-time, clearance
halftone banding

halftone frequency
half-wedged field technique
Hallberg biliointestinal bypass
Haller aberrant duct
Hallermann-Streiff-François syndrome
hallucal pronation
hallux abductovalgus
hallux abductus angle
hallux elevatus
hallux extensus
hallux flexus deformity
hallux interphalangeal joint
hallux interphalangeus angle
hallux limitus (HL)
hallux malleus deformity
hallux migration
hallux rigidus deformity
hallux valgus (HV)
    bilateral
    unilateral
hallux valgus angle (HVA)
hallux valgus deformity
hallux valgus interphalangeus angle
hallux valgus-metatarsus primus varus
    complex
hallux varus deformity
halo cast
halo effect
halogenated thymidine analogue
    (radiosensitizer)
halo ring
halo sign
halo, tumor (on ultrasound image)
halo vest
HAMA (human anti-murine
    antibodies) response
hamartoma
    cardiac
    cartilaginous
    chondromatous
    duodenal wall
    glioneural
    mesenchymal

hamartoma (cont.)
    pancreatic
    pulmonary
    subependymal
    vascular
    ventromedial hypothalamic
hamartomatous lesion
hamartomatous polyp
hamate bone
hamate tail fracture
hamburger sign
hammocking of leaflet
Hamilton-Stewart formula for
    measuring cardiac output
Hamman pneumopericardium sign
Hamman-Rich syndrome (idiopathic
    pulmonary fibrosis)
hammer-marked skull secondary to
    thinning
hammer toe (or hammertoe)
    dynamic
    fixed
hammock mitral valve
hammock valve
hammocking of mitral valve leaflet
Hampton hump
Hampton line
hamstring muscle
Hanafee catheter
hand
    articulations of
    digital artery of
    phalanges of
hand-agitated
hand bone phosphorus
hand-joint synovitis
hand grip exercise
handheld probe
hand injection of imaging agent
handles, jug (zygomatic arches)
Hand-Schüller (Schueller)-Christian
    disease
hangman's fracture

HAP (hepatic arterial-dominant phase)
images (CT scan)
HAPE (high altitude pulmonary
edema)
Hara classification of gallbladder
inflammation
HARC-C wavelet compression
technique
hard disk herniation
hard metal disease
hardening of arteries
hard nodular urinary calculus
harmonic power Doppler ultrasound
harmonization
hardware optimized trapezoid (HOT)
pulse
Hardy-Clapham sesamoid classification
Harkavy syndrome
harmonic imaging
Harris and Beath position
Harris axial projection of the heel
Harrison sulcus
Hartmann closure of rectum
Hartmann point
Hartmann pouch
Hartnup disease
Hartzler ACX-II or RX-014 balloon
catheter
Hartzler angioplasty balloon
Hartzler LPS dilatation catheter
Hartzler Micro XT dilatation catheter
harvester lung
harvesting
bone
graft
vein
Hashimoto thyroiditis
HASTE (half-Fourier acquisition
single shot turbo spin echo) MR
cholangiography
HASTE MRI sequence
HAT-transformed images

Hatcher-Smith cervical fusion
hatchet-head deformity
Hatle method to calculate mitral valve
area
Hausdorff error
Hausdorff metric measure
haustral blunting
haustral fold
haustral indentation
haustral markings
haustral pattern
haustral pouch
haustrations
haustrum (pl. haustra)
haversian canal
haversian gland
Hawkins breast localization needle
with FlexStrand cable
Hawkins classification of talar neck
fractures
Hawkins impingement sign
Hawkins line
Hawkins sign
Hawkins II talar neck fracture
Hayem-Widal syndrome
Hayes view of superior-inferior
sacroiliac joints
Haygarth node
haze
hilar
perihilar
hazy density
hazy infiltrate
HBCT (helical biphasic contrast CT)
HC (head circumference)
HC/AC ratio (head circumference to
abdominal circumference)
HCC (hepatocellular carcinoma)
HCTH (helical CT holography)
HDI (HDTV-interlaced)
HDI (high definition imaging) 3000
ultrasound system
HDI 5000 SonoCT imaging

HD 85 (barium sulfate) imaging agent
HDIC (hepatodiaphragmatic
    interposition of the colon)
HDM bronchial provocation test
HDM challenge
HDR (high dose rate)
HDR (high dose rate) brachytherapy
HD 200 Plus (barium sulfate) imaging
    agent
HE (half scan with extrapolation)
    method/projection
head
    cartilaginous cap of phalangeal
    clavicular head of sternocleido-
        mastoid
    femoral
    first metatarsal (FMH)
    floating
    forward positioning of
    humeral
    long
    metatarsal
    pancreas
    radial
    short
    terminal
    transillumination of
    ulnar
head and neck, femoral
head circumference (HC)
head-first position
head frame distortion
head frame, Riechert-Mundinger (RM)
headhunter catheter
head kidney
head of barium column
head-up tilt
healing infarct
health physics
HealthShield wound drainage catheter
heart
    abdominal
    air-driven artificial

heart *(cont.)*
    alcoholic
    ALVAD (intra-abdominal left
        ventricular assist device)
    artificial
    angiosarcoma of
    aortic opening of
    apex of
    armored
    artificial
    athlete's
    athletic
    axis of
    balloon-shaped
    Baylor total artificial
    beer
    beriberi
    boat-shaped
    bony
    booster
    boot-shaped
    bovine
    bread-and-butter
    bulb of
    cardiogenic shock
    cervical
    chaotic
    conical
    coronary artery of
    crisscross
    degeneration of
    diaphragmatic surface of
    dome-shaped
    donor
    drop
    dynamite
    enlargement of
    elongated
    empty
    encased
    enlarged
    failing
    fat

heart *(cont.)*
  fatty
  fibroid
  fibroma of
  flabby
  flask-shaped
  globoid
  hairy
  hanging (suspended)
  holiday
  horizontal
  hyperdynamic
  hyperkinetic
  hyperthyroid
  hypertrophied
  hypoplastic
  hypothermic
  inferior border of
  inflammation of
  intermediate
  irritable
  ischemic
  left (atrium and ventricle)
  left border of
  left ventricle of
  luxus
  lymphosarcoma of
  malposition of
  massively enlarged
  mildly enlarged
  movable
  myxedema of
  myxoma of
  neurofibroma of the
  nonpenetrating trauma of
  one-ventricle
  ovoid
  ox
  paracorporeal
  parchment
  pear-shaped
  pectoral
  pendulous

heart *(cont.)*
  prostate carcinoma metastatic to
  pulmonary
  Quain fatty
  resting
  rhabdomyoma of
  right (atrium and ventricle)
  right border of
  right ventricle of
  round
  sabot
  semihorizontal
  semivertical
  single outlet
  snowman
  soldier's
  spastic
  sternocostal surface of
  stone
  superior border of
  superoinferior
  suspended
  systemic
  teardrop
  three-chambered
  thrush breast
  tiger
  tiger lily
  tobacco
  total artificial (TAH)
  transplanted
  transverse
  Traube
  triatrial
  trilocular
  univentricular
  University of Akron artificial
  upstairs-downstairs
  Utah artificial
  Utah TAH (total artificial heart)
  venous
  venting of
  vertical

heart *(cont.)*
    wandering
    water-bottle
    wooden shoe
heart and great vessels
heart and lung transplantation
heart apex
heart attack (myocardial infarction)
heart border
heart catheterization (also cardiac)
    femoral
    retrograde
    transseptal
    transvenous
heart in sinus rhythm
heart overload
heart decortication
heart disease, atherosclerotic
heart failure
    acute
    backward
    chronic
    compensated congestive
    congestive
    decompensated congestive
    diastolic
    fetal
    forward
    high output
    left-sided
    low output
    refractory
    right-sided
    systolic
heart-lung transplant (transplantation)
heart motion-adapted magnetic
    resonance velocity mapping
heart power failure
heart prosthesis
heart sac
heart tamponade
heart remnant
Heartscan heart attack prediction test

heart to background ratio
heart to lung ratio (HLR)
HeartView CT cardiac imaging
heat ablation
heat-damaged Tc-RBCs
heat expandable stent
heat fracture
heat-generating source
Heath-Edwards classification of
    pulmonary vascular disease
heating, electromagnetic
heat-transmitting balloon catheter
heave and lift
heaving precordial motion
heavy-particle irradiation
Heberden disease
Heberden nodes
Heberden sign
Hecht pneumonia
Heckathorn disease
Hector, tendon of
Hecht pneumonia
heel bone
heel pad sign
heel tendon
Heerfordt syndrome
Hegglin syndrome
Heim-Kreysig sign
Heinig sternoclavicular view
Helbing sign
helical biphasic contrast-enhanced CT
    (HBCT)
helical coil stent
helical computed tomography (CT)
helical CT holography (HCTH)
helical pattern
helical thin-section CT scan
helical-tip Halo catheter
helicine artery of uterus
Helios diagnostic imaging system
helium-filled balloon catheter
Helix camera
Heller myotomy

Helmholtz coil
Helmholtz configuration
heloma (pl. helomata)
heloma durum
heloma molle
hemal arch
hemangioblastoma tumor
hemangioendothelioma
hemangioma
  cavernous
  hepatic
  infantile
  synovial
  verrucous
hemangiomatosis
hemangiopericytoma
Hemaquet sheath
hematemesis
hematochezia
hematocystic spot (HCS)
hematogenous dissemination
hematogenous spread of metastases
hematologic parameters
hematoma
  aneurysmal
  balancing subdural
  broad ligament
  carotid plaque
  chronic subdural (CSDH)
  cord
  corpus cavernosum
  corpus luteum
  dissecting aortic
  dural
  encapsulated subdural
  epidural (EDH)
  evolving
  extracerebral
  extradural
  gelatinous
  hemispheric
  intracerebral
  intracranial

hematoma *(cont.)*
  intramural
  intraparenchymal
  intrarenal
  intraventricular
  liver
  localized subdural
  mural
  nasal septum
  organized
  parenchymal
  penis
  perianal
  pericardial
  perineal
  perinephric
  perirenal
  posterior fossa
  postoperative pelvic
  primary intracerebral
  rectus sheath
  retromembranous
  retroperitoneal
  scalp
  scrotal
  spinal epidural
  spontaneous spinal epidural
  subcapsular
  subdural
  subepithelial
  subfascial
  subgaleal
  subscapular
  testicular
  vaginal
  vulvar
hematoma cap
  azygos
  left pleural apical
hematoma formation on bowel wall
hematomediastinum (hemomediastinum)
hematopericardium (hemopericardium)

hematopoiesis, extramedullary
hematopoietic stem cell transplantation
hematuria, asymptomatic
hemiagenesis
hemiarch
hemiatrophy
hemiaxial view
hemiazygos vein, accessory
hemibody irradiation
hemic calculus
hemicardium
hemicolon
hemicranium
hemidiaphragm
    attenuation by
    tenting of
hemidiaphragmatic
hemidiaphragmatic mobility
hemidiaphragm depression
hemifacial microsomia
hemihypertrophy
hemipelvis
hemisection of spinal cord
hemispheric mass effect
hemisphere
    cerebellar
    cerebral
    dominant
    left
    mesial
    right
hemisphere atrophy
hemisphere damage
hemisphere lesion
hemisphere stroke
hemithorax (pl. hemithoraces)
hemivertebra
    balanced
    unbalanced
Hemocath catheter
hemodialysis (HD)
    LifeSite
    surgically implanted
    venovenous

hemodialysis access shunt
hemodialysis graft dysfunction
hemodynamic alterations
hemodynamic assessment
hemodynamically significant findings
hemodynamically weighted echo
    planar MR imaging
hemodynamic impotence
hemodynamic penumbra
hemodynamic reserve impairment
hemodynamic response
hemodynamic support
hemodynamics, cardiovascular
hemoglobin tomography
hemomediastinum (hematomedia-
    stinum)
hemoperfusion
hemopericardium
hemoperitoneum
hemophilia, post-traumatic
hemopneumothorax
hemoptysis
hemorrhage
    accidental
    adrenal
    alveolar
    anastomotic
    aneurysmal
    antepartum
    arterial
    bladder wall
    brain stem
    capillary
    central nervous system
    cerebellar
    cerebral
    chronic parenchymal
    concealed
    corpus luteum
    cutaneous
    delayed traumatic intracerebral
        (DTICH)
    diffuse subarachnoid

hemorrhage *(cont.)*
Duret
dysfunctional uterine
eight-ball
epicranial subaponeurotic
epidural
exsanguinating (into pleural space)
external
extradural
extrapleural
fetal-maternal
fetomaternal
focal endocardial
frank
functional uterine
gastrointestinal
hypothalamic
internal
interstitial
intertrabecular
intra-abdominal
intra-alveolar
intracerebral (ICH)
intracranial
intramural arterial
intraocular
intraparenchymal
intrapartum
intraplaque (IPH)
intrapleural
intrapulmonary
intrarenal
intratumoral
intraventricular (IVH)
life-threatening
lobar intracerebral
massive exsanguinating
massive pulmonary
meningeal
neonatal intracranial
nondominant putaminal
nontraumatic epidural
neonatal intracranial

hemorrhage *(cont.)*
nonvariceal gastrointestinal
old
parenchymal
parenchymatous
periaqueductal
peribronchiolar
peripartal vaginal
perirenal
pontine
postoperative mediastinal
postpartum
profuse uterine
prostatic
pulmonary
putaminal
renal
renal artery
retrobulbar
retroperitoneal
salmon-patch
sentinel transoral
slit
spinal epidural (SEH)
spinal subarachnoid
spinal subdural (SSH)
splinter
striate
subacute
subarachnoid (SAH)
subchorionic
subdural (SDH)
subependymal
submucosal
subserosal
thalamic
third stage
traumatic meningeal
umbilical
uterine
variceal
venous
hemorrhage from biopsy site

hemorrhage in ectopic pregnancy
hemorrhagic consolidation
hemorrhagic corpus luteum cyst
hemorrhagic cyst
hemorrhagic cystitis
hemorrhagic disease of newborn
hemorrhagic duodenitis
hemorrhagic dystrophic thrombocyto-
  penia
hemorrhagic gastritis
hemorrhagic infarct
hemorrhagic necrosis
hemorrhagic nephritis
hemorrhagic nodular purpura
hemorrhagic ovarian cyst
hemorrhagic pericarditis
hemorrhagic pleurisy
hemorrhagic pyelitis
hemorrhagic retinitis
hemorrhagic salpingitis
hemorrhagic shearing lesion
hemorrhagic stroke
hemorrhagic zone, pyramidal
hemostatic puncture closure device
  (HPCD)
hemothorax (pl. hemothoraces)
hemotympanum
Henderson-Jones chondromatosis
Henderson-Jones disease
Henke trigone
Henle
  jejunal interposition of
  ligament of
Henle loop
Henle sheath
Henry
  master knot of
  vertebral artery of
Henry and Wrisberg, ligaments of
Henschen view of petrous temporal
  region
Hensing fold
heparin

heparinization
heparinized blood
hepatic abscess
hepatic adrenal rest tumor
hepatic angiogram, angiography
hepatic angiomyolipoma
hepatic arterial dominant phase (HAP)
  images
hepatic arterial phase (HAP)
hepatic arteriovenous fistula
hepatic artery, accessory
hepatic artery pseudoaneurysm
hepatic artery thrombosis
hepatic bed
hepatic cirrhosis
hepatic congestion
hepatic cord
hepatic cyst
hepatic diverticulum
hepatic duct bifurcation
hepatic flexure of colon
hepatic hemangioma
hepatic insufficiency
hepatic involvement
hepatic necrosis
hepatic vein thrombosis
hepatic venography with hemodynamic
  evaluation
hepatic veno-occlusive disease
hepatic venous Doppler wave pattern
hepatic venous outflow
hepatic venous web disease
hepatic web dilation
hepatitis
  fulminant
  fulminant herpes
  infectious (hepatitis A)
  serum (hepatitis B)
hepatization
hepatobiliary disease
hepatobiliary ductal system imaging
  with quantitative measurement of
  gallbladder function

hepatobiliary ductal system imaging
   with pharmacologic intervention
hepatobiliary imaging
hepatobiliary scintigraphy
hepatobiliary tree
hepatoblastoma
hepatocarcinoma
hepatocellular carcinoma (HCC)
hepatocellular dysfunction
hepatoclavicular view
hepatodiaphragmatic interposition of
   colon (HDIC)
hepatoduodenal-peritoneal reflection
hepatofugal flow
hepatofugal portal venous flow
hepatojugular reflux
hepatolithiasis
hepatoma
hepatomalacia
hepatomegaly
hepatopetal flow
hepatopleural fistula
hepatoptosis
hepatopulmonary syndrome
hepatorenal bypass graft
hepatorenal saphenous vein bypass
   graft
hepatorenal syndrome (HRS)
hepatosplenomegaly
hepatotoxicity
herald bleed
Herbert-Fisher fracture classification
   system
Hercules 7000 mobile x-ray unit
Hering canal
Hermodsson fracture
Hermodsson internal rotation view of
   shoulder
Hermodsson tangential view of
   shoulder
hernia (pl. hernias, herniae)
   abdominal
   abdominal wall

hernia *(cont.)*
   axial hiatal
   Barth
   Bochdalek
   cecal
   cerebral
   congenital
   congenital diaphragmatic
   Cooper
   cul-de-sac
   diaphragmatic
   direct
   direct inguinal
   encysted
   epigastric
   esophageal
   external
   femoral
   funicular inguinal
   gastroesophageal
   hiatal
   hiatus
   incarcerated
   incisional
   incomplete
   indirect inguinal
   inguinal
   inguinofemoral
   inguinoscrotal
   intersigmoid
   interstitial
   intrapericardial diaphragmatic
   labial
   mediastinal
   mesocolic
   Morgagni
   oblique
   obturator
   omental
   ovarian
   pantaloon
   paraduodenal
   paraesophageal hiatal

hernia *(cont.)*
  paraileostomal
  parastomal
  perineal
  peritoneal
  properitoneal
  pudendal
  rolling hiatal
  scrotal
  sliding
  sliding hiatal
  sliding-type hiatal
  spigelian
  strangulated
  transmesenteric
  umbilical
  ventral
  vesicle
hernia defect
hernia formation
hernial hydrocele
hernia pouch
hernia sac
herniated abdominal contents
herniated cerebellar tonsil
herniated cervical disk
herniated disk
herniated intervertebral disk (HID)
herniated nucleus pulposus (HNP)
herniated preperitoneal fat
herniation
  ascending colon
  brain
  brain tissue
  central
  cerebellar
  cerebral
  cingulate
  concentric
  disk
  fatal
  foramen magnum
  frank disk

herniation *(cont.)*
  hard disk
  hippocampal
  impending
  internal disk
  intraspongy nuclear disk
  lumbosacral intervertebral disk
  phalangeal
  soft disk
  subfalcine (subfalcial)
  subligamentous disk
  supraligamentous disk
  temporal lobe
  tentorial notch
  thoracic intervertebral disk
  tonsillar
  transtentorial
  uncal
herniation of brain tissue
herniation of nucleus pulposus into
  adjacent vertebral body
HER-2 neu oncoprotein expression
HES (HydroCoil Embolic System)
Heschl convolution
Heschl transverse gyrus
Hesselbach ligament
Hesselbach triangle
heterocyclic free radicals
heterogeneity
heterogeneous appearance
heterogeneous hyperattenuation
heterogeneous isodense enhancement
heterogeneously dense breasts
heterogeneous microdistribution
heterogeneous perfusion pattern
heterogeneous system disease
heterogeneous uptake
heterologous graft
heterotaxy
  abdominal
  visceral
heterotaxy syndrome

heterotopia
 gastric
 gray matter
heterotopic bone formation
heterotopic ectopic pregnancy
 locations
heterotopic gray matter
heterotopic ossification
heterotopic pancreas
heterotopic pregnancy
Hetzel forward triangle method for
 cardiac output
Heubner, recurrent artery of
Hewlett-Packard color flow imager
Hewlett-Packard phased-array imaging
 system
Hewlett-Packard scanner
Hewlett-Packard ultrasound unit
Hexabrix (ioxaglate meglumine;
 ioxaglate sodium) imaging agent
hexadactyly
hexamethylpropyleneamine oxime
 imaging agent
Hey amputation
HFD (high frequency Doppler) ultrasound
HFLA duration
HFU, HIFU (high intensity focused
 ultrasound)
HI (half scan with interpolation)
 method/projection
hiatal hernia
hiatus
 adductor
 diaphragmatic
 esophageal
 popliteal
hiatus hernia
Hibbs metatarsocalcaneal angle
hibernating myocardium
hibernation, myocardial
hibernoma
Hickey profile view of mastoid region

Hickey view of hip
Hickman indwelling right atrial
 catheter
Hickman tunneled catheter
hickory-stick fracture
HID (herniated intervertebral disk)
HIDA ("high-dah")
HIDA (hepato-iminodiacetic acid)
HIDA-CCK scintigraphy (also CCK-
 HIDA)
HIDA scan
Hidalgo catheter
hide-bound bowel sign
hierarchical information
hierarchical scanning pattern
Hieshima coaxial catheter
HIFU (high intensity focused
 ultrasound)
high altitude pulmonary edema
 (HAPE)
high amplitude impulse
high attenuation
high blood pressure (HBP)
high cardiac antimyosin uptake
high contrast film
high defect in atrial septum
high definition imaging (HDI) 3000
 ultrasound system
high definition television (HDTV)
high density barium
high density linear array
high dose film dosimeter
high dose rate (HDR)
high dose rate remote afterloading
high energy imaging
high energy protons
high energy trauma
high field open MRI scanner
high field strength MR imaging
high field strength scanner
high field system
high filling pressure
high flow, low resistance pattern

high flow vascular malformation
high frequency Doppler ultrasound
high frequency miniature probe
high frequency therapeutic ultrasound
high frequency ultrasound imaging
high grade squamous intraepithelial
    lesion (HGSIL)
high grade stenosis
high grade tumor
high impedance circulation
high intensity focused ultrasound
    (HFU, HIFU)
high intensity ultrasound (HIU)
high intensity ultrasound energy
    (HIUE)
high interstitial pressure
high lateral wall myocardial infarction
high left main diagonal artery
high loop ureterostomy
high minute ventilation
Highmore, antrum cardiacum of
high order curve recognition
high osmolar media (HOM)
high output circulatory failure
high output heart failure
High Performance Detach emboliza-
    tion coil
High Performance Detach guidewire
high-pitched signal
high pontine lesion
high power field
high power, thin section quantitative
    MT
high rate detect interval
high rate pacing
high rate ventricular response, atrial
    fibrillation with
high reflectivity
high resolution
    low speed radiography
    transfontanellar ultrasound
high resolution B-mode imaging
high resolution computed tomography
    (HRCT) scan

high resolution coronal cuts on CT
    scan
high resolution CT mammography
high resolution diffraction
high resolution EEG
high resolution infrared (HRI) imaging
high resolution magnification
high resolution storage phosphor
    imaging
high resolution ultrasonography
high resolution ultrasound
high-riding patella (patella alta)
high right atrium
high sensitivity measurement
high signal mass
high spatial frequency reconstruction
    algorithm
high spatial resolution cine CT
    (HSRCCT)
high spatial resolution contrast-
    enhanced MR angiography
high spatial resolution mode
    (volumetric imaging)
high spatial resolution ultrasound
high specificity
high speed rotation dynamic
    angioplasty catheter
high takeoff of left coronary artery
high temperature diffraction
high temporal resolution cine CT
    (HTRCCT)
high temporal resolution mode
    (multitime point imaging)
high torque (see *Hi-Torque*)
high vaginal laceration
high velocity gunshot wound
high velocity jet
hilar area
hilar artery
hilar dance
hilar gland enlargement
hilar haze
hilar lymph node enlargement

hilar mass
hilar plate
hilar prominence
hilar reaction
hilar shadows
hilar structures
hilar vessels
Hilgenreiner acetabular index
Hilight Advantage System CT scanner
Hillock arch
Hill-Sachs deformity
Hill-Sachs shoulder lesion
Hill-Sachs sign
Hill-Sachs view of shoulder
Hill sign
Hilton law
hilum (formerly hilus) (pl. hila)
   hepatic
   kidney
   lips of
   lung
   renal
   splenic
hilus (pl. hili) tuberculosis
hindbrain deformity
hindfoot excursion
hindfoot instability
hindfoot joint complex
hindfoot valgus
hinged implant
hip
   congenital dislocation of (CDH)
   congenital dysplasia of (CDH)
   developmental dysplasia (DDH) of
   dislocated
   hanging
hip axis length (HAL)
hip bone (os coxae)
hip bump
hip capsule constriction, hourglass
hip dislocation
Hippel-Lindau syndrome
hip prosthesis

hip replacement
hippocampal formation
hippocampal gyrus
hippocampal herniation
hippocampal infarction
hippocampal MR volumetry
hippocampal region
hippocampal sclerosis
hippocampal volume
hippocampus
hippocampus-amygdala formation
   (HAF)
hippocratic fingers
hippocratic nails
Hirschsprung-associated enterocolitis
   (HAEC)
Hirtz submentovertex (SMV) projection
His
   angle of
   atrioventricular node of
   atrioventricular opening of
   bundle of
His band
His bundle
His spindle
His-Haas muscle transfer
Hispeed CT scanner
histamine
histiocytic origin
histiocytoma
   angiomatoid
   benign fibrous
   fibrous
   low grade malignant
   malignant fibrous
histiocytosis, Langerhans cell
Hi-Star midfield MRI system
histiocytosis, sinus
histiocytosis X
histogram
   dose-volume
   gaussian dose-volume

histogram *(cont.)*
magnetization transfer ratio
multisectional dose-volume
histogram analysis
histogram-based intensity windowing
histogram equalization algorithms
histologic grading
histology
histopathological subtype
histopathologic comparison
histopathologic-CT correlation
histoplasmoma
histoplasmosis
Hitachi CT scanner
Hitachi MR scanner
Hitachi Open MRI System
Hitachi 2.0 diagnostic ultrasound
system
Hitachi ultrasound
Hi-Torque Floppy (HTF) guidewire
HIU (high intensity ultrasound)
HIUE (high intensity ultrasound
energy)
HIV-related metabolic abnormality
HIV-seronegative
HIV-seropositive
HJB (high jugular bulb)
HL (hallux limitus)
HLA (horizontal-long axial) images
HLHS (hypoplastic left heart
syndrome)
HLR (heart to lung ratio)
H-mode echocardiography
HMPAO (hexamethylpropyleneamine
oxime) for SPECT scan
HNA (hypothalamoneurohypophyseal
axis)
HNP (herniated nucleus pulposus)
HOA (hypertrophic osteoarthropathy)
Hobbs view
HOC or HOCM (hypertrophic
obstructive cardiomyopathy)
hockey-stick appearance of catheter tip

hockey-stick deformity of tricuspid
valve
Hodgkin disease
Hodgkin lymphoma
Hodgkin tumor
Hodgson aneurysmal dilatation of the
aorta
Hodgson disease
Hoffa disease
Hoffmann atrophy
Hofmeister anastomosis
Hohl tibia condylar fracture
classification
Holdsworth classification of spinal
injury
hole burning, selective
hole pattern
holiday heart syndrome
hollow chest syndrome
hollow foot
hollow-point bullet
hollow viscus obstruction
Holly position of the foot
Holmblad method to view the knee
Holmes cortical cerebellar
degeneration
Holmes heart
Holmes syndrome
holmium (Ho) (an element)
holmium-166 imaging agent
holmium:YAG (yttrium aluminum
garnet) laser for angioplasty
holocranial
Hologic QDR 1000W dual energy
x-ray absorptiometry scanner
Hologic 2000 scanner
hologram
holography
medical
MEVH
multiple-exposure volumetric
(MEVH)
3-D

holography *(cont.)*
 volumetric multiplexed transmission
 Voxgram multiple exposure
holoprosencephaly
holosystolic mitral valve prolapse
Holt-Oram syndrome
Holthouse hernia
Holzknecht space
Holzknecht stomach
HOM (high osmolar media)
homoartery
homogeneity
homogeneous appearance
homogeneous echo pattern
homogeneous opacity
homogeneous perfusion
homogeneous soft tissue density
homogeneous thallium distribution
homology mapping
homonuclear spin systems
homotransplantation
Honda sign appearance
H1 (halistatin-1)
 H1 imaging agent
 H1 CSI scan
 H1 MR spectroscopic imaging
 H1 spectroscopy
H_2 ^{15}O (water O-15)
 H_2 ^{15}O PET (positron emission
  tomography)
 H_2 ^{15}O positron emission
  tomography
 H_2 ^{15}O radioactive diagnostic agent
H-1-H (headhunter) catheter
honeycomb degeneration
honeycomb formation
honeycombing, fibrotic
honeycomb lung
honeycomb mucosa
honeycomb pattern
hood, extensor
hooked appearance of soft palate
hooklike osteophyte formation

hook-shaped ureter
hookwire
 Basic II
 Echo-Coat
 Kopans
 spring
 ultrasound-guided
hookwire localization, CT-directed
hoop-shaped loops of bowel
Hoover sign
Hope sign
Horizon nitinol temporary stent
Horizon temporary urinary stent
horizontal fissure
horizontal fissure of lung
horizontal fracture
horizontal gaze
horizontal lie
horizontal long axial images (HLA)
horizontal long axis SPECT image
horizontal plane
horizontal plane loop
horizontal striping
horizontal toit externe angle (HTE
 angle)
horn
 Ammon
 anterior
 central
 dorsal spinal cord
 enlarged frontal
 frontal
 lateral
 meniscal
 occipital
 posterior
 posterior gray (of spinal cord)
 projectile
 spinal cord
 spinal dorsal
 splaying of frontal
 temporal
 uterine

horn *(cont.)*
ventral
ventricular
Horner syndrome
horseshoe abscess (in the hand)
horseshoe appearance
horseshoe configuration on thallium
imaging
horseshoe kidney
horseshoe shape
Horsley anastomosis
Horton disease
hose-pipe appearance of terminal
ileum
host, immunocompromised
hot area
"hot" contrast
hot cross bun skull
hot nodule
hot nose sign
hot spot artifact
hot spot imaging agent
hot spot on scan
hot spot theory
hot-tip laser
Hough projection of sphenoid strut
Hough transform (HT)
Hounsfield calcium density
measurement unit (on CT scan)
Hounsfield unit (HU) (on CT scan)
hourglass bladder
hourglass constriction of gallbladder
hourglass constriction of hip capsule
hourglass contraction of uterus
hourglass deformity on myelogram
hourglass-shaped lesion
hourglass stomach
hourglass uterus
House grading system
housemaid's knee
Howtek Scanmaster DX scanner
Ho:YAG (holmium yttrium aluminum
garnet) laser

HPCD (hemostatic puncture closure
device)
hpf (high power field)
HPGe detector
HRA (high right atrium)
HRCT (high resolution computed
tomography) image
HRI (high resolution infrared)
imaging
HRS (hepatorenal syndrome)
HS (half scan) method/projection
H/S or IISG (hysterosalpingography)
catheter
Hsieh PA oblique projection of the hip
HSS ligament rating scale
HSSG (hysterosalpingosonography)
HT (Hough transform)
HTE (horizontal toit externe [angle])
HTML (hypertext markup language)
HTTP (also http) (hypertext transfer
protocol)
HU (Hounsfield unit)
hub lock
Huchard disease
Hughes-Stovin syndrome
Hughston Clinic classification of
injury
Hughston patella view
human anti-murine antibodies
(HAMA)
human serum-albumin (albumin, iodinated ^{131}I human serum) imaging
agent
human transferrin receptor gene
marker
human visual sensitivity weighting
humeral bone
humeral head-splitting fracture
humeroradial articulation
humeroulnar articulation
humerus
humidifier lung
HUMI uterine catheter

hump
buffalo
hip
dowager's
Hampton
humpback
Hunter canal
Hunter syndrome
Hunter-Sessions balloon occluder
Hunter-Sessions inferior vena cava
balloon occluder
hunterian ligation of aneurysm
Hunt-Hess aneurysm grading system
Hunt-Hess subarachnoid hemorrhage
scale
Hunt-Kosnik classification of
aneurysm
Huppert disease
Hurler syndrome
Hurwitz dialysis catheter
Huschke ligament
Hutchinson-type neuroblastoma
Hutinel-Pick syndrome
HV (hallux valgus)
HVA (hallux valgus angle)
Hx (history)
hyaline-cartilage endplate of the
intervertebral disk
hyaline membrane disease
hyaloid fossa
hybrid MRI imaging agent
hybrid-RARE imaging
hydatid
alveolar
sessile
Virchow
hydatid cyst
hydatidiform mole (molar pregnancy)
HydraCross TLC PTCA catheter
Hydradjust IV table
hydramnios
hydranencephaly
hydrocephalus

hydrated proteoglycan gel of anulus
fibrosus
hydration
hydraulic shear stress
hydrencephalomeningocele
hydrencephaly
hydrocele, hernial
hydrocephalic
hydrocephalocele
hydrocephalus
acquired
acute
asymptomatic
bilateral
chronic
communicating
congenital
delayed
idiopathic
infantile
noncommunicating
normal-pressure (NPH)
normotensive
obstructive
occult
posthemorrhagic
postinfectious
post-traumatic
primary
progressive
secondary
symptomatic
tension
unilateral
unshunted
hydrocephalus ex vacuo
HydroCoil Embolic System (HES)
hydrodynamic potential of disk
hydroencephalocele
hydroencephaly
hydrogen-1 (or 1H) magnetic
resonance spectroscopy
hydrogen peroxide

hydrogen proton imaging
Hydrolyser microcatheter for
    thrombectomy systems
hydroma (see *hygroma*)
hydrometrocolpos
hydrometry, magnetic resonance
hydronephrosis
    chronic obstructive
    giant
    prenatal
hydronephrosis due to ureteral
    obstruction
hydronephrotic kidney
hydropericardium
hydroperitoneum
hydrophilic-coated catheter
hydrophilic-coated urologic stent
hydrophone, needle
hydropic changes
hydropic degeneration
hydropneumothorax
hydrops
    endolymphatic
    gallbladder
    labyrinthine
    semicircular canal
hydrosalpinx
hydrostatic pressure of blood
hydrosyringomyelia
hydrothorax
hydroureter
hydroureteronephrosis
hygroma
    cystic
    subdural
hyoid bone
hyoscyamine butylbromide imaging
    agent
Hypaque (diatrizoate meglumine)
    imaging agent
Hypaque (diatrizoate sodium) imaging
    agent

Hypaque-Cysto (diatrizoate meglu-
    mine) imaging agent
Hypaque Meglumine 60% (diatrizoate
    meglumine iodine) imaging agent
Hypaque myelography
Hypaque-76 (diatrizoate meglumine;
    diatrizoate sodium) imaging agent
Hypaque Sodium 50% (diatrizoate
    sodium) imaging agent
Hypaque swallow
hyparterial bronchi
hyperabduction maneuver
hyperacute renal transplant rejection
hyperacute stroke
hyperaeration
hyperaldosteronism
hyperattenuating ring sign
hyperattenuation, heterogeneous
hypercalcemia-supravalvular aortic
    stenosis
hyperconcentration of imaging agent
hyperdense middle cerebral artery sign
hyperdynamic abductor hallucis
hyperdynamic AV fistulae
hyperechoic area
hyperechoic region
hyperechoicity
hyperemia
    active
    arterial
    collateral
    diffuse
    fluxionary (active)
    mucous membrane
    passive
    reactive
    venous
hyperemic flow
hyperexpanded lobe
hyperexpansion, compensatory lobe
hyperextensibility of joints
hyperextension injury

hyperextension of neck
hyperextension teardrop fracture
hyperfixation
Hyperflex steerable wire
hyperflexion/hyperextension cervical
   injury
hyperflexion injury
hyperflexion teardrop fracture
hyperfractionated radiation therapy
hyperinflation
   dynamic pulmonary
   pulmonary
hyperintense marrow space
hyperintense mass
hyperintense ring sign
hyperintense signal
hyperintensity
   cortical
   white matter signal
hyperkinetic segmental wall motion
hyperlordosis, functional
hyperlucency
hyperlucent lung
hypermetabolic nodule
hypermetabolic region
hypermobile urethra
hypermotility
hypermyelination
hypernephroma
hyperosmotic solution
hyperostosis
   ankylosing spinal
   Caffey
   diffuse idiopathic skeletal (DISH)
   idiopathic cortical (ICH)
   infantile cortical
   senile ankylosing (of spine)
   skull
hyperostosis associated with venous
   malformation
hyperostosis frontalis interna
hyperoxia challenge
HyperPACS system

hyperperistalsis
hyperplasia
   adaptive
   adenomatous (AH)
   adrenal
   adrenocortical
   angiofollicular lymph node
   angiolymphoid
   atypical lobular
   benign prostatic
   compensatory
   congenital adrenal (CAH)
   cortical nodular
   ductal
   endometrial
   epiphyseal
   fibrous tissue
   focal nodular (FNH)
   follicular
   giant follicular
   hematopoietic bone marrow
   intravascular papillary endothelial
   lipoid adrenal
   lung lymphoid
   lymphoid
   mucosal
   multigland
   myointimal
   neoplastic
   nodular adrenal
   nodular lymphoid
   nodular regenerative
   parathyroid
   pituitary
   prostatic
   pseudoangiomatous stromal
   reactive
   sinus
   smooth
   splenic
   Swiss-cheese
   telangiectatic focal
   thymus
   thyroid

hyperplastic adenomatous polyp
hyperplastic lesion
hyperpolarized He-3 (^{3}He) imaging
   agent
hyperpolarized helium
hyperpolarized ^{129}Xe (xenon-129) gas
hyperprolactinemia
hyperreflectile
hyperrugosity
hypersensitivity pneumonia
hypersensitivity pneumonitis
hypersplenism
hypertelorism
hypertension (HTN, Htn)
   benign intracranial (BIH)
   intracranial
   portal
   primary pulmonary (PPH)
   pulmonary artery
   renovascular
   sinistral portal
   striate hemorrhage in intracranial
hypertension injury
hypertensive cardiomegaly
hypertensive cardiopathy
hypertensive contrast concentration
hypertensive crisis
hypertensive diathesis
hypertensive heart disease
hypertensive hemorrhage
hypertensive ischemic ulcer
hypertensive left ventricular
   hypertrophy
hypertensive renal disease
hypertensive stroke
hypertensive vascular degeneration
hypertensive vascular disease
hypersensitivity pneumonia
hypersensitivity pneumonitis
hypertext markup language (HTML)
hypertext transfer protocol (HTTP,
   http)

hyperthermia
   capacitive
   loco-regional
   radiotherapy with
   radiotherapy without
   volumetric interstitial
   whole body
hyperthermia probe
hyperthermia treatment
   deep
   external
   interstitial
   intracavitary
   low energy radiofrequency
      conduction
   microwave
   superficial
   ultrasound
hypertonic airways
hypertonicity
hypertransradiancy
hypertrophic asymmetry
hypertrophic cardiomyopathy (HC)
hypertrophic marginal spurring
hypertrophic nonunion
hypertrophic obstructive cardiomyopathy (HOC or HOCM)
hypertrophic pyloric stenosis
hypertrophic spurring
hypertrophic subaortic stenosis
hypertrophied kidney
hypertrophy
   adaptive
   asymmetric septal (ASH)
   benign prostatic
   biatrial
   bilateral
   biventricular
   bone
   bladder
   breast
   cardiac
   clitoral

hypertrophy *(cont.)*
  compensatory
  compensatory renal
  complementary
  concentric left ventricular
  corpus cavernosum
  eccentric left ventricular
  epiphyseal
  four-chamber
  functional
  glomerular
  labial
  left atrial
  left ventricular (LVH)
  ligamentous-muscular
  lipomatous (of the interatrial
    septum)
  massive pubertal
  muscular
  myocardial
  myocardial cellular
  olivary
  panchamber
  penile
  physiologic
  pyloric
  renal
  right atrial
  right ventricular (RVH)
  scalenus anticus muscle
  smooth muscle
  trigonal
  trilobar
  type A (B or C) right ventricular
  unilateral
  ventricular
  villous
  vulvar
  Wigle scale for ventricular
hypervascular arterialization
hypervascular hepatocellular
  carcinoma
hypervascularization

hypervascular lesion
hypervascular metastasis
hypervolemia
hypervolemic pulmonary edema
hypnosis, adjunct
hypoaeration
hypoattenuating (CT scan)
hypoattenuation
hypocycloidal ankle tomography
hypodense area
hypodense lesion
hypoechogenic
hypoechoic area on ultrasound
hypoechoic band
hypoechoic fluid collection
hypoechoic foci
hypoechoic halo
hypoechoic layer
hypoechoic mantle
hypoechoic rim
hypoechoic tubular structure
hypoechoic ultrasound
hypofractionated radiation therapy
hypofrontality
hypoganglionosis of colon
hypogastric artery
hypogastric region
hypogastrium
hypogenetic lung syndrome
hypoglossal canal
hypoglossal nerve (twelfth cranial
  nerve)
hypointense signal
hypokinesia
  apical
  cardiac
  diffuse
  diffuse ventricular
  global
  inferior wall
  regional
  septal
hypokinetic left ventricle

hypokinetic segmental wall motion
hypolucency of lung
hypometabolic area
hypometabolism, global
hypomobility, facet
hypoparathyroidism
hypoperfused state
hypoperfusion
   acute alveolar
   apical
   global cerebral
   peripheral
   pulmonary
   resting regional myocardial
   septal
   systemic
hypoperistalsis
hypopharyngeal diverticulum
hypopharynx
hypophyseal (or hypophysial)
hypophysial (or hypophyseal)
hypophysial Rathke duct
hypophysis, infundibulum
hypoplasia
hypoplastic aorta syndrome
hypoplastic aortic arch
hypoplastic emphysema
hypoplastic heart
hypoplastic heart ventricle
hypoplastic horizontal ribs
hypoplastic kidney
hypoplastic left (or left-sided) heart
   syndrome (HLHS)
hypoplastic left heart syndrome
hypoplastic left ventricle syndrome
hypoplastic lung
hypoplastic right heart
hypoplastic subpulmonic outflow
hypoplastic tricuspid orifice

hyposensitive carotid sinus syndrome
hyposensitization
hypospadias
hypostatic bronchopneumonia
hypostatic congestion
hypostatic pneumonia
hypostatic pulmonary insufficiency
hypotension, cerebral
hypotensive challenge
hypotensive shock bowel
hypothalamic lesion
hypothalamus tumor
hypothenar eminence
hypothenar muscle groups of hand
hypothermia
hypotonic duodenography
hypotonic patient
hypovolemia
hypovolemic shock
hypoxic brain damage
hypoxic cell sensitizer
hypoxic injury
hypoxic ischemic brain injury
hypoxic ischemic encephalopathy
hypoxic ischemic insults
hypoxic pulmonary hypertension
hypoxic pulmonary vasoconstriction
hypoxic vasoconstriction
Hyskon imaging agent
hysterogram
hysterography
hysterosalpingogram
hysterosalpingography
hysterosalpingosonography (HSSG)
hysteroscopic selective catheterization
hysteroscopy
hysterosonography
hysterotubogram
Hz (hertz or cycles per second)

I, i

I (iodine) (an element)
IAB (intra-aortic balloon) catheter
IABP (intra-aortic balloon pump)
IADSA (intra-arterial digital subtraction angiography)
IAM (internal auditory meatus)
IAS (interatrial septum)
iatrogenic carotid-cavernous fistula
iatrogenic damage
iatrogenic dural tear
iatrogenic injury
iatrogenic pseudoaneurysm
iatrogenic trauma
IBC (inflammatory breast cancer)
IBD (inflammatory bowel disease)
IBM field-cycling research relaxometer
IBM NMR spectrometer
IBM Speech Server clinical reporting system
I-B1 radiolabeled antibody
IBS (irritable bowel syndrome)
ICA (internal carotid artery)
ICAM-1 (intercellular adhesive molecule)
I-Cath catheter
ICE (intracardiac echocardiography)

ICEDP (intracranial epidural pressure)
ICEUS (intracaval endovascular ultrasonography)
ICG (indocyanine green) fluorescein angiography
ice-pick view on M-mode echocardiogram
ICH (intracerebral hemorrhage)
ICP (intracranial pressure)
ICRU 50 radiotherapy
ICS (improved Chen-Smith) coder
ICS (intercostal space)
ictal hyperperfusion
ictal phase study
ictal SPECT
ictal technetium Tc-99m HMPAO brain SPECT
ictus site
ICU (intensive care unit)
ICUS (intracoronary ultrasound)
ICV (internal cerebral vein)
IDD (intraluminal duodenal diverticulum)
identification
    particle
    peak

identification *(cont.)*
  phase
  topographic
idiopathic calcium pyrophosphate
  dihydrate (iCPPD) deposition
  disease
idiopathic cardiomegaly
idiopathic disease
idiopathic fibrosis, pulmonary interstitial
idiopathic fracture
idiopathic hypertrophic subaortic
  stenosis (IHSS)
idiopathic inflammatory bowel
  disease (IBD)
idiopathic intestinal pseudo-
  obstruction
idiopathic megacolon
idiopathic mural endomyocardial
  disease
idiopathic phalangeal acro-osteolysis
idiopathic pleural calcification
idiopathic pulmonary arteriosclerosis
  (IPA)
idiopathic pulmonary fibrosis
idiopathic retroperitoneal fibrosis
idiopathic scoliosis
idiopathic unilobar emphysema
idiopathic varicocele
IDIS (intraoperative digital subtraction) angiography system
IDK (internal derangement of knee)
IDSA (intraoperative digital subtraction angiography)
IDSI (Imaging Diagnostic Systems
  Inc.) scanner
IDXrad radiology information system
IEA (inferior epigastric artery) graft
IgG autoantibodies
IGRT (image-guided radiotherapy)
IHSS (idiopathic hypertrophic
  subaortic stenosis)

^{125}I iothalamate GFR (glomerular
  filtration rate) test
iiRAD DR1000C imaging
IJV (internal jugular vein)
ileal conduit
ileal motility
ileal neobladder
ileal pouch-anal anastomosis
  H-shaped
  J-shaped
  S-shaped
  W-shaped
ileal reservoir
ileal ureter
ileitis
  backwash
  Crohn
  distal
  granulomatous
  obstructive dysfunctional
  prestomal
  regional
  terminal
ileoanal endorectal pull-through
ileocecal fat pad
ileocecal junction
ileocecal region
ileocecal sarcoidosis
ileocecal spots (views)
ileocecal valve
  competent
  incompetent
ileococcygeus muscle
ileocolic disease
ileocolic fold
ileocolic vessel
ileocolitis
ileoconduit
ileogram
ileostogram (loopogram)
ileostomate
ileostomist

ileotransverse colon anastomosis
ileum
  jejunization of the
  terminal
ileus
  adhesive
  adynamic
  adynamic/paralytic
  dynamic
  dynamic/spastic
  gallbladder
  gallstone
  mechanical
  meconium
  occlusive
  paralytic
  postoperative
  spastic
Ilfeld-Holder deformity
iliac angle
iliac artery angioplasty
iliac artery disease
iliac artery stent
iliac atherosclerotic occlusive disease
iliac bone
iliac crest
iliac dowel
iliac fossa
iliac lesion
iliac-renal bypass graft
iliac spine
iliac stenosis
iliac tuberosity
iliac vessel
iliac wing
iliocaval compression syndrome
iliocaval junction
iliocaval thrombolysis
iliocaval tree
iliofemoral bypass
iliofemoral vein thrombosis
iliofemoral venous stenosis
ilioinguinal approach of Letournel

ilioinguinal ring
ilioinguinal syndrome
iliopectineal eminence
iliopectineal line
iliopopliteal bypass
ilioprofunda bypass graft
iliopsoas abscess
iliopsoas muscle
iliopsoas ring
iliotibial band friction syndrome
ilium
Ilizarov ring
ill-defined consolidation
ill-defined mass
Illumen-8 guiding catheter
illuminating catheter
ILP (interstitial laser photocoagulation)
IM (intermetatarsal) joint
IM (intramedullary) rod (rodding)
IMA (inferior mesenteric artery)
IMA (intermetatarsal angle)
IMA (internal mammary artery)
image (see also *imaging*)
  amplitude
  AMT-25-enhanced MR
  anterior planar
  arterial flow phase
  artifact
  attenuated
  axial
  axial gradient echo
  axial proton-density-weighted
  axial T2-weighted
  binary
  blood-pool phase
  BOLD (blood oxygenation level dependent)
  bone phase
  bull's eye
  cockade
  color-coded pulmonary blood flow
  column mode sinogram

image *(cont.)*
  computer-generated
  cone-beam
  contiguous
  coronal
  coronal SPIR
  coronal T1-weighted MR image
    (spin echo)
  cross-sectional
  CT reconstruction
  CT/MRI-defined tumor slice
  CT/MRI-defined tumor volume
  delayed
  distortion-free
  EKG-triggered, flow-compensated
    gradient echo
  excitation-spoiled fat-suppressed
    T1-weighted SE
  exercise
  fast spin echo T2-weighted
  fat- and water-suppressed T2-
    weighted images
  FFT (fast Fourier transform)
  FLASH (fast low-angle shot)
  flawed
  flow
  four-dimensional (4D)
  gadolinium-enhanced T1-weighted
  gradient echo
  gradient echo phase
  gray scale
  GRE (gradient-recalled echo)
  HAP (hepatic arterial-dominant
    phase) (CT scan)
  HAT-transformed
  HLA (horizontal-long axial)
  horizontal long axis SPECT
  HRCT (high resolution computed
    tomography)
  in vivo He-3 MR
  inhomogeneous
  initial
  in-phase

image *(cont.)*
  intermediate
  inversion recovery
  latent
  localizing
  long TR/TE
  maximum intensity projection and
    source
  midsagittal MR
  minimum intensity projection
    (MIP)
  mirror
  misleading
  multiecho axial
  multiecho coronal
  multiplanar reformatted radio-
    graphic and digitally recon-
    structed
  native
  negative
  nonsubtraction
  opposed GRE
  out of phase GRE
  out of plane ultrasound
  overlapping
  panoramic
  parallel hole
  parallel-tagged MR
  phase
  phase-velocity
  pinhole
  plain-paper
  planar LAO
  postinjection
  poststress
  proton density (MRI)
  real-time
  redistribution
  regional ejection fraction (REFI)
  row mode sinogram
  sagittal
  sagittal gradient echo
  sagittal oblique

image *(cont.)*
    sagittal T-1
    sagittal transabdominal
    scout
    scrambled
    SE (spin echo)
    sequential
    serial
    serial static
    short axis
    short TR/TE (repetition time/echo
      time)
    silhouette
    SPECT
    spin lock induced T1rho-weighted
    spot
    static
    stereotactic CT scan
    stop action
    stress
    stress and rest
    stroke volume
    subtraction
    survey-view
    thick slice
    thin-collimation
    thin-slice
    3D
    three-dimensional reformatted
    tomographic
    T1-weighted
    transaxial
    24-bit
    T2-weighted
    ultrasonic tomographic
    ultrasonographic
    unopposed
    variance
    venous-phase
    ventilation
    vertical-long axial (VLA)
    volume-rendered
    volumetric

image acquisition gated examination
image acquisition time
image analysis system
Imagecast imaging management
    system
ImageChecker
ImageChecker M1000
image coder, Chen-Smith
image contrast amplification
image control
imaged (verb)
image edge profile acutance
image fusion
image-guided intraoperative navigation
image-guided radiosurgery
image-guided radiotherapy (IGRT)
image intensification
image intensifier
image matrix
image noise
Imagent GI (perflubron) imaging
    agent
image postprocessing errors artifact
image quality degradation
imager (see also *scanner*)
    digital fundus
    Magnes 2500 WH (whole head)
Imager ac (barium sulfate) imaging
    agent
image reconstruction
image restoration algorithm
image volume
imaging (also *image*; *scan; scanner*)
    abdominopelvic CT
    AC AT (automated computerized
      axial tomography)
    acoustical shadowing
    Acuson Aspen ultrasound system
    Acuson computed sonography
    Add-On Bucky
    Adenoscan
    adenosine echocardiography
    adrenal

imaging *(cont.)*
Advantx LC+ cardiovascular
aerosol ventilation scan
A-FAIR (arrhythmia-insensitive
flow-sensitive alternating
inversion recovery)
air contrast
air enema fluoroscopic
Airis II open MRI system
airway fluoroscopy
Aloka
Aloka color Doppler real-time 2D
blood flow imaging with Cine
Memory
Altaire high-field-performance open
MR imaging system
amplitude
AMT-25-enhanced MR
angiography
angiography for controlling GI
bleeding
angiotensin II, AT_1 receptor
anisotropic 3D
annotated
antegrade pyelography
anterior planar
anthropometric
antifibrin antibody
antegrade
antegrade pyelography
aortography
AP angle cephalad cervical spin
AP coccyx, 10-20° caudad
aperiodic functional MR
AP L5-S1, 30-35° cephalad
lumbar spine
AP open-mouth cervical spine
x-ray
AP sacrum, 15-25° cephalad
AP supine abdomen
AP 10-15° caudad cystography
AP upper airway
AP upright abdomen

imaging *(cont.)*
AquariusNET streaming 2-D/3-D
medical imaging server
arrhythmia-insensitive flow-
sensitive alternating inversion
recovery (A-FAIR)
arterial flow phase
arteriovenous shunt
arthrography
Artoscan MRI
A-scan
ascending contrast phlebography
Aspen ultrasound system
Aspire continuous (CI)
Atlas 2.0 diagnostic ultrasound
system
ATL real-time Neurosector scan
ATL UM 9 HDI Colorflow
ultrasound system
attenuation
auditory and visual functional
AU5 harmonic ultrasound system
Aurora MR breast
automated bolus detection three-
dimensional fast gradient-
recalled echo sequence
AutoSonix system
axial
axial CT with timed excretory
urography
axial grade echo
axial transabdominal
Bak-Pac portable ultrasound
balanced gradient echo cardiac cine
balloon expulsion
balloon test occlusion
barium-based fecal tagging
barium enema
barium swallow
biad SPECT
bilateral whole-breast ultrasound
bile duct scan
biliary tract

imaging *(cont.)*
  biliary tract CT scan
  binary
  biphasic CT with mesenteric CT
    angiography
  biplanar aortography
  BI-RADS (Breast Imaging Report-
    ing and Data System)
  Bisound AP 3000 Colorflow
    ultrasound system
  black blood T2-weighted
    inversion recovery MR
  BladderScan BVI 2500 ultrasound
    scanner
  blood flow
  blood oxygen level dependent
    (BOLD)
  blood pool
  blood pool phase
  BMIPP SPECT scan
  B-mode
  B-mode acquisition and targeting
    (BAT)
  body coil
  body section radiography
  BOLD (blood oxygen level
    dependent) MR
  bolus challenge
  bolus chase three-dimensional MR
    digital subtraction angiography
  bone age
  bone density
  bone length
  bone mineral content
  bone phase
  bone scan
  bone scintiscan
  brain scan
  breast
  breath-hold, contrast-enhanced 3D
    MR angiography scan
  breath-hold fast spin echo or multi-
    shot spin echo echo-planar

imaging *(cont.)*
  breath-hold fast recovery optimized
    fast spin echo
  breath-hold T1-weighted MP-GRE
    MR
  breath-hold ungated
  breath-hold velocity-encoded cine
    MR
  bronchial provocation
  bronchography
  Bruel & Kjaer 3535 ultrasound
    system
  B-scan
  Bucky
  bull's eye
  Captopril-stimulated renal
  cardiac
  cardiac blood pool
  cardiac catheterization
  cardiac MRI for function
  cardiac MRI for morphology
  cardiac MRI for velocity flow
    mapping
  cardiac positron emission
    tomography (PET)
  cardiac radiography
  CAT (computerized axial
    tomography)
  cardiac wall motion
  cardiokymography (CKG)
  cardiovascular radioisotope scan
    and function
  capsule endoscopy
  cardiac short axis MR
  Cardiolite scan
  CardioTek (Cardiotec) scan
  cardiotocography
  carotid duplex
  carotid sinus
  CathScanner ultrasound
  CathTrack catheter locator system
  CC (conventional colonoscopy)
  CDI (color Doppler imaging)

imaging *(cont.)*
CECT (contrast enhancement of
computed tomographic) head
and body
C-11 acetate
celiac and mesenteric
arteriography
cephalogram
cerebral perfusion SPECT
chemical-selective fat saturation
chemical shift
cholangiography
cine
cine CT (computed tomography)
cine gradient-echo
cine mode MR
cine PC (phase contrast)
cineradiography
cine view in MUGA scan
CISS (constructive interference in
steady state) MR
cisternography
Clinical Ultrasonic Bone
Sonometry (CUBA)
coded aperture
cold spot myocardial imaging
collimation
colloid shift on liver-spleen scan
color amplitude
color-coded pulmonary blood flow
color Doppler (CDI)
color flow
color flow duplex
column mode sinogram
combined leukocyte-marrow
combined multisection diffuse-
weighted and hemodynamically
weighted echo planar MR
combined thallium-Tc-HMPAO
Compuscan Hittman computerized
computed axial tomography
(CAT)
computed rotational osteography

imaging *(cont.)*
computed tomographic colonography (CTC)
computed tomography (CT)
computed tomography enteroclysis
computed tomography laser
mammography (CTLM)
computed transmission tomography
chondroitin sulfate iron colloid
(CSIS)-enhanced MR
cone-beam
confocal microscopy
constructive interference in steady
state (CISS) magnetic resonance
contiguous
continuous arterial spin-labeling
perfusion MR
contrast-enhanced coded phase-
inversion harmonic ultrasound
contrast-enhanced in vivo proton
MR spectroscopy
contrast-enhanced magnetization
transfer saturation
contrast enhancement of computed
tomographic (CECT)
contrast epididymogram
contrast material enhanced
contrast vasogram
conventional colonoscopy (CC)
conventional planar (CPI)
conventional spin echo MR
Convergent color Doppler
coronary artery scan (CAS)
corpus cavernosonography
correlative diagnostic
cross-sectional
CRYOguide ultrasound system
CSF-suppressed T2-weighted 3D
MP-RAGE MR
CT (computed tomography)
CTAT (computerized transverse
axial tomography)

imaging *(cont.)*
CTC (computed tomographic
colonography)
CT colonography
CT colonography with teleradiology
CT guidance for cyst aspiration
CT guidance for needle biopsy
CT guidance for placement of
radiation therapy fields
CT pulmonary angiography
CT-LINAC (computed tomography
with linear accelerator)
CT urography
curved-slab maximum intensity
projections (MIPs)
CVIS
cystocolpoproctography
cystography
cystourethroscopy
dacryocystography
deep-inspiration CT angiography
delayed
delayed bone
Delta 32 TACT three-dimensional
breast imaging system
DentaScan
DEXA (dual energy x-ray
absorptiometry) bone density
scan
dexamethasone suppression test
for Cushing syndrome
diagnostic
diffraction-enhanced (DEI)
diffuse near-infrared spectroscopy
diffusion and perfusion magnetic
resonance
diffusion magnetic resonance
diffusion-tensor (DTI)
diffusion-tensor magnetic resonance
diffusion-weighted
diffusion-weighted echo-planar
diffusion-weighted MR

imaging *(cont.)*
digital ICG (indocyanine green)
fluorescein dye) videoangiography
digitally fused CT and radiolabeled
digital radiography
digital subtraction bowel cleansing
with mucosal reconstruction
digital vascular (DVI)
digital x-ray tomosynthesis
Digitizer Director
dipyridamole echocardiography
dipyridamole handgrip
dipyridamole infusion
dipyridamole thallium stress
dipyridamole thallium-201
direct MR arthrography
DirectRay device
DirectView CR 900
Discovery LS
displacement field-fitting MR
diuretic renal scan
Dixon quantitative chemical shift
magnetic resonance
dobutamine stress echocardiography (DSE)
Doppler
Doppler color flow
Doppler tissue
Doppler ultrasonography
Doppler venous
double contrast
double dose gadolinium
double echo chemical shift
in-phase and opposed-phase
FLASH MR
double helical CT
double phase technetium Tc 99m
sestamibi
DSC (dynamic susceptibility
contrast) MR
DTI (diffusion tensor)

imaging *(cont.)*
DTI-FT
dual echo DIET fast SE (spin
echo)
dual energy contrast-enhanced digital subtraction mammography
dual energy x-ray absorptiometry
(DEXA)
dual isotope
dual modality PET/CT
dual phase
dual phase spiral CT scan
duodenography
duplex
duplex carotid
duplex Doppler
DWI (diffusion weighted)
dynamic contrast-enhanced
subtraction MR
dynamic helical scan
dynamic hyperpolarized ^{3}He
(helium) magnetic resonance
dynamic optical breast imaging
(DOBI)
Dynamic PACSPlus system
dynamic scintigraphy
dynamic single photon emission
tomography
dynamic susceptibility contrast
(DSC) MR
dynamic susceptibility-weighted
contrast-enhanced MR
EBCT (electron beam computed
tomography)
E.CAM dual head emission
E.CAM+ coincidence-imaging
ECG-gated reconstructed multidetector row CT coronary
angiography
echocardiography (ECG)
ECG-gated multislice MR
ECG-gated spin echo MR
echo contrast variability

imaging *(cont.)*
echo-enhanced transcranial color-
coded ultrasound
EchoEye 3-D ultrasound
EchoEye ultrasound imaging
system
echo-planar (EPI)
echo-planar FLAIR (fluid attenuated inversion-recovery)
echo-planar MRA
ED (end diastolic)
18-FDG-PET
elasticity
electric joint fluoroscopy
electrocardiogram-gated MRI
electrocardiography-gated echo-
planar
electrocardiography-triggered
navigator cardiac motion
prescanning
electrodiagnostic
electron-beam dynamic CT
electronic portal (EPID)
electron radiography
electromagnetic blood flow
echogenic immunoliposomes
(ELIPs) on ultrasound
elliptic centric contrast-enhanced
magnetic resonance angiography
endoanal MR
endorectal coil MR
endoscopic catheterization of
biliary ductal system
endoscopic catheterization of
pancreatic ductal system
endoscopic optical coherence
tomography (EOCT)
endoscopic ultrasonography
endoscopic ultrasound (EUS)
Doppler
endosonography
Ensemble contrast (ECI)
EnSite 3000

imaging *(cont.)*
enteroclysis procedure
EPI (echo-planar imaging)
epididymography
EPR spatial
equilibrium MUGA
ERCP (endoscopic retrograde
cholangiopancreatography)
esophageal function
esophagography
ETL 3D FSE
EU (excretory urography)
EU-M30S endoscopic ultrasonography receiver
evacuation proctography
Excelart short bore MRI
excitation-spoiled fat-suppressed
T1-weighted ST
excretory urography (EU)
exercise
exercise thallium-201 stress
ex vivo MR
FACT (focused appendix computed
tomography)
falloposcopy (with imaging)
fast cardiac phase contrast cine
fast Fourier transform (FFT)
fast low-angle shot (FLASH)
fast multiplanar spoiled gradient-
recalled (FMPSPGR)
fast phase-contrast MRI
fast SE
fast SE and fast IR (FMPIR)
fast spin echo MR
fast spoiled gradient-recalled MR
fat-suppressed three-dimensional
spoiled gradient-(FDG)
FDDNP-PET scan
FDG myocardial
FDG PET
ferumoxides-enhanced MR
fetal imaging in utero
fetal magnetic resonance

imaging *(cont.)*
fiber tractography (FT)
field-guided CT scan
filmless
511-keV high energy
field of view
50 msec low resolution
first pass myocardial perfusion
FLAIR (fluid-attenuated inversion-
recovery)
FLAIR-FLASH
FLASH (fast low-angle shot)
flawed
flow
fluid-attenuated inversion-recovery
(FLAIR)
fluorescence spectroscopy
FluoroNav virtual fluoroscopy
FluoroPlus angiography
FluoroPlus Cardiac real-time
digital
FluoroPlus Roadmapper digital
fluoroscopy
fluoroscopic
fluoroscopic localization for transbronchial biopsy or brushing
fluoroscopy-guided condylar
lift-off
flush aortogram
FMPIR
FMPSPGR
Fonar Stand-Up MRI
Fonar-360 MRI scanner
four-dimensional (4D)
four-hour delayed thallium
4-row scanner
free-breathing black-blood coronary
MR angiography
free-breathing cardiac MR
free-breathing three-dimensional
coronary MR angiography
free induction decay

imaging *(cont.)*
 frequency domain (FDI) in
  ultrasound
 FS-BURST MR
 fSE (functional SE)
 FT (fiber tractography)
 functional MR (FMR)
 fused PET-CT scan
 gadolinium (Gd) (see *imaging*
  agent)
 galactogram
 gallbladder
 gallium (Ga) (see *imaging agent*)
 gastric emptying
 gastric mucosa
 gastrointestinal motility
 gas ventilation
 gated cardiac CT
 gated cardiac blood pool
 gated MR
 gene delivery
 generalized nephrographic (GNG)
  phase
 GE RT 3200 ADV II ultrasound
 Given diagnostic imaging
 GNG (generalized nephrographic)
  phase
 Gore 1.5-T Torso Array
 graded compression ultrasonography
 gradient-echo
 gradient-echo phase
 gradient-echo sequence
 gradient-recalled-echo (GRE) MR
 GRASS MR (gradient-recalled
  acquisition in steady state)
 gray scale
 GRE (gradient-recalled echo)
 GRE breath-hold hepatic
 GRE gadolinium-chelate enhanced
 GRE-in
 GRE-out
 half-Fourier, three-dimensional

imaging *(cont.)*
 harmonic
 harmonic power Doppler ultrasound
 HAT-transformed
 HBCT (helical biphasic computed
  tomography)
 HCTH (helical CT holography)
 HDI 3000 ultrasound
 HDI 5000 SonoCT
 heart motion-adapted magnetic
  resonance velocity mapping
 HeartView CT cardiac
 helical computed tomography
 Helios diagnostic
 hemodynamically weighted echo
  planar MR
 hepatobiliary scan
 Hercules 7000 mobile x-ray unit
 Hewlett-Packard phased-array
 HIDA (hepato-iminodiacetic acid)
 HIDA-CCK scintigraphy
 high definition (HDI)
 high energy
 high-field-strength MR
 high frequency Doppler ultrasound
 high frequency ultrasound
 high intensity focused ultrasound
  (HIFU)
 high resolution ultrasound
 high resolution B-mode
 high resolution storage phosphor
 high spatial resolution contrast-
  enhanced MR angiography
 Hitachi 2.0 diagnostic ultrasound
 HLA (horizontal long axial)
  SPECT scan
 Hologic QDR 1000W dual energy
  x-ray absorptiometry
 holography
 H-1 CSI (halostatin-1 CSI)
 H-1 MR spectroscopic
 horizontal long axis (HLA)
  SPECT scan

imaging *(cont.)*
  hot spot imaging
  hot spot myocardial imaging
  HRCT (high resolution CT)
  hybrid-RARE
  hydrogen-1 (or 1H) magnetic
    resonance spectroscopy
  hydrogen proton
  hypotonic duodenography
  hysterosalpingography
  IGRT (image-guided radiotherapy)
  iiRAD DR1000C
  image acquisition gated scan
  Imagecast
  ImageChecker
  ImageChecker M1000
  IMiG-MRI
  immunoglobulin (Ig), monoclonal
  indirect MR arthrography
  indium-111 (111In) antimyosin
  infarct avid
  infrared
  initial
  in-phase
  in-phase GRE
  in-phase/opposed-phase
  Intera CV cardiac magnetic
    resonance
  intermediate
  interventional
  intracoronary
  intracranial
  intraoperative
  intraoperative laparoscopic
    cholangiography
  intraoperative MR
  intraoperative ultrasound
  intraperitoneal technetium sulfur
    colloid
  intrarectal ultrasound
  intrathecal gadolinium-enhanced
    MR cisternography

imaging *(cont.)*
  intravenous fluorescein angiog-
    raphy (IVFA)
  intravoxel incoherent motion echo-
    planar MR
  in vivo
  in vivo He-3 MR
  in vivo proton MR spectroscopy
  iodine (see *imaging agent*)
  iodomethylnorcholesterol (^{59}NP)
    scintigraphy
  IRIS (Intensified Radiographic
    Imaging System)
  irreversible compression of MR
  Isocam scintillation
  Isocam SPECT
  IsoStent radioisotope stent
  isotope
  isotope-labeled fibrinogen
  isotope shunt
  isotropic single shot DWI (diffu-
    sion weighted)
  isotropic thin slice CT
  isotropic 3D
  Judkins coronary arteriography
  kidney
  kidney function
  kidneys, ureters, bladder (KUB)
  kinematic MR
  kinematic T2-weighted MR
  kinestatic charge detector (KCD)
  laparoscopic contact ultrasound
    (LCU)
  laparoscopic intracorporeal ultra-
    sound (LICU)
  laparoscopic ultrasound system
    (LUS)
  laser-polarized helium MR
  LAST (large area sensing technol-
    ogy) imager
  lateral upper airway soft tissue
  leukocytes, indium-111-labeled
    leukocytes

imaging *(cont.)*
light reflection rheography
limited
linacography
line
linear scan
lipid-polarized helium MR
lipid sensitive MR
liver-spleen
localizing
Longport Digital Scanner (LDS)
loopogram
lower extremity
lower limb venography
low field MR
low-field-strength
low-mechanical-index continuous-
mode contrast-enhanced ultrasound
low resolution
Luma cervical
lymphangiography
lymphoscintigraphy
macromolecular contrast-enhanced
MR
magic-angle spinning
Magnes 2500 WH (whole head)
magnetic resonance (MR)
magnetic resonance angiography
(MRA)
magnetic resonance cholangiography with HASTE sequence
magnetic resonance cholangiopancreatography (MRCP)
magnetic resonance neurography
(MRN)
magnetic resonance splenoportography
magnetization transfer
magnetoacoustic
MAG 3 dynamic renal scan
mammary ductogram
mammary galactogram

imaging *(cont.)*
MammoReader system
MammoSite RTS
Mammotome ultrasound system
marker transit
mass
Matrix LR3300 laser
maximum intensity projection
Meckel ^{99m}Tc pertechnetate
gastric-mucosa scan
microwave
middle-field-strength MR
midsagittal MR
miniature
minimum intensity projection
Miraluma breast
mirror
misleading
M-mode echocardiogram
molecular coincidence detection
(MCD)
monoclonal antibody
moving-bed infusion-tracking MRA
method for
MRA (magnetic resonance
angiography)
MRI (magnetic resonance
imaging)
MR imaging without MT, triple
dose gadolinium-enhanced
MR pelvimetry
MRSI (magnetic resonance spectroscopic imaging)
MSCT (multislice computed
tomography)
MUGA (multiple gated acquisition) cardiac blood pool
multibreath washout
multicomponent apparent diffusion
coefficient line scan
multidetector computed tomography

imaging *(cont.)*
  multidetector row CT colonog-
    raphy
  multidetector row spiral computed
    tomography
  multiecho
  multiecho coronal
  multi-injection time-resolved MR
    angiography
  multimodality
  multiorgan
  multiphase-multisection T2-
    weighted MR
  multiplanar MR
  multiplanar reformatted radio-
    graphic and digitally recon-
    structed radiographic
  multiple gated acquisition
    (MUGA) cardiac blood pool
  multipulse
  multisection diffuse-weighted
  multisection MR
  multisection proton MR spectro-
    scopic
  multislice computed tomography
    (MSCT)
  multislice first pass myocardial
    perfusion
  multistation MR
  multitime point
  multitracer
  MUSTPAC ultrasound
  myelography
  myocardial perfusion
  Myoscint
  MyoSight cardiology
  native
  native tissue harmonic (NTHI)
  navigated spin echo diffusion-
    weighted MR
  NeatVision
  needle biopsy of intrathoracic
    lesion with follow-up films

imaging *(cont.)*
  nephrographic phase
  nephrostogram
  nephrotomography
  neurodiagnostic
  neuroradiologic
  Nicolet Elite Doppler ultrasound
  noncontrast enhanced
  nondiluted contrast
  nonenhanced true FISP MR
    angiography
  noninvasive
  noninvasive vascular
  nonlinear laser microscopy
  nonsubtraction
  ^{59}NP (iodomethylnorcholesterol)
    scintigraphy
  nuclear bone
  nuclear gated blood pool
  nuclear perfusion
  oblique axial MR
  off-lateral projection
  off-resonance saturation pulse
  Olympus GF-UM130 ultrasound
    gastroscope
  Omnisense ultrasound bone
    sonometer
  one-dimensional chemical shift
    (1D-CSI)
  100 msec high resolution
  on-line portal
  OPART Toshiba open MRI
  Opdima digital mammography
  Open Sky MRI
  opposed GRE
  opposed-phase FLASH MR
  opposed-phase GRE
  opposed-phase MR
  optical
  OptiVu HDVD (high definition
    video display) system
  oral cholecystogram (OCG)
  orbital Doppler sonography

imaging *(cont.)*
　Orca fluoroscopic C-arm
　orthopantogram
　orthoroentgenogram
　OsteoView 2000 digital
　out of phase GRE
　out of plane ultrasound
　overlapping
　oxygenation-sensitive functional
　　MR
　oxygen-enhanced lung MR
　PA axial sternoclavicular joints
　Palpagraph mammography
　pancreas ultrasonography
　pancreatography
　panoramic
　parallel hole
　parallel-tag MR
　parathyroid ultrasonography
　PASTA (polarity-altered spectral-
　　selective acquisition)
　PC (phase contrast)
　PDI
　pelvimetry with placental
　　localization
　pelvimetry without placental
　　localization
　Perception 5000 PC-based ultra-
　　sound scanner
　perchlorate washout
　percutaneous drainage of abscess
　percutaneous intracoronary
　　angioscopy
　percutaneous placement of
　　enteroclysis tube
　percutaneous placement of
　　gastrostomy tube
　percutaneous transhepatic
　　cholangiography
　percutaneous transhepatic dilata-
　　tion of biliary duct stricture
　　with stent placement perfusion
　percutaneous vertebroplasty (PV)

imaging *(cont.)*
　perfusion-ventilation lung
　perfusion MR
　perfusion scintigraphy
　perfusion-weighted
　perineogram
　peritoneogram
　periorbital Doppler
　peripheral vascular
　Persantine-thallium
　PET (positron emission tomog-
　　raphy)
　PET metabolic
　PET myocardial fatty acid
　PET perfusion
　PET perfusion metabolism
　PETT (positron emission trans-
　　axial tomography)
　pharmacodynamic study
　phase
　phase contrast (PC)
　phased-array surface coil MR
　phase encode time reduced
　　acquisition sequence
　phase velocity
　Philips 1.5T Intera magnetic
　　resonance imager
　pinhole
　PIPIDA hepatobiliary
　plain films
　planar (2D)
　planar spin
　planar thallium
　point
　polarity-altered spectral-selective
　　acquisition (PASTA)
　portable transabdominal bladder
　　ultrasound scanner
　portal venous-dominant phase
　　(PVP) images (CT scan)
　POSICAM medical
　positron
　postcontrast MR

imaging *(cont.)*
  postdrainage
  postexercise
  postinjection
  postmetrizamide CT
  postoperative
  postoperative biliary duct stone
    removal
  postoperative cholangiography
  poststress
  power Doppler (PDI)
  power-mode color Doppler imaging
  PowerVision ultrasound system
  pre-contrast
  prenatal MR
  preoperative
  pressure perfusion
  pretherapy
  protodensity MR
  proton density
  proton density-weighted
  pseudodynamic MR
  pullback
  pulmonary perfusion
  pulmonary ventilation
  pulsed electron paramagnetic
  pulsed magnetization transfer MR
  pulsed ultrasound
  pulse inversion harmonic
  pulse inversion ultrasound
  pyelography
  PYP (pyrophosphate) technetium
    myocardial
  pyrophosphate (PYP)
  QCT (quantitative computed
    tomography) (for bone loss)
  quantitative
  quantitative fluorescence
  quantitative spirometrically
    controlled CT
  radioactive fibrinogen
  radioactive iodine uptake (RAIU)
  radioaerosol scintigraphy

imaging *(cont.)*
  radiographically normal
  radioimmunoluminography
  radioisotope bone
  radioisotope
  radioisotope cisternography
  radioisotope gallium
  radioisotope indium-labeled white
    blood cell scan
  radioisotope lung scan
  radioisotope technetium
  radioisotope uptake in bone
  radioisotope uptake in vascular
    brain tumor
  radioisotope voiding cystography
  radionuclide
  radionuclide gated blood pool
  radionuclide milk
  radionuclide renal
  radionuclide renography
  radionuclide thyroid
  rapid axial MR
  rapid-sequence
  RARE MR
  real-time
  real-time echocardiogram
  real-time spatial compound
    (SonoCT)
  real-time ultrasound
  real-time 2D blood flow
  reconstructed radiographic
  rectilinear bone scan
  redistributed thallium
  redistribution
  redistribution myocardial
  redistribution thallium-201
  reflectance spectroscopy
  regional cerebral blood flow
  regional ejection fraction (REFI)
  registration and alignment of 3D
  renal
  renal angiography
  renal circulation

imaging *(cont.)*
renal computed tomography (CT)
renal cyst
renal duplex
renal perfusion
renal ultrasonography
renal venography
renogram
rest (resting)
rest-dobutamine stress myocardial
   perfusion study
resting MUGA
rest myocardial perfusion
rest-redistribution
rest thallium-201 myocardial
retrograde
retrograde cystography
retrograde urethrography
retrograde ureteropyelography
Reveal XVI PET/CT
ring-type
rose bengal sodium ^{131}I biliary
Rotograph Plus panoramic dental
   tomography imaging system
row mode sinogram
RPO and LPO 30° intravenous
   urography
RPO 30° voiding cystogram
R to R
sagittal
sagittal gradient echo
sagittal oblique
sagittal T1
sagittal transabdominal
sagittal ultrasound
saline-enhanced MR
scanned projection radiography
   (SPR)
scanogram
scintigraphic scan
scintillation
scintimammography
scintirenography

imaging *(cont.)*
scout
scrambled
SE (spin echo)
sector scan echocardiography
segmented k-space turbo gradient
   echo breath-hold sequence
segmented true fast
segmenting dual echo MR
selective
selenium (^{75}Se)-labeled bile acid
Senographe 2000D digital
   mammography system
SenoScan mammography
Sens-A-Ray digital dental
sequential
sequential CT imaging
sequential plane
sequential point
sequential quantitative MR
Sequoia ultrasound
serial
serial contrast MR
serial static
serial duplex
serialography
sestamibi stress scan
shaded surface display (SSD)
shuntogram
sialography
SieScape ultrasound
Signa Special Procedures (SP)
silhouette
simultaneous volume
sincalide cholescintigraphy
single dose gadolinium
single shot fast spin echo and
   gadolinium-enhanced fat-
   suppressed spoiled gradient-
   echo MR
single slab three-dimensional pulse
   sequence

imaging *(cont.)*

single voxel proton brain
  spectroscopy (PROBE)
sinus tract
Site-Rite, Site-Rite 2, Side-Rite 3
  ultrasound systems for vascular
  imaging
16–detector row computed tomography
16-row scanner
Skylight system
slab
sliding-thin-slab maximum
  intensity projection CT
slip-ring
small field of view (FOV)
SmartSpot high resolution digital
Softscan laser scanner
somatostatin receptor scintigraphy
  (SRS)
Sonablate 200 ultrasound system
Sones coronary arteriography
SonoCT (real-time spatial
  compound imaging)
Sonopsy 3-D
SonoSite 180 handheld ultrasound
sonourethrography
source
SPECT (single photon emission
  CT)
SPECT/MRI imaging system
SPECT thallium
spectroscopic
spectroscopy
SPIDER (steady state projection
  imaging with dynamic echo
  train readout)
spike-related functional MR
spine CT with contrast
spine CT without contrast
spin echo (SE)
spin echo cardiac
spin echo MR

imaging *(cont.)*

spin lock
spin lock induced T1rho weighted
SPIO (superparamagnetic iron
  oxide)
spirometrically controlled CT
splanchnic vascular
spleen ultrasonography
splenoportography (transsplenic
  portography)
split-brain
split-echo diffusion-weighted MR
spot
spot-film
SPR (scanned projection radiography)
SRS (somatostatin receptor scintigraphy)
SSD (shaded surface display)
stacked scans
standard-dose enhanced conventional MR
static
static 3D FLASH (fast low-angle
  shot)
steady state projection imaging
  with dynamic echo train readout
  (SPIDER)
stent placement
step-oblique mammography
stepping-table gadolinium-enhanced
  digital subtraction MR angiography
stereotactic localization for breast
  biopsy
STIR (short T1 inversion
  recovery)
stop action
strain-rate MR
stress
stress redistribution
stress thallium-201 myocardial
stroke volume

imaging *(cont.)*
subtraction
Subtraction Ictal SPECT co-registered to MRI (SISCOM)
superparamagnetic iron oxide-
enhanced
SureStart
Surgi-Vision prostate MRI microcoil
survey-view
susceptibility-weighted MR
swallowing dysfunction
Synergy ultrasound system
Synthetic Aperture Focusing
Technique (SAFT) in intravascular ultrasound imaging
tagging cine MR
TDMS (Trex digital mammography
system)
TDOG (tissue Doppler gated)
TechneScan MAG3
technetium (see *imaging agent*)
technetium-labeled sulfur colloid
Technos ultrasound system
TEE (transesophageal echocardiography)
tesla
thallium (Tl) (an element)
^{201}Tl exercise
^{201}Tl myocardial
^{201}Tl SPECT brain
thallium myocardial perfusion
thallium rest-redistribution
thallium scintigraphy
thallium stress
thermoacoustic CT with radio
waves
thick slice
thin-collimation
thin-collimation multidetector row
spiral CT
thin section excretory phase CT
thin slice

imaging *(cont.)*
three-dimensional (3D, 3-D)
3D CISS MR
3D CT densitometry
3D Fourier transform (3DFT)
3DFT GRASS MR
3DFT SPGR MR
3D H-1 MR spectroscopic
3D reformations of MR
3D turbo SE (spin echo)
three-phase
three phase helical
3-Scape real-time 3-D
three-time-point contrast-enhanced
MR
ThromboScan
thyroid
thyroid ultrasonography
thyroid ultrasound
time of flight (TOF)
timed
TIPS (transjugular intrahepatic
protosystemic shunt)
tissue Doppler
tissue Doppler gated (TDoG)
dynamic three-dimensional
ultrasound
tissue harmonic
TOF (time of flight)
tomographic
T1FS (T1-weighted fat-suppressed)
Toshiba EccoCee ultrasound system
Toshiba 270 ultrasound system
total body scan
T1-weighted
T1-weighted coronal
T1-weighted sagittal
Toshiba Aspire continuous
TrakBack ultrasound catheter
transabdominal
transabdominal ultrasound
transaxial
transaxial fat-saturated 3-D images

imaging *(cont.)*
  transcervical catheterization of
    fallopian tube
  transcranial Doppler ultrasound
  transesophageal Doppler color
    flow
  transluminal atherectomy
  transluminal balloon angioplasty
  transperineal ultrasonography
  transperineal ultrasound
  transrectal ultrasound
  TransScan 2000 breast mapping
    device
  transthoracic 3DE
  Trex digital mammography system
    (TDMS)
  triple dose gadolinium
  triple phase bone scan
  triple phase helical CT
  TRON 3 VACI cardiac
  true fast
  TSPP (technetium stannous pyro-
    phosphate) rectilinear bone
  T-Scan 2000 transpectral imped-
    ance scanner
  TS2000 (TransScan 2000)
  T2-QMRI (T2-quantitative
    magnetic resonance imaging)
  T2-weighted
  T2-weighted coronal
  T2-weighted turbo SE images
  turboFLAIR (fluid-attenuated
    inversion recovery)
  turboFLASH (fast low-angle shot)
  turbo STIR images
  two-dimensional (2D, 2-D)
    2D Fourier transform
    2D gradient-recalled echo
  two-frame gated
  two-phase CT
  ultrafast
  ultrafast CT
  ultracardiography

imaging *(cont.)*
  ultrasonic tomographic
  ultrasound backscatter microscopy
    (UBM)
  ultrasonography
  unenhanced MR
  unenhanced helical CT
  unsuppressed
  upper GI and small bowel series
  ureteral reflux
  urethrocystography
  urography
  vaginogram
  variance
  vascular flow
  vectorcardiography
  velocity-encoded cine MR
  velocity-encoded magnetic
    resonance
  velocity-encoded MR
  venography
  venous
  venous enhanced subtracted peak
    arterial MR venography
  ventilation
  ventilation-perfusion (V-Q, VQ)
  VersaLab ultrasonic medical device
  vertical-long axial (VLA)
  vesiculography
  videofluoroscopic
  videoradiography
  virtual reality
  Virtuoso portable three-dimensional
  VisCath fiberoptic
  Vitrea 3D
  VLA (vertical-long axial)
  voiding cystourethrography
  volume-rendered
  volumetric
  V-Q, VQ (ventilation-perfusion)
  VScore with AutoGate cardiac
  VScore with AutoGate high quality
    cardiac

imaging *(cont.)*
  wall motion
  water-selective SE (spin echo)
  water-specific three-point Dixon
    gradient echo
  whole body bone scintigraphy
  white blood cell
  whole body scan
  whole body thallium
  wide-beam scan
  xenon 133 (^{133}Xe) SPECT
  xenon washout
  xeroradiography
  Xillix LIFE-GI fluorescence
    endoscopy
  Xplorer digital radiography
  Xplorer filmless high resolution
    digital radiography
  Xplorer 1000 digital x-ray
  x-ray sensitive vidicon
imaging agent (including contrast
    media, radioactive drugs,
    radioisotopes, and technetium)
    (see also *radiotherapy agents*)
  AcuTect (technetium Tc 99m
    apcitide
  Adenoscan (adenosine injection)
  aerosolized technetium Tc 99m
    DTPA
  aggregated albumin with
    technetium Tc 99m
  aggregated iodinated ^{131}I serum
    albumin
  Albunex ultrasound (human
    albumin, sonicated)
  Altropane ^{123}I-based
  AMI 121
  Anatrast (barium sulfate)
  anti-D-dimer antibodies, radio-
    labeled
  antifibrin antibody, radiolabeled
  antimyosin monoclonal antibody,
    Fab fragment

imaging agent *(cont.)*
  arcitumomab (CEA-Scan) (tech-
    netium Tc 99m arcitumomab)
  baby formula with ferrous sulfate
  Baricon (barium sulfate)
  barium sulfate
  Barobag (barium sulfate)
  Baro-Cat (barium sulfate)
  Baros Effervescent Granules
    (sodium bicarbonate and
    tartaric acid)
  Barosperse (barium sulfate)
  Bear-E-Yum CT (bubble-gum
    flavored barium sulfate)
  Bear-E-Yum GI (bubble-gum
    flavored barium sulfate)
  Bexxar Dosimetric Package
    (tositumomab; iodine I 131
    tositumomab)
  Bexxar Therapeutic Package
    (tositumomab; iodine I 131
    tositumomab)
  Bilivist (ipodate sodium)
  bubble-gum flavored barium
    sulfate
  C (carbon) (an element)
  CA15-3 antigen radioimmunoassay
  calcium (Ca) (an element)
    ^{45}Ca
    ^{47}Ca
  carbogen radiosensitizer
  carbon (C) (an element)
    ^{11}C acetate
    ^{11}C butanol
    ^{11}C carbon monoxide
    ^{11}C carfentanil
    ^{11}C deoxyglucose
    ^{11}C flumazenil
    ^{11}C-labeled cocaine
    ^{11}C-labeled fatty acids
    ^{11}C L-159
    ^{11}C L-884
    ^{11}C L-methylmethionine

imaging agent *(cont.)*
 carbon *(cont.)*
  ^{11}C methionine
  ^{11}C methoxystaurosporine
  ^{11}C N-methylspiperone
  ^{11}C N-methylspiroperidol
   (NMS)
  ^{11}C nomifensine
  ^{11}C palmitate
  ^{11}C palmitic acid radioactive
  ^{11}C raclopride
  ^{11}C thymidine
 carbonated saline solution
 carcinoma-specific monoclonal
  antibody
 Cardiografin (diatrizoate
  meglumine)
 Cardiolite (technetium Tc 99m
  sestamibi)
 Ceretec (technetium Tc 99m
  exametazime)
 cerium (Ce) (an element)
 cerium silicate
 Choletec (^{99m}Tc mebrofenin)
 Cholografin Meglumine
  (iodipamide meglumine)
 chromium (Cr) (an element)
 chromium-labeled red blood cells
 CO labeled with O-15
 CO_2 negative
 Combidex (ferumoxtran-10)
 Conray
 Conray 30; 43
 copper (Cu) (an element)
  ^{62}Cu PTSM
  ^{67}Cu (copper-67)
  Cu/Zn-SOD (copper-zinc
   superoxide dismutase)
 corn oil and ferric ammonium
  citrate
 Cr (chromium) (an element)
 Cs (cesium) (an element)
 Cu (copper) (an element)

imaging agent *(cont.)*
 cyanocobalamin (vitamin B_{12})
 Cysto-Conray (now Conray-43)
  (iothalamate meglumine
  injection 43%)
 Cysto-Conray II (iothalamate
  meglumine injection 17.2%)
 Cystografin (diatrizoate meglu-
  mine)
 Definity (perflutren)
 degassed tap water
 denatured technetium Tc 99m
  RBCs
 depreotide (technetium Tc 99m
  depreotide)
 diatrizoate meglumine
 diatrizoate sodium
 dihydroxyphenylalanine [DOPA],
  C-11-labeled
 DOPA (C-11-labeled dihydroxyphenylalanine)
 DTPA
 Enecat CT (barium sulfate)
 Enhancer (barium sulfate)
 Entero Vu (barium sulfate for
  suspension)
 Entrobar (barium sulfate)
 Epi-C (barium sulfate)
 Ethiodol (ethiodized oil)
 Evans blue
 exametazime
 F (fluorine) (an element)
 FAC (ferric ammonium citrate)
 Feridex (ferumoxides)
 ferric ammonium citrate
 ferric ammonium citrate-cellulose
  paste
 ferric chloride
 FerriSeltz (ferric ammonium
  citrate [FAC]
 ferromagnetic
 ferumoxsil
 ferumoxtran (ferumoxtran-10)

imaging agent *(cont.)*
  Fibrimage technetium Tc 99m
  5-iodoacetamidofluorescein
  5-iodo-2-deoxyuridine
  Flo-Coat (barium sulfate)
  fludeoxyglucose (^{18}F)
  fluorine (F) (an element)
    ^{18}F estradiol (FES)
    ^{18}F fludeoxyglucose (^{18}FDG)
    ^{18}F fluoro-DOPA (6FD)
    ^{18}F fluorodeoxyglucose
      (^{18}FDG)
    ^{18}F fluoromisonidazole
    ^{18}F-labeled HFA-134a
    ^{18}F-labeled polyfluorinated
      ethyl
    ^{18}F L-DOPA
    ^{18}F N-methylspiperone
    ^{18}F spiperone
  fluorocarbon-based ultrasound
  fluorodeoxyglucose (FDG)
  Ga (gallium) (an element)
  gadobenate dimeglumine
  gadobenic acid
  gadobutrol (neutral gadolinium
    chelate)
  gadodiamide
  gadolinium (Gd) (an element)
  gadolinium oxide imaging agent
  gadolinium zeolite
  gadofosveset trisodium
  Gadolite oral suspension (gado
    linium zeolite)
  gadopentetate dimeglumine
  gadoteridol
  gadoversetamide
  galactose
  galactose-based ultrasound
  gallium (Ga) (an element)
    ^{67}Ga bone scan
    ^{67}Ga citrate scan
    ^{68}Ga-EDTA

imaging agent *(cont.)*
  GastroMark or GastroMARK
    (ferumoxsil)
  Gd (gadolinium) (an element)
  Glofil-125 (iothalamate sodium
    I 125)
  glucagon
  glucarate ^{99m}Tc hot spot
  glucarate tracer
  gold Au-198 (^{198}Au)
  gold-195m
  H_2 ^{15}O (water O-15) radioactive
  hand-agitated
  HD 85 (barium sulfate)
  HD 200 Plus (barium sulfate)
  Hexabrix (ioxaglate meglumine;
    ioxaglate sodium)
  hexamethylpropyleneamine oxime
    (HMPAO), Tc 99m
  high density barium
  high osmolar
  holmium (Ho) (an element)
  hot spot
  human serum-albumin (albumin,
    iodinated ^{131}I
  hydrogen peroxide
  hybrid MRI
  Hypaque (diatrizoate meglumine)
  Hypaque (diatrizoate sodium)
  Hypaque-Cysto (diatrizoate
    meglumine)
  Hypaque-50
  Hypaque Meglumine 60% (diatri-
    zoate meglumine iodine)
  Hypaque-76 (diatrizoate meglu-
    mine; diatrozate sodium)
  Hypaque Sodium 50% (diatrizoate
    sodium)
  hyperpolarized ^{3}He gas
  hyperpolarized ^{129}Xe
  Hyskon
  I (iodine) (an element)

imaging agent (cont.)
  iodized oil
  Iodo-Gen
  iodohippurate sodium
  iodomethamate sodium
  iodophenyl pentadecanoic acid
    (I-123 IPPA)
  Iodotope (sodium iodide ^{131}I)
  iodoxamate meglumine
  iodoxamic acid
  iohexol
  ionic
  ionic paramagnetic
  iopamidol 200, 250, 300, 370
  iopanoic acid
  iopentol
  iopentol nonionic
  iopydol
  iopydone
  iosefamic acid
  iotetric acid
  iothalamate
  iothalamate meglumine
  iothalamate sodium
  iothalmic acid
  iotrolan
  iotroxic acid
  ioversol
  ioxaglate meglumine
  ioxaglate sodium
  ioxilan with iohexol
  ipodate
  ipodate calcium
  ipodate sodium
  Ir (iridium) (an element)
  iridium (Ir) (an element)
    ^{192}Ir (iridium-192)
  isoflurane
  Isovue-200; 300; 370 (iopamidol)
  Isovue-M 200; 300
  K (potassium) (an element)
  kinase C antiglioma monoclonal
    antibody

imaging agent (cont.)
  Kinevac
  krypton-81m (^{81m}Kr) radioactive
  LeuTech
  Levovist ultrasound
  Lipiodol
  Lipiodol myelographic
  lipophilic
  liposomal doxorubicin
  Liqui-Coat HD (barium sulfate)
  Liquipake
  L-methyl ^{11}C-methionine
  L-[1-^{11}C] tyrosine
  long scale
  low osmolality
  low osmolar
  L-tyrosine (^{11}C)
  LumenHance (manganese chloride
    tetrahydrate)
  lymphangiographic
  Lymphazurin 1% (isosulfan blue)
  MAA (macroaggregated albumin)
  macromolecular
  Macroscint (indium In 111 IGIV
    pentetate)
  Macrotec (technetium Tc 99m
    MAA)
  Magnevist (gadopentetate dimeglu-
    mine)
  mangafodipir trisodium
  manganese (Mn) (an element)
    MnCl (manganese chloride)
    Mn DPDP (dipyridoxal
      diphosphonate) chelate
    MnPcS4
    Mn-SOD
    Mn TPPS4
  manganese chloride tetrahydrate
  mannitol and saline 1:1 solution
  MD-Gastroview (diatrizoate
    meglumine; diatrizoate
    sodium)
  MDP

imaging agent *(cont.)*
 Medebar Plus (barium sulfate)
 Medescan (barium sulfate)
 meglumine
 meglumine diatrizoate
 meglumine iocarmate
 meglumine iodipamide
 meglumine iothalamate
 meglumine iotroxate
 meso-HMPAO
 mespiperone C 11
 metabolic 8-hydroxyquinolyl-
  glucuronide
 metaiodobenzylguanidine (MIBG)
 methiodal sodium
 methylene blue
 methyl methacrylate
 metrizamide
 metrizoate
 metrizoate sodium
 metrizoic acid
 MIBG (metaiodobenzylguanidine)
 MIBI (2-methoxy isobutyl
  isonitrile)
 microbubble contrast
 mineral oil
 Miraluma (technetium ^{99m}Tc
  sestamibi fit)
 MMCM (macromolecular contrast
  media)
 Mn (manganese)
 monoclonal (MOAB, MoAb)
  antibody
 monoclonal antibody 7E3
 monoclonal antibody B72.3
  labeled with indium
 motexafin gadolinium
 MultiHance (gadobenate dimeglumine)
 myelographic
 Myoscint
 Myoview (technetium Tc 99m
  tetrofosmin)

imaging agent *(cont.)*
 N (nitrogen) (an element)
 ^{13}N (nitrogen-13 ammonia)
 naloxone
 nanoparticulate
 negative contrast
 NeoTect (technetium Tc 99m
  depreotide)
 NeoTect disease-specific
 nephrotropic MR
 Neurolite (technetium Tc 99m
  bicisate)
 neurotropic
 NeutroSpec (technetium Tc 99m)
  fanolesomab kit
 nicotinamide
 nimodipine
 nitrogen-13 ammonia (^{13}N)
 nitrogen-13 ammonia radioactive
  tracer
 nitrous oxide
 no-carrier-added ^{18}F
 nofetumomab merpentan
 nonionic
 nonionic paramagnetic contrast
 nonsteroidal antiphlogistics
 normal human serum albumin
 ^{59}NP (iodomethylnorcholesterol)
 O (oxygen) (an element)
 OctreoScan 111 (^{111}In pentetreotide)
 oil emulsion
 oil-soluble contrast medium
  (OSCM)
 olsalazine sodium
 Omnipaque (iohexol)
 Omnipaque (nonionic)
 Omniscan (gadodiamide)
 OncoScint breast
 OncoScint CR/OV (^{111}In satumomab pendetide)
 OncoScint CR372
 OncoScint-NSC (OncoScint-NSC
  lung)

imaging agent *(cont.)*
OncoScint PR356
OncoTrac
OptiMark (gadoversetamide
  injection)
Optiray 320, 350 (ioversol)
Optiray nonionic
Optison
Oragrafin
Oragrafin Calcium
Oragrafin Sodium
oral
oral contrast
Oxilan-300, Oxilan-350 (ioxilan)
oxygen (O) (an element)
  inhaled (MR contrast)
  ^{15}O (oxygen-15)
  ^{15}O carbon dioxide (inhaled)
  ^{15}O carbon monoxide
  ^{15}O labeled water
  ^{17}O NMR spectroscopy
  ^{15}O oxygen
P (phosphorus) (an element)
palladium (Pd) (an element)
  ^{103}Pd radioactive
paramagnetic
paramagnetic Cr-labeled red
  blood cells
Pb (lead)
^{212}Pb-labeled monoclonal antibody
Pentagastrin
pentavalent DMSA
pentetreotide ^{111}I
peppermint oil (with barium
  enema)
peptide
Perchloracap
perflubron
perfluorocarbon
perfluorocarbon ^{19}F
perfluoroctylbromide (PFOB)
pertechnetate sodium
phenobarbital

imaging agent *(cont.)*
phosphoric acid
phosphorus (P)
  ^{32}P chromic phosphate
  ^{32}P sodium phosphate
PMT (pyridoxyl-5-methyl
  tryptophan)
polygelin colloid
positive GI contrast agent
potassium (K) (an element)
  ^{43}K (potassium-43)
  ^{81}Kr-m (krypton-81m) radioactive
Prepcat (barium sulfate)
ProHance (gadoteridol) nonionic
  gadolinium
propyliodone
Prostascint (CYT-356 radiolabeled
  with ^{111}In) diagnostic
Prostascint monoclonal antibody
P623-Gd (gadolinium)
P-32
Quantison (human serum albumin
  microcapsule)
radioactive iodinated serum
  albumin (RISA)
radioactive isotope
radiolabeled anti-D-dimer antibodies
radiolabeled antifibrin antibody
radiolabeled MoAb
radiolabeled peptide alpha-M2
radiopaque
Rb (rubidium) (an element)
  ^{82}Rb-based cardiac
Re (rhenium)
RenoCal-76 (diatrizoate meglumine)
Reno-Dip (diatrizoate meglumine)
Renografin-60
Reno-M-30
Reno-M-60

imaging agent *(cont.)*
 Reno-30, Reno-60 (diatrizoate
  meglumine)
 residual
 reticuloendothelial
 rhenium (Re) (an element)
  [186]Re hydroxyethylidene
  diphosphonate (HEDP)
 Ringer irrigation
 Ringer solution
 rose bengal sodium ^{131}I radioactive
  biliary agent
 rubidium (Rb) (an element)
 rubidium chloride ([82]Rb)
  [82]Rb (rubidium-82)
  [86]Rb (rubidium-86)
  [82]Rb-based cardiac
  [86]Rb-35S-33P
 Rubratope-57 (cyanocobalamin
  Co 57)
 samarium (Sm) (an element)
  [153]Sm ethylene diamine tetramethylene phosphoric
  (EDTMP) acid
 satumomab pendetide (OncaScint
  CR/OV)
 selenium (Se) (an element)
  [75]Se (selenium-75)
 sestamibi (technetium Tc 99m
  sestamibi)
 7E3 monoclonal antiplatelet
  antibody
 7-methoxy ^{11}C methoxystauro-
  sporine
 sincalide
 Sinografin
 Sitzmarks (polyvinyl chloride)
 6FD ([^{18}F] 6-fluoro-L-dopa)
 Sm (samarium) (an element)
 sodium amidotrizoate
 sodium bicarbonate and tartaric
  acid
 sodium bicarbonate solution

imaging agent *(cont.)*
 sodium chloride 0.9%
 sodium diatrizoate
 sodium diatrizoate with
  menaquinone
 sodium iodide ring
 sodium iodine (^{123}I); sodium
  iodide I 123
 sodium iodipamide
 sodium iodohippurate
 sodium iodomethamate
 sodium iothalamate
 sodium ioxaglate
 sodium ipodate
 sodium methiodal
 sodium pertechnetate Tc 99m
 sodium tyropanoate
 Somatostatin
 sonicated
 sonicated meglumine sodium
 sonicated Renografin-76
 SonoRx (simethicone-coated
  cellulose suspension)
 SonoVue
 sorbitol 70%
 SPIO (superparamagnetic iron
  oxide)
 spontaneous echo
 SPP (superparamagnetic particle)
 sprodiamide
 Sr (strontium) (an element)
 stannous sulfur colloid
 strontium (Sr) (an element)
  [82]Sr (strontium-82)
  [85]Sr (strontium-85)
  [89]Sr (strontium-89)
 sucrose polyester
 sulesomab (technetium Tc 99m
  sulesomab)
 sulfobromophthalein (BSP)
 sulfur colloid labeled with Tc 99m
 superparamagnetic iron oxide
  (SPIO)

imaging agent *(cont.)*
  tantalum (Ta) (an element)
  ^{183}Ta (tantalum Ta 183)
  Tc (technetium) (an element)
  TcHIDA (technetium HIDA)
  Tc 99m tetrofosmin (technetium
    Tc 99m tetrofosmin)
  Tc O_4
  teboroxime
  Technescan Gluceptate (technetium
    Tc 99m gluceptate)
  TechneScan MAG3 (^{99m}Tc mertia-
    tide) renal diagnostic
  technetated aggregated human
    albumin
  technetium (Tc, ^{99m}Tc) (an
    element)
  ^{99m}Tc aggregated albumin
  ^{99m}Tc albumin
  ^{99m}Tc albumin aggregated
  ^{99m}Tc albumin colloid
  ^{99m}Tc albumin microspheres
  ^{99m}Tc anti-granulocyte mono-
    clonal murine antibody Fab
    fragments
  ^{99m}Tc antimelanoma murine
    monoclonal antibody
  ^{99m}Tc antimony-trisulfide
    colloid
  ^{99m}Tc apcitide
  ^{99m}Tc arcitumomab
  ^{99m}Tc biciromab
  ^{99m}Tc bicisate (Neurolite)
  ^{99m}Tc BIDA
  ^{99m}Tc colloid
  ^{99m}Tc colloid albumin
  ^{99m}Tc DIEDA
  ^{99m}Tc-diethylenetriamine-
    pentaacetic acid
  ^{99m}Tc dimercaptosuccinic acid
  ^{99m}Tc DISIDA
  ^{99m}Tc disofenin
  ^{99m}Tc DMSA

imaging agent *(cont.)*
  technetium *(cont.)*
  ^{99m}Tc DTPA
  ^{99m}Tc DTPA aerosol
  ^{99m}Tc DTPA-galactosyl-human
    serum-albumin
  ^{99m}Tc DTPA-HSA
  ^{99m}Tc ECD
  ^{99m}Tc ethylene dicysteine (EC)
  ^{99m}Tc etidronate
  ^{99m}Tc exametazime
  ^{99m}Tc Fab fragment of anti-
    CEA antibody IMMU-4
  ^{99m}Tc ferpentetate
  ^{99m}Tc furifosmin
  ^{99m}Tc GH (glucoheptonate)
  ^{99m}Tc GHP
  ^{99m}Tc glucarate hot spot
  ^{99m}Tc gluceptate
  ^{99m}Tc GSA
  ^{99m}Tc HDP
  ^{99m}Tc HIDA
  ^{99m}Tc HMPAO (hexamethyl-
    propylamine oxime)
  ^{99m}Tc human serum albumin
  ^{99m}Tc IDA (iminodiacetic acid)
  ^{99m}Tc IMMU-4 monoclonal
    antibody
  ^{99m}Tc iron-ascorbate-DTPA
  ^{99m}Tc-labeled A.C. (albumin
    colloid)
  ^{99m}Tc labeled anti-alpha-
    fetoprotein
  ^{99m}Tc-labeled anti-CEA MoAb
  ^{99m}Tc-labeled antifibrin DD-
    3B6/22 Fab monoclonal
    antibody fragments
  ^{99m}Tc-labeled antigranulocyte
    antibodies
  ^{99m}Tc-labeled fibrinogen
  ^{99m}Tc-labeled human serum
    albumin
  ^{99m}Tc-labeled red blood cells

imaging agent *(cont.)*
 technetium *(cont.)*
  99mTc-labeled stannous methylene diphosphonate
  99mTc lidofenin
  99mTc MAA (macroaggregated
   albumin)
  99mTc MAG3 (mercaptoacetyl-
   triglycerine)
  99mTc MDP
  99mTc mebrofenin
  99mTc medronate
  99mTc medronate disodium
  99mTc mertiatide
  99mTc MIBI uptake
  99mTc microaggregated albumin
  99mTc MISO
  99mTc murine monoclonal antibody IgG2a to B cell
  99mTc murine monoclonal antibody to human alpha-feto-
   protein
  99mTc murine monoclonal antibody to human chorionic
   gonadotropin
  99mTc Myoview
  99mTc nitrido complex
  99mTc NUBI
  99mTc oxidronate
  99mTc pentetate sodium
  99mTc pentetate calcium trisodium
  99mTc pentetic acid
  99mTc PIPIDA
  99mTc PMT
  99mTc polyphosphate
  99mTc PYP (pyrophosphate)
  99mTc RBC (red blood cells)
  99mTc SC (sulfur colloid)
  99mTc sestamibi
  99mTc siboroxime
  99mTc sodium
  99mTc sodium gluceptate

imaging agent *(cont.)*
 technetium *(cont.)*
  99mTc sodium pertechnetate
  99mTc SPP (stannous pyrophosphate)
  99mTc succimer
  99mTc sulesomab
  99mTc sulfur colloid
  99mTc sulfur microcolloid
  99mTc teboroxime
  TechneScan MAA (99mTc
   macroaggregated albumin)
  TechneScan MAA (99mTc
   pyrophosphate)
  99mTc TBI
  99mTc tetrofosmin
  99mTc tin-pyrophosphate
  99mTc TMCHI
  99mTc triisocyanide
  99mTc trimetaphosphates
 technetium antimony trisulfide
  colloid
 technetium bound to DTPA
 technetium bound to serum
  albumin
 technetium bound to sulfur colloid
 technetium ethylene cysteine
  diethylester
 technetium pertechnetate sodium
 technetium-tagged RBCs
 Telepaque (topanoic acid)
 Teslascan (mangafodipir trisodium)
 Tesuloid
 tetrofosmin (technetium Tc 99m
  tetrofosmin)
 thallium (Tl) (an element)
 201Tl (thallium-201)
 thallous chloride
 tissue
 Tl (thallium) (an element)
 TmDOTP-5
 Tomocat (barium sulfate)

imaging agent *(cont.)*
  Tonopaque (barium sulfate)
  tyropanoate sodium
  tositumomab (iodine I 131
    tositumomab)
  triisocyanide ^{99m}Tc
  triiodinated
  Tru-Scint AD (technetium Tc 99m
    MAb-170)
  TSPP (technetium stannous
    pyrophosphate)
  tyropanoate
  tyropanoate sodium
  U (uranium) (an element)
  ^{235}U (uranium-235)
  ultrasmall particle superpara-
    magnetic iron oxide (USPIO)
  Ultravist (iopromide)
  uniphasic
  urokinase
  USPIO (ultrasmall superparamag-
    netic iron oxide)
  Verluma (nofetumomab merpen-
    tan)
  Visipaque (iodixanol) intravascular
    injection
  Visipaque 270 (iodixanol)
  visualization of
  water-soluble
  water-soluble iodinated
  water-soluble nonionic positive
  whole blood monoclonal antibody
  Xe (xenon) (an element)
  xenon (Xe) (an element)
  ^{127}Xe (xenon-127)
  ^{133}Xe (xenon-133)
  ZK44012
imaging anatomic correlation
imaging-based stereotaxis in tumor
  neurosurgery
imaging contrast enhancement
imaging-directed 3D volumetric information on intracranial lesion

imaging pathologic correlation
imaging plane
imaging renogram
imaging system (see *scanner*)
imaging workstation
Imatron C-100 scanner
Imatron C-100 ultrafast CT scanner
Imatron C-100XL CT Scanner
Imatron C-150L EBCT scanner
Imatron Fastrac C-100 cine x-ray CT
  scanner
Imatron Ultrafast CT scanner
imbalance of phase or gain artifact
imbricate
imbrication, capsular
imciromab pentetate imaging agent
IMED intravenous infusion device
IMI (inferior myocardial infarction)
^{131}I-MIBG (metaiodobenzylguanidine)
  imaging agent
IMiG-MRI
immediate intervention
immediate postictal period
immersion B-scan ultrasound
imminent death
imminent demise
immobilization
immobilized
immune electron microscopy
immune globulin intravenous pentate
immune inflammation
immunoblastic
immunocompetency
immunocompromised patient
immunoelectrophoresis
immunoglobulin G (^{111}I-IgG)
immunolymphoscintigraphy
Immunomedics system
immunoscintigraphy
immunoscintimetry
immunosuppressive therapy
IMPA cephalometric measurement
IMP SPECT scan

impacted fracture
impacted subcapital fracture
impacted urethral stones
impacted valgus fracture
impaction
  fecal
  stone
impaired renal function
impaired venous return
impaired ventilation-perfusion
impairment
  circulatory
  functional
  functional aerobic impairment
    (FAI)
  functional tubular impairment
  hemodynamic reserve impairment
  inspiratory muscle function
  mild cognitive
  motor
  renal function
  sensory
ImpaxPACS system
impedance phlebography
impedance plethysmography (IPG)
impedance, renovascular
impending myocardial infarction
impede filling
impediment
impending myocardial infarction
imperfect regeneration
imperforate aneurysm
imperforate anus
impinge
impinged upon
impingement
  dural
  lateral
  ligamentous (ankle)
  nerve root
  talar
  talofibular
impingement exostosis

impingement syndrome
impinging
implant (see also *prosthesis*)
  BrachySeed I-125
  BrachySeed Pd-103
  BEBIG iodine-125 seed implant
  biodegradable
  cochlear
  double lumen breast
  double stem silicone
  double stem silicone lesser MP
  epidural
  hinged
  hydroxyapatite
  IMR (interventional magnetic
    resonance)
  interstitial
  iodine I-125 interstitial radiation
  iridium-192 endobronchial
  iridium-192 wire
  mammary
  methyl methacrylate beads
  open cord tendon
  otologic
  palladium (^{103}Pd) prostate
  palladium 103 (^{103}Pd) ultrasound-
    guided transperineal
  permanent interstitial
  PMMA (poly-methyl methacry-
    late)
  synthetic bone
  prostate
  retropectoral mammary
  silicone
  silicone elastomer rubber ball
  silicone wrist
  single lumen breast
  temporary interstitial
  Theraseed (palladium Pd 103)
  total knee
  VDS (ventral derotating spinal)
implantable bone growth stimulator,
  Osteo Stim

implant abutment
implantation, IMR (interventional
magnetic resonance) (see also
implant)
implantation of radioactive sources
implantation theory of endometriosis
implanted imaging-opaque marker
implanted pacemaker
impression
cardiac (on liver)
colic
digastric
duodenal
esophageal
gastric
liver
renal
suprarenal
improved Chen-Smith (ICS) coder
improvement, interval
impulse, apical
I-MRI (interventional MRI)
IMR-image-guided general surgery
IMRT (intensity-modulated radiation
therapy)
inactive mode
inadequate cardiac output
inadequate ovarian function
inadequate runoff
inadequate visualization
inadvertent penetration
inanition
incarcerated gravid uterus
incarcerated hernia
incarceration
incarial bone
incidentaloma (on sonography)
incisional hernia
incisural sclerosis
inciting event
inciting factors
inclination of treadmill
inclinometer

incoherence, magnetic resonance spin
incompetence
aortic
aortic valve
chronotropic
communicating vein
deep venous
mitral valve
postphlebitic
pulmonary
sphincter
traumatic tricuspid
tricuspid valve
valve
valvular
incompetence of pelvic fundus
incompetent leaflet
incompetent valve
incomplete border sign
incomplete closure
incomplete dislocation
incomplete filling
incomplete resolution of pneumonia
incomplete fracture of bone
incomplete Kartagener syndrome
incomplete pulmonary fissure
incomplete resolution of pneumonia
incomplete stroke
incongruity, angle of
incontinence
incorporation of new-bone formation
increased activity, surrounding halo
of
increased AP (anterior/posterior)
diameter of chest
increased attenuation
increased basilar cisterns
increased central venous pressure
increased cerebral vascular resistance
increased density
increased echo signal on ultrasound
increased extracellular fluid volume
increased interstitial fluid

indium *(cont.)*
[111]In pentetreotide (OctreoScan)
[111]In satumomab pendetide monoclonal antibody
[111]In scintigraphy
[111]In white blood cell imaging
indocyanine dilution curve
indocyanine green (ICG)
indocyanine green angiography
indocyanine green dye for detection
of intracardiac shunt
indocyanine green dye method for
cardiac output measurement
indocyanine green fluorescein angiography
indolent radiation-induced rectal ulcer
indolent ulcer
induced thrombosis of aortic
aneurysm
inducibility basal state
inducible
inductance
induction anesthesia
induction chemotherapy
indurated mass
indurated tissue
induration
indurative pneumonia
indurative pleurisy
indwelling catheter
indwelling Foley catheter
indwelling nonvascular shunt
indwelling stent
indwelling ureteral stent
indwelling urinary bladder catheter
inelastic collision
inelastic pericardium
inequality, limb-length
inexorable progression
in extremis
Inf (infarction)
infant, profoundly obtunded
infantile hemangioma

infantile hydrocephalus
infantile lobar emphysema
infantile-onset spinocerebellar ataxia
infantile pelvis
infantile pneumonia
infantile syndrome
infantile thoracic dystrophy
infarct (see *infarction*)
infarct avid imaging (hot spot scan,
technetium pyrophosphate scan)
infarcted heart muscle
infarcted lung segment
infarct expansion
infarction (also *infarct*)
acute myocardial (AMI)
age indeterminate
anemic
anterior communicating artery
distribution
anterior myocardial (AMI)
anterior wall myocardial
anteroinferior myocardial
anterolateral myocardial
anteroseptal myocardial
apical myocardial
arrhythmic myocardial
atherothrombotic
atherothrombotic brain
atrial
bicerebral
bland
bleeding into the
bone
border zone-region
brain stem
capsular
capsulocaudate
capsuloputaminal
capsuloputaminocaudate
cardiac
cerebellar
cerebral
cerebral artery

infarction *(cont.)*
concomitant
cortical
diaphragmatic myocardial (DMI)
dominant-hemisphere
embolic
evolving myocardial
extensive anterior myocardial
focal skin
frontal lobe
full thickness
gyral
healing
hemispheric
hemorrhagic
high lateral myocardial
hippocampal
hyperacute myocardial
impending
impending myocardial
inferior myocardial (IMI)
inferolateral myocardial
inferoposterolateral myocardial
intestinal
intraoperative myocardial
ischemic brain stem
lacunar brain
lateral myocardial
livedo reticularis, digital
medullary
mesencephalic
mesenteric
multifocal
multiple cortical
muscle
myocardial (MI)
nonarrhythmic myocardial
nonembolic
nonfatal myocardial
non-Q wave myocardial
nonseptic embolic brain
nontransmural myocardial
occipital lobe

infarction *(cont.)*
old myocardial
omental
papillary muscle
paramedian
parenchymal
pituitary
pontine
posterior cerebral territory
posterior myocardial
posteroinferior myocardial
postmyocardial
pulmonary
Q wave myocardial
red
recent myocardial
renal
right ventricular
segmental bowel
septal myocardial
septic pulmonary
severe
silent myocardial
sinoatrial node
spinal cord
subacute myocardial
subcortical
subendocardial (SEI)
subendocardial myocardial
temporal lobe
territorial
testicular
thalamic
thrombotic
transmural
transmural myocardial
uninfected
ventral pontine
watershed
white matter
infarct avid imaging (hot spot scan,
    technetium pyrophosphate scan)
infarcted heart muscle

infarcted lung segment
infarcted segment of lung
infarctoid cardiomyopathy
infarct size limitation
infected pseudoaneurysm
infected thrombosed graft
infection calculus
infection, opportunistic
infectious disease
infectious diskitis
infectious hepatitis (hepatitis A)
infective thrombosis (or thrombus)
inferior basal segment
inferior border
inferior border of heart
inferior border of lung
inferior border of rib
inferior cerebellar peduncle
inferior dorsal radioulnar ligament
inferior epigastric artery
inferior facet
inferior frontal gyrus
inferior ligaments
inferior lobe of lung
inferior margin of superior rib
inferior mediastinum
inferior mesenteric artery
inferior (diaphragmatic) myocardial
  infarction
inferior parietal lobule
inferior pubic ramus (pl. rami)
inferior pulmonary ligament
inferior pulmonary vein
inferior quadriceps retinaculum
inferior temporal gyrus
inferior temporal lobule
inferior thyroid vein
inferior tip of scapula
inferior vena cava (IVC) orifice
inferior vena cava syndrome
inferior vena caval filter
inferior wall akinesis
inferior wall hypokinesis

inferior wall MI (myocardial
  infarction)
inferiormost
inferoapical wall
inferobasal
inferolateral displacement of apical
  beat
inferolateral wall myocardial
  infarction
inferolaterally
inferomedial
inferomedially
inferoposterior wall myocardial
  infarction
inferoposterolateral
INFH (ischemic necrosis of femoral
  head)
infiltrate (also infiltration)
  active
  aggressive interstitial
  aggressive perivascular
  alveolar
  apical
  basilar
  basilar zone
  bilateral interstitial pulmonary
  bilateral upper lobe cavitary
  bronchocentric inflammatory
  butterfly pattern of
  calcareous
  calcium
  cavitary
  circumscribed
  confluent
  consolidated
  diffuse
  diffuse aggressive polymorphous
  diffuse alveolar interstitial
  diffuse bilateral alveolar
  diffuse interstitial
  diffuse perivascular
  diffuse reticulonodular
  eosinophilic

infiltrate *(cont.)*
  epituberculous
  fatty
  fibronodular
  fluffy
  focal interstitial
  focal perivascular
  ground glass
  hazy
  infiltration
  interstitial
  interstitial nonlobar
  invasive angiomatous interstitial
  leukemia
  linear
  lung
  lung base
  lymphocytic
  marrow
  massive
  meningeal
  micronodular
  migratory
  mononuclear
  multifocal aggressive
  mural
  neoplastic marrow
  parasitic
  patchy
  peribronchial
  perihilar
  peripheral
  perivascular
  plasmacytic
  pneumonic
  pulmonary
  pulmonary eosinophilic
  pulmonary parenchymal
  pulmonic
  punctate
  reticular
  reticulonodular
  retrocardiac

infiltrate *(cont.)*
  strandy
  sulfasalazine-induced pulmonary
  transient
  tuberculous
infiltrating lesion
infiltration (see *infiltrate*)
infiltration of pulmonary parenchyma
infiltration pattern
infiltrative
Infinion scanner
infinitesimal Z spectrum
Infiniti catheter from Cordis
inflamed edematous medium-sized
  bronchi
inflamed mainstem bronchial mucosa
inflamed pericardium
inflamed pleura
inflammation
  acute phase of
  adhesive
  adnexa uteri
  airway
  allergic airway
  alveolar septal
  atrophic
  Bartholin gland
  bladder
  bursal
  calcaneal bursa
  cardiac muscle
  cell-mediated immune
  chronic
  cirrhotic
  diffuse
  disseminated
  fibrosing
  fibrinous
  focal
  granulomatous (of bronchi)
  hyperplastic
  hypertrophic
  immune

inflammation *(cont.)*
 interstitial
 meningeal
 metastatic
 mucosal
 necrotic
 obliterative
 parenchymatous
 patchy
 perivesical
 polyarticular symmetric
  tophaceous joint
 proliferative
 pseudomembranous
 sclerosing
 spleen
 subacute
 subtle
 suppurative
 thyroid gland
 tubulointerstitial
 urinary tract
 vulvovaginal
 vein
inflammation caused by
 burning
 crushing
 cutting
 foreign body
 fungus
 parasite
 radiation
inflammatory adhesions
inflammatory bowel disease (IBD)
inflammatory breast cancer (IBC)
inflammatory breast carcinoma
inflammatory carcinoma of breast
inflammatory disease
inflammatory fracture
inflammatory lesion
inflammatory myocarditis
inflammatory myofibroblastic tumor
inflammatory paranasal sinus disease

inflammatory polypoid mass
inflammatory process
inflammatory reaction
inflammatory response syndrome
inflammatory response, whole body
inflate
inflation
 air
 balloon
 sequential balloon
 simultaneous balloon
inflow
 aortic
 blood
inflow cuff
inflow disease progression
In-Flow intraurethral valved catheter
inflow tract of left ventricle
influenza
information, hierarchical
infra-apical
infra-auricular
infracardiac type total anomalous
 venous return
infraclavicular pocket
infracoccygeal approach
infracolic midline
infracristal ventricular septal defect
infradiaphragmatic vein
infragastric
infragenicular popliteal artery
infragenicular position
infrageniculate artery
infraglenoid tuberosity
infragluteal crease
infrainguinal
infrahepatic vena cava
infrainguinal bypass stenosis
infrainguinal revascularization
infrainguinal vein bypass graft
inframammary crease
inframammary syndrome
inframyocardial

infrapatellar contracture syndrome
(IPCS)
infrapatellar fat pad
infrapopliteal artery occlusion
infrapopliteal vessel
infrapulmonary position
infrared imaging
infrared light-emitting diode
infrarenal abdominal aortic aneurysm
infrarenal aorta
infrarenal aortic stenosis
infrarenal stenosis
infrascapular
infraspinatus muscle atrophy
infraspinous fossa
infrasternal angle
infratemporal fossa
infratentorial approach
infratentorial compartment
infratentorial Lindau tumor
infraumbilical mound
infravesical obstruction
infundibular atresia
infundibular chamber
infundibular pulmonary stenosis
infundibular septum
infundibular stalk
infundibular subpulmonic stenosis
infundibuloventricular crest
infundibulum
   bile duct
   cerebral
   gallbladder
   hypophysis
   os
   right ventricular
   sandwiched
   tumor of
Infuse-a-port catheter
infusion line, peripheral intravenous
infusion transcatheter therapy
Ingram-Bachynski classification of
   hip fracture

ingrowth, bone
inguinal bulge
inguinal crease
inguinal floor
inguinal fold
inguinal hernia
inguinal ligament syndrome
inguinal node
inguinal region
inguinal ring
inguinal trigone
inguinoscrotal hernia
inhalational injury
inhalation by slow inspiration
inhalation of krypton-77 to measure
   cerebral blood flow on PET scan
inhalation of radioactive xenon gas
inhalation pneumonia
inhalation study
inhalation technique
inhalation tuberculosis
inhaled oxygen brain MR contrast
   agent
inhaled radionuclide
inherently unstable condition
inherited multicentric osteolysis
inhomogeneity correction
inhomogeneity, off-axis dose
inhomogeneous distribution
inhomogeneous echo pattern
inhomogeneous image
inhomogeneous tracer distribution
inion bump
initial delay in appearance time of
   contrast material
initial image
initial shock
initial staging evaluation
initiation
injection
   air
   barium (through colostomy)
   bolus

injection *(cont.)*
  contrast medium
  CT-guided transthoracic percuta-
    neous ethanol
  double
  extrathecal
  hand (done by hand)
  imaging agent
  intra-amniotic
  intra-arterial
  intramuscular (I.M., IM)
  intramuscular fetal
  intraperitoneal fetal
  intrathecal
  intravascular
  intravenous (I.V., IV)
  intravenous bolus
  intravenous fetal
  machine (done by machine)
  manual
  Omnipaque (iohexol) intrathecal
  opacifying
  percutaneous ethanol
  percutaneous thrombin
  periradicular corticosteroid
  plasmid DNA
  power
  rest
  sclerosing
  selective arterial
  serial
  sonographically guided human
    thrombin
  straight AP pelvic
  ultrasound-guided percutaneous
    thrombin
  venous
injection port
injection test for pneumoperitoneum
injector
  auto
  Hercules power
  Medrad power angiographic

injector *(cont.)*
  power
  pressure
  PulseSpray
injured kidney
injury (pl. injuries)
  acute inhalational
  acute stretch
  axial compression (of spine)
  ballistic
  barked
  bilateral incomplete ureteral
  blunt
  brachial plexus
  burst
  cervical spine
  closed head (CHI)
  cocking
  compression flexion
  compression-plus-torque theory of
    cervical
  compressive hyperextension
  concomitant tracheal
  crush
  crushing
  decelerative
  degloving
  discoligamentous
  distraction hyperflexion
  Erb (to brachial plexus)
  Erb-Duchenne-Klumpke
  extension (of spine)
  extensive head
  extrapulmonary
  flexion-distraction
  flexion-rotation
  forced flexion
  growth plate
  head (HI)
  high caliber, low velocity handgun
  hyperextension
  hyperflexion
  hyperflexion/hyperextension
    cervical

injury *(cont.)*
  hypertension
  hypoxic
  hypoxic-ischemic
  iatrogenic ureteral
  immunologic
  intercostal nerve
  intraperitoneal
  inversion
  ischemic
  Klumpke (to brachial plexus)
  lateral bending (of spine)
  Lisfranc
  low back
  matrix
  meniscal
  mild head
  motor vehicle (MVI)
  nerve
  obstetrical
  penetrating lung
  perinatal
  peripheral nerve
  physeal
  plexus
  postcatheterization
  postnatal
  prenatal
  pronation-external rotation (P-ER)
  pulmonary parenchymal
  radial vascular thermal
  radiation induced skin
  rapid deceleration
  repetitive strain (RSI)
  repetitive stress (RSI)
  ring-sparing
  seat belt
  severe head
  skier's
  snowboard (or snowboarding)
  soft tissue
  softball sliding
  spinal cord (SCI)

injury *(cont.)*
  straddle (of urethra)
  strain-sprain
  subendocardial
  subtle
  supination-outward rotation
  three-column (spinal column)
  through and through
  throwing-arm
  transcutaneous crush
  traumatic
  traumatic brain (TBI)
  traumatic head
  two-column
  ultrasonic assessment of
  unilateral cervical root avulsion
  vertical shear
  vesical
  weightbearing rotational
  whiplash
  windup
Injury Scale, Abbreviated
Injury Severity Score (ISS)
injury to nerve roots
inlay graft
inlet
  esophageal
  pelvic
  thoracic
inlet and outlet views of pelvis
inlet contraction of pelvis
inner adrenal cortex
inner table
innermost intercostal muscles
InnerVasc sheath
Innervision MR scanner
innocuous
innominate (*not* innominant)
innominate aneurysm
innominate angiography
innominate artery buckling
innominate artery kinking
innominate artery stenosis

innominate bone
innominate vein
Innovante balloon
Innovante catheter
Innovante dilator
Innovante filter
Innovante guidewire
Innovante introducer
Innovante occluder
Innovante retrieval device
Innovante sheath
Innovante stent
Innovator Holter system
inoperable brain tumor
inoperable disease
Inoue balloon catheter
in-phase GRE imaging
in-phase image
in-phase/opposed-phase imaging
in-phase sequence
in-plane vessels
Inrad HiLiter ultrasound-enhanced
    stylet
Insemi-Cath catheter
insertion
    anomalous
    Bosworth bone peg
    ligamentous
    percutaneous (via femoral vein)
    percutaneous pin
    tendinous
insidious onset
insidious progression
in situ
in situ bypass
in situ grafting
in situ pinning
insonation, Doppler
insonifying wave field
inspiration, inhalation by slow
inspiration phase
inspiratory effort
inspiratory flow

inspiratory flow rates
inspiratory flow volume, tidal
inspiratory increase in venous
    pressure
inspiratory phase
inspiratory reserve volume (IRV)
inspiratory retraction
inspiratory spasm
inspired air
inspissated mucus
inspissation of feces
instability
    anterolateral rotary knee
    articular
    atlantoaxial
    chronic functional
    dorsal intercalary segment (DISI)
    first ray
    hindfoot
    inversion
    joint
    lateral rotatory ankle
    ligamentous
    osseous
    postlaminectomy
    rotary
    rotary ankle
    rotational
    rotatory
    shoulder joint
    spinal
    subtalar
    temporal
    truncal
    varus-valgus
    volarflexed intercalated segment
        (VISI)
instantaneous enhancement rate
instantaneous gradient
InstaScan scanner
in-stent balloon redilation
InStent CarotidCoil stent
InStent self-expanding and balloon
    expandable stent

instillation, subarachnoid
insufficiency
   acute cerebrovascular
   acute coronary
   aortic (AI)
   aortic valve
   arterial
   autonomic
   basilar
   basilar artery
   brachial-basilar
   cardiac
   cardiopulmonary
   cerebrovascular
   chronic venous
   congenital pulmonary valve
   coronary
   gastric
   hepatic
   hypostatic pulmonary
   ileocecal
   mitral (MI)
   muscular
   myocardial (MI)
   nonocclusive mesenteric arterial
   nonrheumatic aortic
   parathyroid
   postirradiation vascular
   post-traumatic pulmonary
   pulmonary (PI)
   pulmonary arterial flow
   pulmonary valve
   pyloric
   renal
   respiratory
   Sternberg myocardial
   thyroid
   transient ischemic carotid
   tricuspid (TI)
   uterine
   valvular
   valvular aortic
   velopharyngeal

insufficiency (cont.)
   venous
   vertebrobasilar arterial
insufficiency fracture
insufficiency of aortic valve
insufficient pulmonary arterial flow
insufflation
   air
   CO_2
   gas
   tubal
insular gyrus
insular lobe
insula, roof of
insular region of brain
insulative development
insulin ^{125}I
insulin ^{131}I
insulinoma
insult
   aortic
   bihemispheric
   cerebrovascular
   infectious
   mechanical (to spine)
   myocardial
   occlusive cerebrovascular
   toxic
intact valve cusp
intact ventricular septum
integral, Choquet fuzzy
integral dose
integrated bipolar sensing
integrated dual head coincidence
   camera and x-ray based attenuation
   maps
integrated parallel acquisition technique (IPAT)
integration, telecom
Integris 3-D RA (rotational angiography)
Integris 3000 scanner
Integris V3000 imager

integrity, spinal
integrity and alignment
Intel PC Link2 board
Intel Plink Ethernet card
intensified radiographic imaging
  system (IRIS)
intensifier, image
intensifying screen artifact
intensity
  angina with recent increase in
  beam
  CIDNP signal
  decreased
  equal in
  fat-signal
  low signal
  maximal
  radiation
  segmental high (SHI)
  signal (SI)
  variable
intensity-modulated photon beams
intensity-modulated radiation therapy
  (IMRT)
intensity windowing
intensive care unit (ICU)
intentional reversible thrombosis
interacquisition variability
interaction splitting
interactive premasking
Intera CV cardiac magnetic resonance
  imager
interactive electronic scalpel
interactive MR-guided biopsy
interactive visual approach
interarticular disk
interarticularis, pars
interatrial baffle
interatrial communication
interatrial groove
interatrial septal defect
interatrial septum, lipomatous
  hypertrophy of the

interatrial transposition of venous
  return
interbody fusion
interbronchial mass
intercalary defect
intercarpal articulation
intercarpal coalition
intercarpal joints
intercaudate distance
intercaval band
intercavernous anastomosis
intercellular adhesive molecule
  (ICAM-1)
intercellular edema
intercellular space
Intercept prostate microcoil
Intercept urethra microcoil
Intercept Vascular 0.030-inch Internal
  MR Coil
Intercept Vascular guidewire
interchondral joint
interchordal space fenestration
interclavicular notch
intercollicular groove
intercom, noise reduction
intercomparison measurement
  technique
intercondylar eminence
intercondylar fossa
intercondylar fracture
intercondylar groove
intercondylar notch
intercondyloid eminence
intercondyloid fossa
intercondyloid notch
intercoronary anastomosis
intercoronary collateral flow
intercoronary steal syndrome
intercostal artery
intercostal muscle
intercostal nerve injury
intercostal retraction on inspiration
intercostal space (ICS)

intercostal vein
intercostal vessels
intercostobrachial nerve
intercristal diameter
interdigital clavus
interdigital ligament
interdigital neoplasm
interdigital neuroma
interdigitating coil stent
interdigitation of vastus lateralis with
    fascia
interface
    acetabular-prosthetic
    acoustic
    air
    air-tissue
    bone-implant
    bony
    catheter-skin
    DICOM
    fat-water
    joint
    media-adventitia
    muscle-fat
    socket/residuum
    socket stump
interface spacing, multiple-beam
interference dissociation
interferometry, phase shifting
interfraction interval
interfragmental compression
interfragmentary plate
intergluteal cleft
interhemispheric asymmetry
interhemispheric cyst
interhemispheric fissure
interhemispheric tracer activity
interictal PET FDG study
interictal phase
interictal SPECT study
interictal spiking
interlabial orifice
interlaminar

interleaf thickness
interleaved axial slabs
interleaved notched saturation
interleaved GRE sequence
interleaved imaging passes
interleaved inversion-readout segment
interlobar empyema
interlobar fissure
interlobar pleurisy
interlobar septum (pl. septa)
interlobar veins of kidney
interlobular emphysema
interlobular pleurisy
interlobular septal thickening
interlobular vasculature
interlobular veins of kidney
interlobular vessels
interlocking detachable coils
interloop abscess
intermaxillary spine
intermediate artery
intermediate bursa
intermediate coronary syndrome
intermediate cuneiform fracture-
    dislocation
intermediate heart
intermediate images
intermediate part of urethra
intermediate signal mass
intermediate slices
intermediolateral gray column
intermesenteric abscess
intermetacarpal articulation
intermetatarsal angle (IMA)
intermetatarsal angle-reducing
    procedure
intermetatarsal joint (IM)
intermetatarsal ligament
intermetatarsal space
intermetatarsophalangeal bursa
intermittent diffuse esophageal spasm
intermittent occlusion
intermittent self-catheterization

intermittent venous claudication
intermuscular septum
internal auditory meatus
internal caliber
internal capsule and basal ganglia
   tumor
internal capsule intracerebral hemorrhage
internal carotid artery (ICA)
internal clot
internal conjugate diameter
internal cyclotron target
internal derangement of knee (IDK)
internal disk herniation
internal echogenicity
internal-external drainage catheter
internal femoral rotation
internal iliac artery
internal intercostal muscles
internal intermuscular septum
internal jugular approach for cardiac
   catheterization
internal jugular bulb
internal jugular triangle
internal jugular vein
internal jugular venous cannula
internal mammary artery (IMA)
internal pudendal artery
internal retention mechanism
internal rotation in extension (IRE)
internal rotation in flexion (IRF)
internal snapping hip syndrome
internal thoracic artery
internal thoracic vein
internal tibial torsion (ITT)
internal tibiofibular torsion
internuclear distance
interopercular distances
interorbital distance
interosseous ligament
interosseous membrane
interosseous muscle groups of hand
interosseous nerve

interosseous space
interosseous talocalcaneal ligament
interparietal bone
interpedicular distance
interpediculate
interpeduncular cistern
interpeduncular notch
interpeduncular space
interperiosteal fracture
interphalangeal (IP)
interphalangeal dislocation
interphalangeal fusion
interphalangeal joint
interpleural space
interpolate cues
interpolation
   color space
   cubic convolution
   linear
   nearest neighbor
   prism
   trilinear
interpolation algorithm
interpolation kernel
Interpore bone replacement material
interposed colon segment
interposition graft
interposition, soft tissue
interpretive criteria
interpretive error
interpretive variability
interpulse time
interrogation
   color-duplex
   pulse Doppler
   radiation
   transtelephonic ICD
interrupted aortic arch
interruption, aortic arch
interscalene space
intersection gap
intersegmental aberration
interseptal region

intersesamoid ligament
intersigmoid hernia
intersigmoid recess
interslice distance
interslice gap
interspace
  ballooning of vertebral
  disk
  vertebral disk
  wedging of vertebral
intersperse
intersphincteric abscess
interspinal ligament
interspinous distance
interspinous ligament
interspinous process
interspinous widening
interstices, bone
interstitial boost
interstitial brachytherapy
interstitial changes
interstitial diffuse pulmonary fibrosis
interstitial ectopic pregnancy locations
interstitial edema
interstitial emphysema
interstitial fibrosis
interstitial fluid
interstitial heat generating source
interstitial hyperthermia treatment
interstitial implant
  permanent
  temporary
interstitial infiltrate
  diffuse alveolar
  invasive angiomatous
interstitial insertion of temperature
  sensors
interstitial laser photocoagulation
  (ILP)
interstitial lung disease (ILD)
interstitial markings, increased
interstitial meniscal tear
interstitial MR lymphography

interstitial nonlobar infiltrates
interstitial plasma cell
interstitial pneumonia
interstitial pneumonia air leak
interstitial pneumonitis
interstitial prematurity fibrosis
interstitial probe
interstitial prominence
interstitial pulmonary edema
interstitial pulmonary fibrosis
interstitial radioactive colloid therapy
interstitial radioelement application,
  ultrasonic guidance for
interstitial radiotherapy
interstitial scarring
interstitial shadowing
interstitial space
interstitial template irradiation
interstitial thermoradiotherapy
interstitial thickening, intralobular
interstitial tissues
intertarsal
interthalamic bridge
intertrabecular hemorrhage
intertrabecular soft tissue
intertrochanteric plate
intertubercular diameter
interval
  acromiohumeral (AHI)
  atlantoaxial
  atlantodens (ADI)
  supracricoid
interval change
interval development
interval improvement
interval intra-atrial conduction
interval progression
interval resolution
intervention
  immediate
  surgical
  therapeutic
interventional limb salvage

interventional magnetic resonance
(IMR)
interventional MRI (I-MRI)
interventional radiology (IR)
interventional neuroradiology
interventional procedure
interventional radiography
interventional radiology
interventricular (IV)
interventricular foramen
interventricular groove
interventricular septal defect
interventricular septum
interventricular sulcus, posterior
interventricular vein, posterior
intervertebral disk narrowing
intervertebral disk space
intervertebral foramen
intervertebral joint
intervertebral ligament
intervertebral vacuum cleft sign
intervillous space
interzone
intestinal atresia
intestinal diverticulum
intestinal emphysema
intestinal endometriosis
intestinal follicle
intestinal hypoperistalsis syndrome
intestinal infantilism
intestinal malrotation
intestinal transit time, abnormal
intestinal ureter, construction of
intestinal villous architecture
intestinal web
intestine
   blind
   coils of
   kink in
   large
   malrotation of
   small
intestinovesical fistula

"in the magnet" (in magnetic
   resonance imaging)
intima
   arterial
   diffuse thickening of arterial
   friable thickened degenerated
   hypertrophied
   tunica
intimal attachment of diseased
   vessel
intimal atherosclerotic disease
intimal debris
intimal dissection
intimal flap
intimal irregularity
intimal plaque
intimal proliferation
intimal remodeling
intimal tear
intimal thickening
intimal-medial dissection
intimomedial thickness
in toto
intra-abdominal abscess
intra-abdominal endometriosis
intra-abdominal arterial bypass graft
intra-abdominal fat
intra-acetabular
intra-acinar pulmonary arteries
intra-alveolar fibrosis
intra-alveolar hemorrhage
intra-aneurysmal thrombus
intra-aortic balloon assist
intra-aortic balloon counterpulsation
intra-aortic balloon double lumen
   catheter
intra-aortic balloon pump(ing) (IABP)
intra-arterial chemotherapy
intra-arterial digital subtraction
   angiography (IADSA)
intra-arterial DSA
intra-aortic endovascular sonography
intra-arterial filling defects

intra-arterial injection of water-
soluble iodinated contrast agent
intra-arterial intracerebral thrombolysis
intra-articular mass
intra-arterially
intra-arterial superselective
nimodipine
intra-arterial thrombosis
intra-arterial thrombus
intra-articular adhesion
intra-articular body
intra-articular calcaneal fracture
intra-articular fracture
intra-articular ligament
intra-articular loose body
intra articular radiopharmaccutical
therapy
intra-atrial baffle
intra-atrial filling defect
intra-atrial reentry
intra-atrial thrombi
intra-axial brain tumor
intra-axial cyst
intra-axial varix
Intrabeam intraoperative radiotherapy
(IORT) system
intracanalicular
intracapsular fracture
intracardiac baffle
intracardiac calcium
intracardiac echocardiography (ICE)
intracardiac mass
intracardiac pressure
intracatheter pressure
intracardiac pressure in Doppler
echocardiogram
intracardiac right to left shunt
intracardiac shunt(ing)
intracardiac thrombus
Intracath catheter
intracatheter
intracatheter pressure

intracaval endovascular ultrasonography (ICEUS)
intracavitary afterloading applicators
intracavitary brachytherapy
intracavitary clot formation
intracavitary extension of tumor
intracavitary filling defect
intracavitary hyperthermia treatment
intracavitary prostate ultrasonography
intracavitary prostate ultrasound
intracavitary radiation source
intracavitary radioactive colloid
therapy
intracavitary radioelement application
intracavitary radiotherapy
intracellular lipid
IntraCoil self-expanding nitinol stent
intracoronary Doppler flow wire
intracellular DNA double strand
intracerebral hematoma
intracerebral hemorrhage
basilar
bulbar
cerebellar
cerebral
cerebromeningeal
cortical
internal capsule
intrapontine
pontine
subcortical
ventricular
intracerebral lesion
intracerebral lymphoma
intrachondrial bone
intracompartmental ischemia and
edema
intracoronary imaging
intracoronary stent placement
intracoronary stenting
intracoronary ultrasound (ICUS)
intracortical osteogenic sarcoma
intracranial air

intracranial aneurysm
  arteriosclerotic
  congenital
  dissecting
  mycotic
  traumatic
intracranial berry aneurysm
intracranial calcification
intracranial circulation
intracranial cyst
intracranial electroencephalography
intracranial fat prolapse
intracranial germinoma
intracranial glioma
intracranial hemorrhage
intracranial imaging
intracranial malformation
intracranial mass
intracranial neoplasm
intracranial sinus thrombosis
intracranial tuberculoma
intracranial tumor
intracranial vascular lesion
intracranial vascular occlusion
intracranial vessel
intractable bleeding disorder
intractable heart failure
intractable ulcer
intracystic papillary carcinoma
intradecidual sign
intradermal injection of Tc-HSA
intradiaphragmatic aortic segment
intradiskal
intraductal mucin-producing tumor
intraductal papilloma, benign
intraductal pressure
intradural abscess
intradural anastomosis
intradural arteriovenous fistula
intradural extramedullary tumor of
  spinal cord
intradural nerve root

intradural retromedullary arteriovenous fistula
intradural vessels
intraesophageal stent
intraforaminal approach
intraglandular granulomatous
  lymphadenopathy
intrahepatic abscess
intrahepatic atresia (IHA)
intrahepatic bile duct dilatation
intrahepatic biliary drainage catheter
intrahepatic biliary duct dilatation
intrahepatic biliary radicles
intrahepatic biliary tract dilatation
intrahepatic biliary tree
intrahepatic cholestasis
intralabyrinthine
intralaminar thalamus
intraligamentous ectopic pregnancy
  locations
intralobular fibrosis
intraluminal air
intraluminal brachytherapy
intraluminal defect
intraluminal dilation
intraluminal dimension
intraluminal duodenal diverticulum
  (IDD)
intraluminal filling defect
intraluminal flow
intraluminal foreign bodies
intraluminal low dose rate
  brachytherapy
intraluminal mass
intraluminal meconium
intraluminal membranes
intraluminal Silastic esophageal stent
intraluminal sutureless prosthesis
intraluminal thrombus, laminated
intramammary adenopathy
intramedullary epidermoid cyst
intramedullary fixation

intramedullary osteosclerosis
intramedullary rod (rodding)
intramedullary spinal cord
  germinoma
intramedullary spinal cord tumor
intramedullary spinal lesion
intramesenteric abscess
intramural air in colon
intramural arterial hemorrhage
intramural clot
intramural colonic air
intramural coronary artery aneurysm
intramural diverticulum
intramural ectopic pregnancy
  locations
intramural gas
intramural hematoma
intramural portion of distal ureter
intramural thrombus
intramural tunnel
intramuscular aortic segment
intramuscular hemangioma
intramyocardially
Intran disposable intrauterine
intraneural ganglion cyst
intraneuronal neurofibrillary tangles
intranodal architecture
intranuclear diskogram
intraocular hemorrhage
intraoperative arteriography
intraoperative cholangiography (IOC)
intraoperative digital subtraction
  angiography (IDSA)
intraoperative electrocortical stimulation (IOECS) mapping
intraoperative gamma probe
intraoperative high dose rate
  (IOHDR) brachytherapy
intraoperative high dose rate
  brachytherapy (IOHDR)
intraoperative imaging
intraoperative laparoscopic cholangiography

intraoperative laser ablation
intraoperative laser photocoagulation
  of ventricular tachycardia
intraoperative MR cholangiography
intraoperative MR imaging
intraoperative myocardial infarction
intraoperative navigation (iON)
  system
intraoperative pancreatography
intraoperative radiation therapy
  (IORT)
intraoperative radiography
intraoperative radiolymphoscintigraphy
intraoperative radiotherapy (IORT)
intraoperative scanning technique
intraoperative transmyocardial revascularization (ITMR)
intraoperative ultrasonography
  (IOUS)
intraoperative ultrasound
intraoperative x-ray visualization of
  fixation devices
intraoral periapical radiograph
intraorbital air
intraosseous abscess
intraosseous ganglia
intraosseous vascular malformations
intraosseous venography
intraosseous wiring
intrapapillary terminus
intraparenchymal cyst
intrapartum hemorrhage
intrapedicular fixation
intrapericardial bleeding
intrapericardial pressure
intraperiosteal fracture
intraperitoneal abscess
intraperitoneal air
intraperitoneal cavity
intraperitoneal exposure
intraperitoneal fluid
intraperitoneal injury

intraperitoneal rupture
intraperitoneal Tc-sulfur colloid scan
intrapixel sequential processing
(IPSP)
intrapleural fibrinolysis
intrapleural pressure
intrapleural hemorrhage
intrapleural pressure
intrapleurally
intrapontine intracerebral hemorrhage
intraportal endovascular ultrasonography (IPEUS)
intrapulmonary arteriovenous malformation
intrapulmonary barotrauma
intrapulmonary disease
intrapulmonary hemorrhage
intrapulmonary pressure
intrapulmonary shunt(ing)
intrarenal collecting system
intrarenal hematoma
intrarenal hemorrhage
intrarenal pelvis
intrarenal reflux
intrarenal stenosis
intraretinal microangiopathy (IRMA)
intrasellar Rathke cleft cyst (RCC)
intrasellar tumor
intraspinal adenoma
intraspinal lesion
intraspinal tumor
IntraStent DoubleStrut LD stent
IntraStent DoubleStrut renal artery
stent
IntraStent DoubleStrut XS renal artery
stent
intrastitial afterloading nylon tubes
intrastitial radiation source
intratendinous fluid collection
intratentorial lipoma
intrathecal gadolinium-enhanced MR
cisternography

intrathecal imaging
intrathecal injection of metrizamide
intrathecal injection of radiopharmaceutical
intrathecal ionics
intrathecal roots
intrathecal space
intrathoracic adenopathy
intrathoracic airway obstruction
intrathoracic airway pressure
intrathoracic dimension
intrathoracic dislocation of shoulder
intrathoracic goiter
intrathoracic Kaposi sarcoma
intrathoracic pressure
intrathoracic rib
intrathoracic stomach
intrathoracic thyroid
intrathoracic upper airway
obstruction
intratracheal
intratumoral agent
intratumoral necrosis
intratumoral structure
intraurethral coil
intrauterine cardiac failure
intrauterine catheter
intrauterine cytomegalic inclusion
disease
intrauterine fetal transfusion, ultrasonic guidance for
intrauterine fossa
intrauterine fracture of fetus
intrauterine growth retardation
(IUGR)
intrauterine heart failure
intrauterine pregnancy
intrauterine pressure catheter
intrauterine sac
intravaginal ultrasound
intravascular clotting process
intravascular coagulation of blood
(ICD), disseminated

intravascular contents, secondary
  extravasation of
intravascular contrast
intravascular filling defect
intravascular gas
intravascular guidewire
intravascular loopless antenna
  guidewire
intravascular mass
intravascular MRI technique
intravascular prosthesis
intravascular radiopharmaceutical
  therapy
intravascular sickling, lung
intravascular signal intensity in MR
  angiography
intravascular space
intravascular stenting
intravascular thrombosis
intravascular tumor thrombus
intravascular ultrasound (IVUS)
intravascular ultrasound catheter
intravascular ultrasound elastography
intravascular volume depletion
intravascular volume status
intravenous (I.V. or IV)
intravenous bolus injection of imaging
  agent
intravenous cholangiography (IVC)
intravenous coronary thrombolysis
intravenous DSA (digital subtraction
  angiography)
intravenous fetal injection
intravenous fluorescein angiography
  (IVFA)
intravenous infusion line, peripheral
intravenous injection of isotope as
  bolus
intravenous line
intravenous pyelogram (IVP)
intravenous pyelography
  excretory
  rapid-sequence

intravenous urogram (IVU)
intravenous urography
intravenously enhanced CT scan
intraventricular aberration
intraventricular conduction block
intraventricular conduction defect
intraventricular conduction delay
intraventricular cryptococcal cyst
intraventricular hemorrhage (IVH)
intraventricular meningioma
intraventricular pressure
intraventricular rerouting
intraventricular right ventricular
  obstruction
intraventricular systolic tension
intraventricular tunnel repair
intravesical lesion
intravesical obstruction
intravesical stone
intravesical ureter
intravoxel dephasing
intravoxel incoherent motion echo-
  planar MR imaging
intravoxel phase dispersion (IVPD)
  MRE
Intrepid PTCA catheter
intrinsic deflection
intrinsic disease
intrinsic foot muscles
intrinsic lesion
intrinsic minus deformity (clawhand)
intrinsic minus hallux
intrinsic plus deformity
intrinsic positive end expiratory
  pressure (PEEP)
intrinsic pulmonary disease
intrinsic sick sinus syndrome
intrinsic stenotic lesions
intrinsic vein graft stenosis
introducer
  Arrow-Flex percutaneous sheath
  AVA HF
  AVA 3XI

introducer *(cont.)*
  Avanti angiographic catheter
  BD Introsyte-N Autoguard
    shielded
  Becton-Dickinson
  Bentson
  BriteMax sheath
  Cath-Lock
  Check-Flo
  Ciaglia percutaneous tracheostomy
  Cook
  Desilets-Hoffman catheter
  Guidant
  Hemaquet catheter
  Hemaquet sheath
  Innovante
  Introsyte-N Autoguard shielded
  Littleford-Spector
  LPS Peel-Away
  Mullins catheter
  Outcomes by Design sheath
  Pacesetter
  peel-away
  Prelude vascular
  Razi cannula
  Schwartz
  Swartz SL S
  Terumo sheath
  Tuohy-Borst
introducer sheath
Introsyte-N Autoguard shielded
  introducer
introitus
intubated small bowel series
intubation
  endotracheal
  esophagogastric (EG)
  nasal
  nasogastric (NG)
  nasotracheal
  oral
  orotracheal

intussusception
  appendiceal
  bowel
  gastroduodenal
  intestinal
  retrograde
  self-limiting adult small bowel
  vein
  venous
in utero echocardiogramF
invagination
  basilar
  ligament into joint
  stomal
invasion
  aspergillus
  arterial
  chest wall
  depth of
  exogenous
  local
  mediastinal
  metastatic
  neoplastic (of meninges)
  neoplastic (of roots)
  perineural
  tumoral
  vascular
invasion of margins
invasive angiomatous interstitial
  infiltration
invasive ductal tumor
invasive lesion
invasive lobular tumor
invasive malignancy
invasive malignant sheath tumor
invasive radiological vascular
  procedures
inverse radiotherapy technique
inversion-eversion
inversion injury of the ankle
inversion recovery (IR)
inversion recovery image

inversion recovery sequence
inversion recovery technique
inversion sprain
inversion time (TI)
inversus, situs
inverted Meckel diverticulum
inverted pear-shaped uterus
inverted pelvis
inverted V sign
inverted Y block
inverted Y complex
inverted Y configuration
in vitro evaluation of coils
in vitro labeling
in vivo balloon pressure
in vivo correlation
in vivo disposition study
in vivo He-3 MR images
in vivo imaging
in vivo labeling
in vivo proton MR spectroscopy
involucrum
involuntary guarding
involuted uterus
involvement
  arcuate fiber
  bone
  bone marrow
  bowel
  cardiac
  cranial nerve
  extracutaneous intrathoracic
  hepatic
  lymph node
  medullary
  meningeal
  metastatic
  myelomatous
  no
  pleural
  possible
  spinal
  surgical margin

involvement *(cont.)*
  thalamotegmental
  tumor
  unilateral
  vascular
  vertebral
  visceral
INVOS 2100 optical spectroscopy
Ioban prep
iobenzamic acid imaging agent
iocarmic acid imaging agent
IOC (intraoperative cholangiography)
iocetamic acid imaging agent
IOCM (isosmolar contrast medium)
iodamine meglumine contrast
  medium
iodinated contrast medium
iodinated ^{125}I radioactive
iodinated ^{131}I human serum albumin
  (albumin, iodinated I 131 serum)
iodinated imaging agent
iodinated nanoparticles
iodine (I) (an element)
  ^{123}I ABZM
  ^{123}I BMIPP SPECT
  ^{125}I brachytherapy
  ^{125}I fibrinogen scan
  ^{123}I heptadecanoic acid
  ^{123}I IBZM
  ^{192}I high dose rate remote after-
    loader
  ^{131}I murine MAb to alpha-fetopro-
    tein (AFP) imaging agent
  ^{125}I interstitial radiation implant
  ^{131}I iodocholesterol
  ^{125}I iodopyracet
  ^{131}I iofendylate
  ^{123}I iofetamine HCl
  ^{123}I IPPA (phenylpentadecanoic
    acid)
  ^{131}I-labeled anti-CEA MoAb
    (CC49) and IFN-alpha

iodine *(cont.)*
   ^{131}I-labeled cis-11-beta-methyoxy-
    17-iodovinyl estradiol scintig-
    raphy
   ^{131}I-labeled human MoAb
   ^{131}I-labeled monoclonal Fab
    fragment directed against a
    tumor antigen
   ^{131}I-MIBG
   [131]I 6B-iodomethyl-19-norcholes-
    terol
   [131]I tositumomab
iodine-based imaging agent
iodine-deficiency goiter
iodine dose
iodine 123–labeled cis-11ß-methoxy-
   17-iodovinyl estradiol scintigraphy
iodine-based imaging agent
iodine radioactive source
iodipamide meglumine imaging agent
iodixanol imaging agent
iodized oil imaging agent
iodoform gauze
Iodo-Gen imaging agent
iodohippurate sodium
iodophenyl pentadecanoic acid (I-123
   IPPA) imaging agent
iodomethamate sodium
iodophthalein sodium
Iodotope (sodium iodide ^{131}I) imaging
   agent
iodoxamate meglumine
iodoxamic acid
ioglycamic acid imaging agent
IoGold radioactive seeds
IOHDR (intraoperative high-dose-
   rate) brachytherapy
iohexol imaging agent
IOM (interosseous membrane)
ion exchange chromatography
ionic imaging agent
ionic paramagnetic imaging agent
ionic potassium

ionic property
ionics, intrathecal
ionization chamber
ionizing radiation
iontophoresis, transtympanic
iopamidol 200, 250, 300, 370
   imaging agent
iopanoic acid imaging agent
iopentol nonionic imaging agent
iopydol
iopydone imaging agent
IORT (intraoperative radiotherapy),
   Intrabeam
iosefamic acid
iotetric acid
iothalamate imaging agent
iothalamate meglumine imaging agent
iothalamate sodium imaging agent
iothalmic acid
Iotrex liquid brachytherapy source
Iotrex imaging agent
iotrolan
iotroxic acid
ioversol imaging agent
IOUS (intraoperative ultrasonography)
ioversol imaging agent
ioxaglate meglumine imaging agent
ioxaglate sodium imaging agent
ioxilan with iohexol imaging agent
IPA (idiopathic pulmonary arteriosclerosis)
IPAT (integrated parallel acquisition
   technique)
IPCS (infrapatellar contracture
   syndrome)
IPEUS (intraportal endovascular ultrasonography)
IPG (impedance plethysmography)
IPH (idiopathic portal hypertension)
IPH (intraplaque hemorrhage)
IPHP (intraperitoneal hyperthermic
   perfusion)
IP (interphalangeal) joint

I-Plant radioactive iodine-125
ipodate calcium imaging agent
ipodate imaging agent
ipodate sodium imaging agent
IPPA (iodine-123 phenylpentadecanoic acid)
IPPB (intermittent positive pressure
breathing)
ipsilateral antegrade site
ipsilateral approach
ipsilateral basal ganglia
ipsilateral cerebellar signs
ipsilateral cortical diaschisis
ipsilateral corticospinal tract signs
ipsilateral downstream arteries
ipsilateral hemisphere activation
ipsilateral hemispheric carotid TIA
(transient ischemic attack)
ipsilateral iliac fossa
ipsilateral nonreversed greater
saphenous vein bypass
ipsilateral pleural effusion
ipsilesional
IPSP (intrapixel sequential processing) neuron evaluation method
iPTH (immunoreactive parathyroid
hormone)
IR (interventional radiology)
IR-guided pigtail catheter place
ment
IR (inversion recovery)
Ir (iridium) (an element)
IRA (ileorectal anastomosis)
IRBBB (incomplete right bundle
branch block)
Irex Exemplar ultrasound
iridium (^{192}Ir) (an element)
^{192}Ir endobronchial implant
^{192}Ir-loaded stent
^{192}Ir seed therapy
iridium radioactive source
iridium ribbon
iridium seed

iridium wire implant
IRIS (intensified radiographic imaging system)
IRMA (intraretinal microangiopathy)
iron overload artifact
iron overloading
iron storage disease
irradiate
irradiated zinc
irradiation
convergent beam (CBI)
curative
external beam
gamma
heavy-particle
hemibody
interstitial template
low intensity laser (LILI)
neutron
palliative
partial brain
phosphorus-32 intracavitary
proton
stereotactic proton
template
total body
whole brain
irradiation chamber
irradiation pneumonia
irreducible dislocation
irreducible dorsal dislocation of the
metatarsophalangeal joint
irreducible fracture
irregular blocks
irregular bone
irregular gallbladder wall thickening
irregular hazy luminal contour
irregularity
diffuse
intimal
luminal
irregular mass, polypoid calcified
irreversible airways obstruction

irreversible compression of MR
  image
irreversible ischemia
irreversible narrowing of bronchioles
irreversible organ failure
irrigation, saline
irritability
  atrial
  muscle
  myocardial
  nerve root
  ventricular
irritable bowel syndrome (IBS)
irritable colon
ISAH stereotactic immobilization
  frame
ISAH stereotactic immobilizing mask
ischemia
  brachiocephalic
  brain
  brain stem
  cardiac
  carotid artery
  cerebral
  chronic cerebral
  coronary
  exercise-induced myocardial
  exercise-induced transient
    myocardial
  global myocardial
  hypoxia-
  irreversible
  limb-threatening
  mesenteric
  myocardial
  neonatal intracranial
  nonlocalized
  peri-infarction
  provocable
  regional myocardial
  regional transmural
  remote

ischemia *(cont.)*
  reversible
  segmental
  silent
  silent myocardial
  subendocardial
  transient cerebral
  transient myocardial
  vertebral-basilar
  vertebrobasilar
  zone of
ischemic area
ischemic brain damage
ischemic changes, persistence of
ischemic colitis
ischemic contracture
ischemic decompensation
ischemic disease
ischemic epiphysis
ischemic episode
ischemic event
ischemic heart disease (IHD)
ischemic hypoxia
ischemic infarction
ischemic injury
ischemic instability
ischemic kidney
ischemic necrosis
ischemic reperfusion injury
ischemic segment (on echocardiogram)
ischemic time
ischemic ulcer, hypertensive
ischemic viable myocardium
ischemic zone
ischial bone
ischial spine
ischial tuberosity
ischioacetabular fracture
ischiogluteal bursa
ischiorectal abscess
ischiorectal fossa plane

ischium
    ascending ramus of
    ramus of
ISDN connection
ISG medical imaging workstation
Isherwood projection of subtalar joint
    region
Ishida coaxial catheter
ISIS spectroscopy
island
    bone
    bony
    mucosal
    tissue
    Reil
isoattenuation
Isocam scintillation imaging system
Isocam SPECT imaging system
isocapnic hyperventilation-induced
    bronchoconstriction
isocenter placement error
isocenter shift method
isocenter, single
isoclosed curve
isodense appearance
isodense enhancement
isodense mass
isodensity
isodose contour
isodose line
isodose plan
isodose width
isoechoic
isoeffective bronchial mucosa
isoelectric at J point
isoelectric line
isoelectric period
isoflurane
isointense soft tissue on MRI
isolated clustered calcifications of
    breast
isolated dislocation of semilunar bone
isolated heat perfusion of extremity

isolated ventricular inversion
isomerism, atrial
isometric exercise stress test
isometric heart contraction
isoperistaltic ileal reservoir
isoproterenol infusion
IsoStent radioisotope stent
isosulfan blue imaging agent
isotope (see *imaging agent*)
isotope bone scan
isotope cisternography
isotope injected intravenously as
    bolus
isotope meal
isotope radiation therapy, intensity-
    modulated (IMRT) radioactivity
    in lungs
isotope scan (scanning)
isotope, stable
isotope venogram
isotopic bone scanning
isotopic cisternography
isotopic dilution
isotopic ratio
isotopic skeletal survey
isotropic lung scan
isotropic imaging
isotropic lung scan
isotropic single shot DWI (diffusion
    weighted imaging)
isotropic thin slice CT imaging
isotropic 3D or volume study
isotropic voxels
isotropy, liver diffusion
isovolumetric contraction
isovolumetric period
isovolumic contraction time
isovolumic period
isovolumic relaxation
Isovue contrast series (200, 300,
    370) (iopamidol)
    intrathecal injection
    parenteral injection

Isovue-M contrast series (200, 300)
Isovue (iopamidol, injectable) nonionic contrast agent
Israel camera
ISS (inferior sagittal sinus)
ISS (Injury Severity Score)
ISSI (interspinous segmental spinal
  instrumentation)
isthmic coarctation, congenital
isthmic tubal ectopic pregnancy
  locations
isthmus
  aortic
  stenotic
  temporal
isthmus aneurysm
isthmus of aorta
isthmus of femur
isthmus of uterus
isthmus of Vieussens
IT (iliotibial) band
ITA (internal thoracic artery) graft
ITC (Interventional Therapeutics
  Corporation)
  ITC balloon catheter
  ITC radiopaque balloon catheter
iterative algorithm
iterative gradient optimization
iterative halftoning
iterative reconstruction
ITMR (intraoperative transmyocardial
  revascularization)
IUdR (idoxuridine, iododeoxyuridine)
  halogenated thymidine analogue, a
  radiosensitizer

IUGR (intrauterine growth retarda-
  tion)
^{131}I uptake (thyroid function) test
IVM vascular occluder
IV, I.V. (intravenous) bolus
IV (interventricular) septum
Ivalon embolization
Ivalon particles
Ivalon sponge
IVB (intraventricular block)
IVC (inferior vena cava)
IVC (intravenous cholangiogram)
IVC filter, percutaneous
IVDSA (intravenous digital subtrac-
  tion angiography)
Ivemark syndrome
IVFA (intravenous fluorescein angiog-
  raphy)
IVH (intraventricular hemorrhage)
ivory phalanx sign
ivory vertebra sign
IVP (intravenous pyelogram)
IVR (idioventricular rhythm)
IVS (interventricular septum)
IVSD (interventricular septal defect)
IVST (interventricular septal thick-
  ness)
IVU (intravenous urogram)
IVUS (intravascular ultrasound)
IVUS (intravascular ultrasound)
  catheter
ivy sign

J, j

J (joule)
jackknife position
Jackman orthogonal catheter
Jackson bronchoscope
Jackson-Olympus bronchoscope
Jackson-Pratt catheter
jackstone calculus
Jaffe-Lichtenstein disease
jagged bone fragments
jagged osteophytes
Jahss classification of metatarso-
    phalangeal joint dislocation
jamming, facet
Janeway lesion
Jansen-Anderson intrauterine catheter
Jansen disease
Janus syndrome
Janus twins
Jarcho-Levin syndrome
Jaroschy projection of the patella
Javid carotid artery clamp
Javid endarterectomy shunt
jaw bone
JB1 catheter
JB3 catheter
J-coupled spins
J-curve movable core guidewire

Jedmed/DGH A-scan
Jefferson burst fracture
Jefferson cervical fracture
Jefferson fracture of atlas
Jeffery classification of radial fracture
jejunal loop interposition of Henle
jejunal motility
jejunization of the ileum
jejunoileal bypass (JIB)
jejunostomy tube
Jelco intravenous catheter
jeopardize
jet area (JA)
jet, high velocity
jet length (JL)
jet lesion
jet nebulizer
Jeune asphyxiating thoracic dystrophy
Jeune-Tommasi syndrome
Jewett bladder carcinoma classification
J guidewire
J-hook deformity of distal ureter
JIB (jejunoileal bypass)
JL (jet length)
JL4 (Judkins left 4) catheter
JL5 (Judkins left 5) catheter
J loop technique on catheterization

Jobert fossa
Jocath coronary balloon catheter
Jocath diagnostic catheter
Jocath graft connector
Jocath guidewire
Jocath stent
Jocath stent-graft
Jod-Basedow phenomenon
Jography angiographic catheter
Jography balloon catheter
Jography diagnostic catheter
Jography graft connector
Jography guidewire
Jography stent
Joguide balloon catheter
Joguide coronary guiding catheter
Joguide diagnostic catheter
Joguide graft connector
Joguide guidewire
Joguide stent
Joguide stent-guide
Johner shoulder view
Johns Hopkins coarctation clamp
Johnson and Dutt view
Johnson axiolateral projection of the
    femoral head and neck
Johnson-Jahss classification of
    posterior tibial tendon tear
joint
    AC (acromioclavicular)
    atlantoaxial
    bail-lock knee
    ball-and-socket
    basal
    calcaneocuboid
    capitate hamate
    capitolunate
    carpometacarpal (CMC)
    carpophalangeal
    Charcot
    Chopart
    chronic recurrent dislocation of
    condyloid

joint *(cont.)*
    costochondral
    costotransverse
    costovertebral
    cubonavicular
    cuneiform
    distal interphalangeal (DIP)
    distraction of
    ellipsoid
    facet
    flail
    free knee
    Gaffney
    Gillette
    glenohumeral
    gliding
    hallux interphalangeal (IP)
    hinge
    hip capsule
    hyperextensibility of
    immovable
    intercarpal
    interchondral
    intermetatarsal (IM)
    interphalangeal (IP)
    intervertebral
    lesser metatarsophalangeal
    Lisfranc
    lunotriquetral (LT)
    Luschka
    manubriosternal
    metacarpal-phalangeal (MCP, MP)
    metacarpophalangeal (MCP, MP)
    metatarsal-phalangeal (MTP)
    metatarsocuneiform (MC)
    metatarsophalangeal (MPJ, MTP)
    midcarpal
    midtarsal
    mortise
    naviculocuneiform
    neuropathic tarsal-metatarsal
    occipital-axis
    occipitoatlantoaxial

joint *(cont.)*
  pisotriquetral
  pivot
  proximal interphalangeal (PIP)
  radiocapitellar
  radiocarpal
  radioscaphoid
  radioulnar
  Regnauld degeneration of MTP
  sacroiliac (SI)
  saddle
  scaphocapitate
  scapholunate
  scaphotrapezoid
  scaphotrapezoid-trapezial (STT)
  secondary cartilaginous
  sesamoidometatarsal
  SI (sacroiliac)
  Silastic finger
  SL (scapholunate)
  sternal
  sternoclavicular
  sternocostal
  STT (scaphotrapezoid-trapezial)
  subtalar
  surgeon's tarsal joint
  Swanson finger
  synovial
  talocalcaneal
  talocrural
  talofibular
  talonavicular
  tarsal-metatarsal
  tarsometatarsal
  temporomandibular
  thoracic
  tibiofibular
  tibiotalar
  transverse tarsal
  trapeziometacarpal
  trapezioscaphoid
  trapeziotrapezoid
  triquetrohamate

joint *(cont.)*
  uncovertebral
  unstable
  weightbearing
  xiphisternal
joint arthrography
joint capsule
joint congruency
joint congruity
joint debris
joint depression fracture
joint dislocation
joint effusion
joint erosions
joint fluid extravasation
joint fracture
joint fulcrum
joint hyperextendability
joint incongruity
joint interface
joint kinematics
joint laxity
joint mice (or mouse)
joint morphology
joint photographic experts group
  (JPEG) algorithms
joint play, excessive
joint segment
joint space
  cartilage
  narrowing
  widened
joint space narrowing (JSN)
joint space width (JSW)
joint survey
joint swelling
Joliot method for sorption studies
Jones classification of diaphyseal
  fractures
Jones fracture
Jones position (elbow in flexion)
Joubert syndrome
joule (J)

joule shocks
JPEG (joint photographic experts
    group)
JPEG algorithms
JPEG compression
J pouch, two-loop ileal
J-shaped tube
J-shaped ureter
JSN (joint space narrowing)
JSW (joint space width)
J-tipped spring guidewire
Judet oblique views of acetabulum
Judet pelvic x-ray
Judkins cardiac catheterization
Judkins coronary angiography
Judkins coronary arteriography
Judkins femoral catheterization
Judkins 4 diagnostic catheter
Judkins left 4 coronary catheter (JL4)
Judkins right 4 coronary catheter
    (JR4)
Judkins selective coronary
    arteriography
Judkins USCI catheter
jug handle view
jug handles (zygomatic arches)
jugular bulb, internal
jugular catheter
jugular foramen syndrome
jugular triangle, internal
jugular vein distention (JVD)
jugular veins filled from above
jugular veins filled from below
jugular venous distention (JVD)
jugular venous excursions
jugular venous impulse
jugular venous pressure (JVP)
jugular venous pressure collapse
jugular venous pulsation (pulse)
jugulodigastric chain
jugulodigastric node
jugulovenous distention (JVD)
jump vein graft

jumped facet
jumper's knee
junction
    anorectal
    aortic sinotubular
    atriocaval
    atrioventricular
    cardioesophageal (CE)
    cardiophrenic
    caval-atrial
    cervicomedullary
    cervicothoracic
    cervicouterine
    cervicovaginal
    choledochopancreatic ductal
    chondrosternal
    corticomedullary
    costochondral
    craniocervical
    craniovertebral
    cystic-choledochal
    duodenojejunal (DJJ)
    esophagogastric (EG)
    fundic-antral
    gastrocnemius-soleus
    gastroesophageal (GE)
    gray-white matter
    ileocecal
    iliocaval
    J
    meniscosynovial
    metaphyseal-diaphyseal
    mucocutaneous
    musculotendinous
    myoneural
    myotendinous
    neuromuscular
    occipitocervical
    pancreaticobiliary ductal
    pelviureteral
    pelviureteric
    penoscrotal
    pharyngoesophageal

junction *(cont.)*
  phrenovertebral
  pontomedullary
  pontomesencephalic
  pyloroduodenal
  QRS-ST
  saphenofemoral
  sinotubular
  squamocolumnar
  sternoclavicular
  subclavian
  sylvian/rolandic
  temporal-occipital
  tracheoesophageal (TE)
  ureteropelvic (UPJ)
  ureterovesical (UVJ)
  uterotubal
junctional defect
junctional focus (pl. foci)
junctional zone thickness
junction separation, costochondral
juvenile idiopathic arthritis
juvenile ossifying fibroma
juvenile Paget disease
juvenile rheumatoid arthritis

juvenile Tillaux fracture
juxta-anastomotic stenoses
juxta-arterial ventricular septal defect
juxta-articular osteoid osteoma
juxta-articulation
juxtacaval fat collection
juxtacortical chondroma
juxtacortical sarcoma
juxtacrural
juxtaductal coarctation of aorta
juxtapapillary diverticulum
juxtaphrenic peak
juxtaposed leftward
juxtaposed rightward
juxtaposition
juxtapyloric ulcer
juxtarenal aortic aneurysm
juxtarenal aortic atherosclerosis
juxtarenal cava
juxtatricuspid ventricular septal defect
juxtavesical
JVD (jugulovenous or jugular venous
  distention)
JVP (jugular venous pressure)
J wire

K, k

K (potassium) (an element)
KAAT II Plus intra-aortic balloon
   pump
Kager triangle
Kahler disease
Kalamchi-Dawe classification of
   congenital tibial deficiency
Kalman filter
Kandel projection to demonstrate club-
   foot
Kaplan-Meier method
Kaposi sarcoma
   endobronchial
   epicardial
   intracolonic
   intrathoracic
   myocardial infiltration by
   pulmonary
Karl Storz bronchoscope
Karplus sign of pleural effusion
Kartagener syndrome
Kartagener triad
Kasabach-Merritt phenomenon
Kasabach oblique projection of the
   odontoid process
Kashin-Bek disease
Kast syndrome

Katayama hysteroscopic catheter
Katayama syndrome
Katzman infusion of radionuclide
   cisternography
Katz-Wachtel phenomenon
Kawai bioptome
Kawasaki disease
Kaye tamponade balloon catheter
Kayexalate enema
k-capture
KCD (kinestatic charge detector)
KDA profile
Kearns-Sayre syndrome
keel of glenoid component
keel-like ridge
keeled chest
Keith bundle of fibers in heart
Keith-Flack sinoatrial node
Kellock sign of pleural effusion
Kellogg-Speed lumbar spinal fusion
Kelly-Goerss Compass stereotactic
   system
keloid scar
Kemp-Elliot-Gorlin syndrome
Kemp-Harper submentovertex (SMV)
   projection of the jugular foramina
Kennedy area-length method

Kennedy ligament technique
Kennedy method for calculating
   ejection fraction
Kensey atherectomy catheter
Kent-His bundle
keratocyst
Kerckring fold
Kerckring nodule
Kerley A lines
Kerley B lines
Kerley C lines
kernel size
Kernig sign
Kernohan classification of astro-
   cytomas and glioblastomas
Kernohan notch phenomenon
Keshan disease
Kety equation
keV or kev (kiloelectron volt)
keV gamma ray
keyboard, Cherry
keyhole deformity
keystone of calcar arch
kg (kilogram)
kHz (kilohertz)
kick, atrial (AK)
kidney
   abdominal
   absence of
   afferent vessels of
   arcuate artery of
   Armanni-Ebstein
   arteriolosclerotic
   arteriosclerotic
   artificial
   Ask-Upmark
   atrophic
   autotransplantation of
   bilateral small
   biopsy of
   blunt trauma to
   cake
   carbuncle of

kidney *(cont.)*
   cicatricial
   clear cell of
   congenital absence of
   congested
   contracted
   contralateral
   cortical scarring of
   crossed ectopic
   cross-fused ectopic
   crush
   cyanotic
   cystic
   decapsulation of
   decortication of
   dialysis
   disk
   displacement of
   distended
   donor
   double
   doughnut (also donut)
   dromedary
   duplex
   duplication of left
   duplication of right
   dysfunctional
   ectopic
   edematous
   enlarged
   fatty
   fibrotic
   fibrous capsule of
   flea-bitten
   floating
   Formad
   fracture of
   fused
   Gambro Lundia Minor artificial
   Goldblatt
   granular
   head of
   hilum of

kidney *(cont.)*
  hilus of
  horseshoe
  hydronephrotic
  hypermobile
  hypertrophied
  hypoplastic
  infundibulum of
  injured
  interlobar veins of
  interlobular artery of
  interlobular veins of
  irregular
  ischemic
  lacking
  large red
  lateral border of
  lobe of
  lobulated
  long axis of
  lower pole of
  lumbar
  malacoplakia of
  medial border of
  medulla of
  medullary cystic
  medullary sponge
  middle
  mobile
  mortar
  movable
  multicystic dysplastic
  mural
  myelin
  myeloma
  native
  nonfunctioning
  pancake
  pelvic
  pelvis of
  pole of
  polycystic
  porous

kidney *(cont.)*
  ptotic
  putty
  pyelonephritic
  Rose-Bradford
  sacciform
  scarred
  sclerotic
  shriveled
  sigmoid
  small
  small atrophic
  solitary
  solitary functioning
  sponge
  stab wound to
  straight veins of
  supernumerary
  suspension of
  tenderness over
  thoracic
  transplanted
  tuberculosis of
  unilateral small
  venous segments of
  wandering
  water-bottle
  waxy
  wedge resection of
kidney abscess
kidney arteriovenous fistula
kidney atrophy
kidney calculus
kidney carbuncle
kidney carcinoma
kidney donor
kidney fracture
kidney function study
kidney hypertrophy
kidney imaging
kidney internal splint/stent (KISS)
kidney laceration
kidney lobe

kidney machine
kidney malignancy
kidney medulla
kidney pain
kidney-pancreas transplant
kidney parenchyma
kidney pinked up immediately
kidney pole
kidney rest
kidney scan
kidney shadow
kidney-shaped placenta
kidney stone forceps
kidney stone, passing of
kidney tenderness
kidney to background ratio
kidney tomography
kidney transplant
kidney transplantation
kidney transport anomaly
kidney trauma
kidney tubule
kidney tumor
kidneys, ureters, and bladder (KUB)
Kienböck disease
Kienböck dislocation
Kiernan spaces in liver
Kikuchi-Fujimoto disease
Kilfoyle classification of condylar
    fracture
Kilian line
Kilian pelvis
Killip-Kimball classification of heart
    failure
kiloelectron volt (keV or kev)
kilohertz (kHz)
Kim-Ray Greenfield inferior vena
    caval filter
Kimura disease
kinase C antiglioma monoclonal anti-
    body
kinase, thymidine
kinematic MRI studies

kinematic T2-weighted MR imaging
kinestatic charge detector (KCD)
kinetic energy
kinetic parameter analysis
kinetic perfusion parameters
kinetics
    elimination
    sorption
    washout
kinetocardiogram
Kinevac (sincalide) imaging agent
King multipurpose coronary graft
    catheter
kink artifact
kinked innominate artery
kinking
    arterial
    blood vessel
    bowel
    carotid artery
    catheter
    colon
    graft
    innominate artery
    intestinal
    Lane
    patch
kinking of ureter
kinking of vessels secondary to shift
    of intrathoracic structures
kinky-hair syndrome
Kinnier-Wilson disease
Kinsbourne syndrome
Kinsey atherectomy catheter
Kirchner diverticulum
Kirk distal thigh amputation
Kisch method (hip)
Kish urethral illuminated catheter
KISS (kidney internal splint/stent)
    catheter
kissing atherectomy technique
kissing balloon technique
kissing-type artifact

Kistler classification of subarachnoid
hemorrhage
kite projections to demonstrate club-
foot
Klatskin tumor
Klauder syndrome
Klebsiella pneumoniae pneumonia
Klein-Waardenburg syndrome
Klippel-Feil sequence
Klippel-Trénaunay-Weber syndrome
K-L transform
K-means clustering algorithm
K-means clusters
knee
    anterior cruciate deficit of
    breaststroker's
    Brodie
    corner of
    dislocated
    floating
    housemaid's
    internal derangement of the (IDK)
    jumper's
    locked
    motorcyclist's
    runner's
    wrenched
kneecap
knee-chest position
knee knob of Osgood-Schlatter disease
knee-like bend in a structure
kneeling position
knee view
knife
    roentgen
    UltraCision ultrasonic
knob, blurring of aortic
knobby process
knock-knee (genu valgum) deformity
knuckle bone
knuckle, boxer
knuckle of colon

knuckle-shaped
knuckle sign
Knutson view (skyline patella)
Koala intrauterine pressure catheter
Kocher anastomosis
Kocher fracture
Kocher lateral J approach
Kocher-Lorenz classification of
    capitellum fracture
Kocher maneuver
Koch sinoatrial node
Koch triangle, apex of
Kock pouch
Kodak software
Koerber-Salus-Elschnig syndrome
Köhler disease
Köhler lines
Köhler-Pellegrini-Stieda disease
Kohlrausch fold
Kohn, pores of
Kohonen self-organizing mapping
    (SOM)
Komai stereotactic head frame
Kommerell diverticulum
Konica scanner
Konstram angle
Kontron balloon catheter
Kopans needle
Kopans needle/hookwire system
Korányi-Grocco sign
Korányi-Grocco triangle
Korotkoff method in Doppler
    cerebrovascular examination
Korsakoff syndrome
Korotkoff test for collateral circulation
Kouchoukos method
Kovacs method (to view lowermost
    lumbar intervertebral foramen)
Krabbe disease
Krabbe diffuse sclerosis
Krukenberg tumor

krypton (^{81m}Kr) (an element)
^{81}Kr-m (krypton-81m) radioactive
  imaging
Kr-81m (krypton) imaging agent
k-space
k-space matrix
k-space sampling
k-space velocity mapping
KUB (kidneys, ureters, and urinary
  bladder)
Kubelka-Munk theory
Kuchendorf oblique PA projection of
  the patella
Kugel anastomosis
Kugel artery
Kugelberg-Welander juvenile spinal
  muscle atrophy
Kugel collaterals
Kümmell disease
Kupffer cell function
Kurzbauer unobstructed lateral
  projection of the sternoclavicular
  articulation

Kussmaul-Maier disease
Kveim test
kVp (kilovolts peak) meter
Kwart AQ Retro-Inject stent
Kwart Retro-Inject stent
Kyle fracture classification system
kyllosis (clubfoot)
kymography
kyphoscoliosis
kyphoscoliotic heart disease
kyphosis
  Cobb method of measuring
  loss of
  lumbar
  lumbosacral
  postlaminectomy
  Scheuermann juvenile
  thoracic
kyphotic angulation
kyphotic pelvis

L, l

L (liter)
L (lumbar vertebra)
LA (left atrium)
LAA (left atrial appendage)
LAA (left auricular appendage)
LA/AR (left atrium/aortic root) ratio
LABA (laser-assisted balloon
    angioplasty)
Labbé triangle
Labbé, vein of
Labcath catheter
label
    double
    long wavelength photolabel
    radioactive
    radionuclide
    single
    triple
labeled antibodies
labeled fibrinogen
labeled positron
labeled RBCs
labeled red blood cell sequestration
labeling
    antibody
    arterial spin (ASL)
    [111]In (indium-111) WBCs

labeling *(cont.)*
    in vitro
    in vivo
    in vivo/in vitro
    microglobulin
    radioactive
    radioisotope
    site-specific
    technetium Tc-human serum
        albumin
    Tc 99m red cell
    Tc-tagged RBCs
    white blood cell
labial hernia
labial hypertrophy
labile blood pressure
labral injury
labral variant
labrum
    acetabular
    articular
    glenoid
    glenoidal
labyrinth
    artery of
    bony
    cochlear

labyrinth *(cont.)*
  ethmoidal
  Ludwig
  membranous
  osseous
  renal
  Santorini
  vestibular
labyrinthine artery
labyrinthine hydrops
labyrinthine structures
LACD (left apexcardiogram,
  calibrated displacement)
laceration
  anal sphincter
  bladder
  bowel
  broad ligament
  central
  cervical
  high vaginal
  kidney
  pelvic floor
  perineal
  perineal muscle
  periurethral
  uterine
  vaginal
laciniate ligament of ankle
lacking a kidney
lack of clear-cut cerebral dominance
lacrimal bone
lacrimal canaliculus obstruction
lacrimal duct stent
lacrimal scintigraphy
lactating adenoma
lacteal fistula
lactiferous duct
lactulose enema
lacuna (pl. lacunae)
  bone
  cartilage
  intervillous

lacuna *(cont.)*
  osseous
  penis
  resorption
lacunar abscess
lacunar infarct
lacunar ligament
lacunar stroke
lacy trabecular pattern
LAD (left anterior descending)
  coronary artery
Ladder diagram
LAE (left atrial enlargement)
lag, motion
LAID (left anterior internal diameter)
LAIS excimer laser for coronary
  angioplasty
Laitinen CT guidance system
Laitinen stereotactic head frame
lake
  bile
  capillary
  mucous
  lipid
  venous
Laks method
lambdoid suture
Lambert projection
lamella (pl. lamellae)
  articular
  circumferential
  concentric
  enamel
lamellar body density (LBD) count
lamellated bone
lamina
  medullary
  osseous spiral
lamina propria
laminar flow
laminated calcification
laminated intraluminal thrombus
lamination of gyrus

laminography, cardiac
Lancisi muscle
landmark
    anatomic
    bony
    bony skull
landmark registration
Landolfi sign
Landsmeer ligament
Lane disease
Lane kink
Lanex medium screen
Langenbeck triangle
Langerhans cell histiocytosis
Langer line
language reorganization
Lanier clinical reporting system
lanthanide-induced shifts
Lanz point
LAO (left anterior oblique)
    LAO position
    LAO projection
    LAO view
LAP (left atrial pressure)
laparoscopic adrenalectomy
laparoscopic contact ultrasonography
    (LCU)
laparoscopic Doppler probe
laparoscopic intracorporeal ultrasound
    (LICU)
laparoscopic Roux-en-Y gastric bypass
    surgery
laparoscopic ultrasonography (LUS)
laparoscopic ultrasound (LUS)
L/A (liver/aorta) peak ratio
Lapiné ("la-pee-NAY")—see
    Chassard-Lapiné
Laplace effect
Laplace law
Laplace mechanism
Laquerriere and Pierquin ulnar groove
    projection

large bladder capacity
large bladder rupture
large bore catheter
large caliber coronary guiding catheter
large capacity bladder
large cell carcinoma
large clothing artifact
large clots
large colloidal particles
large core needle biopsy
large field radiotherapy
large hinge angle electron fields
large obtuse marginal branch
large thymus shadow obscuring
    cardiac silhouette
large venous tributaries
large vessel disease of diabetic foot
large vessel thrombosis
Larmor equation
Larmor frequency
Larmor precession
Larsen-Johansson disease
laryngeal cartilage
laryngeal fracture
laryngeal keel
laryngeal nodule
laryngeal vestibule
laryngeal web
laryngogram
laryngography
    contrast
    double contrast
larynx
    appendix of ventricle of
    glottic
    infraglottic
    laryngeal
    supraglottic
    ventricle of
    vestibule of
laser
    coagulative interstitial
    Nerve Fibre Analyzer GDx, The

laser-assisted balloon angioplasty
  (LABA)
laser-assisted microvascular
  anastomosis (LAMA)
laser balloon angioplasty (LBA)
laser biomicroscopy
laser correlational spectroscopy (LCS)
laser desiccation of thrombus
laser Doppler velocimetry
Laserflo Doppler probe
laser-induced thermotherapy (LITT)
laser-polarized helium MRI
laser printer, Ektascan
Laserprobe-PLR Plus
laser thermal ablation
LASH (left anterior superior
  hemiblock)
Lasix renography
LAST (large area sensing technology)
  imager
last menstrual period (LMP)
Lastac System angioplasty laser
lata, fascia
Latarjet, nerve of
late effect analysis
late effects of normal tissues (LENT)
  scoring system
late effects toxicity scoring
late film
late graft occlusion
late liver phase
late normal tissue sequelae
latent image
latent pleurisy
late-phase termination
lateral angle of uterus
lateral aspect
lateral bending views of spine
lateral border of kidney
lateral bronchi
lateral cervical spine film
lateral column calcaneal fracture
lateral condyle

lateral corticospinal tract
lateral costotransverse ligament
lateral decubitus position
lateral decubitus view
lateral displacement
lateral entrapment
laterality
lateralization
lateralizing deficit
lateralizing finding
lateralizing sign
laterally displaced fracture
lateral-medial view
lateral oblique projection
lateral opposed beam
lateral position
lateral projection
lateral recumbent position
lateral reticular formation
lateral spring ligament of foot
lateral sulcus
lateral tomography
lateral ulnar collateral ligament
lateral upper airway, soft tissue x-ray
lateral upright chest x-ray
lateral ventricle
lateral view
lateral wall of urinary bladder
lateral web
lateral wedge fracture of vertebral
  body
lateroconal fascia
late systolic posterior displacement on
  echocardiogram
latex allergy
LaTeX device-independent
latissimus dorsi muscle
LATS (long-acting thyroid stimulator)
lattice, fibrovascular
lattice model
lattice relaxation time
lattice vibrations
latticework

Laubry-Pezzi syndrome
Lauenstein and Hickey lateral hip
    projection
Lauenstein projection
Laue pattern
Laue photographic technique
Lauge-Hansen classification of ankle
    fracture
Laurence-Moon-Biedl-Bardet
    syndrome
Laurin angle
Laurin x-ray view
Lausanne stereotactic robot
law
    Bragg
    Courvoisier
    Hilton
Law method to demonstrate petrous
    temporal region
Law projection to demonstrate floor
    and posterior wall of antrum
Lawrence method to view the
    humerus
Law view
laxa, cutis
laxity
    joint
    ligament
    varus stress
layer
    bright
    circumferential echodense
    echodense
    echo-free
    hypoechoic
    inner bright
    sonolucent
layered periosteal reaction
layering calcification
layering effusion
layering of contrast material
layering of gallstones
lazaroid U74389G

LBA (laser balloon angioplasty)
L/B (lesion to brain) ratio
LBBB (left bundle branch block)
LBCD (left border of cardiac
    dullness)
LBP (low back pain)
LC-DCP (low contact dynamic
    compression plate)
LCA (left coronary artery)
LCF or LCX (left circumflex)
    coronary artery
LCL (lateral collateral ligament)
LCP (Legg-Calvé-Perthes disease)
LCS (laser correlational spectroscopy)
LCT (liquid crystal thermography)
LCU (laparoscopic contact ultra-
    sonography)
LDF (laser-Doppler flowmetry) probe
LDR (low dose radiation) seed
    brachytherapy
LDS (Longport Digital Scanner)
lead apron
lead eye shield
lead pellet marker
lead-pipe colon
lead-pipe fracture
lead-pipe rigidity
lead points
lead shielding
leaf alignment
leaflet
    anterior mitral (AML)
    anterior motion of posterior mitral
        valve
    aortic valve
    arching of mitral valve
    ballooning of
    billowing mitral (BML)
    calcified
    cleft
    coaptation of
    commissural
    conjoined

leaflet *(cont.)*
  degenerated
  doming of
  doughnut-shaped prolapsing
  flail mitral
  floating
  fluttering of valvular
  fused
  hammocking of
  incompetent
  mitral valve
  mural
  myxomatous valve
  nodularity of
  noncalcified mitral
  noncoronary
  paradoxical motion of
  poorly mobile
  posterior mitral (PML)
  posterior mitral valve
  posterior tricuspid (PTL)
  prolapse of
  prolapsed
  prolapsed mitral valve
  pseudomitral
  redundant aortic
  redundant mitral valve
  sail-like anterior
  septal
  thickened
  tricuspid valve
  valve
leaflet fusion
leaflet incompetence
leaflet motion
leaflet prolapse
  anterior
  posterior
leaflet tip
leaf of diaphragm
leak
  air
  aortic paravalvular

leak *(cont.)*
  baffle
  blood
  capillary
  cerebrospinal fluid (CSF)
  chyle
  contained (of aortic aneurysm)
  current
  generalized capillary
  interatrial baffle
  light
  mitral
  paraprosthetic
  paravalvar
  paravalvular
  periprosthetic
  perivalvular
leakage
  blood-tumor-barrier
  cerebrospinal fluid (CSF)
  contrast media
  radiocolloid
leaking abdominal aortic aneurysm
leaking vein
leak point pressure in bladder
leaky valve
lean mass
leapfrog position
least-squares (LS) algorithms
leather bottle stomach
leaves of diaphragm
leaves of mesentery
Le Fort (I, II, or III) fracture
left anterior descending (LAD) artery,
  superdominant
left anterior descending coronary
  artery takeoff
left anterior oblique (LAO) projection
left atrial active emptying fraction
left atrial appendage
left atrial cannulation
left atrial chamber
left atrial contraction

left atrial diameter
left atrial end diastolic pressure
left atrial enlargement
left atrial maximal volume
left atrial myxoma
left atrial pressure (LAP)
left atrial tension
left atrial thrombosis
left atrial to aortic (root) ratio
    (LA/Ao, LA-Ao)
left atrium, giant
left auricle
left auricular appendage (LAA)
left biliary duct system
left border of heart
left bundle branch block (LBBB)
left bundle branch hemiblock
left circumflex (LCX) coronary artery
left common femoral artery
left coronary artery arising from
    pulmonary artery
left coronary cusp
left coronary plexus (of heart)
left flank position
left frontoanterior (LFA) position
left frontoposterior (LFP) position
left frontotransverse (LFT) position
left heart failure
left heart pressure
left iliac system
left internal mammary artery (LIMA)
left Judkins catheter
left lateral decubitus position
left lower lobe
left lower lobe collapse
left main coronary artery (LMCA)
left main stem bronchus
left mentotransverse (LMT) position
left middle lobe
left mid lung
left occipitoposterior (LOP) position
left occipitotransverse (LOT) position
left posterior oblique (LPO) position

left pulmonary artery
left pulmonary cusp
left respiratory nerve (phrenic)
left-right asymmetry
left sacroposterior (LSP) position
left-sided bladder diverticulum
left-sided heart failure
left-sided heart pressure
left side down decubitus position
left-sided reflux
left sternal border
left to right cardiac shunt
left to right shift
left to right ventricular shunt
left upper lobe
left ureter
left ventricle
    double inlet
    hypoplastic
    morphologic
left ventricular afterload
left ventricular assist device (LVAD)
left ventricular chamber
left ventricular ejection fraction
    (LVEF)
left ventricular ejection fraction by
    acoustic quantification
left ventricular end diastolic pressure
    (LVEDP)
left ventricular end-diastolic volume
left ventricular end-systolic volume
left ventricular hypertrophy (LVH)
left ventricular hypoplasia
left ventricular loading
left ventricular maximal volume
left ventricular outflow tract
left ventricular preload
left ventricular pressure
left ventricular pseudoaneurysm
left ventricular stroke volume
left ventricular regional wall motion
    abnormality
left ventricular segmental contraction

left ventricular stroke work (LVSW)
left ventricular stroke work index
  (LVSWI)
left ventricular systolic pump function
left ventricular systolic time interval
  ratio
left ventriculogram
left ventriculography
leg (legs)
  baker
  bayonet
  champagne-bottle
  postphlebitic
Legg-Calvé-Perthes disease
Legg-Calvé-Waldenström disease
Lehman ventriculography catheter
Lehr-Par collimator
Leiner disease
leiomyosarcoma, gastrointestinal
Leitner syndrome
Leksell D-shaped stereotactic frame
Leksell-Elekta stereotactic frame
Leksell stereotaxic device used with
  CT scanner
LeMaitre Glow 'N Tell tape
lemon sign
length
  crown-heel
  crown-rump
  echo train
  limb
  track cone
LENI (lower extremity noninvasive)
lens-distortion compensation
LENT (late effects of normal tissues)
  scoring system
lenticular bone of hand
lenticular nucleus
lenticulostriate artery
lentiform nucleus
Leonard-George method to view
  femoral head and neck
LEOPARD syndrome

leptomeningeal cyst
leptomeningeal disease
leptomeningeal ivy sign
leptomeninges
Lequesne, center-edge angle of
Lequesne view (faux profil view)
Leriche syndrome
LEs (lower extremities)
LES (lower esophageal sphincter)
Lesgaft hernia
Lesgaft triangle
lesion (see also *disease*)
  ablation
  acanthotic
  accessible
  acquired
  acute cerebellar hemispheric
  adrenal
  afferent nerve
  aneurysmal
  angulated
  annular
  anterior parietal
  anterochiasmatic
  Antopol-Goldman
  aortic arch
  apical
  apple core
  areolar
  Armanni-Ebstein
  artifactual
  atheromatous
  atherosclerotic
  atrophic
  Baehr-Lohlein
  Bankart shoulder
  Bennett
  bifurcation
  bilateral
  biparietal
  bird's nest
  blastic
  bleeding

lesion *(cont.)*
  Blumenthal
  Bracht-Wachter
  brain stem
  Brown-Séquard
  bull's-eye
  calcified
  callosal
  cardiac valvular
  cartilaginous
  cavernous sinus
  caviar
  cavitary
  central
  cerebral
  cervical cord
  chiasmal
  chiasmatic
  circular
  circular cherry-red
  circumscribed
  coin (of lungs)
  cold
  complete nerve
  complex
  concentric
  constricting esophageal
  constrictive
  conus medullaris
  coronary artery
  coronary branch ostial
  cortical
  corticospinal pathway
  critical
  cryosurgical
  culprit
  cyclops
  cystic
  cystic renal
  deep
  de novo
  deep-seated
  dendritic

lesion *(cont.)*
  de novo
  desmoid
  destructive
  Dieulafoy
  diffuse
  discrete
  disk
  dominant hemisphere
  dorsal root entry zone
  doughnut
  DREZ (dorsal root entry zone)
  dumbbell
  Duret
  Ebstein
  eccentric
  eccentric restenosis
  echogenic
  ellipsoid
  endobronchial
  enhancing
  epicortical
  epileptogenic
  equivocal
  esophageal
  excitatory
  expansile lytic
  extra-axial
  extracapillary
  extrinsic
  fibro-osseous
  fibromuscular
  fingertip
  florid duct
  flow-compromising
  flow-limiting
  fluctuant
  focal
  focal hemispheric
  focal ischemic
  frank
  friable
  frontal lobe

lesion *(cont.)*
  fungating
  genital
  geographic
  Ghon primary
  glomerular tip
  gross
  gummatous
  hamartomatous
  hemodynamically significant
  hemorrhagic
  hemorrhagic shearing
  high cervical spinal cord
  high density
  high grade obstructive
  high grade squamous intraepithelial
    (HGSIL)
  high pontine
  high signal
  Hill-Sachs shoulder
  homogeneous
  hot
  hourglass-shaped
  hyperintense
  hyperplastic
  hypervascular
  hypodense
  hypothalamic
  impaction
  indeterminate
  indiscriminate
  infiltrating
  infiltrative
  infranuclear
  intra-axial brain
  intracerebral
  intracranial vascular
  intramedullary spinal
  intrasellar
  intraspinal
  intravesical
  intrinsic stenotic
  invasive

lesion *(cont.)*
  irregular-shaped
  irregularly shaped
  ischemic
  isointense
  Janeway
  jet
  Kidner
  lateral temporal epileptogenic
  left lower lobe (LLL)
  left upper lobe (LUL)
  lipomatous
  local
  localized
  Lohlein-Baehr
  low density
  lower motor neuron
  low grade squamous intraepithelial
    (LGSIL)
  lytic (osteolytic) bone
  malignant
  Mallory-Weiss
  mass
  medial longitudinal fasciculus
    (MLF)
  median nerve
  mesenteric vascular
  mesial temporal epileptogenic
  metabolic
  metadiaphyseal
  metaphyseal
  metastatic bone
  midbrain
  midline
  mixed
  mongolian spot-like
  Monteggia
  mucocutaneous
  multifocal
  multiple focal
  multiverrucous friable
  muscular
  nail bed

lesion *(cont.)*
  napkin-ring annular
  necrotic
  neoplastic
  neurogenic
  neurologic bladder
  neuropathic GU tract
  nidus of
  nipple
  nodular
  nondominant hemisphere
  nonenhancing
  noninfective endocardial
  noninvasive
  nonpalpable
  nucleus basalis
  obstructive (of the CSF pathways)
  occipital
  occlusive
  occult
  onion scale
  onionskin
  organic
  osseous
  osteoblastic
  osteocartilaginous
  osteochondral (of the talar dome)
  osteochondral (of the talus)
  ostial
  outcropping of
  oval cherry-red raised
  papillary
  papular
  papulonecrotic
  parasagittal
  parasellar
  parietal cortex
  parietal lobe
  parieto-occipital
  partial
  pedunculated
  periapical
  peripheral

lesion *(cont.)*
  peripheral nerve
  periventricular
  permeative
  Perthes-Bankart
  photon-deficient
  plaquelike
  polyostotic bone
  polypoid
  pontine
  posterior column
  posterior compartment
  posterior fossa-foramen magnum
  posterior language area
  preinvasive
  premalignant
  pretectal
  primary
  pulmonary
  purulent
  questionable
  radial sclerosing
  radiofrequency
  radiographic stability of
  radiopaque
  rectal
  rectosigmoid polypoid
  recurrent
  regurgitant
  renal mass
  resectable
  retrochiasmal
  retrochiasmatic
  rheumatic
  rib
  right lower lobe (RLL)
  right upper lobe (RUL)
  ring-enhancing (on CT)
  root
  root entry-zone
  sampling of mammographic
  satellite
  secondary

lesion *(cont.)*
  segmental
  serial
  sessile
  sharply demarcated circumferential
  signal characteristics of
  skip
  SLAP (superior labrum anterior
    posterior)
  slowly developing
  solid renal
  solitary
  sonolucent
  sonolucent cystic
  space-occupying
  spherical
  spinal cord
  spontaneous
  squamous intraepithelial (SIL)
  stacked ovoid
  stellate
  Stener
  stenosing
  stenotic
  striatal
  structural
  subchondral
  subcortical intracranial
  submucosal
  subtentorial
  subtle
  subtotal
  superficial
  supranuclear
  suprasellar
  supratentorial
  suspicious
  synchronous
  systemic
  tandem
  target
  tectal
  telangiectatic

lesion *(cont.)*
  temporal
  temporal lobe
  thalamic
  thymic
  tight
  total
  transfer
  transmural linear
  transverse cord
  treated premalignant
  trophic
  tuberculoid
  tuberculous
  tubular
  tubulointerstitial
  type A, B, or C
  ulcerated
  ulcerating
  ulcerative
  ulnar nerve
  uncommitted metaphyseal
  unilateral
  unresectable
  unstable
  upper motor neuron
  valvular regurgitant
  vascular
  vasculitic
  vegetative
  wedge-shaped
  well-defined
  white matter
  wide field
  wire-loop
  Wolin meniscoid
lesion depth
lesion in posterior fossa–foramen
  magnum
lesion in spinal cord
lesion localization
lesion of rapidly progressive
  glomerulonephritis

lesion to background ratio
lesion to cerebrospinal fluid noise
lesion to muscle ratio
lesion to nonlesion count ratio
lesion to white matter noise
lesion with increased blood pool
lesion with poorly defined margins
LESP (lower esophageal sphincter
   pressure)
lesser atrophy of disuse
lesser curvature of stomach
lesser metatarsophalangeal joint
lesser multangular (trapezoid) bone
lesser omentum
lesser sac abscess
lesser saphenous vein
lesser sciatic notch
lesser trochanter
lethal consequences
lethal midline granuloma
lethal myocardial injury
Letournel and Judet classification
   and column theory of acetabular
   fracture
Letournel iliac wing view
Letterer-Siwe disease
lettering artifact
leukemia infiltrate
leukocytes, indium-111-labeled
leukoencephalopathy
   multifocal
   progressive multifocal
leukomalacia, periventricular (PVL)
leukopenia, radiogenic
Leung coaxial catheter
Leung thumb loss classification
LeuTech infection imaging agent
LeuTech radiolabeled antibody kit
LeuTech radiolabeled imaging agent
levator ani muscle
LeVeen catheter
LeVeen plaque-cracker

level
   absorbance
   air-fluid
   fluid
   fluid-fluid
   gas-fluid
   pontine-medullary levels
   ring shadows with air-fluid
   stairstep air-fluid levels
   window
   Zielke derotation level
levoposition
levorotatory
levoscoliosis
levotransposition (L-transposition)
levoversion
Levovist ultrasound imaging agent
Lewis angle
Lewis method to view sesamoid bones
   of first metatarsal
Leydig duct
L5-S1 vertebral interspace
LFV (large field of view)
LGA (low grade astrocytoma)
LGV (lymphogranuloma venereum)
Lhermitte-Duclos disease
Lhermitte sign
LHV (left hepatic vein)
Libman-Sacks endocarditis disease
Lichtman radiographic classification of
   Kienböck disease
licked candy stick appearance
LICS (left intercostal space)
LICU (laparoscopic intracorporeal
   ultrasound)
Liddle syndrome
lidocaine
Lido-Pen Auto-Injector
lie
   horizontal
   longitudinal
   posterior
   transverse

Liebel-Flarsheim CT 9000 contrast
 delivery system
Lieberkühn (Lieberkuehn) crypt
lienography
LiF (lithium fluoride)
 LiF thermoluminescence dosimeter
Life-Pack 5 cardiac monitor
LifeSite hemodialysis (HD)
Lifestream coronary dilatation catheter
ligament
 accessory
 acromioclavicular
 acromiocoracoid
 alar
 annular
 anococcygeal
 apical (of dens)
 Arantius
 arcuate
 arterial
 atlantal
 attenuated
 auricular
 avulsed
 axis
 Bardinet
 Barkow
 beak
 Bellini
 Berry
 Bertin
 Bichat
 bifurcated
 Bigelow
 Botallo
 Bourgery
 broad (of uterus)
 Brodie
 Burns
 calcaneoclavicular
 calcaneocuboid
 calcaneofibular (CF)
 calcaneonavicular

ligament *(cont.)*
 calcaneotibial
 Caldani
 Campbell
 Camper
 capsular
 Carcassonne
 cardinal
 caroticoclinoid
 carpometacarpal
 Casser
 casserian
 caudal
 ceratocricoid
 cervical
 check
 check rein
 cholecystoduodenal
 chondroxiphoid
 ciliary
 Civinini
 Clado
 Cleland
 Cloquet
 collateral
 Colles
 congenital laxity of
 conjugate
 conoid
 conus
 coracoacromial
 coracoclavicular
 coracohumeral
 corniculopharyngeal
 coronary
 costoclavicular
 costocolic
 costotransverse
 costoxiphoid
 cotyloid
 Cowper
 cricopharyngeal
 cricosantorinian

ligament *(cont.)*
  cricothyroid
  cricotracheal
  cross
  crucial
  cruciate
  cruciatum cruris
  cruciform
  Cruveilhier
  cuboideonavicular
  cuneocuboid
  cuneonavicular
  cystoduodenal
  deep collateral
  deltoid (of shoulder, of ankle)
  Denonvilliers
  dentate
  denticulate
  Denucé
  diaphragmatic
  Douglas
  duodenal
  duodenorenal
  epididymal
  epihyal
  extracapsular
  extrinsic carpal
  falciform
  fallopian
  femoral
  Ferrein
  fibular collateral
  fibulotalar
  fibulotalocalcaneal
  flaval
  floating
  Flood
  fundiform
  gastrocolic
  gastrodiaphragmatic
  gastrohepatic
  gastrolienal
  gastropancreatic

ligament *(cont.)*
  gastrophrenic
  gastrosplenic
  genital
  genitoinguinal
  Gerdy
  Gillette suspensory
  Gimbernat
  gingivodental
  glenohumeral
  glenoid
  glossoepiglottic
  Grayson
  Günz (Guenz)
  Günzberg (Guenzberg)
  hammock
  Helmholtz axis
  Henle
  Hensing
  hepatic
  hepatocolic
  hepatocystocolic
  hepatoduodenal
  hepatoesophageal
  hepatogastric
  hepatogastroduodenal
  hepatophrenic
  hepatorenal
  hepatoumbilical
  Hesselbach
  Hey
  Holl
  Hueck
  Humphry
  Hunter
  Huschke
  hyalocapsular
  hyoepiglottic
  iliofemoral
  iliolumbar
  iliopectineal
  iliopubic
  iliotibial (of Maissiat)

ligament *(cont.)*
iliotrochanteric
infrapatellar
infundibulo-ovarian
infundibulopelvic
inguinal
intercapital
intercarpal
interclavicular
interclinoid
intercornual
intercostal
intercuneiform
interdigital
interfoveolar
intermetatarsal
internal collateral
interosseous
intersesamoid
interspinal
interspinous
intertransverse
intervertebral
intra-articular
intrascapular
ischiocapsular
ischiofemoral
Jarjavay
jugal
Krause
laciniate
lacunar
Landsmeer
Lannelongue
lateral arcuate
lateral collateral (LCL)
lateral ulnar collateral
Lauth
lienophrenic
lienorenal
ligation reversal surgery
limited proteoglycan matrix of
Lisfranc

ligament *(cont.)*
Lockwood
longitudinal
LTC (lateral talocalcaneal)
lumbocostal
lunotriquetral
Luschka
Mackenrodt
macroscopic hemorrhage
Maissiat
Mauchart
Meckel
medial collateral (MCL)
median arcuate
meniscofemoral
meniscotibial
metacarpoglenoidal
metacarpophalangeal
microscopic hemorrhage of
mucosal suspensory
natatory
naviculocuneiform
nuchal
occipital-atlas-axis
occipitoaxial
odontoid
orbicular
ovarian
palmar
pectinate
pectineal
peridental
periodontal
peritoneal
Petit
Pétrequin
petroclinoid
phalangeal glenoidal
phrenicocolic
phrenicoesophageal
phrenicolienal
phrenicosplenic
phrenoesophageal

ligament *(cont.)*
  phrenogastric
  phrenosplenic
  pisohamate
  pisometacarpal
  pisounciform
  pisouncinate
  plantar
  posterior cruciate (PCL)
  posterior longitudinal (PLL)
  posterior oblique (POL)
  Poupart
  pterygomandibular
  pterygospinal
  pterygospinous
  pubocapsular
  pubocervical
  pubofemoral
  puboprostatic
  pubovesical
  pulmonary
  quadrate
  radial collateral
  radial metacarpal
  radiate sternocostal
  radiocarpal
  radiolunotriquetral
  radioscaphocapitate
  radioscaphoid
  radioscapholunate
  reflected inguinal
  reflecting edge of
  retinacular
  Retzius
  rhomboid
  right triangular
  ring
  Robert
  round
  Rouviere
  sacrodural
  sacrospinous
  sacrotuberous

ligament *(cont.)*
  Santorini
  Sappey
  scapholunate
  Schlemm
  serous
  sesamoid
  sesamophalangeal
  sheath
  Simonart
  Soemmerring
  sphenomandibular
  spinoglenoid
  spiral
  splenocolic
  splenorenal
  spring
  Stanley cervical
  stellate
  sternoclavicular
  sternopericardial
  stretched out
  Struthers
  stylohyoid
  stylomandibular
  stylomaxillary
  superficial dorsal sacrococcygeal
  superficial posterior sacrococcygeal
  superficial transverse metacarpal
  superficial transverse metatarsal
  superior costotransverse
  superior pubic
  superior transverse scapular
  suprascapular
  supraspinous
  suspensory
  sutural
  syndesmotic
  synovial
  talocalcaneal
  talofibular
  talonavicular
  tarsal

ligament *(cont.)*
  tarsometatarsal
  tectoral
  temporomandibular
  Teutleben
  Thompson
  thyroepiglottic
  thyrohyoid
  tibial collateral
  tibial sesamoid
  tibiocalcaneal
  tibiofibular
  tibionavicular
  torn meniscotibial
  transverse atlantal
  transverse carpal
  transverse crural
  transverse genicular
  transverse humeral
  transverse intertarsal
  transverse metacarpal
  transverse metatarsal
  transverse perineal
  transverse tibiofibular
  trapezoid
  Treitz
  triangular
  triquetrohamate
  Tuffier inferior
  ulnar collateral (UCL)
  ulnocarpal
  ulnolunate
  ulnotriquetral
  umbilical
  urachal
  uterine
  uterosacral
  uterovesical
  vaginal (of fingers and toes)
  venous
  ventral sacrococcygeal
  ventral sacroiliac
  ventricular

ligament *(cont.)*
  vertebropelvic
  vesicoumbilical
  vesicouterine
  vestibular
  vocal
  volar
  volar carpal
  Walther oblique
  Weitbrecht
  Winslow
  Wrisberg
  xiphicostal
  xiphoid
  Y-shaped
  Zaglas
  Zinn
ligament laxity
ligamentous bouncing
ligamentous box
ligamentous complex
ligamentous disruption
ligamentous impingement
ligamentous insertion
ligamentous instability
ligamentous laxity
ligamentous luxation
ligamentous support
ligamentous thickening
ligand, neuroreceptor
lightbox, CCD
light leak
light microscopy
light reflection rheography imaging
light source, fiberoptic
LILI (low intensity laser irradiation)
Lilienfeld superoinferior projection of
  the pubic and ischial bones and
  symphysis pubis
Lilienfeld coalition view of calcaneum
Lilienfeld posterolateral projection of
  ileum and acetabulum
Liliequist membrane

LIMA (left internal mammary artery)
  graft
limb absence
limb asymmetry
limb bud
limb length asymmetry
limb of artery
limb of bifurcation graft
limb of vein
limitation of joint motion
limitations, bandwidth
limited compression
limited films
limited view
limits, amplitude
linacography
Lindblom AP lordotic chest view
line
  acetabular
  anorectal
  anterior axillary (AAL)
  anterior humeral
  aortic
  arterial
  axillary
  branching
  calcification
  central sacral (CSL)
  Correra
  costoclavicular
  costophrenic septal
  curvilinear subpleural
  CVP (central venous pressure)
  demarcation
  Ellis
  Ellis-Garland
  epiphyseal
  fat
  Feiss
  Fleischner
  fracture
  gas density
  gluteal

line *(cont.)*
  growth arrest
  iliopectineal
  isodose
  isoelectric
  isopotential
  joint
  Kerley A
  Kerley B
  Kerley C
  Kilian
  Köhler
  lateral joint
  Linton
  Lorentzian
  lower lung
  low intensity
  lucent
  medial joint
  median
  metaphyseal lucent
  Meyer
  midaxillary
  midclavicular (MCL)
  midscapular
  midspinal
  midsternal
  Moyer
  Nélaton
  orthogonal tag
  parallel pitch
  pectinate
  Perkins
  photon therapy beam
  pleural
  popliteal
  posterior axillary
  pubococcygeal
  radiocapitellar
  raster
  reference
  resonance
  Schoemaker

line *(cont.)*
  scorbutic white
  semilunar
  Shenton
  soleal
  subcutaneous fat
  subpleural curvilinear
  trough
  vertebral body
  Wagner
  white (linea alba)
linea alba
linear absorption coefficient
linear accelerator isocenter motion
linear accelerator (LINAC, linac)
  radiosurgery
linear amplifier
linear and depressed skull fracture
linear array
  Acuson 5 MHz
  convex
  high density
linear-array-hydrophone assembly
linear artifact
linear atelectasis
linear attenuation coefficient
linear band of maximal radiolucency
linear calcification
linear defect
linear density
linear erosion
linear fracture
linear infiltrate
linear interpolation
linearity
linearization, perceptual
linear lucency
linear markings
linear opacity
linear phased arrays
linear radiolucency in the disk space
linear scanning
linear scar in lungs

linear shadow
linear skull fracture
linear streaks en face
linear tear
linear tomography
line imaging
line placement
line saturation
  gaussian
  Lorentzian
line scanning
line shadow
line shape sensitivity
line width
lingual bone
lingual thyroid
lingual vascular canals of the mandible
linguine sign in breast
lingula pulmonis
lingular artery
lingular bronchus
lingular mandibular bony defects
  (LMBD)
lingular nodule
lingular orifice
linitis plastica
link, musculotendinous-osseous
Linton shunt
Linx exchange guidewire
lipid, intracellular
lipid-laden plaque
lipid-lowering therapy
lipid-rich material
lipid-sensitive MR
lipid signal
lipid zone
Lipiodol (iodized poppy seed oil)
  myelographic imaging agent
liplike projections of cartilage
lipofibroma
lipoid pneumonia
lipoid pneumonitis

lipoma
  cardiac
  filar
  intratentorial
  uterine
lipoma arborescens
lipomatous hypertrophy of interatrial
  septum
liponecrosis
lipophilic contrast agents
lipophilic sequestration system
liposarcoma of heart
liposomal doxorubicin imaging agent
liposomes, antibody-conjugated
  paramagnetic (APCLs)
lipping, osteophytic
liquefactive emphysema
Liqui-Coat HD (barium sulfate)
  imaging agent
liquid crystal thermogram
liquid crystal thermography (LCT)
liquid pleural effusion
liquid scintillation analysis
liquid scintillation spectrometer
Liquipake imaging agent
Lisfranc dislocation
Lisfranc fracture
Lisfranc joint
Lissauer column
lissencephaly, cobblestone
list mode data collection
Lister tubercle
liters per minute per meter squared
  (L/min./m²)
Litespeed catheter
Litespeed stent
Litespeed wire
lithiasis
  renal (also renolithiasis)
  testicular microlithiasis
lithium
lithium nephropathy
lithogenic bile

litholysis
Lithostar nonimmersion lithotriptor
lithotomy position
lithotripsy
  laser
  ultrasonic
lithotriptor (also lithotripter)
lithotriptor with fluoroscopic and
  ultrasound localization
LITT (laser-induced thermotherapy)
Litten diaphragm phenomenon
Littmann stethoscope
littoral cell angioma
Littré gland abscess
Littré hernia
Litwak cannula
Litzmann obliquity
liver
  alcoholic fatty
  biliary cirrhotic
  capsule of
  caudate lobe of
  centrilobular region of
  cirrhosis of
  cirrhotic
  degenerative
  degraded
  diaphragmatic surface of
  dome of
  duodenal impression on
  echogenic
  enlarged
  fatty
  floating
  frosted
  hobnail
  infantile
  large droplet fatty
  left lobe of
  metastasis to
  nodular
  noncirrhotic
  polycystic

liver *(cont.)*
  polylobar
  potato
  prominent
  pyogenic
  quadrate lobe of
  renal impression on
  right lobe of
  shrunken
  small droplet fatty
  stasis (in cirrhosis)
  undersurface of
  visceral surface of
  wandering
  waxy
liver abscess
liver/aorta (L/A) peak ratio
liver attenuation
liver bed
liver coil
liver diffusion isotropy
liver edge
liver flap
liver function
liver hematoma
liver hydatid disease
liver-jugular sign
liver, kidneys, and spleen (LKS)
liverlike lung
liver/liver peak (L/LP) ratio
liver parenchyma
liver scan, radionuclide
liver scintiphotograph
liver span
liver-spleen scan
Livingston triangle
LKS (liver, kidneys, and spleen)
LLD (leg length discrepancy)
LLD (limb length discrepancy)
LLE (left lower extremity)
LLQ (left lower quadrant)
L-loop heart
L-looping

L-loop ventricular situs
L/LP (liver/liver peak) ratio
L-malposition of aorta
LMCA (left main coronary artery)
L-methyl ^{11}C-methionine
L/min./m^2 (liters per minute per
  meter squared)
LMP (last menstrual period)
LMR (localized magnetic resonance)
LNV (last normal vertebra)
loading
  differential
  peripheral
  spike
  uniform
loading dose
load, T2-lesion
lobar bile duct
lobar bronchus (pl. bronchi)
lobar cavitation
lobar consolidation
lobar emphysema
lobar lung atrophy
lobar pneumonia
lobe
  accessory
  accessory hepatic
  anterior tip of temporal
  azygos vein
  caudate (of liver)
  collapsed
  cuneiform
  falciform
  fetal
  flocculonodular (of cerebellum)
  frontal
  inferior
  insular
  kidney
  left
  left lower
  left middle
  left upper

lobe *(cont.)*
  limbic
  lower
  mammary gland
  medial temporal
  middle
  occipital
  orbital aspect of frontal
  parietal
  polyalveolar
  prostatic
  pulmonary
  pyramidal
  quadrate
  renal
  Riedel
  right
  right lower
  right middle
  right upper
  sequestered (lung)
  superior
  temporal
  thyroid
  uncus of temporal
  upper
lobe of azygos vein
lobectomy
lobster-claw deformity
lobular architecture of liver
lobular carcinoma in situ
lobular pneumonia
lobulated border
lobulated filling defect
lobulated saccular appearance
lobule
local compression fracture
local invasion
localization
  autoradiographic
  carpal-tarsal
  computerized tomography guidance
    for stereotactic

localization *(cont.)*
  confirmatory needle
  CT-directed hookwire
  fluoroscopic
  hookwire
  lesion
  lithotriptor with fluoroscopic and
    ultrasound
  off-axis point
  pelvimetry with placental
  pelvimetry without placental
  percutaneous (of pulmonary
    nodules using suture-ligated
    microcoils)
  placental
  point
  protein kinase C (brain)
  pulse sequence, single shot
    adiabatic
  radiopharmaceutical
  seizure
  single shot adiabatic
  stereotactic
  surface coil
  wire
localization grid
localized H1 spectroscopy
localized magnetic resonance (LMR)
localized mass effect
localized mediastinal fluid
localized obstructive emphysema
localized subdural hematoma
localizer, breast
localizing images
local recurrence
lock, hub
lock washer configuration
loco-regional hyperthermia
loco-regional recurrence
locomotor pattern
Loc-Sure single pass catheter
loculated effusion on chest x-ray
loculated fluid collection

loculated pleural effusion
locules, multiple
locus, scanning
Lodge Moor lateral oblique projec-
   tions to demonstrate cervical
   articular facets (no hyphen)
Loeffler (Löffler)
Loeffler bacterial pneumonia
Loeffler endocarditis
Löffler (Loeffler)
Löfgren syndrome
Lohlcin-Baehr lesion
Lohlein diameter
LOM (low osmolar media)
L1-L5 (five lumbar vertebrae)
L1-APo cephalometric measurement
L1-L6 intervertebral disks
L1-NB cephalometric measurement
long ACE fixed-wire balloon catheter
long-acting thyroid stimulator (LATS)
long axial oblique view
long axis acquisition
long axis parasternal view
long axis slice
long axis view
Long Beach stereotactic robot
long bone
long bone fracture
long bore collimator
Longdwel Teflon catheter
long echo train fast spin echo
   sequence
long fibers of the posterior talofibular
   ligament
longitudinal arch of foot
longitudinal arteriography
longitudinal B-mode
longitudinal blood supply to ulnar
   nerve
longitudinal fasciculus, medial (MLF)
longitudinal fissure
longitudinal fracture
longitudinal lie

longitudinally
longitudinal magnetization
longitudinal muscles
longitudinal narrowing
longitudinal relaxation
longitudinal taenia musculature
longitudinal ultrasonic biometry
Longport Digital Scanner (LDS)
long scale
long segment femoropopliteal stent
   placement
long segment narrowing
Long Skinny over the wire balloon
   catheter
long-standing
long taper/stiff shaft Glidewire used in
   coronary artery imaging
long term patency
long TR, short TE
long TR/TE (T2 weighted image)
long tract signs
long tube decompression
long wavelength photolabel
loop
   afferent
   air-filled
   alpha sigmoid
   bowel
   capillary
   cervical
   closed
   closed conducting
   colonic
   contiguous
   diathermic
   dilated bowel
   double reverse alpha sigmoid
   duodenal
   efferent
   flow volume
   gamma transverse colon
   Gerdy interatrial
   Gerdy interauricular

loop *(cont.)*
  Henle
  intestinal
  J (on catheterization)
  jejunal
  lenticular
  Meyer
  Meyer-Archambault
  N-shaped sigmoid
  P (on vectorcardiography)
  peduncular
  pressure volume
  puborectalis
  reentrant
  rubber vessel
  sentinel
  sigmoid
  small bowel
  Stoerck
  subclavian
  T (on vectorcardiography)
  tendon
  transverse cFolon
  vector
  ventricular
  vessel
  Vieussens
looped ureter
loopless (dipole) antenna (of catheter
  or guidewire)
loopogram (ileostogram)
loop ostomy bridge
loose fracture
loose joint body
Looser-Milkman syndrome
Lo-Por tracheal tube
Lo-Profile and Lo-Profile II balloon
  catheter
Lo-Profile steerable dilatation catheter
Lorad M-II D mammographic system
Lorad StereoGuide stereotactic breast
  biopsy system

lordosis
  cervical
  lumbar
  reversal of
  thoracic
lordotic curve
lordotic pelvis
lordotic position
lordotic view
Lorentzian line saturation
Lorenz method (hip view)
loss, electron equilibrium
loss of definition
loss of sigmoid curve
loss of thoracic kyphosis
lossy algorithm
lossy compression of transverse source
  images
lossy compression on the diagnostic
  accuracy of CT colonography for
  detecting colonic polyps
lossy wavelet compression
Louis, sternal angle of
low acoustic pressure harmonic
  software
low angle scattering
low-angle shot (flash) technique
low attenuation pulsation artifact
Low-Beers parietotemporal projection
Low-Beers projection
Low-Beers view
low cardiac output syndrome
low contrast film
low contrast structure
low density lesion
low density structure
low dose film mammographic
  technique
low dose folinic acid
low dose radiation (LDR) seed
  brachytherapy
low dose screen-film technique
low dose mammography

low energy collimator
low energy photon attenuation
  measurement
low energy radiofrequency conduction
  hyperthermia treatment
lower esophageal sphincter (LES)
lower extremity noninvasive (LENI)
lower left sternal border
lower lobe lung mass
lower lung field
lower lung line
lower pole collecting system
lower pole of kidney
lower pole of patella
lower pole ureter
Lower (Richard Lower)
  Lower rings
  Lower tubercle
lower soft tissue attenuation of the
  accordion sign
lower tract obstruction
lower ureter and vagina fistula
low field MR angiography
low field MR imaging
low field strength MR imaging
low flow syndrome
low flow vascular malformation
low frequency shear waves
low grade squamous intraepithelial
  lesion (LGSIL)
low intensity laser irradiation (LILI)
low intensity pulsed ultrasound
low level echo
Lown-Ganong-Levine syndrome
  (LGL)
low mechanical index continuous-
  mode contrast-enhanced ultrasound
low mechanical index harmonic
  software
low osmolality
low osmolar contrast media
low output heart failure
low pressure cardiac tamponade

low sensitivity
low signal intensity
low specificity
low speed rotational angioplasty
  catheter
low temperature diffraction
low urethral pressure (LUP)
low velocity flow
low wedge pressure
LPA (left pulmonary artery)
LPO (left posterior oblique) position
LPS balloon catheter
LPS Peel-Away introducer
LPV (left pulmonary vein)
LRA (low right atrium)
LS (lumbosacral) spine
LSB (lower sternal border)
LSC background prediction
LSCVP (left subclavian central venous
  pressure)
LSD-image (line scan diffusion
  imaging)
LSe Kwart Retro-Inject stent
LSO (lutetium oxy-ortho-silicate)
L-transposition (levotransposition)
  of great arteries
L-tyrosine (^{11}C) imaging agent
Lubinus acetabular cup, cemented
Lubri-Flex urologic stent
lucency
  interspersed
  linear
lucent defect
lucent line, metaphyseal
Lucey-Driscoll syndrome
Lucite beam spoiler
Ludovici angle
Ludwig angle
Luer-Slip IAB catheter
luetic aortitis
luetic arteritis
Lugol solution

Lukes-Collins classification of
lymphoma
Luma cervical imaging system
Lumaguide catheter
lumbar artery
lumbar facet joint synovial cyst
lumbar pneumencephalography
lumbar scoliosis
lumbar spine view
lumbar transverse process
lumbar vertebra
lumbarization
lumbosacral kyphosis
lumbosacral series
lumbosacral spine
lumen (pl. lumens, lumina)
  aortic
  arterial
  attenuated
  bile duct
  bowel
  bronchial
  clot-filled
  cloverleaf-shaped
  crescentic
  cystic duct
  D-shaped vessel
  double barrel
  duct
  duodenal
  eccentrically placed
  elliptical
  empty
  esophageal
  false
  gastroduodenal
  intestinal
  obstructive thrombus within the
  occluded
  patent
  slitlike
  slit-shaped vessel
  star-shaped vessel

lumen *(cont.)*
  true
  vascular
lumen boundary
LumenHance (manganese chloride
  tetrahydrate) imaging agent
lumen-intimal interface
lumenogram
lumina (pl. of lumen)
Lumina guidewire
luminal area
luminal caliber
luminal configuration, scalloped
luminal contour, irregular hazy
luminal cross-sectional area
luminal diameter
luminal dimension
luminal encroachment
luminal irregularity
luminal morphology
luminal narrowing
luminal plaquing
luminal silhouette
luminal stenosis
luminal thrombosis
luminance
luminogram, air
Luminol
Lumiscan 150 scanner
Lumiscan scanner
lumpy appearance of lung
Lunar DPX densitometer
Lunar Expert densitometer
Lunar scanner
lunate bone
lunate dislocation
lunatomalacia
Lunderquist guidewire
Lunderquist-Ring torque guide
lung
  accessory
  acquired unilateral hyperlucent
  air-conditioner

lung *(cont.)*
airless
arc welder's
artificial
atelectatic
bauxite
bird breeder's
bird fancier's
bird handler's
black
brown
bubbly
budgerigar-fancier's
cardiac
cheese handler's
cheese washer's
coal miner's
coal worker's
coffee worker's
collapsed
consolidated
cork handler's
cork worker's
corundum smelter's
dark and mottled
drowned
dynamic
emphysematous
empty collapsed
eosinophilic
expanded
farmer's
fibrinoid
fibroid
fibrosis of
fish-meal worker's
fissures of
flock worker's
fresh
furrier's
gangrene of
grain handler's
hardened

lung *(cont.)*
harvester's
hemorrhagic consolidation of
hen worker's
hilum of
honeycomb
humidifier
hyperlucent
hypogenetic
hypoplastic
infarcted segment of
inferior border of
light pink
liverlike
lumpy appearance of
malt worker's
maple bark-stripper's
mason's
meat wrapper's
mediastinal part of medial surface
   of
miller's
mottled gray
mushroom worker's
native
periphery of the lung
pigeon-breeder's
pigeon-fancier's
posterior border of
premature infant's
pseudocysts of
pump
radioactivity in
rheumatoid
root of
rudimentary
septic
shock
shrunken
silicotic
silo-filler's
silver finisher's
silver polisher's

lung *(cont.)*
  smoker's
  static
  stiff noncompliant
  stretched
  subsegment of
  thatched roof worker's
  thresher's
  tropical eosinophilic
  underventilated
  unilateral hyperlucent
  vanishing
  welder's
  well-inflated
  wet
  white
lung abscess
lung agenesis
lung air spaces
lung apex (pl. apices)
lung architecture
lung architecture distortion
lung base
lung calculus
lung carcinoma
lung cirrhosis
lung collapse, massive
lung consolidation
lung count curve
lung disease, interstitial
lung endometriosis
lung expansion
lung field
lung fissure
lung/heart ratio of thallium 201
  activity
lung hemangioma
lung hepatization
lung hypoplasia
lung infiltrate (infiltration)
lung inflammation
lung injury, penetrating
lung lobule

lung lymphoid hyperplasia
lung markings
lung mass with mediastinal invasion
lung necrosis
lung opacity
lung overexpansion
lung overinflation
lung parenchyma consolidation
lung periphery
lung reexpansion
lung scan, perfusion and ventilation
lung segment, infarcted
lung segmentation
lung stiffness
lung transplantation
lung underinflation
lung volume asymmetry (on x-ray)
lung volume reduction surgery
lung washout
lung zone
lunula (pl. lunulae)
LUP (low urethral pressure)
lupus erythematosus (LE)
LUQ (left upper quadrant)
Luque rod used in spinal fusion for
  scoliosis
Luque sublaminar wire used in spinal
  fusion for scoliosis
LUS (laparoscopic ultrasonography)
LUS (laparoscopic ultrasound)
Luschka crypts of gallbladder mucosa
Luschka, joint of
Luschka muscle
Lutembacher complex
Lutembacher syndrome
lutetium oxy-ortho-silicate (LSO)
luxated bone
luxation
Luxtec fiberoptic system for diagnostic
  and surgical visualization
luxury perfusion
LV (left ventricular) function pressure

LV (left ventricular) function wall
motion
LVAD (left ventricular assist device),
HeartMate
LVAS (left ventricular assist system),
Novacor
LVdd (left ventricular diastolic dimen-
sion)
LVD (left ventricular dysfunction)
LVEDD (left ventricular end diastolic
dimension)
LVEDI (left ventricular end diastolic
volume index)
LVEDP (left ventricular end diastolic
pressure)
LVEF (left ventricular ejection
fraction)
LVESD (left ventricular end systolic
dimension)
LVESVI (left ventricular end systolic
volume index)
LVET (left ventricular ejection time)
LVFS (left ventricular functional
shortening)
LVFW (left ventricular free wall)
LVG (left ventriculogram)
LVgram (slang for left ventriculogram)
LVH (left ventricular hypertrophy)
with strain
LVID (left ventricular internal
diameter) (or dimension)
LVIDd (left ventricular internal
dimension at end diastole)
LVIDD (left ventricular internal
diastolic dimension)
LVIDs (left ventricular internal dimen-
sion at end systole)
LVIV (left ventricular inflow volume)
LVM (left ventricular mass)
LVMI (left ventricular mass index)
LVOT (left ventricular outflow tract)
LVOTO (left ventricular outflow tract
obstruction)

LVOV (left ventricular outflow
volume)
LVP (left ventricular pressure)
LVP1 and LVP2 (left ventricular pressure on apex cardiogram)
LVPW (left ventricular posterior wall)
LVs (left ventricular systolic)
dimension
LVS (left ventricular support) system
LVS (left ventricular systolic)
pressure
LVSW (left ventricular stroke work)
LVSWI (left ventricular stroke work
index)
LVW (left ventricular wall)
lym-1 monoclonal antibody labeled
with iodine-131 (^{131}I)
Lyme carditis
Lyme disease
lymphadenectomy, pelvic
lymphadenopathy
intraglandular granulomatous
mesenteric
lymphangiectasia
congenital renal
renal
lymphangiographic contrast
lymphangiography
lymphangioleiomyomatosis
lymphangioma, cardiac
lymphangitic carcinomatosis
lymphangitic metastasis
lymphatic cachexia
lymphatic channels
lymphatic drainage
lymphatic duct
lymphatic malformation (LM)
lymphatic mapping
lymphaticovenous malformation
(LVM)
lymphatic system
lymphatic vessel

Lymphazurin (isosulfan blue) imaging
  agent
lymph capillaries
lymph gland
lymph node (see *node*)
lymph node enlargement
lymph node involvement
lymph node metastases
lymph node syndrome
lymph node, tumor-infiltrated
lymphoblastoma
lymphocele
lymphocytic infiltrate
lymphocytic interstitial pneumonitis
  (LIP)
lymphocytic splenomegaly,
  postcardiotomy
lymphogenous dissemination
lymphogenous metastasis
lymphography
  interstitial MR
  time-lapse quantitative computed
    tomography
lymphoid interstitial pneumonia
lymphoma
  adult T-cell
  African
  B-cell
  B-cell monocytoid
  Burkitt
  centrocytic
  cleaved cell
  diffuse
  diffuse large cell
  diffuse mixed small and large cell
  diffuse small cleaved cell
  follicular
  follicular center cell
  follicular mixed small cleaved
  follicular predominantly large cell
  follicular predominantly small cell
  giant follicle
  granulomatous

lymphoma *(cont.)*
  histiocytic
  Hodgkin
  infiltrative
  intermediate lymphocytic
  large cell, immunoblastic
  large cleaved cell
  large noncleaved cell
  Lennert
  lymphoblastic
  lymphocytic plasmacytoid
  lymphocytic poorly differentiated
  lymphocytic well-differentiated
  malignant
  mantle zone
  mediastinal
  Mediterranean
  mixed lymphocytic-histiocytic
  multifocal
  nodular
  noncleaved cell
  non-Hodgkin
  peripheral T-cell
  pleomorphic
  polypoid
  primary diffuse large B-cell
  primary of central nervous system
  small B-cell
  small cleaved cell
  small lymphocytic
  small noncleaved cell
  T-cell
    convoluted
    cutaneous
    small lymphocytic
  U-cell (undefined)
  ulcerative
  undefined
  undifferentiated
lymphonodular hyperplasia
lymphoproliferative disorder, intrathoracic
lymphosarcoma

LymphoScan nuclear imaging system
lymphoscintigraphic
lymphoscintigraphy, radiocolloid
lymph vessels of thymus gland
lyoluminescence
Lysholm method to view the petrosa,
    internal auditory meatus (IAM),
    and mastoid cells

lytic (osteolytic)
lytic area
lytic bone lesion
lytic change
lytic lesion

M, m

m (meta-stable) (in technetium ^{99m}Tc)
m (meter)
mA (milliampere)
MAA (^{99m}Tc MAA) (macroaggregated
  albumin)
Mab-170 monoclonal antibody
MAC (mitral annular calcium)
Macalister muscle
MacCallum patch
machine, parallel virtual
Machlett collimator
Mackenzie point
MacLean-Maxwell disease
Macleod syndrome
MacNab view of the patella
macroadenoma, prolactin-secreting
  pituitary
macroaggregated albumin
macrocolon
macrodacryocystography, digital
  subtraction
macrofistulous AV (arteriovenous)
  communications
macrometastasis
macromolecular contrast-enhanced
  MR imaging
macromolecular drugs

macronodular pattern
Macroscint (indium ^{111}In IGIV
  pentetate)
macros copically evident tumor
macroscopic magnetization vector
Macrotec (technetium Tc 99m MAA)
  imaging agent
MacSpect real-time NMR station
Maddahi method of calculating right
  ventricular ejection fraction
Madelung deformity
Maffucci syndrome
Magendie, foramen of
magic angle artifact
magic angle effect
magic angle spinning NMR
Magic Wallstent
Magna-SL scanner
Magnes biomagnetometer system
Magnes 2500 WH (whole head)
  imager
magnet
  doughnut
  GE Signa 1.5T
  Magnex
  nonenclosed
  open

magnet *(cont.)*
Oxford
pancake MRI
passively shimmed superconducting
shim
shimmed
short bore
superconducting
tubular
2 T large bore
magnet mode
magnet rate
magnet response
magnetic dipole
magnetic field gradients (MFG)
magnetic field, oscillating
magnetic moment
magnetic particulates
magnetic resonance (MR) (see also
magnetic resonance imaging)
magnetic resonance angiography
(MRA)
echo planar
gated inflow
low field
magnetic resonance angiography-
directed bypass procedure
magnetic resonance arthrography
magnetic resonance bursography
magnetic resonance catheter imaging
and spectroscopy system
magnetic resonance cholangiography
(MRC)
magnetic resonance cholangiography
with HASTE
magnetic resonance cholangiopancreatography (MRCP)
magnetic resonance cystometry
magnetic resonance elastography
(MRE)
intravoxel phase dispersion (IVPD)
phase-contrast
steady state

magnetic resonance enhancement
pattern
magnetic resonance epidurography
magnetic resonance H-1 stimulated-
echo acquisition mode spectroscopy
magnetic resonance hydrometry
magnetic resonance imaging (MRI)
(see *imaging; MRI terms*)
MRI-guided breast biopsy
MRI-guided focused ultrasound
transducer
MRI-guided laser-induced interstitial
MRI-guided thermotherapy
MRI mapping
MRI morphometry
MRI prescan
MRI probe head
MRI segmentation
MRI transducer
magnetic resonance mammography
(MRM)
magnetic resonance myelography
magnetic resonance needle tracking
magnetic resonance neurography
(MRN)
magnetic resonance pancreatography
(MRP)
magnetic resonance phase velocity
mapping
magnetic resonance phlebography
magnetic resonance receptor agents
magnetic resonance renography
magnetic resonance sialography
magnetic resonance signal
magnetic resonance simulator
magnetic resonance spectroscopic
imaging (MRSI)
magnetic resonance spectroscopy
(MRS)
magnetic resonance spin incoherence
magnetic resonance splenoportography

magnetic resonance system, open-
configuration
magnetic resonance tomography
(MRT)
magnetic resonance urography (MRU)
magnetic resonance velocity mapping
magnetic resonance venography
magnetic resonance volume estimation
magnetic source imaging (MSI)
magnetic susceptibility artifact (MRI)
magnetism
magnetization
longitudinal
net tissue
spatial modulation
magnetization and spin lock transfer
imaging
magnetization imaging
magnetization-prepared rapid gradient
echo-water excitation
(MRPRAGE-WE)
magnetization-prepared 3D gradient-
echo (MP-RAGE) sequences
magnetization transfer (MT)
high power, thin section quantitative
quantitative
magnetization transfer contrast
magnetization transfer effect
magnetization transfer ratio (MTR)
magnetization transfer ratio histogram
magnetization transfer saturation
magnetoacoustic MRI
magnetoencephalogram
magnetoencephalography (MEG)
magnetogyric ratio
Magnetom 1.5T scanner
Magnetom SP MRI imager
Magnetom SP63 scanner
Magnetom Vision MR system
magnetometer probe
magnetoresistive sensor circuit

Magnevist (gadopentetate dimeglumine) imaging agent
Magnex Alpha MR system
Magnex MR scanner
magnification
high resolution
signal
magnification and spot compression
magnification error
magnification mammography
magnitude
MAG 3 dynamic renal scan
Mahaim and James fibers
Mahaim bundles
Mahler sign
mahogany flush
main bronchus
main energy substrate
main fissure
main glow peak
main magnetic field inhomogeneity
artifact
main portal vein peak velocities
(MPPv)
main pulmonary artery
main sac
main stem bronchus
main stem carina
Maisonneuve fibular fracture
Majocchi disease
major calices
major fracture fragment
major histocompatibility complex class
II antigen (MHC-2)
mA/kV (milliamperes per kilovolt)
Mal de Meleda syndrome
maladie de Roger (Roger disease)
malaligned atrioventricular septal
defects
malalignment
malangulation
malacoplakia of kidney

malar bone
malaria
malarial pneumonitis
Malcolm-Lynn C-RXF cervical
  retractor frame
maldevelopment
maldistribution of ventilation and
  perfusion
Malecot catheter
male urethra
male urethral stricture
malformation
  adenomatoid
  angiographically occult intracranial
    vascular malformation
  angiographically occult vascular
    (AOVM)
  anorectal
  Arnold-Chiari
  Arnold-Chiari (type II)
  arterial
  arteriovenous (AVM)
  cavernous
  Chiari II
  congenital
  congenital cardiac
  congenital vascular
  conotruncal
  coronary artery
  costosternal
  cystic adenomatoid
  dancer foot
  Dandy-Walker
  Dieulafoy vascular
  Ebstein
  embolization of vascular
  endocardial cushion
  extracardiac
  familial cavernous
  fast flow
  high flow vascular
  hyperostosis associated with venous
  intraosseous vascular

malformation *(cont.)*
  intrapulmonary arteriovenous
  low flow vascular
  septal
  sink-trap
  slow flow vascular
  submucosal arterial
  truncular venous
  valve
  vascular
malformed phlebectasia in the calf
Malgaigne fracture
malignancy
  aggressive
  bladder
  borderline
  cervical
  endometrial
  grading of
  high grade
  invasive
  kidney
  low grade
  metastatic
  penile
  primary
  prostatic
  renal
  secondary
  staging of
  uterine
  vulvar
malignancy-associated nephropathy
malignancy threshold
malignant acetabular osteolysis
malignant airway obstruction
malignant breast mass
malignant degeneration
malignant effusion
malignant fibrous histiocytoma
malignant glomerulonephritis
malignant hemangioendothelioma
malignant lesion

malignant lymphoma
malignant melanoma
malignant mesothelioma
malignant mixed tumor
malignant nephroangiosclerosis
malignant nephrosclerosis
malignant osteoid
malignant osteopetrosis
malignant ovarian teratoma
malignant peripheral nerve sheath
   tumor
malignant pleomorphic adenoma
malignant pleural implants
malignant pleural mesothelioma
   (MPM)
malignant renal neoplasm
malignant teratoma
malignant teratoma tumor
malignant transformation
malignant tumor
malignant-type calcification
malleolar
malleolus (pl. malleoli)
   lateral
   medial
malleolus fibulae
malleolus tibiae
mallet finger
Mallinckrodt angiographic catheter
Mallinckrodt imaging agent
Mallinckrodt scanner
Mallory-Weiss mucosal tear
malperfused
malperfusion
malpighian follicle
malpighian vesicle
malpositioned fetus
malposition of colon
malposition of heart
malposition of uterus
malrotation of intestine
malt worker's lung
malum coxae senile

malum perforans pedis
malunion of fracture fragments
malunited
Mamex DC mammography
mamillary body
mammillation
mammary abscess
mammary calculus
mammary-coronary artery bypass
mammary duct
mammary ductal ectasia
mammary ductogram
mammary fistula
mammary galactogram
mammary gland lobe
mammary implant
mammary lymph node metastasis
mammary tuberculosis
Mammex TR computer-aided
   mammography diagnosis system
Mammo QC mammography
mammogram (see *mammography*)
mammogram-guided biopsy
mammogram-guided core biopsy
mammographer
mammographically guided needle
   localization
mammographic features
mammographic findings
mammographic-histopathologic correlation
mammographic lesion, sampling of
mammographic measurement
mammographic parenchymal patterns,
   Wolfe
mammographic view
mammography (also mammogram)
   annual
   baseline
   bilateral
   clustered calcifications on
   computed tomographic
   computed tomography laser
     (CTLM)

mammography *(cont.)*
contoured tilting compression
crablike lesion on
CT laser (CTLM)
diffraction-enhanced imaging (DEI)
digital
dual energy contrast-enhanced
digital subtraction
Egan
full field digital
GE Senographe 2000D digital
high resolution CT
ImageChecker
low dose
magnetic resonance (MRM)
magnification
Mammex DC
Mammex TR computer-aided
Mammo QC
Mammomat B
microfocal spot
nonpalpable mass on
postbiopsy
radionuclide
retromammary space view in
scintimammography (SMM)
screen-film
screening
Selenia full-field digital
SenoScan full-field digital
SoftScan laser
step-oblique
ultra-high magnification (UHMM)
ultrasound augmented
xero-
x-ray (XMG)
mammography grid
Mammography Quality Standards Act
(MQSA)
Mammomat B mammography
Mammomat Novation full-field digital
mammography system
MammoReader imaging system

MammoSite catheter
MammoSite RTS imaging
Mammotest breast biopsy system
Mammotome handheld minimally
invasive breast biopsy device
Mammotome ultrasound system
mandible
alveolar border of
angle of
mandibular canal
mandibular incisor angle, Frankfort
mandibular notch
mandibuloacral dysplasia
mandibulofacial dysostosis
maneuver (pl. maneuvers)
Adson
costoclavicular
displacement
flexion
Heineke-Mikulicz
hyperabduction
Kocher
McRoberts
Müller (Mueller)
Osler
Rivero-Carvallo
scalene
squatting
transabdominal left lateral
retroperitoneal
Valsalva
mangafodipir trisodium imaging agent
manganese (Mn) (an element)
Mn Cl (chloride) imaging agent
Mn-DPDP (dipyridoxal diphosphonate) chelate imaging agent
Mn PcS4 imaging agent
Mn-SOD
Mn-TPPS4
manganese chloride tetrahydrate
imaging agent
manganese pneumonitis
mangofodipir trisodium imaging agent

Mani catheter
manifest
manifestations, extrapulmonary
Mann-Bollman fistula
mannitol and saline 1:1 solution
Mannkopf sign
Mann-Whitney test
manofluorography (MFG)
manometer-tipped cardiac catheter
manometric pattern
manometry
  anal
  aneroid
  anorectal
  biliary
  ERCP
  esophageal
  rectosigmoid
  sphincter of Oddi
Mansfield Atri-Pace catheter
Mansfield orthogonal electrode
  catheter
Mansfield Scientific dilatation balloon
  catheter
Manson schistosomiasis-pulmonary
  artery obstruction syndrome
mantle
  anechoic
  hypoechoic
mantle block
mantle complex
mantle field
manual computed method
manual intensity windowing
manual pressure over carotid sinus
manual subtraction films
manubriosternal joint
manubriosternal syndrome
manubrium
map
  acceleration
  bull's-eye
  bull's-eye polar

map *(cont.)*
  color flow
  cylindrical
  cylindrical projection
  decimalized variance
  end diastolic polar
  end systolic polar
  sestamibi polar
  spherical
MAP (mean arterial pressure)
MAPCath catheter
map-guided partial endocardial
  ventriculotomy
maple bark stripper's lung
maple bark worker's suberosis
maple syrup urine disease
mapper, brain
mapping
  activation-sequence
  apparent diffusion coefficient
    (ADC)
  body surface
  body surface potential
  brain
  catheter
  Doppler color flow
  electrophysiologic
  endocardial activation
  endocardial catheter
  epicardial
  FMRI
  heart motion-adapted magnetic
    resonance velocity
  homology
  ice
  intramural
  intraoperative electrocortical
    stimulation
  Kohonen's self-organizing (SOM)
  k-space velocity
  lymphatic
  MR (magnetic resonance) velocity
  MRI (magnetic resonance imaging)

mapping *(cont.)*
    pace
    parallel analog
    phase-shift velocity
    precordial
    retrograde atrial activation
    sinus rhythm
    spatial
    straight-line Hough transform (HT)
    2D pulsatility index
    2D resistance index mapping
mapping algorithms
mapping of cerebral sulci
mapping probe, hand-held
Marable syndrome
marantic clot
marantic thrombus
Marathon guiding catheter
march foot (fracture)
march fracture
Marconi Infinion scanner
Mardis firm stent with HydroPlus
    coating
Marex MRI system
Marfan syndrome
marfanoid hypermobility syndrome
margin
    cardiac
    colon
    convex
    cortical
    costal
    delineation of
    disk
    obtuse
    scapular
    stomach
marginal artery of Drummond
marginal branch
marginal circumflex bypass
marginal invasion
marginal osteophyte formation
marginal placenta

marginal serration
marginal spur
marginal ulcer
marginal vein
Marie-Bamberger disease
Marie-Strümpell disease
Marie-Tooth disease
Marine-Lenhart syndrome
markedly accentuated pulmonic
    component
marker
    implanted imaging opaque
    lead pellet
    nipple
    radioactive string
    radiopaque
    serum tumor
    subtle
    tantalum
marker-channel diagram
marker migration
marker transit study
markings
    bronchovascular
    bronchovesicular
    coarse bronchovascular
    haustral
    increased pulmonary vascular
    linear
    peribronchial
    pulmonary vascular
    vascular
Markov chain
Markov random field
Markov source model
Mark II Kodros radiolucent awl
Maroteaux-Lamy syndrome
marrow, bone
marrow edema pattern
marrow infiltration
Marrs intrauterine catheter
Marrs laparoscopic catheter
Marshall, vein of

Martin disease
Martorell aortic arch syndrome
Martorell-Fabre syndrome
Martorell hypertensive ulcer
Mary Allen Engle ventricle
mAs (milliampere-second)
MAS (Morgagni-Adams-Stokes)
  syndrome
masculinizing tumor
mask (pl. masks)
  convolution
  ISAH stereotactic immobilizing
  Orfit
mask-based approach
masking, unsharp
mask ventilation
mason's lung
masquerading effect
mass
  abdominal
  adjacent soft tissue
  adnexal
  airless
  appendiceal
  apperceptive
  calcified
  cavitary
  cavitary lung
  conical
  cordlike
  cystic
  dirty
  discrete
  dominant
  doughy
  echogenic
  elongated
  encapsulated
  enhancing
  exophytic
  expansile
  extraovarian
  fecal

mass *(cont.)*
  firm
  fixed
  fleecy
  fluctuant
  fluid
  fluid-filled
  focal
  freely movable
  groin
  high signal
  hilar
  hyperdense
  hyperintense
  hypervascular
  hypodense
  ill-defined
  inflammatory polypoid
  injection
  interbronchial
  intermediate signal
  intra-abdominal
  intra-articular
  intracardiac
  intracavity
  intraluminal
  intraventricular
  irregular
  left ventricular (LVM)
  lobulated
  low attenuation
  low density
  lower lobe lung
  low signal
  malignant breast
  mastectomy
  mastotomy
  mediastinal
  mixed echogenic solid
  mixed signal
  molar
  mushy
  nodular

mass *(cont.)*
  nonpulsatile abdominal
  paracardiac
  parenchymal tumor
  perirenal
  polypoid calcified irregular
  pulsatile
  relativistic
  right ventricular (RVM)
  saccular
  signal
  soft tissue
  solid
  solitary
  space-occupying
  spherical
  spiculated
  stony
  suspicious
  ventricular
  woody
mass attenuation coefficient
mass balance
mass effect
massive ascites
massive edema
massive effusion
massive embolism (embolization)
massive genital prolapse
massive lung collapse
massive pneumonia
massive pubertal hypertrophy
massive pulmonary hemorrhage
mass lesion
masslike configuration
masslike densities simulating
  neoplasms
Massachusetts (General Hospital)
  Utility Multiprogramming System
  (MUMPS)
massage, carotid sinus
masseter muscle
mastectomy

Master syndrome
Master two-step exercise stress test
masticator muscle
masticator space
mastitis, carcinomatous
mastoid polytomography
mastoid sinus
mastopathy, diabetic
mastotomy
match
  nontransmural
  transmural
  triple
matching
  atlas
  electron-photon field
  general pattern
matched V/Q defect
match-line wedge
Match 35 PTA catheter
mater (not *matter*)
  dura
  pia
material
  atheromatous
  contrast
  inspissated
maternal pelvis
matrix (pl. matrices)
  acquisition
  bone
  calcific
  cartilage
  chondroid
  germinal
  ground-glass
  image
  solid
  transformation
Matrix LR3300 laser imaging
matter
  cortical gray
  cortical white

matter *(cont.)*
  dysplastic white
  gray
  white
maturation, disk
mature pseudocyst of pancreas
Maugeri syndrome
Maverick Monorail balloon catheter
Maverick over the wire balloon
  catheter
Maverick PTCA catheter
Maverick2 Monorail catheter
Maverick XL PTCA catheter
Max Force balloon catheter
maxillary alveolus
maxillary sinus
maxillary spine
maximal respiratory pressure
maximal volume (of left atrium)
maximal voluntary ventilation (MVV)
maximum amplitude constants
maximum diameter to minimum
  diameter ratio
maximum intensity pixel (MIP)
maximum intensity projection (MIP)
maximum intensity projection and
  source images
maximum likelihood algorithms
maximum predicted heart rate
  (MPHR)
maximum slew rate ramps
Max Plus MR scanner
Maxwell 3D Field Simulator
Mayer view to demonstrate petrous
  temporal region
May view to demonstrate zygomatic
  arch
Mazer stent
mazoplasia, cystic
MBF (myocardial blood flow)
MBIH catheter
MBq (megabecquerel)
McArdle syndrome

MCAT (myocardial contrast
  appearance time)
McBurney point
McCort sign
MCD (molecular coincidence detec-
  tion) imaging
MCE (myocardial contrast
  echocardiography)
McGoon coronary perfusion catheter
McHenry treadmill exercise protocol
McIntosh double lumen catheter
MCL (midclavicular line)
MCLS (mucocutaneous lymph node
  syndrome)
MCP (metacarpophalangeal) joint
McRoberts maneuver
MCS (middle coronary sinus)
MCTC (metrizamide CT cisternogram)
MDCT (multidetector computed
  tomography)
MD-50 imaging agent
MD-Gastroview (diatrizoate meglumine; diatrizoate sodium) imaging
  agent
MD-60 imaging agent
MDP, technetium Tc 99m-labeled
Meadows syndrome
meal
  barium
  Boyden test
  double contrast barium
  Ewald test
  fatty
  isotope
  motor
  motor test
  opaque
  retention
  small bowel
  test
mean aortic pressure
mean arterial pressure (MAP)

mean atrial pressure
mean blood pressure
mean cardiac vector
mean circulatory filling pressure
mean circumferential fiber shortening
  rate (MCFSR)
mean free path
mean left atrial pressure
mean maximal expiratory flow
  (MMEF)
mean mitral valve gradient
mean pulmonary artery (MPA)
  pressure
mean pulmonary capillary pressure
  (MPCP)
mean pulmonary transit time
mean rate of circumferential
  shortening
mean right atrial pressure
mean-square error
mean time
mean transit time (MTT), esophageal
mean vectors
mean venous pulsation
Meary metatarsotalar angle
measurable endpoint
measure
  Hausdorff metric
  linear
  prophylactic
  root-mean-squared gradient
measured absorbance
measurement
  attenuation (of photon)
  blood flow volume
  cardiac output
  cerebrospinal fluid flow
  Cerenkov
  diode
  excitation function
  4 T
  high sensitivity
  intercomparison

measurement *(cont.)*
  low energy photon attenuation
  mammographic
  morphometric
  nutation angle
  polarographic needle electrode
  proximal fragment ratio (PFR)
  regional washout
  rocking curve
  semiquantitative
  topographic
measurement and depiction in vivo
MEA syndromes IIa and IIb
meatal segment
meatal stenosis
meat wrapper's lung
mechanical augmentation
mechanical counterpulsation
mechanical dottering effect
mechanical insufflation
mechanical small bowel obstruction
mechanical thrombolysis
mechanical valve
mechanics, intramural
mechanism
  check valve
  deglutition
  flap-valve
  Frank-Starling
  humeral
  internal retention
  pinchcock
  propulsive
  sphincteric
  swallowing
Meckel cave
Meckel diverticulitis
Meckel diverticulum
Meckel scan (scanning)
meconium
  calcified
  intraluminal
meconium obstruction

meconium plug
MEDDARS analysis system for
  cardiac catheterization
Medebar Plus (barium sulfate)
  imaging agent
Medelec DMG 50 Teflon-coated
  monopolar electrodes
Medescan (barium sulfate) imaging
  agent
Medgraphics body plethysmograph
media (see *medium*)
media-adventitia interface
medial border of kidney
medial compartment
medial-lateral view
medially
medial oblique projection
medial rotation of viscera to right of
  midline
median arcuate ligament of diaphragm
median lethal dose
median level echoes
median line
median sacral artery
mediastinal adenopathy
mediastinal air
mediastinal border
mediastinal edema
mediastinal emphysema
mediastinal fat
mediastinal fibrosis
mediastinal fistula
mediastinal hernia
mediastinal invasion
mediastinal lung surface
mediastinal lymph node
mediastinal mass
mediastinal metastasis
mediastinal neoplasm
mediastinal node
mediastinal part of medial surface of
  lung
mediastinal pleura

mediastinal prominence
mediastinal septum
mediastinal shift
mediastinal structures
mediastinal surface of lung
mediastinal thickening
mediastinal tumor
mediastinal wedge
mediastinal widening
mediastinitis, purulent
mediastinodiaphragmatic pleural
  reflection
mediastinum
  anterior
  deviated
  inferior
  middle
  posterior
  superior
  widened (or widening of)
mediastinum cerebelli
mediastinum cerebri
mediastinum displacement
medical cyclotron
medical holography
Medical Image Resource Center
  (MIRC)
Medinvent stent
medical linear accelerator
medication (see also *bowel prep;*
    enemas; imaging agents; radio-
    therapy agents)
  ACE inhibitor
  bromophenol blue
  Captopril
  Colonlite bowel prep
  CoLyte bowel prep
  dihydroxyphenylalanine [DOPA]
  Dulcolax bowel prep
  EDTMP
  Emulsoil bowel prep
  enalaprilat ACE inhibitor
  Ethiodol (ethiodized oil)

medication *(cont.)*
Evac-Q-Kit bowel prep
Evac-Q-Kwik bowel prep
ferric ammonium citrate-cellulose
paste
Fleet bowel prep
furosemide
glucagon
GoLytely bowel prep
HalfLytely bowel prep
indomethacin
isoflurane
methyl methacrylate
naloxone
nicotinamide
nimodipine
nitrous oxide
nonsteroidal antiphlogistics
OCL bowel prep
olsalazine
Pentagastrin
phenobarbital
radiopharmaceutical
somatostatin
Suppocire C
tetramethylene
Tridrate bowel prep
urokinase
X-Prep bowel prep
medicine, photonic
Medigraphics analyzer
MedImage scanner
mediolateral oblique view
mediolateral stress
mediopatellar
MediPort implanted vascular access
device
Medison scanner
Medi-Tech balloon catheter
medium (pl. media) (see *imaging
agent*)
contrast
high osmolar (HOM)
ionic contrast

medium *(cont.)*
low osmolar (LOM)
nonionic contrast media
radiopaque
tunica
Medrad imaging agent injector
Medrad MRInnervu endorectal colon
probe coil
medronate scan
Medspec MR imaging system
Medtronic balloon catheter
Medtronic Minix
Medtronic radiofrequency (RF)
receiver
medulla (pl. medullas, medullae)
adrenal
lymphatic
ovarian
renal
spinal
medulla oblongata
medulla of kidney
medullaris, conus
medullary abscess
medullary canal
medullary cystic kidney
medullary involvement
medullary nephrocalcinosis
medullary pyramids
medullary sponge kidney
medullary tumor
medulloblastoma
Medweb clinical reporting system
MEDX gamma camera
Mees lines
MEG (magnetoencephalography)
megabecquerel (MBq)
megacolon
acquired
congenital
idiopathic
toxic
megacystis

megacystis-megaureter association
megaduodenum
megaelectron volt (MeV)
megaesophagus of achalasia
megahertz (MHz)
megalocystis
megaloureter
megarectum
megaureter, refluxing
megavolt (MV)
megavoltage grid therapy
megavoltage radiation therapy
megavoltage treatment beams
meglumine diatrizoate imaging agent
meglumine iocarmate imaging agent
meglumine iodipamide imaging agent
meglumine iothalamate imaging agent
meglumine iotroxate imaging agent
Meige lymphedema
Meigs capillaries
Meigs-Cass syndrome
Meigs disease
Meigs syndrome
Meissner plexus
melanin, leptomeningeal
melanoma
   malignant
   metastatic
melanosarcoma
melanosis, parenchymal neurocutaneous
melorheostosis of Leri
Melrose solution
Meltzer sign
membrane
   acoustically induced rupture of
   atlantoaxial posterior membrane
   atlanto-occipital membrane
   Bichat membrane
   cricothyroid membrane
   glomerular basement membrane
   interosseous (IOM)
   intraluminal membranes

membrane *(cont.)*
   Liliequist
   microporous
   mucous
   premature rupture of membranes
   pseudomembrane
   rupture of (ROM)
   serous
   synovial
   vernix
membranous septum
membranous subvalvular aortic
   stenosis
membranous urethra
membranous ventricular septal defect
memory-intensive algorithms
Memory-Vu angiographic catheter
MEN (multiple endocrine neoplasia)
Ménétrier disease
Mengert index in pelvimetry
meningeal abscess
meningeal involvement
meningeal hemorrhage
meningeal myelomatosis
meningioma
   cerebellopontine angle
   clival
   convexity
   cystic
   falcine
   falx
   fibroblastic
   fibrous
   malignant
   meningotheliomatous
   parasagittal
   posterior fossa
   suprasellar
   tentorial
   transitional
meniscal bridge
meniscal cleft
meniscal horn

meniscal injury
meniscal tear
meniscus
   articular
   diverging
meniscus (crescent) of contrast-saline
   mixture
meniscus articularis
meniscus lateralis
meniscus medialis
meniscus sign on upper GI study
meniscus (pl. menisci)
Menkes kinky-hair syndrome
menses
menstrual age
menstrual date
mensuration algorithm
mental spine
mentoanterior (MA) position
mentoposterior (MP) position
mentotransverse position
mentum
Mercator projection
Mercedes Benz sign, reversed
mercury artifact
mercury-in-Silastic strain gauge
Meridian echocardiography
Merkel cell carcinoma cell lines
meroacrania
mesencephalic reticular formation
mesenchymal hamartoma
mesenchymoma
mesenteric adenopathy
mesenteric apoplexy
mesenteric arterial thrombosis
mesenteric artery occlusion
mesenteric infarction
mesenteric ischemia
mesenteric lymph nodes
mesenteric lymphadenopathy
mesenteric node
mesenteric rupture

mesenteric sclerosis
mesenteric panniculitis
mesenteric thickening
mesenteric tear
mesenteric venous thrombosis
mesenteritis, sclerosing
mesenterium commune
mesentery
   fan-shaped
   fatty
   leaves of
   root of
   segmental misty (SSM)
   small intestine (SIM)
   ventral
mesial aspect
mesial hyperperfusion
mesial temporal sclerosis
mesiotemporal atrophy
mesoappendix
mesoblastic nephroma
mesocardia
mesocaval anastomosis
mesocaval H-graft shunt
mesocolic hernia
mesocolon
mesocolonic fat
mesocolonic vessels
mesocuneiform bone
mesoderm
   extraembryonic
   gastral
mesodermal
meso-HMPAO, technetium Tc 99m
meson
mesonephric duct
mesonephric tubule
mesonephros
mesorectum
mesosigmoid colon
mesosternum
mesothelial

mesothelioma
  malignant pleural (MPM)
  multicystic
mesoversion of heart
mespiperone C 11
Mester test for rheumatic disease
meta-analysis
metabolic 8-hydroxyquinolyl-
  glucuronide
metabolic rate of oxygen
metabolic response
metabolic tracer uptake
metabolism
  cerebral
  fat
  fatty acid
  myocardial
metabolite
  CMRO$_2$ glucose
  phosphorus
metacarpal bone
metacarpal-phalangeal (or metacarpophalangeal) (MCP) joint
metacarpophalangeal (or metacarpal-
  phalangeal) (MCP) joint
metachronous lung cancer
metadiaphyseal lesion
metaiodobenzylguanidine (MIBG)
  imaging agent
metal technetium target
metallic foreign body
metallic stent
metalloporphyrins
metanephric duct
metaphyseal abscess
metaphyseal lesion
metaphyseal lucent line
metaphyseal dysostosis
metaphyseal-epiphyseal angle
metaphyseal lucent bands
metaphysis (pl. metaphyses)
  agnogenic myeloid
  apocrine (of breast)

metaphysis *(cont.)*
  autoparenchymatous
  celery stalk
  celomic
  columnar
  fundic
  intestinal
  metaphyseal
  myeloid
  primary myeloid
  secondary myeloid
  squamous
metaplasia
  cartilaginous
  osteocartilaginous
  urethral adenomatoid
metapneumonic empyema
metastasis (pl. metastases)
  advanced
  air-space
  breast skin satellite
  calcareous
  cardiac
  CX-1
  drop
  hematogenous
  hypervascular
  local
  lymph node
  lymphangitic
  lymphatic
  mammary lymph node
  mediastinal
  micronodular
  neuroendocrine hepatic
  nodal
  occult
  osteoblastic
  osteolytic
  pulsating
  retrograde
  satellite
  skeletal

metastasis *(cont.)*
　white
　widespread
metastatic abscess
metastatic deposit
metastatic disease, occult distant
metastatic invasion
metastatic involvement
metastatic malignancy
metastatic pneumonia
metastatic skeletal survey
metastatic tumor
Metastron (strontium chloride Sr 89)
　radiotherapeutic agent
metasynchronous tumor
metatarsal break angle
metatarsal-phalangeal (or metatarso-
　phalangeal) (MTP) joint
metatarsal protrusion distance
metatarsal bone
metatarsal head
metatarsocuneiform joint
metatarsophalangeal (or metatarso-
　phalangeal) (MTP) joint
metatarsus adductocavus deformity
metatarsus adductus angle
metatarsus adductus deformity
metatarsus atavicus deformity
metatarsus latus deformity
metatarsus primus varus deformity
metatarsus varus deformity
meter (m), rate
meter per second (m/sec; also mps)
　velocity
methicillin-resistant *Staphylococcus*
　aureus (MRSA, pronounced
　"mer-suh")
methiodal sodium
methionine
method (see also *technique*)
　absorbed-fraction
　acoustic reflection
　Ahlback

method *(cont.)*
　Alexander (for viewing optic canal)
　Ball AP (pelvimetry view)
　Ball lateral (pelvimetry view)
　Beclere
　Blackett-Healy
　Brattstrom
　Causton
　Cleaves
　Clements-Nakayama
　Coyle
　Danelius Miller
　Danelius-Miller modification
　　of Lorenz
　Deneer
　Duncan Howe (no hyphen; first
　　and last name)
　Dunlap, Swanson, and Penner
　Dunlap-Rippstein
　Eraso
　Feist-Mankin
　Fisk
　Friedman
　Fuchs
　Fürmaier
　Gaynor-Hart
　Grandy
　Grashey
　Holmblad
　Hough
　Hsieh
　Isherwood
　Jaroschy
　Johnson
　Kandel
　Kasabach
　Kemp-Harper
　Kisch
　Kovacs
　Kuchendorf
　Kurzbauer
　Laquerriere and Pierquin
　Lauenstein

method *(cont.)*
  Lauenstein and Hickey
  Lauenstein and Hickey (modified)
  Law
  Lawrence
  Leonard-George
  Lewis
  Lorenz
  Lysholm
  Miller
  modified Fuchs
  Nolke
  parallax motion
  Pawlow
  Pearson
  Quesada
  Rippstein
  Risser-Ferguson
  Rosenberg
  Sansregret modification of
    Chausse III
  Schneider
  Settegast
  Staunig
  Stecher
  stork
  Swanson
  Sweet
  Tarrant
  Taylor
  Thoms
  Valdini
  Viehweger
  Wigby-Taylor
method/projection
  full scan (FS)
  full scan with interpolation (FI)
  half scan (HS)
  half scan with extrapolation (HE)
  half scan with interpolation (HI)
  simulated annealing
  under scan (US)

methoxypolyethylene glycol-L-lysine-
  DTPA imaging agent
methylene blue imaging agent
methyl methacrylate
methyl protons
Metricath catheter and transducer
metrizamide cisternography
metrizamide computed tomographic
  cisternogram (MCTC)
metrizamide imaging agent
metrizamide myelography
metrizoate acid imaging agent
metrizoate sodium imaging agent
metrology
metroperitoneal fistula
"mets" (metabolic equivalents)
"mets" (slang for *metastases*)
Mevatron 74 linear accelerator
MeV (megaelectron volt) dose
MEVH (multiple exposure volumetric
  holography)
MFG (magnetic field gradients)
MFG (manofluorography)
mGy/MBq (milligray per megabecquerel)
MHC-2 (major histocompatibility
  complex class II antigen)
MHV (middle hepatic vein)
MHz (megahertz)
MI (mitral insufficiency)
MI (myocardial infarction)
MI adenosine thallium imaging
MIBG (metaiodobenzylguanidine)
    imaging agent
  MIBG scintigraphy
  MIBG SPECT scan
MIBI (2-methoxy isobutyl isonitrile)
micelle
microabscess
microadenoma
microaneurysm
microangiopathy, intraretinal (IRMA)

microbubble contrast imaging agent
   for color Doppler ultrasound on
   breast masses
microbubble resonance frequency
microbubbles
   Renografin-76
   sonicated albumin
microcalcifications
   breast
   clustered
   subtle
microcardia
Micro-CAST collimator
microcatheter (see also *catheter*)
   AngiOptic
   flow-directed
   Hydrolyser
   Revelation
   UltraLite flow-directed
   UroLume flow-directed
   Wanderer
microcavitation
microcirculation, pulmonary
microcirculatory blood flow
microclusters, biodegradable magnetic
microcoils, suture-ligated embolization
microcolon
microcyst
microdactylia
microdistribution, heterogeneous
microdosimetry
Micro-Driver balloon catheter
Micro-Driver stent
microemboli
microencapsulated cisplatin
microerosion
microfiche
microfistulous AV (arteriovenous)
   shunt
microfluidization
microfocal spot mammogram
microfracture
microglobulin labeling

micrognathia
Micro-Guide catheter
Micro-Imager high resolution digital
   camera
microimaging
microinfarct
microlithiasis
MicroLYSUS ultrasound-enhanced
   drug delivery system
micromanometer-tip catheter
micromelena
micrometastases
micronodular infiltrates
micronodular metastases
micronodular pattern
micronodule, centrilobular
microperforation
microporous membrane
microscope, scanning electron (SEM)
microscopic cortical dysplasia
microscopic imaging
microscopy
   differential interference contrast
      (DIC)
   electron
   in vivo
   light
   three-dimensional magnetic
      resonance (3D MR)
   ultrasound backscatter (UBM)
microsecond pulsed flashlamp pumped
   dye laser
Microsoft Access program
microsphere
   trisacryl gelatin
   ytterbium-90 (^{90}Yb)
   technetium ^{99m}Tc albumin
microsphere perfusion scintigraphy
MicroStent II over the wire PTCA
   stent
microtomography
Microtron, MM50 Racetrack
microvascular anastomosis

microvascular circulation
microvascular retrieval
microvasculature
Microvasive Glidewire
Microvasive Rigiflex TTS balloon
 catheter
Microvasive stiff piano wire guidewire
microvenoarteriolar fistula
microvesicular fat
microvillus (pl. microvilli)
microwave hyperthermia treatment
microwave imaging
microwave thermal balloon
 angioplasty
micturition, aberrant
MID (minimum interbone distance)
MID (multi-infarct dementia)
midabdominal wall
midaortic arch
midaortic syndrome
midaxillary line
midbody
midbrain reticular formation (MRF)
MIDCAB (minimally invasive direct
 coronary artery bypass) procedure
midcircumflex
midclavicular line (MCL)
midcolon
mid-diastole
mid-distal
middle aortic syndrome
middle cardiac vein
middle kidney
middle lobe syndrome
middle third of the thoracic esophagus
middle-field-strength MR imaging
middorsal
midepigastrium
midesophageal diverticulum
midesophagus
midface, fetal
midface retrusion
midfemur

midfoot
midget MRI scanner
midgraft stenosis
midgroove portion of lumina
midgut volvulus with malrotation
midlateral course
midleft sternal border
midline, infracolic
midline mucosa-sparing blocks
midline shift
midline structures
midlung field
midlung zone
midmarginal branch of artery
midpelvis
midpole
midportion
midriff
midsagittal MR image
midsagittal slice
midscapular line
midshaft fracture
midshunt peak velocities (MSPv)
midsternum
midsystolic notching of velocity
 spectrum
midventricular short axis slice
midzone
migrational anomaly
migration of clip
migration of marker
migratory patchy infiltration
migratory pneumonia
Mikro-tip micromanometer-tipped
 catheter
Mikulicz angle
Mikulicz syndrome
miliary aneurysm
miliary embolism
miliary granuloma
miliary lung disease
miliary pattern
miliary shadowing

miliary tuberculosis
milieu, therapeutic
milk duct
milk leg syndrome
milk of calcium sign
milk scan
Milkman syndrome (also Looser-
Milkman)
milky effusion
Millar catheter-tip transducer
Millar MPC-500 catheter
Miller-Abbott tube
Miller-Dieker syndrome
Miller disease
miller's lung
Miller projection of hypoglossal canal
Miller view to demonstrate shoulder
dislocation
milliampere (mA)
milliampere-second (mAs)
millijoule (mJ)
Millikan-Siekert syndrome
millimeter (mm)
millimeters of mercury (mmHg)
Millenia balloon catheter for percutaneous transluminal coronary angioplasty
milliseconds (ms, msec)
millivolt (mV)
Milroy disease
Milton angioedema disease
mimic
mimicked
mimicking
mineral oil contrast
mineralization, bone
miner's lung
Ming classification of gastric
carcinoma
miniature uterus
Mini C-arm device
MINI Crown stent
minimal luminal diameter (MLD)

minimally displaced fracture
minimal radiographic distortion
minimal volume
minimum blood pressure
minimum intensity projection (MIP)
image
minimum interbone distance (MID)
mini-PACS
minipapillotome
Mini-Profile dilatation catheter, USCI
minor calices
Minot–von Willebrand syndrome
minuscule
minute-sequence study
minute vessels
minute volume
MION (monocrystalline iron oxides)
MION-gene complex
MIP (maximum intensity pixel)
MIP (maximum intensity projection)
algorithms
MIPcor (coronal maximum-intensity
projection)
Mirage over the wire balloon catheter
Miraluma (technetium ^{99m}Tc sestamibi
kit)
Miraluma breast imaging
Miraluma nuclear breast imaging
MIRC (Medical Image Resource
Center)
MIRI (myocardial infarction recovery
index)
mirror image breast biopsy
mirror image reversal
mirror-imaging
mirror, polygon
MIS (minimally invasive surgery)
misalign
misdiagnosis
Miser tube
misery perfusion
misleading images

mismatch
  perfusion-metabolism
  ventilation-perfusion
misonidazole (radiosensitizer)
misregistration artifact
missile wound
Mistique catheter
misty mesentery
mitochondrial uncoupler CCCP
mitral annular calcification
mitral anulus
mitral apparatus
mitral arcade
mitral atresia
mitral configuration of cardiac shadow
mitral deceleration slope
mitral inflow velocities
mitral insufficiency
mitral leaflets
mitral leak
mitral orifice
mitral regurgitant signal area
mitral regurgitation
  congenital
  pansystolic
mitral regurgitation artifact
mitral regurgitation-chordal elongation
  syndrome
mitral ring calcification
mitral stenosis
  congenital
  relative
  true
mitral valve
  billowing
  cleft
  hammock
  parachute
  prosthetic
mitral valve atresia
mitral valve calcification
mitral valve commissures
mitral valve configuration, fish-mouth

mitral valve echogram
mitral valve leaflet
mitral valve leaflet tip
mitral valve myxomatous degeneration
mitral valve obstruction
mitral valve prolapse, holosystolic
mitral valve regurgitation
mitral valve replacement
mitral valve septal separation
mitral valve stenosis (MVS)
Mitsubishi angioscopic catheter
mixed connective tissue disease
mixed echogenic solid mass
mixed lesion
mixed mesodermal tumor
mixed petal-fugal flow
mixed restrictive-obstructive lung
  disease
mixed signal mass
mixed tumor
mixed venous saturation
mixture model intensity windowing
ml/min/100 g (milliliters per minute
  per 100 grams)
MLC (multileaf collimator)
MLD (minimal luminal diameter)
mm (millimeter)
mm Hg *or* mmHg (millimeters of
  mercury)
MM50 Racetrack Microtron
MMCM (macromolecular contrast
  media) imaging agent
M-mode Doppler echocardiography
M-mode echocardiogram
M-mode echophonocardiography
M-mode transducer
M-mode ultrasound
mmol (millimoles)
mmol/kg (millimoles per kilogram)
mmol/L (millimoles per liter)
Mn (manganese) (an element)
MnCl2 (manganese chloride 2)
  imaging agent

MNP10 protocol
MO (mitral orifice)
MOAB, MoAb (monoclonal antibody), radiolabeled
Mobetron electron beam system
mobile kidney
mobile magnetic resonance (MR)
imager
mobile pedunculated left atrial tumor
mobile thrombus
mobility
Mobius vascular stent
mode
A-
AAI (noncompetitive atrial
demand)
AAI rate responsive
active
asynchronous transfer (ATM)
atrial triggered and ventricular
inhibited
atrial burst
atrioventricular dual demand
B-
bipolar pacing
blink
byte
cine (high frame rate)
committed
DDD pacing
dual demand pacing
DVI (digital vascular imaging)
fixed rate
full to empty VAD
inactive
inhibited pacing
M-mode
multiplanar
noncommitted
pacing
road-mapping
semicommitted
sequential
64 x 64 byte

mode (cont.)
stimulation
triggered pacing
underdrive
unipolar pacing
VAD (ventricular assist device)
VVI (noncompetitive demand
ventricular)
mode abandonment
model
figure of 8
lattice
leading circle
Markov source
Renkin
ring
Shames
xerography
modeler, solid
modeling
Monte Carlo
three-dimensional
vascular and airway
moderately dilated ureter
Modic disk abnormality classification
modification, Young-Burgess (of
Tile-Pennal classification system)
modified Ball pelvimetry
modified birdcage coils
modified Cleaves view (hip)
modified dorsal lithotomy position
modified electron-beam CT scanner
modified Fuchs projection of temporal
styloid process
modified Lauenstein and Hickey
method (frogleg)
modified vessel image processor
(mVIP) software
modiolus
modulation
amplitude
off-center
print reflectance

module, E-TOF detecting
Modulith SL 20
Moenckeberg ((Mönckeberg)
Mohr syndrome
moiré artifact
moiré fringes
molar absorptivity
molar pregnancy
molecular genetics
molecular recognition unit (MRU)
molecule
   ICAM-1
   intercellular adhesive (ICAM-1)
molecular coincidence detection
   (MCD) imaging
mole, hydatidiform
Molina needle-catheter
molybdenum cofactor deficiency
molybdenum-99 generator
moment, magnetic
Mönckeberg arteriosclerosis
Mönckeberg degeneration
Mönckeberg medial sclerosis
M1 (marginal branch #1)
monitor
   cardiac
   radiation
   virtual labor (VLM)
monitoring electrode
monitoring, ultrasound
monitoring wire
monoarticular
monochromatic radiation
monochromatic synchrotron radiation
monoclonal antibody (MOAB, MoAb)
   imaging agent
monoclonal antibody B72.3 labeled
   with indium
monoclonal antibody 7E3
monocrystalline iron oxide nanoparticles (MION)
monocular
monocusp valve

monodactylism
monodisk for septal defect closure
monoenergetic
monomalleolar ankle fracture
mononuclear infiltrate
monopolar RF electrocautery
Monorail balloon catheter
Monro bursa
Monro, foramen of
Monte Carlo algorithm
Monte Carlo calculation
Monte Carlo modeling
Monte Carlo technique
Monteggia fracture-dislocation
Montercaux fracture
Moore fracture
Morand spur
Morel syndrome
Morgagni
   appendix of
   column of
   crypt of
   foramen of
   hyperostosis of
Morgagni hernia
Morgagni-Stewart-Morel syndrome
Morison pouch
morphine-augmented study
morphological and physiological image
   coregistration
morphological changes
morphological correlation
morphologic criteria
morphology
   enhancement
   morphologic
morphometric measurements
morphometry
   magnetic resonance imaging
   voxel-based
Morquio syndrome
Morris point
mortar kidney

mortise, ankle
mortise joint
Morton neuroma
Morton toe
MOS capacitator
mosaic attenuation pattern
mosaic pattern of duodenal mucosa
mosaic perfusion
Moschcowitz thrombotic thrombo-
   cytopenic purpura
MoSearch
Moss staging system for gastric
   adenocarcinoma
motexafin gadolinium imaging agent
moth-eaten appearance
moth-eaten pattern
motility
   colonic
   esophageal
   ileal
   jejunal
   small bowel
motility disorder
motility study
motion
   akinetic segmental wall
   anterior wall
   apical wall
   brisk wall
   catheter tip
   cusp
   discernible venous
   dyskinetic segmental wall
   forceful parasternal
   heaving precordial
   hyperkinetic segmental wall
   hypokinetic segmental wall
   inferior wall
   leaflet
   left ventricular regional wall
   linear accelerator isocenter
   paradoxical (of chest wall)
   paradoxical leaflet

motion *(cont.)*
   paradoxical septal
   photoreceptor
   posterior wall
   posterolateral wall
   regional hypokinetic wall
   regional wall
   rocking precordial
   segmental wall
   septal wall
   shear wave
   sustained anterior parasternal
   systolic anterior (SAM)
   3D time-resolved
   trifid precordial motion
   ventricular wall
   visible anterior
   wall
motion artifact
motion-compensating format converter
motion lag
motor cortex
motor meal barium GI series
motor task activation
mottled density
mottled echo texture
mottled gray lung
mottled pattern
mottled thickening
Mounier-Kuhn syndrome
movable kidney
movement
   basal
   bowel (BM)
   pendulum
   propulsive
   spontaneous fetal
movement artifact
movement pattern
moving-bed infusion-tracking MRA
   method for imaging
moya moya ("puff of smoke") disease
Moynahan syndrome

MPM (malignant pleural mesothelioma)

MPNST (malignant peripheral nerve sheath tumor)

mPower PET scanner by Positron

MP-RAGE (magnetization prepared 3D gradient-echo) sequences

MPA (main pulmonary artery)

MPAP (mean pulmonary artery pressure)

MPD (main pancreatic duct)

MPF catheter

MPGR (multiplanar gradient-recalled) echo

MPHR (maximum predicted heart rate)

MPPv flow

MPR (multiplanar reformation)

MPR (myocardial perfusion reserve)

mps (meters per second)

MQSA (Mammography Quality Standards Act)

MR (magnetic resonance), 3D

MR (mitral regurgitation)

MRA (magnetic resonance angiography)

MRC (magnetic resonance cholangiography)

MR-cholangiography, intraoperative

MRCP (abdominal MRI/magnetic resonance cholangiopancreatography)

MRCP (magnetic resonance cholangiopancreatography)

MRCP using HASTE with a phased array coil

MRE (magnetic resonance elastography)

MRF (midbrain reticular formation)

MRI (see *magnetic resonance imaging*; *MRI terms*; also *imaging*)

MR imaging without MT, triple dose gadolinium-enhanced

MRI-guided breast biopsy

MRI terms (see also *imaging*; *magnetic resonance imaging*)

active biplanar MR imaging guidance

attenuation coefficient on MRI scan

black blood magnetic resonance angiography (MRA)

black blood T2-weighted inversion-recovery MR imaging

BOLD (blood oxygen level dependent) functional MR imaging

bolus chase technique in angiography and MRI scan

bolus chase three-dimensional MR digital subtraction angiography

breath-hold cine MR

breath-hold contrast-enhanced 3D MR angiography

breath-hold fast spin echo or multishot spin echo echo-planar imaging

breath-hold fast recovery optimized fast spin-echo

breath-hold GRE sequences

breath-hold MR cholangiography

breath-hold MR imaging

breath-hold T1-weighted MP-GRE MR imaging

breath-hold ungated imaging

breath-hold velocity-encoded cine MR imaging

CISS (constructive interference in steady state) MR imaging

combined multisection diffuse-weighted and hemodynamically weighted echo planar MRI

continuous arterial spin-labeling perfusion MR imaging

conventional spin-echo MRI vs. breath-hold fast spin echo or multishot spin echo echo-planar imaging

MRI terms *(cont.)*
  coronal T1-weighted MR image
    (spin echo)
  CSF-suppressed T2-weighted 3D
    MP-RAGE MR imaging
  diffusion tensor MRI
  diffusion-weighted echo-planar
    imaging
  diffusion-weighted imaging
  diffusion-weighted pulse sequence
  displacement field-fitting
  double echo chemical shift
    in-phase and opposed-phase
    FLASH
  dynamic susceptibility contrast
    (DSC)
  dynamic susceptibility-weighted
    contrast-enhanced
  dynamic tagging magnetic
    resonance angiography
  echo FLASH
  excitation-spoiled fat-suppressed
    T1-weighted SE
  fast PC cine MR sequence with
    echo planar gradient
  fast spoiled gradient-recalled MR
  fat-suppressed 3D spoiled
    gradient-(FDG)
  fast STIR (short tau inversion
    recovery)
  flow-compensated 2D T1-weighted
    spin echo
  flow-compensated respiratory-
    triggered 3D turbo spin echo
  FMPIR (fast SE and fast IR)
  free-breathing black-blood coronary
    MR angiography
  free-breathing 3D coronary MR
    angiography
  FS (full scan)-BURST MR imaging
  FSPGR (fast spoiled gradient-
    recalled)
  gradient-recalled echo (GRE) MR

MRI terms *(cont.)*
  GRASS MR (gradient-recalled
    acquisition in steady state)
  half dose enhanced MRI with MT
    (magnetization transfer)
  HASTE (half Fourier acquisition
    single shot turbo spin echo)
  HASTE MRI sequence
  hemodynamically weighted echo
    planar
  high-spatial-resolution contrast-
    enhanced MR
  intravascular signal intensity in MR
  intravoxel incoherent motion echo-
    planar MRI
  intravoxel phase dispersion (IVPD)
  MRE
  kinematic T2-weighted MRI
  multi-injection time-resolved MR
  multiple region MRI (mrMRI)
  multisection diffuse-weighted
  multisection MRI
  multisection multirepetition
    acquisition
  navigated spin echo diffusion-
    weighted MR imaging
  navigator echo-based real-time
    respiratory gating and triggering
  navigator echo motion correction
    technique
  NEX (number of excitations)
  nontriggered phase-contrast MR
    angiography
  oblique axial MR imaging
  opposed loop-pair quadrature MR
    coil
  opposed-phase MRI
  opposed-phase sequence
  oversampling (on MRI)
  oxygenation sensitive functional
    MR
  parallel-tagged MR images and
    field-fitting analysis

MRI terms *(cont.)*
  perfusion-weighted MRI
  phosphorus nuclear magnetic
    resonance spectroscopy (P-MRS)
  poor shimming of MRI magnet
  postcontrast MR imaging
  protodensity MRI image
  proton density images
  proton density-weighted images
  proton MR spectroscopy
  pseudodynamic MR imaging of the
    temporomandibular joints
  pulsed magnetization transfer
    contrast MRI
  rapid axial MRI
  RARE (rapid acquisition with
    relaxation enhancement)
  RARE-derived pulse sequence
  real-time MR imaging tracking
  reformatted planar "Christmas
    tree" MR appearance of
    endolymphatic sac
  saline-enhanced MR arthrography
  segmented k-space time of flight
    MR angiography
  segmented k-space turbo gradient
    echo breath-hold sequence
  segmenting dual echo MR head
    scan
  selective presaturation MR
    angiography
  sequential quantitative MR imaging
  short inversion time inversion
    recovery (STIR) (MRI)
  single photon emission CT with
    MR
  single shot fast spin echo and
    gadolinium-enhanced fat-
    suppressed spoiled gradient-
    echo MR
  single slab 3D pulse sequence
  single shot MR cholangiography
  small field of view (FOV) MR
    imaging

MRI terms *(cont.)*
  SPIDER (steady state projection
    imaging with dynamic echo
    train readout)
  split echo diffusion-weighted MR
  stepping-table gadolinium-enhanced
    digital subtraction MR
  susceptibility-weighted MR
  tagged red blood cell nuclear scan
  3D CEMRA (contrast-enhanced
    MR)
  3D phase contrast MR (3D-PCA)
  3D heavily T1-weighted dynamic
    gradient-echo sequence
  THRIVE (T1 high resolution
    isotropic volume examination)
  T2-QMRI (T2-quantitative MRI)
  turboFLAIR (fluid-attenuated
    inversion recovery)
  turboFLASH (fast low-angle shot)
  weighted spin echo column
MRM (magnetic resonance mammography)
MRM (magnetic resonance myelogram)
mrMRI (multiple region magnetic
  resonance imaging)
MRN (magnetic resonance neurography)
MRP (magnetic resonance pancreatography)
MR peritoneography
MRS (magnetic resonance spectroscopy)
MRSA (pronounced "mer-suh")
  (methicillin-resistant *Staphylococcus
  aureus*)
MRSI (magnetic resonance spectroscopic imaging)
MRT (magnetic resonance tomography)
MRU (magnetic resonance urography)
MRU (molecular recognition unit)

ms (milliseconds)
MS (mitral stenosis)
MS (morphine sulfate)
MSAD (multiple scan average dose)
MSA (multiple system atrophy)
   syndrome
MSAFP (maternal serum alpha
   fetoprotein)
MS Classique balloon dilatation
   catheter
MSCT (multislice computed tomog-
   raphy)
MSCTA (multislice computed tomo-
   graphic angiography)
m/sec (meters per second)
msec (millisecond)
MS (multiple sclerosis) plaquing
M-shaped pattern of mitral valve
MSI (magnetic source imaging), 3D
MSO$_4$ (morphine sulfate)
MS-325 imaging agent
MT (magnetization transfer)
MTEs (main timing events)
MTP (metatarsophalangeal) joint
MTR (magnetization transfer ratio)
MT (magnetization transfer) saturation
MTT (mean pulmonary transit time)
MTT (mean transit time), esophageal
M2A capsule
M2A Swallowable Imaging Capsule
mucinous cystadenoma
mucinous tumor
mucocele
mucocutaneous lesion
mucocutaneous tumor
mucoid degeneration
mucoid impaction
mucoid plugging of airways
mucosa
   "burned out"
   cobblestone
   friable
   frothy

mucosa *(cont.)*
   honeycomb
   inflamed mainstem bronchial
   isoeffective
   muscularis
mucosal abnormality
mucosal crinkling
mucosal enhancement
mucosal folds
mucosal inflammation
mucosal island
mucosal pattern
mucosal relief
mucosa of ureter
mucosa of urethra
mucosa-sparing blocks
mucous fistula
mucous lake of stomach
mucous membrane
mucus hypersecretion
mucus plugging
Mueller (Müller) fibers
MUGA (multiple gated acquisition)
   blood pool radionuclide scan
MUGA gating
mulberry calculus
mulberry gallstones
mulberry-type calcification
Müller (Mueller)
Müller duct
Müller fibers
mullerian cyst
mullerian duct
Müller (Mueller) sign (aortic regurgitation)
Mullins catheter introducer
Mullins sheath
Mullins sheath in transseptal catheterization
Mullins transseptal catheter
multangular bone, accessory
multangular ridge fracture
multangulum

multiagent chemotherapy
multiangle, multislice acquisition
magnetic resonance imaging
multibreath washout study
multibubble cavitation
multibubble sonoluminescence
Multicath catheter
multicentric lytic lesions
multicentricity
multichannel analyzer
multicolor flow cytometry
multicompartment clearance
multicoupled loop gap resonator
multicrystal gamma camera
multicystic dysplasia
multicystic dysplastic kidney
multicystic mesothelioma
multicystic ovaries with thickened
capsule
multidetector computed tomography
(CT; MDCT)
multidetector, ECG-triggered
multidetector system
multiecho axial
multiecho coronal image
multiecho image
multiecho sequence
multi-elemental neutron activation
analysis
multiexponential relaxation
multifiber catheter
multifield beam
Multi-Flex urologic stent
multifocal aggressive infiltrate
multifocal lesions
multifocal lymphoma
multifocal short stenosis
multiform ventricular complexes
multiforme, glioblastoma
multigated pulsed Doppler flow
system
multigland hyperplasia of thyroid
multigravida

MultiHance (gadobenate dimeglumine)
CNS imaging agent
multi-interval
multi-illuminant color correction
multi-infarct dementia (MID)
multilaminar bodies
multileaf collimator (MLC)
multilesion angioplasty
Multilink Duet noncoated coronary
stent
Multilink Penta coronary stent system
Multilink Tetra coronary stent system
Multi-Link Vision RX and OTW (over
the wire) coronary stent system
multilocular cyst
Multi-Med triple lumen infusion
catheter
multimodal image fusion technique
multimodality imaging
multinodular goiter
multinuclear magnetic resonance
imaging
multiorgan imaging
multipara
multiparametric color composite
display
multiparous
multiparticle cyclotron
multiphase acquisition
multiphasic multislice magnetic
resonance imaging technique
multiplanar gradient-recalled (MPGR)
echo
multiplanar magnetic resonance
imaging
multiplanar mode
multiplanar reformation (MRP) view
multiplanar reformatted radiographic
and digitally reconstructed images
multiplanar transesophageal echocardiography
multiplane dosage calculations
multiple beam interface spacing

multiple chord, center-line technique
in echocardiogram
multiple endocrine adenomatosis
multiple endocrine neoplasia (MEN)
multiple exposure volumetric
holography (MEVH)
multiple fractures
multiple-gated acquisition (MUGA)
blood pool radionuclide scan
multiple-gated acquisition (MUGA)
scan
multiple hamartoma syndrome
multiple jointed digitizer
multiple locules
multiple organ failure
multiple plane imaging
multiple region magnetic resonance
imaging (mrMRI)
multiple scan average dose (MSAD)
multiple sclerosis plaquing
multiple slice acquisition
multiple trauma
multipulse nuclear magnetic resonance
(NMR) imaging
multipurpose catheter
Multipurpose-SM catheter
multirod collimator
multiscale image contrast amplification
(MUSICA)
multisectional dose-volume histogram
multisection diffuse-weighted magnetic
resonance imaging
multisection magnetic resonance
imaging
multisection multirepetition acquisition
multisensor structured light range
digitizer
multiseptate appearance
multiseptate gallbladder
multishot echoplanar imaging
multislab and cine techniques for
single breath-hold cardiac-synchro-
nized angiography

multislab magnetic resonance
angiography
multislice computed tomographic
angiography (MSCTA)
multislice computed tomography
(MSCT)
multislice first pass myocardial
perfusion imaging
multislice FLASH 2D
multislice mode
multislice multiphase spin echo
imaging technique
multislice spin echo sequence
multispin relaxation
multitracer study
multiverrucous friable lesion
multivessel angioplasty
MUMPS (Massachusetts [General
Hospital] Utility Multiprogramming
System)
Münchmeyer disease
mural aneurysm
mural architecture
mural clot
mural degeneration
mural dilatations
mural endomyocardial fibrosis
mural infiltration
mural leaflet of mitral valve
mural nodule
mural thrombosis
mural thrombus formation
mu (μ) rhythm (μ, twelfth Greek
letter)
muscle (pl. muscles)
   accessory
   adductor magnus
   Aeby
   Albinus
   anterior
   auricular
   axillary
   bipennate

muscle *(cont.)*
Bochdalek
Bovero
Bowman
Braune
Brücke (Bruecke)
bulbocavernosus
canine
cardiac
Casser
casserian
cervical
Chassaignac
chin
circular
Coiter
conal papillary
Crampton
deep
detrusor
digastric
dorsal
Dupré
Duverney
electrically conditioned and driven
    skeletal
external
fixation
fixator
Folius
fused papillary
Gantzer
gastrocnemius
Gavard
greater
Guthrie
Hilton
Horner
Houston
iliococcygeal
iliocostal
infarcted heart
inferior

muscle *(cont.)*
intercostal
internal
interosseous
interspinal
intertransverse
intra-auricular
ischiocavernosus
Jung
Klein
Lancisi
lateral
latissimus dorsi
left ventricular
lesser
levator
longitudinal
Luschka
Macalister
major
Marcacci
masticator
medial
medial papillary
Merkel
middle
minor
Müller (Mueller)
multipennate
nonstriated
oblique
Ochsner
Oddi
Oehl
omohyoid
opposing
organic
papillary
pectoralis major
pectoralis minor
peroneal
peroneus quartus
Phillips

muscle *(cont.)*
  plantaris
  platysma
  posterior
  Pozzi
  pubococcygeal
  quadrate
  Reisseisen
  rhomboideus major
  ribbon
  rider
  Riolan
  Rouget
  round
  Ruysch
  sacrospinalis
  Santorini
  sartorius
  Sebileau
  semimembranous
  semispinal
  semitendinous
  serratus anterior
  short
  Sibson
  skeletal
  smaller
  Soemmerring
  soleus
  somatic
  sphenomandibularis
  spindle-shaped
  sternocleidomastoid
  sternohyoid
  sternothyroid
  strap
  subaortic
  sucking (Bovero)
  superficial
  synergic
  tailor's
  Theile
  Tod

muscle *(cont.)*
  Toynbee
  transverse
  trapezius
  Treitz
  triangular
  trigonal
  true back
  two-bellied
  unipennate
  Valsalva
  vastus medialis
  ventral
  vertical
  visceral
  vocal
  vocalis
  voluntary
  Wilson
  wrinkler
muscle artifact
muscle-fat boundary
muscle-fat interface
muscle uptake PET artifact
muscular atrioventricular septum
muscular branch
muscular bridging
muscular crus (of diaphragm)
muscularis mucosae
muscular layer of spongy urethra
muscular layer of ureter
muscular layer of urethra
muscular subaortic stenosis
muscular venous pump
musculature
musculophrenic artery
musculophrenic branch
mushroom-shaped mass
mushroom picker's (or worker's)
  disease (or lung)
mushy mass
Musset sign (aortic aneurysm)
Mustang steerable guidewire

MUSTPAC (medical ultrasound 3D portable, with advanced communications) imaging
mutation, c-Ki-ras
MV (megavolt; not to be confused with mV, millivolt)
mV (millivolt)
MV (mitral valve)
MVA (mitral valve area)
MVD (mitral valve dysfunction)
MVO (maximum venous outflow)
MVO (mitral valve opening [or orifice])
MVO$_2$ (myocardial oxygen consumption)
MVP (mitral valve prolapse)
MVP over the wire balloon catheter
MVR (mitral valve replacement)
MVS (mitral valve stenosis)
myasthenia gravis
mycetoma
mycoplasmal pneumonia
mycoplasmal pneumonitis
mycotic aneurysm
myelin kidney
myelin pallor
myelodysplasia
myelodysplastic syndrome
myelogram
myelography (with and without contrast)
    air
    cervical
    complete
    lumbar
    lumbosacral
    magnetic resonance (MRM)
    metrizamide
    positive contrast
    thoracic
myelographic imaging agent
myelolipoma

myeloma
    indolent
    localized
    multiple
    sclerosing
    solitary
myelomatous involvement
myelomeningocele
myeloscopy, spinal
myenteric plexus of Auerbach
Myler catheter
mylohyoid ridge
myoblastoma, granular cell
myocardial blood flow (MBF)
myocardial blush
myocardial bridging
myocardial contractile dysfunction
myocardial contractility
myocardial contrast appearance time (MCAT)
myocardial contusion
myocardial degeneration
myocardial depression
myocardial dysfunction
myocardial fibers degeneration
myocardial fibrosis
myocardial granulomatous disease
myocardial hibernation
myocardial hypoperfusion, resting regional
myocardial incompetency
myocardial infarct imaging
myocardial infarction
    anterior
    anterior wall
    anteroapical wall
    anterobasal
    anterolateral wall
    anteroseptal wall
    apical
    apical lateral wall
    basal lateral wall
    diaphragmatic wall

myocardial *(cont.)*
  esophageal spasm mimicking
  high lateral wall
  impending
  inferior (diaphragmatic)
  inferolateral wall
  inferoposterior wall
  intraoperative
  nontransmural
  perioperative
  posterior wall
  posterobasal wall
  posteroinferior
  posterolateral wall
  posteroseptal
  stuttering
  subendocardial
  transmural
  true posterior wall
  uncomplicated non-Q-wave
  uncomplicated Q-wave
myocardial infiltration by Kaposi
  sarcoma
myocardial injury
  lethal
  nonlethal
myocardial insufficiency, Sternberg
myocardial ischemia, exercise-induced
  transient
myocardial muscle
myocardial necrosis
myocardial oxygen consumption
myocardial oxygen demand
myocardial perfusion defect
myocardial perfusion scan
myocardial perfusion tomography
myocardial preservation
myocardial protection
myocardial recovery
myocardial reperfusion injury
myocardial revascularization
myocardial rupture
myocardial scan

myocardial shortening, fractional
myocardial specific marker
myocardial stunning
myocardial tagging
myocardial thickening
myocardial tissue viability
myocardial tumor, metastatic
myocardial uptake of thallium
myocardial work
myocarditis, inflammatory
myocardium
  ablation of
  asynergic
  calcification of
  dilated
  hibernating
  hyperreflectile granular sparkling
    appearance of the
  hypertrophied
  ischemic reperfused
  ischemic viable
  jeopardized
  myxomatous degeneration of
  noninfarcted
  nonperfused
  perfused
  reperfused
  rupture of
  senile
  stunned
  ventricular
  viable
myofibril volume fraction
myofibroma
myogenic bladder failure
myointimal proliferation
myoma
  pedunculated subserous
  submucous
  uterine
myometrial endometriosis
myometrium

Myoscint (monoclonal antibody Fab to
   myosin, labeled with indium-111)
MyoSight cardiology imaging system
myositis ossificans (MO)
myotendinous junction
myotomy, Heller
Myoview (technetium Tc 99m tetrofosmin) imaging drug in scintigraphy
Mystic Mongoose PTCA catheter
myxofibroma
myxoma
   atrial
   biatrial
   cardiac
   familial (of the heart)

myxoma *(cont.)*
   heart
   left atrial
   pedunculated
   vascular
   ventricular
myxomatous degeneration
myxomatous degeneration of mitral
   valve
myxomatous degeneration of myocardium
myxomatous degeneration of valve
myxomatous proliferation
myxomatous valve leaflet

N, n

N (nitrogen) (an element)
   ^{13}N (nitrogen-13 ammonia)
NAA (N-acetyl aspartate)
NAA metabolite signal
nabothian follicle
N-acetyl aspartate (NAA)
Nagele obliquity
Nagele pelvis
Nager acrofacial dysostosis
naloxone
nanoparticles
nanoparticulate contrast agent
napkin-ring annular stenosis
napkin-ring annular tumor
Narco esophageal motility machine
naris (pl. nares)
narrow-band spectral-selective 90 RF
   pulse
narrow-beam geometry
NarrowFlex intra-aortic balloon
   catheter
NarrowFlex prewrapped double lumen
   IAB catheter
narrow gating tolerance
narrowing
   arterial
   atherosclerotic

narrowing (cont.)
   diffuse
   disk space
   focal
   high grade
   joint space (JSN)
   large airway
   luminal
   neural foramen
   residual luminal
   subcritical
narrowing asymmetry
narrowing of the lumen due to
   scarring
nasal sinus
nasal spine
nasion recession
nasobiliary drainage catheter
nasogastric (NG) tube
nasolabial cyst
nasopharyngeal atresia
nasopharyngeal carcinoma (NPC)
nasopharyngeal craniopharyngioma
nasotracheal tube
National Institutes of Health (NIH)
   catheter

457

National Institute of Neurological
   Disorders and Stroke (NINDS)
native aortic valve, preservation of
native atherosclerosis
native coronary artery
native dilated ureter
native images
native kidney
native tissue harmonic imaging
   (NTHI)
native ventricle
native vessel
natural neon gas
Naughton-Balke treadmill protocol,
   modified
Navarre interventional radiology
   devices
navel string
navicular
   carpal
   tarsal
navicular fossa of urethra
navicular view
naviculocapitate fracture
navigable echo signal
navigated spin echo diffusion-weighted
   MR imaging
navigating heart structures
navigation, image-guided intraoperative
navigator echo-based real-time
   respiratory gating and triggering
navigator echo motion correction
   technique
navigator pulse
navigator shifts
Navi-Star diagnostic/ablation deflectable tip catheter
Navi-Star mapping catheter
Navius catheter
Navius guidewire
Navius stent
NB200 vascular access device

NCC (normalized cross-section)
NCL-PGR monoclonal antibody
   imaging agent
NCPF (noncirrhotic portal fibrosis)
NC Ranger PTCA catheter
NC Raptor PTCA dilatation catheter
Nd:YAG (neodymium:yttrium-
   aluminum-garnet) laser
near anatomic position of joint
near field
near-infrared spectroscopy (NIRS)
near-resonance spin lock contrast
nearest neighbor interpolation
NeatMed radiology toolkit software
NeatVision imaging
neck
   aneurysmal
   bone
   dental
   femoral
   Madelung
   pancreatic
   surgical
   uterine
   wry
neck vessel engorgement
necrobiotic xanthogranulomatosis
necroscopy, perinatal
necrosed tissue
necrosis
   acute sclerosing hyaline (ASHN)
   acute tubular (ATN)
   alveolar septal
   aorta idiopathic
   arteriolar
   aseptic
   avascular
   bilateral cortical
   biliary piecemeal
   bloodless zone of
   blood vessel
   bowel
   bridging

necrosis *(cont.)*
  caseous
  centrilobular
  coagulation
  colliquative
  colonic
  contraction band
  cystic medial
  diffuse
  embolic
  epiphyseal
  epiphyseal ischemic
  Erdheim cystic medial
  fat
  fatty
  fibrinoid
  fibrosing piecemeal
  focal
  focal hepatic
  frank
  heart muscle
  hemorrhagic
  hepatic
  hyaline
  indurative
  intestinal
  ischemic
  liquefaction
  localized
  lung
  massive
  massive hepatic
  medial cystic
  midzonal
  mucosal
  myocardial
  Paget quiet
  pancreatic
  papillary
  peripheral
  piecemeal
  postoperative
  postpartum pituitary

necrosis *(cont.)*
  pressure
  progressive emphysematous
  prostatic
  radiation
  renal cortical
  renal tubular
  septic
  soft tissue
  strangulation
  stromal
  subacute hepatic
  subcutaneous fat
  subendocardial
  submassive hepatic
  superficial
  talar avascular
  total
  tracheobronchial mucosal
  tumor
  ventricular muscle
  Zenker
necrotic fluid-filled nodes
necrotic myocardium
necrotic tumor
necrotizing emphysema
necrotizing fasciitis
necrotizing pneumonia
necrotizing respiratory granulomatosis
necrotizing thrombosis
needle
  Brockenbrough
  Colapinto transjugular liver biopsy
  Echo-Coat biopsy
  Echo-Coat localization
  Echo-Coat ultrasound biopsy
  Kopans
  nonferromagnetic
  Quincke spinal
  SampleMaster biopsy
  stabilization
  Tru-Cut liver biopsy
  Whitacre spinal

needle biopsy, CT-scan directed
needle hydrophone
needle tracking, real-time biplanar
Neer shoulder fractures (I, II, III
  classification)
NEFA (nonesterified fatty acid)
  scintigraphy
Nefertiti sniff position
negative contrast agent
negative image of pulmonary edema
negative predictive value
negligible artifacts
negligible pressure gradient
Nélaton dislocation
Nélaton fold
NEMD (nonspecific esophageal
  motility disorder)
neoadjuvant chemotherapy
neoadjuvant hormonal therapy
neoaorta
neoaortic valve
neobreast
neocerebellum
neocholangiole
neocortical neurodegeneration
neodymium:yttrium-aluminum-garnet
  (Nd:YAG) laser
neofornix, vaginal
neonatal adrenal ultrasound
neonatal intracranial hemorrhage
neointimal hyperplasia
neointimal proliferation
neonatal adrenal ultrasound
neonatal cystic pulmonary emphysema
neonate
neon particle protocol
neopallium
Neo PICC neonatal peripherally
  inserted central catheter
neoplasia, multiple endocrine (MEN)
neoplasm (see also *lesion; tumor*)
  benign
  encapsulated

neoplasm *(cont.)*
  endobronchial
  extracranial
  firm
  functioning
  gonadal
  intracranial
  lethal
  low grade
  malignant
  malignant renal
  mediastinal
  ovarian
  paratesticular
  primary
  primary lung
  spherical
  trophoblastic
  well-circumscribed
neoplastic fracture
neoplastic invasion
neoplastic lesion
neoplastic stenosis
Neoprobe radioactivity detector
neorectum
NeoSpect diagnostic imaging agent
Neostar vascular access catheter
NeoTect disease-specific imaging
  agent
NeoTect (technetium Tc 99m
  depreotide) imaging agent
neovaginal prolapse
neovagina stenosis
neovascularity
nephralgia
nephritic calculus
nephroangiosclerosis, malignant
nephroblastoma
nephrogenic adenoma
nephrogram
nephrographic phase (NP)
nephrolithiasis
nephrolithotripsy, percutaneous (PNL)

nephroma, cystic
nephropathy
  contrast agent-induced
  radiocontrast-induced
nephroptosis
nephrosclerosis
  arterial
  malignant
  senile
nephrosis, functional
nephrotic
nephrostogram
nephrostomy balloon catheter
nephrostomy, percutaneous
nephrostomy-type catheter
nephrotic edema
nephrotomogram
nephrotomography
nephrotropic MR imaging contrast
nephrotoxic imaging agent
nephrotoxicity
nephroureterectomy
Neptune trident appearance
Nernst equation
Nerve Fibre Analyzer GDx, The
nerve root compression
nerve root edema
nerve root sheath
nervous heart syndrome
net magnetization factor
net tissue magnetization
network
  articular
  lymphatic
  neural
  venous
network architecture
NEUGAT (neutron/gamma
  transmission) method
neural arch
neural crest origin
neural evaluation algorithm
neural foramen (pl. foramina)

neural network
neural tube defect
neurenteric cyst
neurinoma
neuritic plaque
neuritic plaquing
neuroangiography
neuroblastoma
neuroblockage
neurodegeneration, neocortical
neurodiagnosis
NeuroEcho software
neuroendocrine carcinoma
neuroendocrine tumor
neuroendovascular interventional
  procedures
neurofibrillary tangles
neurofibroma of the heart
neurofibromatosis, plexiform
neurofibromatosis type 1 (NF1)
Neuroform microdelivery stent system
neurogenic bladder
neurogenic dysfunction of the bladder
neurogenic fracture
neurogenic pulmonary edema
neurogenic sarcoma
neurogenic tumor
neurography, magnetic resonance
  (MRN)
neuroholography
neurohypophysis
neuroimaging
neurointerventional radiology
neuroleptic
Neurolite (technetium Tc 99m
  bicisate) imaging agent
neuropathic GU tract lesion
NeuroSector ultrasound
Neuro Lobe software
neurologic signs, focal
neuroma
  Morton
  multicystic acoustic

neuromorphometry
neuromuscular blockade
Neuropac
neuropathic bladder
neuroradiologic examination
neuroradiology
   interventional
   pediatric
neuroreceptor ligand
NeuroScan 3D imager
NeuroSector ultrasound system
neurosonogram
neurosonology
Neuro SPGR software
neurosurgery, stereotactic
neurotoxic effect
neurotropic MR imaging contrast
   agents
neurovascular bundle
neurovascular compression
neutron activation analysis
neutron capture therapy
neutron/gamma transmission
   (NEUGAT) method
neutron
   slow
   thermal
neutron-deficient nuclei
neutron irradiation
neutron-rich biomedical tracer
neutron therapy
NeutroSpec (technetium ^{99m}Tc fanolesomab) imaging agent
nevus (pl. nevi)
new bone formation
NEX (number of excitations) (on MRI
   scan)
NexStent carotid stent
Nexus 2 linear ablation catheter
NF1 (neurofibromatosis type 1)
NG (nasogastric) tube
NH region of AV (atrioventricular)
   node

Niagara temporary dialysis catheter
niche
   Barclay
   Haudek
Nicoladoni-Branham sign
Nicolet Elite Doppler ultrasound
Nicolet NMR spectrometer
nicotinamide radiosensitizer
nidus demarcation
nidus, thrombus
Niemann-Pick disease
Niemeier gallbladder perforation
NIH (National Institutes of Health)
NIH cardiomarker catheter
NIH left ventriculography catheter
Nikaidoh translocation of aorta
Nikolsky sign
nimodipine, intra-arterial superselec-
   tive
NINDS (National Institute of Neuro-
   logical Disorders and Stroke)
NINDS-AIREN criteria
ninety-degree (or 90°) RF pulse (on
   MR spectroscopy)
91-41 MeV proton
Ninja FX PTCA dilatation catheter
nipple abscess
nipple lesion
nipple marker
NIPS (noninvasive programmed
   stimulation)
NIRflex coronary stent
NIR ON stent
NIRoyal Elite Monorail coronary stent
   system
NIR premounted stent delivery system
NIR Prince (or NIR pRINce) stent
NIR with SOX over the wire coronary
   stent system
NIRS (near-infrared spectroscopy)
Nishimoto Sangyo scanner
Nissen antireflux operation
nitinol stent

nitrofuran delivery catheter
nitrogen (N) (an element)
^{13}N ammonia radioactive tracer
^{13}N ammonia uptake on PET scan
nitrogen, body
nitrogen-nipple sign, aortic
nitrogen-13 ammonia radioactive
    tracer
nitrogen washout
nitrous oxide synthetase
NMIS (nuclear medicine information
    system)
NMR (nuclear magnetic resonance)
    imaging (see *imaging*)
NO (nitrous oxide)
no-carrier-added fluorine-18 (^{18}F)
    imaging agent
nociceptive
nodal conduction
nodal contractions
nodal escape
nodal impulse
nodal metastases
nodal point
nodal premature contraction
nodal recurrence
nodal rupture
node
    abdominal lymph
    accessory lymph
    anorectal lymph
    aortic lymph
    aortic window
    apical lymph
    appendicular lymph
    Aschoff
    Aschoff-Tawara
    atrioventricular (AV, AVN)
    auricular lymph
    AV (atrioventricular)
    axillary lymph
    bifurcation lymph
    Bouchard

node *(cont.)*
    brachial lymph
    bronchopulmonary lymph
    buccal lymph
    buccinator lymph
    cardiac
    caval lymph
    celiac lymph
    central lymph
    cervical lymph
    cervical paratracheal lymph
    Cloquet inguinal lymph
    common iliac lymph
    companion lymph
    coronary
    cubital lymph
    cystic lymph
    Delphian lymph
    deltopectoral lymph
    diaphragmatic lymph
    Dürck
    epicolic lymph
    epigastric lymph
    epitrochlear lymph
    Ewald
    external iliac lymph
    facial lymph
    fibular lymph
    Flack
    Flack sinoatrial
    foraminal
    gastric lymph
    gastroduodenal lymph
    gastroepiploic lymph
    gastro-omental lymph
    gluteal lymph
    gouty
    Haygarth
    Heberden
    hemal
    hemolymph
    Hensen
    hepatic lymph

node *(cont.)*
hilar lymph
ileocolic lymph
iliac circumflex lymph
iliac lymph
infraclavicular
infrahyoid lymph
inguinal lymph
intercostal lymph
interiliac lymph
interpectoral lymph
intramammary
jugular lymph
jugulodigastric lymph
jugulo-omohyoid lymph
juxtaintestinal
Keith
Keith-Flack sinoatrial
Koch sinoatrial
lacunar
lumbar lymph
lymph
malar lymph
mandibular lymph
mastoid lymph
medial supraclavicular
mediastinal lymph
mesenteric lymph
Meynet
nasolabial lymph
necrotic fluid-filled
NH region of AV (atrioventricular)
obturator lymph
occipital lymph
Osler
pancreatic lymph
pancreaticoduodenal lymph
pancreaticolienal lymph
pancreacticosplenic
paracardial lymph
paracolic lymph
paramammary lymph
pararectal lymph

node *(cont.)*
parasternal lymph
paratracheal lymph
parauterine lymph
paravaginal lymph
paravesicular lymph
parietal lymph
parotid lymph
Parrot
pectoral lymph
pelvic lymph
peribronchial
pericardial lymph
peroneal
phrenic lymph
popliteal lymph
postaortic lymph
postcaval lymph
posterior mediastinal
postvesicular lymph
preaortic lymph
precaval lymph
prececal lymph
prelaryngeal
prepericardial lymph
pretracheal lymph
prevertebral lymph
prevesicular lymph
pulmonary juxtaesophageal lymph
pulmonary lymph
pyloric lymph
Ranvier
rectal lymph
regional lymph
retroaortic lymph
retroauricular lymph
retrocecal lymph
retropharyngeal lymph
retropyloric
retrorectal lymph node
Rosenmüller (Rosenmueller)
Rotter
SA (sinoatrial)

node *(cont.)*
  sacral lymph
  satellite
  scalene
  Schmorl
  sentinel
  shotty lymph
  sick sinus
  sigmoid lymph
  signal
  singer
  sinoatrial (SAN)
  sinoauricular
  sinus
  Sister Mary Joseph
  solitary lymph
  splenic lymph
  subcarinal
  submandibular lymph
  submental lymph
  subpyloric
  subscapular lymph
  superficial inguinal lymph
  supraclavicular lymph
  suprapyloric
  supratrochlear lymph
  syphilitic
  Tawara
  teacher
  thyroid lymph
  tibial
  tracheal lymph
  tracheobronchial lymph
  Troisier
  tumor-infiltrated lymph
  vesicular lymph
  vestigial left sinoatrial
  Virchow
  visceral lymph
no discernible findings
nodo-Hisian (nodohisian) bypass tract

nodosum
  erythema
  polyarteritis (PAN)
nodoventricular bypass fiber
nodoventricular bypass tract
nodoventricular pathway
nodoventricular tachycardia
nodular aneurysm
nodular density
nodular enhancement
nodular fibrosis
nodular goiter
nodularity
  calcified
  coarse
  diffuse
  noncalcified
  surface
  vein
nodularity of leaflet
nodular-like
nodular lymphoid hyperplasia (NLH)
nodular mass
nodular pattern
nodular proliferation
nodule (pl. nodules)
  AH (adenomatous hyperplasia)
  air-space
  Albini
  aortic valve
  Arantius
  Aschoff
  autonomous
  Bianchi
  cold
  cortical
  Cruveilhier
  cutaneous
  Dalen-Fuchs
  discordant
  enhancing
  fibrous
  Fränkel (Fraenkel) typhus

nodule *(cont.)*
functioning
Gamna
Gamna-Gandy
Gandy-Gamna
Hoboken
hot
hypermetabolic
Kerckring
Koeppe
Morgagni
mural
noncavitary
nondelineated
nonenhancing
nonfunctioning thyroid
ossific
peripheral
Picker
regenerative
rheumatic
rheumatoid
Schmorl
semiautonomous
siderotic (in the spleen)
silicotic
singer's
Sister Mary Joseph
solitary
surfer's
teacher's
tobacco
toxic
tuberculous
typhoid
typhus
warm
nodule uptake of intravenous ^{131}I or
^{99m}Tc technetium
nodulus Arantii (pl. noduli Arantii)
nodus arcus venae azygos
nofetumomab merpentan imaging
agent

no-gap technique
no involvement
noise
lesion to cerebrospinal fluid
lesion to white matter
pixel
respiratory
subtractive
white
noise amplification
noise distribution, spectral
noise reduction intercom
Nolke projection of upper sacral canal
NOMOS correction factor
nonablative heating
nonarticular radial head fracture
nonasbestos pneumoconiosis
nonassessable segment
nonbacterial pneumonia
nonballoon therapies (atherectomy,
excimer laser angioplasty, stents)
noncalcified mitral leaflets
noncalcified nodule
noncardiac pulmonary edema
noncardiogenic pulmonary edema
noncaseating granuloma
noncaseating tubercles
noncavitary nodule
noncircularity degree
noncoaxial catheter tip position
noncolinear
noncollagenous pneumoconiosis
noncommunicating cyst
noncommunicating hydrocephalus
noncompensatory pause
noncompliant plaque
noncompressible appendix
noncontact imaging technology
noncontractile scar tissue
noncontrast-enhanced imaging
noncontrast-enhanced scan
noncontrast phase (NCP)
non-coplanar arc technique

non-coplanar multiple static port
non-coplanar therapy beams
noncoronary cusp
noncoronary leaflet
noncoronary sinus
nondecremental
nondelineated nodule
nondependent lung
nondiluted contrast
nondisplaced fracture
nondistensible balloon
nondistensible pericardium
nondominant vessel
nonduplex collecting system
nonenclosed magnet
nonenhanced CAT scan
nonenhancing nodule
nonenhancing lesion
nonferromagnetic needle
nonfilarial chylocele
nonfilling venous segment
nonforeshortened angiographic view
nonfunctioning thyroid nodule
non-Hodgkin lymphoma
nonhomogeneous consolidation
nonhyperfunctioning adrenal adenoma
nonimmunological fetal hydrops
noninducible tachycardia
noninfarcted segment
noninfective endocardial lesion
noninteger period
noninflammatory fluid accumulation
    in pleural cavity
noninvasive diagnosis
noninvasive imaging study
noninvasive vascular imaging tech-
    nique
nonionic imaging agent
nonionic paramagnetic imaging agent
nonisotropic gradient
nonlethal myocardial ischemic injury
nonlinear excitation profile

nonlingular branches of upper lobe
    bronchus
nonmyeloablative transplant recipient
Nonne-Milroy lymphedema
non-neurogenic gastrointestinal
    mesenchymal tumor
non-nodular fibrosis
non-nodular silicosis
nonocclusive mesenteric arterial
    insufficiency
nonopaque calculus
nonopaque stone
nonopaque urine
nonpalpable mass on mammogram
nonpancreatic pseudocyst
nonpenetrating trauma to heart
nonpeptide angiotensin II antagonist
nonpolarized
nonpuerperal breast abscess
nonpulsatile abdominal mass
nonpulsatile mass
nonpyogenic thrombosis
nonradiopaque foreign body
nonresonance Raman spectroscopy
nonresponsive to TSH manipulation
nonrheumatic valvular aortic stenosis
nonsegmental areas of opacification
nonselective angiography
nonseminomatous germ cell tumor
nonseminomatous tumor
nonseminomatous-type testicular
    tumor
non-single harmonic wave
non-small cell lung cancer (NSCLC)
nonspecific bowel gas pattern
nonspecific changes
nonspecific esophageal motility
    disorder (NEMD)
nonspecific phenomenon
nonsteroidal antiphlogistics
nonstress test (NST)

nonstructural curves (inscoliosis) with
uncoil with bending to the convex
side
nonstructural scoliosis
nonsubtraction images
nonsyndromic bicoronal synostosis
nonsyndromic unicoronal synostosis
nontrabeculated atrium
nontransmural myocardial infarction
nontransmural match
nontraumatic dislocation
nontraumatic epidural hemorrhage
nontraumatic rupture of urethra
nontraumatizing catheter
nontriggered phase-contrast MR
angiography
nonuniform attenuation
nonuniform rotational defect (NURD)
nonunion of fracture fragments
nonunion of operated sternum
nonunion, torsion wedge
nonvalved conduit
nonviable scar from myocardial
infarction
nonvisualization of gallbladder
nonweightbearing view
"noo-kul" (phonetic for *nuchal*)
Noonan syndrome
noose occluder
NoProfile balloon catheter
no-reflow phenomenon
Norfolk intrauterine catheter
Norgaard projection of both hands
Norland bone densitometry
Norland pQCT XCT2000 scanner
Norland XR26 bone densitometer
normal
   borderline
   high
   low
normal anatomic variation
normal-appearing bronchi
normal fundus

normal human serum albumin
normalized average glandular dose
normalized cross-section (NCC)
normal-pressure hydrocephalus
normal-region pixel
normokalemic reperfusion
normotensive
normothermia
normovolemia
normovolemic
normoxia
NOS (not otherwise specified)
nose cone
nosocomial pneumonia
nosocomial TB (tuberculosis)
transmission
notch
   acetabular
   anacrotic
   angular
   antegonial
   aortic
   auricular
   cardiac
   cerebellar
   clavicular
   coracoid
   costal
   cotyloid
   craniofacial
   dicrotic
   digastric
   ethmoidal
   fibular
   frontal
   greater sciatic
   interclavicular
   intercondylar
   intercondyloid
   intervertebral
   Kernohan
   lesser sciatic
   radial sigmoid

notch *(cont.)*
  scapular
  sciatic
  sigmoid
  spinoglenoid
  sternal
  suprasternal
  trochlear
  ulnar
notched aortic knob
notching of pulmonic valve on echocardiogram
notching, rib
notch view
no therapy zone
Nothnagel syndrome
not so subtle differences
NovaCath multilumen infusion
  catheter
Novoste Beta-Cath brachytherapy
  system
Novoste Beta-Cath bubble study
  (contrast echocardiography)
Novy cornual cannulation catheter
NOX (number of excitations) on MRI
NP (nephrographic phase)
[59]NP (iodomethylnorcholesterol)
  scintigraphy
NPC (nasopharyngeal cancer)
NPC (nodal premature contraction)
NRH (nodular regenerative
  hyperplasia)
NSCLO (non-small cell lung cancer)
NT (nuchal translucency)
NTHI (native tissue harmonic
  imaging)
N-13 ammonia uptake on PET scan
nubbin sign
nuchal translucency (NT)
Nuck
  canal of
  diverticulum of
nuclear bone imaging

nuclear density
nuclear electric quadripole relaxation
nuclear gated blood pool testing
nuclear hepatobiliary imaging
nuclear magnetic resonance (NMR)
  (see also *imaging*)
NMR imaging
NMR magnetometer probe
NMR quadrature detection array
NMR scan
NMR spectography
NMR spectrometer
NMR spectroscopy
NMR spectrum
NMR station, MacSpect real-time
NMR tomography of breast
nuclear medicine information system
  (NMIS)
nuclear parameters
nuclear perfusion imaging
nuclear relaxation
nuclear renal scintigraphy
nuclear signal
nuclear spin
nuclear spin quantum number
nuclear-tagged red blood cell bleeding
  study
nucleonics
nucletron applicator
nucleus (pl. nuclei)
  caudate
  dentate
  Kölliker
  lenticular
  lentiform
  neutron-deficient
  residual
nucleus globosus
nucleus pulposus
nuclide analysis
null point
number, clonogen
number of excitations (NEX) on MRI

NURD (nonuniform rotational defect)
nursemaid's elbow
nutation angle measurement
nutcracker esophagus

nutmeg appearance of liver
Nycore angiography catheter
Nydex catheter

O, o

O (oxygen) (an element)
OA (osteoarthritis)
OBD (organic brain disease)
object-film distance (OFD)
oblique axial MR imaging
oblique diameter
oblique, extension, and flexion
   (position extremity in)
oblique fissure of lung
oblique foot projection
oblique hernia
oblique fracture
oblique radiograms
oblique vein
oblique view
obliquity
   Litzmann
   Nägele
   Roederer
   Solayrès
obliterans, atherosclerosis
obliteration
   costophrenic angle
   nidus
   psoas shadow
   surgical
obliterative arteriosclerosis

O'Brien classification of radial
   fracture
obscure
obscuration
obstetrical trauma
obstetric ultrasound
obstipation
obstructed calices
obstructing embolus
obstruction
   acute abdominal
   adynamic intestinal
   airway
   aortic arch
   aortic outflow
   aortoiliac
   arterial
   Bartholin gland
   bilateral
   bile flow
   biliary
   bladder neck
   bladder outlet
   bowel
   bronchial
   cardiac
   cerebrospinal fluid

471

obstruction *(cont.)*
  chronic airway
  closed-loop
  closed-loop intestinal
  colon
  colonic
  common bile duct
  common duct
  complete bowel
  congenital left-sided outflow
  congenital subpulmonic
  cornual
  cowl-shaped
  duct
  efferent duct
  endobronchial
  esophageal
  extrahepatic
  extrinsic malignant ureteral
  false colonic
  fecal
  fixed airway
  fixed coronary
  food bolus
  foreign body
  functional
  functional ureteral
  gastric
  gastric outlet
  hepatic
  hepatic venous outflow
  high grade
  high small bowel
  hollow viscus
  hydrocephalic
  hydronephrosis due to ureteral
  idiopathic
  increased pulmonary
  infravesical
  interposed colon segment
  intestinal
  intrathoracic airway
  intraventricular right ventricular

obstruction *(cont.)*
  intravesical
  irreversible airway
  lacrimal canaliculus
  large bowel
  lower tract
  low small bowel
  lymphatic
  malignant airway
  mammary duct
  mechanical
  mechanical biliary
  mechanical duct
  mechanical extrahepatic
  mechanical intestinal
  mechanical small bowel
  meconium
  mitral valve
  neurogenic intestinal
  otic
  outflow
  outlet
  pancreatic duct
  paralytic colonic
  partial bowel
  partial ureteral
  preocclusive
  prostatic
  pulmonary artery
  pulmonary outflow
  pulmonary vascular
  pulmonary venous
  pyloric outlet
  pyloroduodenal
  rectal
  recurrent bladder neck
  renal
  renal artery
  respiratory
  respiratory tract
  right ventricular outflow
  secondary
  secretory duct of Bartholin gland

obstruction *(cont.)*
  simple mechanical
  small bowel (SBO)
  strangulated bowel
  strangulation
  subclavian artery
  subpulmonic
  subvalvular aortic
  subvalvular diffuse muscular
  superior vena caval
  supravesical
  tubal
  tubular
  upper airway
  upper tract
  ureteral
  ureteric
  ureteropelvic junction (UPJ)
  ureteropelvic junction
  ureterovesical
  urethral
  urinary
  urinary tract
  vascular
  venous
  ventricular outflow
  ventricular outflow tract
  vesical outlet
obstructive
obstructive abnormality
obstructive airway disease
obstructive atelectasis
obstructive component
obstructive emphysema
obstructive hydrocephalus
obstructive hypertrophic cardiomyopathy
obstructive hypopnea
obstructive jaundice
obstructive lesion
obstructive pneumonia
obstructive pulmonary disease (OPD)
obstructive pulmonary overinflation

obstructive renal dysplasia
obstructive thrombus
obstructive thrombus within the lumen
obstructive-type atelectasis
obstructive ventilatory defect
obturating embolus
obturator fossa
obturator hernia
obturator internus muscle
obturator nodal chain
obturator node
obturator sign
obtuse marginal (OM) coronary artery
obtuse marginal branch (OMB)
occipital-atlas-axis ligaments
occipital-axis joint
occipital bone
occipital condyle
occipital fissure
occipital fracture
occipital gyrus
occipital lesion
occipital lobe
occipital pole
occipital-temporal sulcus
occipital tip
occipital vessels
occipital view of skull
occipitoanterior
occipitoanterior (OA) position
occipitoatlantoaxial fusion
occipitocervical articulation
occipitofrontalis muscle
occipitoposterior
occipitoposterior position
occipitotemporal gyrus
occipitotemporal sulcus
occipitotemporopontine tract
occiput
occiput anterior (OA) position
occiput left anterior (OLA) position
occiput posterior (OP) position
occlude

occluded graft
occluder
  ameroid
  Amplatzer ductal
  CardioSEAL septal
  Clamshell
  Flo-Rester vessel
  Hunter-Sessions balloon
  Innovante
  IVM vascular
  noose
  radiolucent plastic
  Rashkind
  Rashkind double disk
  Sarns
  Stockert/Shiley venous
occluder button component folded and
  introduced into sheath
occluder delivered into left atrium
  under fluoroscopic control
occluding spring emboli
occluding thrombus
occlusal plane
occlusal segment
occlusion
  acute mesenteric artery
  anterior descending artery
  aqueductal
  arterial
  ASD transcatheter
  balloon
  basilar
  bilateral
  coil
  complete
  coronary
  deep venous
  ductus arteriosus
  embolic
  fallopian tube
  fenestration
  graft
  intermittent

occlusion *(cont.)*
  intracranial vascular
  late graft
  percutaneous ureteral
  pressure-controlled intermittent
    coronary
  renal artery
  side branch
  snowplow
  subtotal
  tapering
  total
  traumatogenic
  unilateral
  ureteral
  vascular
  vein graft
  vertebrobasilar
  vessel
occlusion measurement
occlusion of blood supply
occlusion of breast duct
occlusion of ureter
occlusive arterial thrombus
occlusive cerebrovascular insult
occlusive impedance phlebography
occlusive lesion
occult cerebral vascular malformation
  (OCVM)
occult distant metastatic disease
occult mammary lymph node
  metastasis
occult mediastinal metastasis
occult metastasis
occult spinal dysraphism
occult fracture
occult lesion
occult, roentgenographically
occult subluxation
OCD (osteochondral defect) of the
  glenoid fossa
OCG (oral cholecystogram)
ochronosis

Ochsner graft
OCL bowel prep
O'Connor finger dexterity test
OCT (optical coherence tomography)
octagon board
octapolar catheter
OctreoScan 111 (^{111}In pentetreotide)
  radiologic imaging agent
octreotide acetate radiotherapy agent
ocular globe topography
ocular pneumoplethysmography (OPG)
oculoauriculovertebral (OAV)
oculomotor apparatus
oculomotor nerve (third cranial nerve)
oculomotor-trochlear nucleus
oculopharyngeal dystrophy
oculoplethysmography (OPG)
oculoplethysmography/carotid
  phonoangiography (OPG/CPA)
oculopneumoplethysmography
oculosubcutaneous syndrome of Yuge
Oddi, sphincter of
Oden classification of peroneal tendon
  subluxation
odontogenic fibromyxoma
odontoid bone
odontoid fracture
odontoid process
odontoid view of cervical spine
odontoma
odor stimulation
ODQ (opponens digiti quinti) muscle
OEC Series 9600 cardiac system
OFD (object-film distance)
off-axis dose inhomogeneity
off-axis factor
off-axis point localization
off-center cut
off-center modulation
off-pump aneurysmectomy
off-pump beating heart revascularization

off-pump coronary artery bypass
  (OPCAB)
off-pump coronary artery bypass graft
  (OPCABG)
off-resonance saturation pulse imaging
off-resonance spin-locking
offset, frequency
Ogden classification of epiphyseal
  fracture
Ogilvie syndrome (pseudo-obstruction
  of colon)
Ogston line
ohm (pl. ohms)
oil-aspiration pneumonia
oil embolism
oil emulsions contrast
oil, peppermint (used with barium
  enema)
oil-soluble contrast medium (OSCM)
OKT4 monoclonal antibody imaging
  agent
OKT8 monoclonal antibody imaging
  agent
Okuda transhepatic obliteration of
  varices
Olbert catheter
olecranon
olecranon fossa
olecranon process
olecranon tip fracture
oleothorax
Olcrud and Molander fracture
  classification
olfactory cleft
oligemic lobe
oligoclonal IgG bands in cerebrospinal
  fluid
oligodactylia
oligodendroglioma tumor
oligodendroma
oligohydramnios
Oligon Foley catheter

olisthesis
olisthetic vertebra, wedging of
olive catheter tip
olive ring
Oliver-Cardarelli sign
olive-tipped catheter
olivopontocerebellar atrophy
olivopontocerebellar degeneration
Ollier disease
olsalazine sodium
Olsen cholangiogram clamp
Olympus angioscope
Olympus CF-1T100L forward-viewing
   video colonoscope
Olympus EU-M30S endoscopic ultrasonography receiver
Olympus EVIS Q-200V video endoscope
Olympus Gastrocamera GTF-A
Olympus GF-UM130 ultrasound
   gastroscope
Olympus GF-UM3 and CF-UM20
   ultrasonic endoscope
Olympus UM-1W transendoscopic
   ultrasound probe
Olympus VU-M2 and XIF-UM3
   echoendoscope
OM (obtuse marginal) coronary artery
OMB (obtuse marginal branch)
OMB1 (obtuse marginal branch #1)
omental cake
omental infarction
omental thickening
omentum
   colic
   gastric
   gastrocolic
   gastrohepatic
   gastrosplenic
   greater (omentum majus)
   incarcerated
   lesser (omentum minus)
   pancreaticosplenic
   splenogastric

omentum majus
omentum minus
OmniCath atherectomy catheter
Omniflex balloon catheter
OmniFlow vascular graft
Omni Flush shape Accu-Vu catheter
OmniMesh ablation catheter
OmniMesh bidirectional catheter
OmniMesh braided-tip catheter
Omnipaque (iohexol) nonionic
   imaging agent
Omnir stent
Omniscan (gadodiamide) nonionic
   imaging agent
Omnisense ultrasound bone sonometer
OmniStent
omohyoid muscle
omphalic
omphalocele
omphaloma
omphalomesenteric duct
oncology (see also *radiotherapy agent;*
   radiation therapy)
   PACSRO (picture archiving and
      communications systems in
      radiation oncology)
   PortalVision radiation oncology
   VARIS radiation oncology
on-column preparation
On-Command catheter
OncoScint breast imaging agent
OncoScint CR/OV (^{111}In satumomab
   pendetide) imaging agent
OncoScint CR372 imaging agent
OncoScint-NSC (non-small cell) lung
   imaging agent
OncoScint PR356 imaging agent
OncoTrac imaging agent
one-part fracture
one-dimensional chemical shift
   imaging (1D-CSI)
1.5 tesla scanner
one-dimensional transient elastography

one-shot echo planar imaging
onion bulb appearance of myelin
    sheaths
onion bulb changes on biopsy
onion peel appearance on x-ray
onion-shaped dilatation of duodenum
onionskin configuration of collagenous
    fibers
onionskin periosteal reaction
onlay graft
on-line anion exchange purification
on-line portal imaging
opacification
opacified
opacify
opacifying
opacity (pl. opacities)
    air-space
    alveolar
    bubbly
    diffuse
    ground-glass
    homogenous
    increased
    linear
    lung
    patchy alveolar
    pleural-based area of increased
    reticular
opaque calculus
opaque media
opaque stone
opaque wire suture
OPART open MRI with access to all
    four sides
OPCAB (off-pump coronary artery
    bypass)
OPCABG (off-pump coronary artery
    bypass graft)
OPD (obstructive pulmonary disease)
OPD4 monoclonal antibody imaging
    agent
Opdima digital mammography system

open architecture system
open beam
open break fracture
open configuration magnetic
    resonance system
open dislocation
open end ureteral catheter
open fontanelle
open fracture
open heart CPR
open heart endocardial radiofrequency
    ablation
open magnet
open magnetic resonance imaging
open-mouth odontoid view
open neural tube defect
open pneumothorax
OpenSail balloon catheter
open systems interconnect (OSI)
open tuberculosis
opening, buttonhole
OpenPACS system
Open Sky MRI (trademarked) scanner
opera glass hand
operation (see *procedure*)
operative cholangiography
opercular
operculum, cerebral
OPG (ophthalmoplethysmography)
OPG/CPA (oculoplethysmography/
    carotid phonoangiography)
ophthalmic biometry by ultrasound
    echography
ophthalmoplethysmography (OPG)
opiate μ (mu) receptor
opiate receptor binding
opisthotonic position
Opitz thrombophlebitic splenomegaly
OPLL (opacification of posterior
    longitudinal ligament)
opportunistic fungal pneumonia
opportunistic infection
opposed GRE images

opposed loop-pair quadrature MR coil
opposed-phase GRE imaging
opposed-phase imaging
opposed-phase MRI
opposed-phase sequence
opposing pleural surfaces
Opta catheter
optic chiasm
optic glioma
optic globe
optic nerve compression
optic pathway
optic recess
optic strut
optical coherence tomography (OCT)
optical imaging
optical isomer
optical localization fiber
optical surface imaging (OSI)
optimal imaging planes
optimally
Optical Tracking System
Opticon catheter
Opti-Flow angiography catheter
Opti-Flow catheter
OptiMark (gadoversetamide
    injection)
Opti-Plast XT balloon catheter
optimization, interactive gradient
optimization parameters
Optiray nonionic
Optiray 320 imaging agent
Optiray 350 (ioversol) imaging agent
Optiscope catheter
Optison contrast agent
Optistat power contrast injector
Optiva intravenous catheter
OptiVu HDVD (high definition video
    display) imaging system
optokinetic nystagmus (OKN)
opulent dinner
Orabilex imaging agent
Oracle Focus PTCA catheter

Oracle Focus ultrasound imaging
    catheter
Oracle Megasonics high pressure
    PTCA catheter
Oracle Megasonics PTCA catheter
Oracle Micro Plus PTCA catheter
Oracle Micro Plus ultrasound imaging
    catheter
Oragrafin sodium (ipodate sodium)
    imaging agent
oral cholecystogram (OCG)
oral contrast agent
oral enhanced CT scan
oral magnetic particles
orbit
    angular process of
    bony
orbital abscess
orbital apex
orbital bone
orbital mass compression
orbital pseudotumor
Orbiter PV catheter
orbital rim stepoff
orbit artifacts due to body contour
orbitofrontal region
orbitosphenoidal bone
Orca fluoroscopic C-arm
Oreopoulos-Zellerman peritoneal
    dialysis catheter
organ
    accessory
    annulospiral
    circumventricular
    Corti
    critical
    extraperitoneal
    floating
    poles of
    retroperitoneal
    Zuckerkandl
organic brain disease (OBD)
organic granulomatosis

organic liquid scintillator
organification defect
organizing (BOOP)
organoaxial
organomegaly
orientation
  coronal
  disk to magnetic field
  disturbed
  sagittal
  slice
  spatial
  temporal
  transverse
ORIF (open reduction and internal
  fixation)
orifice
  anal
  aortic
  atrioventricular
  cardiac
  coronary
  coronary sinus
  double coronary
  esophagogastric
  external urethral
  gastroduodenal
  golf-hole ureteral
  hypoplastic tricuspid
  ileocecal
  inferior vena cava
  interlabial
  internal urethral
  lingular
  mitral
  narrowed
  pharyngeal
  pulmonary
  pyloric
  rectal
  regurgitant
  segmental
  slitlike

orifice *(cont.)*
  tricuspid
  ureteral (or ureteric)
  urethral
  vaginal
  valve
orifice to anulus ratio
origin
  anomalous
  muscle
origin of artery
origin of vessel
Orion balloon catheter
oroendotracheal tube
orogastric tube
oropharyngeal airway
oropharynx
orotracheal intubation
Orthacor material
orthocephalic
Orthoclone
orthogonal angiographic projection
orthogonal RF coil
orthogonal tag lines
orthogonal view on angiography
orthonormal diameter
orthopantogram
orthopantomography
  antemortem
  postmortem
orthopnea position
orthoroentgenogram
Orthoset radiopaque bone cement
orthostatic stress
orthotopic ureter
orthovoltage radiation therapy
Ortner syndrome
os (pl. ossa) (see also *bone*)
  cervical
  coronary sinus
  external cervical
  internal cervical
os acetabuli (acetabulum)

os calcis (calcaneus)
OSCAR ultrasonic bone cement
    removal system
oscillating magnetic field
oscillations, bubble
oscillography
oscilloscope tuning station
OSCM (oil-soluble contrast medium)
os coxae (hip bone; ilium, ischium,
    pubis)
os cuboides secondarium (cuboid
    bone)
Osgood-Schlatter disease
OSI (open systems interconnect)
OSI (optical surface imaging)
Osler disease
Osler-Libman-Sacks syndrome
Osler nodes
Osler sign
Osler triad
Osler-Weber-Rendu telangiectasia
Osm (osmole)
osmotic blood-brain barrier disruption
osmotic demyelination syndrome
osmotic edema
osmotic effect
os naviculare (navicular bone)
os pubis (pubic bone)
osseous bridge
osseous destructive process
osseous dysplasia
osseous graft
osseous metastases
osseous outgrowth
osseous remodeling
osseous spiral lamina
osseous structure
osseous survey
osseous union
ossicle, Riolan
ossiferous
ossific nodule
ossific nucleus of navicular

ossification
    abnormal
    enchondral
    endochondral
    heterotopic
    intracartilaginous
    intramembranous
    irregular enchondral
    muscle
    periarticular heterotopic (PHO)
    peripheral
    primary center of
    secondary center of
    soft tissue
ossification center, accessory
ossification variant
ossified body
ossifying fibroma of long bone
osteal stenoses
ostealgia
ostemia
ostempyesis
OsteoAnalyzer device
osteoaneurysm
osteoarthritic change
osteoarthritic spur
osteoarthritis (OA)
    degenerative
    erosive
    generalized
    post-traumatic
    traumatic
osteoarthritis radiographic grading
    (I-V)
osteoarthropathy, primary hypertrophic
osteoarticular
osteoblastic bone regeneration
osteoblastic metastasis
osteoblastic tumor
osteocachexia
osteocalcin
osteocartilaginous body
osteocartilaginous lesion

osteochondral defect (OCD) of the
  glenoid fossa
osteochondral lesion of the talar dome
osteochondral fracture
osteochondral lesion
osteochondritic loose body
osteochondritic separation of
  epiphyses
osteochondritis dissecans (OD)
osteochondrofibroma
osteochondrolysis
osteochondroma
  epiphyseal
  soft tissue
osteochondromatosis
  multiple
  synovial
osteochondromatous dysplasia,
  epiarticular
osteochondrophyte
osteochondrosarcoma
osteochondrosis deformans juvenilis
osteochondrosis dissecans
osteoclasis
osteoclastic erosion
osteo condensans ilii
osteocystoma
osteocyte
osteodiastasis
osteodystrophy
osteoenchondroma
osteofibrochondrosarcoma
osteofibromatosis
osteogenesis, distraction
osteogenesis imperfecta
osteogenesis imperfecta tarda
osteogenic sarcoma
Osteo-Gram bone density test
osteohalisteresis
osteoid osteoma
osteolipochondroma
osteolipoma

osteolysis
  acetabular
  inherited multicentric
  malignant acetabular
  scalloping
osteolytic metastases
osteoma
  juxta-articular osteoid
  osteoid
  parosteal
  spongy
  ulcer
osteomalacia
  hematogeneous
  renal tubular
  senile
osteomatosis
osteomesopyknosis
osteomyelitic sinus
osteomyelitis
osteonal bone
osteonecrosis
  dysbaric
  Ficat classification of femoral head
  radiation
osteopenia
osteopetrosis
osteophyte
  bony
  bridging
  cervical
  fringe of
  horseshoe
  jagged
  marginal
osteophyte formation
  beaklike
  hooklike
  marginal
  nipplelike
osteophytic bone lip
osteophytic lipping

osteophytic proliferation
osteophytosis
osteoporosis
   corticosteroid-induced
   disuse
   juvenile
   post-traumatic
   postmenopausal
   senile
osteoporotic atrophy
osteoporotic bone
osteoporotic skeleton
osteoradionecrosis
osteosarcoma
   cardiac
   classical
   extraosseous
   fibroblastic
   intracortical
   intraosseous
   juxtacortical
   osteoblastic
   parosteal
   periosteal
   telangiectatic
osteosclerosis
osteosis
osteospongioma
osteothrombosis
OsteoView desktop hand x-ray system
OsteoView 2000 digital imaging
   system
ostia (pl. of ostium)
ostial lesion
ostial stenosis
ostiomeatal stent
ostium (pl. ostia)
   aortic
   artery
   atrioventricular
   coronary
   coronary sinus

ostium abdominale tubae uterinae
   (abdominal orifice of uterine tube)
ostium primum defect
ostium secundum defect
os trigonum (triangular bone of
   tarsus)
os zygomaticum
Ott intrauterine catheter
Otto pelvis dislocation
Outback reentry catheter
outcome, clinical
outcomes (radiology outcomes data)
Outcomes by Design balloon
Outcomes by Design catheter
Outcomes by Design sheath introducer
Outcomes by Design steerable
   guidewire
Outcomes by Design stent
outer table
Outerbridge ridge
Outerbridge scale (articular damage)
outflow
   hypoplastic subpulmonic
   maximum venous (MVO)
   subpulmonic
outflow cardiac patch
outflow anastomosis
outflow cannula
outflow obstruction
outflow of ventricle
outflow tract
outgrowth, osseous patellar
outlet
   pelvic
   pyloric
   thoracic
   ventricular
   widened thoracic
outlet chamber, rudimentary
outlet contraction of pelvis
outlet view of pelvis
out of phase GRE images
outpocketings of mucosa

outpouching of portion of wall of
  artery
outpouchings of the bowel wall
output
  adequate cardiac
  augmented cardiac
  assumed Fick cardiac
  cardiac (CO)
  Dow method for cardiac
  Fick method for cardiac
  Gorlin method for cardiac
  Hetzel forward triangle method
    for cardiac
  inadequate cardiac
  low cardiac
  pulmonic
  reduced systemic cardiac
  stroke
  systemic
  thermodilution cardiac
  ventricular
output amplitude
output point
OV (ovarian)
Ovadia-Beals classification of tibial
  plafond fracture
oval cherry-red raised lesion
ovale, foramen
ovalis
  anulus
  fossa
  limbus fossae
ovarian abscess
ovarian adenosarcoma
ovarian carcinoma
ovarian cyst, functional
ovarian ectopic pregnancy locations
ovarian endometriosis
ovarian follicle
ovarian function
ovarian granulosa cell tumor
ovarian hernia
ovarian tumor

ovary (pl. ovaries)
  accessory
  atrophied
  cystic
  embryonic
  ligament of
  mulberry
  polycystic
  suspensory ligament of
Ovation Falloposcopy System
overaeration
over couch view
overdistention
  alveolar
  pulmonary
overdrive suppression
overexpansion, pulmonary
overgrowth, bony
overhanging edges or margins
Overhauser effect
overhead film
overhead oblique view
overinflation
  pulmonary
  unilateral
overlapping images
overlapping structures, angiographically
overlie
overlying epicardial fat
overload (overloading)
  acute hemodynamic
  cardiac
  chronic hemodynamic
  diastolic
  fluid
  pressure
  right ventricular
  systolic ventricular
  volume
overlying attenuation artifact
over-read (noun)
overrelaxation factors

over-responsive programming
overriding great artery
overriding great vessel
overriding of anulus
overriding of fracture fragments
overriding of tricuspid valve
overriding toes
overriding ventricular septum of aorta
oversampling (on MRI)
overstaged
over the wire balloon catheter
overuse injury
overuse syndrome
overventilation, alveolar
ovoid heart
ovoids, external beam with
ovoid-shaped
ovoid-shaped calcific density
ovum (pl. ova)
Owen view
oxalate calculus
oxalosis
Oxford magnet

"ox heart" (cor bovinum)
oxidation, Baeyer-Villiger
oxidative metabolism
oxidized complex
Oxilan-300, Oxilan-350 (ioxilan)
  imaging agent
oximetry, transcranial cerebral
oxycel
oxygen (O) (an element)
  ^{15}O (oxygen-15)
  ^{15}O carbon dioxide (inhaled)
  ^{15}O carbon monoxide
  ^{15}O inhaled
  ^{15}O labeled water
  ^{15}O NMR spectroscopy
oxygenation-sensitive functional MR
oxygen cisternography
oxygen extraction fraction (OEF)
oxygen, inhaled (MR contrast agent)
oxygen-15 labeled water (^{15}O-labeled
  water)
oxygen-17 NMR spectroscopy

P, p

P (phosphorus) (an element)
P (posterior)
PA (posteroanterior or posterior-
    anterior)
  PA and lateral films
  PA and lateral views
  PA axial sternoclavicular joints
    x-ray
  PA projection
  PA upright chest x-ray
PA (pulmonary artery)
Paas disease
PABP (pulmonary artery balloon
    pump)
pacchionian
pacemaker
pace mapping
Pace Plus System scanner
Paceport catheter
pack-a-day smoking history
packing
  cubic
  extraction, and calculation
    technique
  periodic
pack-year smoking history
pack years of cigarette smoking

PACS (picture archive and communi-
    cation system)
PACS, PBT Technologies
PACSRO (picture archiving and
    communications systems in
    radiation oncology)
pad
  abdominal
  antimesenteric fat
  fat
  fibrocartilaginous
  padding
  UltraEase ultrasound
paddle, compression
PADP-PAWP (pulmonary artery
    diastolic and wedge pressure)
  gradient
pad sign of aortic insufficiency
PAEDP (pulmonary artery end
    diastolic pressure)
Paget abscess
Paget-associated osteogenic sarcoma
Paget disease, "fluffy rarefaction" of
pagetoid bone
Paget osteitis deformans
Paget-Schroetter venous thrombosis of
    axillary vein

485

Paget-von Schroetter syndrome
pain, flank
pair production
Pais fracture
PALA enhancement
palatal
palate
  bony
  Byzantine arch
  cleft
  hard
  high arched
  soft
palatine bone
palatopharyngeal fold
paleopathologic and radiologic study
palisade formation
palladium (Pd) (an element)
  ^{103}Pd isotope used in brachy-
    therapy
  ^{103}Pd prostatic implant
  ^{103}Pd radioactive material
  ^{103}Pd implantation brachytherapy
  ^{103}Pd ultrasound-guided trans
    perineal implantation
palladium 103 (^{103}Pd) radiotherapy
  agent
palliation of pain
palliative irradiation
palliative radiation therapy
pallidus—see *globus pallidus*
palmitic acid
pallor
  myelin
  subtle myelin
palmar metacarpal ligament
palmar plate
Palmaz balloon-expandable iliac stent
Palmaz-Schatz coronary stent
Palmaz-Schatz stent (PSS)
Palmaz vascular stent
palmitic acid imaging agent
palpability

Palpagraph mammography device
palpation
palpatory
palpebral fissure
PAM (pulmonary artery mean)
  pressure
panacinar emphysema
panaortic
pancake kidney
pancake MRI magnet
pancake vertebra
pancarpal destructive arthritis
panchamber enlargement
Pancoast syndrome
Pancoast tumor
pancreas
  aberrant
  accessory
  annular
  anterior surface of
  Aselli
  CT scan of
  degeneration of
  dorsal
  head of
  heterotopic
  interior surface of
  lesser
  neck of
  posterior surface of
  tail of
  uncinate process of
  ventral
  Willis
  Winslow
pancreas divisum
pancreatic acinar cell carcinoma
pancreatic adenoma
pancreatic adenomatosis
pancreatic angiography
pancreatic duct, accessory
pancreatic ductal dilatation
pancreatic pseudoaneurysm

pancreatic duct
  accessory
  disruption of
  duodenal end of dorsal
  duodenal end of main
  main
  obstruction of
  proximal part of dorsal
pancreatic duct cannulation,
  endoscopic retrograde
pancreatic-enteric continuity
pancreatic fistula
pancreaticobiliary common channel
pancreaticohepatic syndrome
pancreatic pseudocyst
pancreatic scan
pancreatitis
pancreatoblastoma
pancreatocholangiogram, retrograde
pancreatogram
pancreatography
  endoscopic retrograde
  intraoperative
  magnetic resonance (MRP)
  retrograde
pancreatolithiasis
panda sign
panfacial fracture
panlobular emphysema
panmural fibrosis
panniculitis, mesenteric
pannus deformity of odontoid
pannus of synovium
panoramic CT scan
panoramic image
panoramic radiography
Panorex x-ray
pansystolic mitral regurgitation
pantalar fusion
pantaloon embolus
pantaloon hernia
PAP (pulmonary artery pressure)

papilla
  acoustic
  bile
  duodenal
  ectopic
  major duodenal
  minor duodenal
  renal
  Santorini
  urethral
  Vater
papillary epithelial neoplasm
papillary fibroelastoma
papillary proliferation
papillary tumor
papilloma
  choroid plexus
  cockscomb
  Hopmann
  ventricular tumor
Papillon-Lefevre syndrome
PAPVR (partial anomalous pulmonary
  venous return)
para-aortic region
para-articular bone remodeling
para-articular calcification
parabola, metatarsal
paracardiac mass
paracardiac-type total anomalous
  venous return
paracentral lobule
paracervical instillation catheter
paracervical region
parachute deformity of mitral valve
paracicatricial emphysema
paracoccidioidomycosis
paracolic gutter
paracorporeal
paracostal
paradoxical embolus
paradoxical hyperconcentration of
  imaging agent

paradoxical motion
paradoxical motion of leaflet
paradoxical suppression
paraduodenal hernia
paraesophageal hernia
paraesophagogastric devascularization
parafascicular nucleus
paraganglioma
paragangliomatosis
Paragon coronary stent
paragonimiasis
parahilar (also perihilar)
paraileostomal hernia
parallax motion method for localization of foreign bodies in the orbit
parallel analog mapping
parallel and spiral flow patterns
parallel hole image
parallel hole medium sensitivity collimator
parallel opposed ports
parallel opposed unmodified ports
parallel-tagged MR images and field-fitting analysis
parallel tag planes
parallel track sign
Parallel virtual machine
paralysis of diaphragm
paralytic chest
paralytic ileus
paramagnetic artifact
paramagnetic contrast media
paramagnetic Cr-labeled red blood cells
paramagnetic relaxation
paramagnetic shift
paramagnetic substances
paramagnetism
paramalleolar arteries
paramedian pontine reticular formation (PPRF)
paramedian position
paramedian sagittal plane

paramediastinal glands
parameningeal
parameter
  clinical
  hematologic
  kinetic perfusion
  nuclear
  optimization
  parameters
  physiologic
  scan
  sonographic
  thermal treatment
  ventricular function
parametrial abscess
parametric abscess
paranasal sinus
paraneoplastic cerebellar degeneration
paraneoplastic hypercalcemia
paraneoplastic process
parapatellar plica
parapelvic (also peripelvic)
parapelvic gutter
parapharyngeal abscess
parapharyngeal space
parapharyngeal space abscess
parapneumonic effusion
paraprosthetic-enteric fistula
paraprosthetic leakage
pararenal abscess
pararenal aortic aneurysm
pararenal aortic atherosclerosis
parasagittal head region
parasagittal intracranial mass
parasagittal meningioma
parasagittal region
parasellar mass
paraseptal emphysema
paraseptal position
paraspinal abnormality
paraspinal muscles
paraspinal musculature
paraspinal pleural stripe

paraspinal soft tissue mass
paraspinal soft tissue shadowing
paraspinous musculature
parasternal bulge
parasternal long axis view
parasternal lymph nodes
parasternal motion
parasternal short axis view
parasternal view of heart
parasternal window
parasympathetic nervous system
paratesticular neoplasm
paratracheal soft tissues
paratracheal stripe
paratrooper fracture
paravalvar leak
paravalvular
paravertebral gutter
paravertebral musculature
paravertebral nerve plexus
paravertebral region
paravertebral venous plexus
ParCA (Parodi balloon catheter for
   angiography)
parcellate, parcellated
parcellation
parchment heart syndrome
parchment right ventricle
parenchyma
   breast
   cerebral
   infiltration of pulmonary
   liver
   lung
   pulmonary
   renal
   spinal cord
parenchymal collaterals
parenchymal consolidation
parenchymal echogenicity
parenchymal fibrous band
parenchymal hematoma
parenchymal infarct

parenchymal infiltrates, pulmonary
parenchymal lung disease
parenchymal neurocutaneous
   melanosis
parenchymal tracer accumulation
parenchymal transit
parenchymal tumor mass
parenchymatous atrophy
parenchymatous cerebellar
   degeneration
parenchymatous hemorrhage
parenchymatous neurosyphilis
parenchymatous phase
parenchymatous pneumonia
parent vein
paresis, hemilingual
parietal band
parietal bone
parietal branches
   paired
   unpaired
parietal cephalohematoma
parietal cortex lesion
parietal cortex, post-rolandic
parietal extension of infundibular
   septum
parietal gyrus
parietal layer
parietal lobe lesion
parietal lobe sign
parietal pericardial calcification
parietal pericardium
parietal pleura
parietocanthal view
parieto-occipital lesion
parieto-occipital sulcus
parietotemporal area
Paris system
Park Medical Systems scanner
Parks bidirectional Doppler flowmeter
Parks ileal reservoir
Parodi balloon catheter for angiography (ParCA)

Parona space
parosteal chondrosarcoma
parosteal osteogenic sarcoma
parosteal osteosarcoma
parotid gland
parotid pleomorphic adenoma
paroxysmal crisis, hypertensive
parrot-beak meniscus tears
parry fracture
pars interarticularis
Parsonnet probe
Parsons, third intercondylar
    tubercle of
partial anomalous pulmonary venous
    return (PAPVR)
partial-brain radiation therapy
partial collapse of lung
partial dislocation
partial dislodgement
partial flexion position
partial k-space sampling
partial liquid ventilation with
    perflubron
partial obliteration of a lateral
    ventricle (on scan)
partial obstruction of ureter
partial ossicular replacement
    prosthesis (PORP)
partial pericardial absence
partial saturation and spin echo pulse
    sequence
partial saturation technique
partial thickening
partial-thickness tear
partial ureteral obstruction
partial volume averaging
partial volume effect, artifact due to
particle (pl. particles)
    beta
    bone
    calcium/oxyanion-containing
    charged
    Ivalon

particle beam
particle debris
particle identification
particle masks
particle size determination
particulate debris
particulates, magnetic
partition
    atrial
    gastric
partition coefficient
parts, fetal small
PAS (pulmonary artery systolic)
    pressure
pascals of force (SI units)
Passage hemostasis valve (used in
    angiography)
passage of renal stone
passage of blind catheter
Passager introducing sheath
passages, narrowing of bronchiolar
passive clot
passive filling
passively congested lung tissue
passively shimmed superconducting
    magnet
passive pneumonia
passive track detector
passive tracking and visualization
passive vascular congestion
passive venous distention
PASTA (polarity-altered spectral-
    selective acquisition) imaging
patch
    atriopulmonary
    autologous pericardial
    CardioFix Pericardium
    Carrel
    CV Peri-Guard
    Dacron Sauvage
    Dura-Guard
    epidural blood
    Fluoropassiv thin-wall carotid

patch *(cont.)*
  Gore-Tex cardiovascular
  Gore-Tex soft tissue
  gusset-type
  kinking of
  MacCallum
  outflow cardiac
  pericardial
  Peri-Guard
  periosteal
  Peyer
  RapiSeal
  small defibrillating
  Supple Peri-Guard
  Teflon intracardiac
  Telectronics defibrillator
  transannular
  Vascu-Guard
  vein
patch crinkling
patch electrodes placed outside the
  pericardium
patch graft, Dacron onlay
patch graft of outflow tract
patchy air-space consolidations
patchy alveolar opacities
patchy atelectasis
patchy atrophy of renal cortex
patchy consolidation
patchy distribution of the tracer
patchy endometriosis
patchy infiltrate
patchy inflammation
patchy migratory infiltrates
patchy zones
patella
  apex of head of
  bipartite
  dislocated
  floating
  high-riding
  lower pole of
  skyline view of

patella *(cont.)*
  subluxing
  undersurface of
  patella alta (high-riding)
  patella baja
  patellar button
  patellar chondromalacia
  patellar contour
  patellar dislocation
  patellar edge
  patellar entrapment
  patellar fat pad
  patellar fossa
  patellar groove
  patellar subluxation
  patellar tendinosis
  patellofemoral articular cartilage
  patellofemoral joint space
  patellofemoral region
patency
  arterial
  coronary artery
  coronary bypass graft
  ductus arteriosus
  graft
  long term
  short term
  vein
patency and valvular reflux of deep
  veins
patency of vein graft
patency of vessel
patency rate
patent bifurcation
patent bronchus sign
patent ductus arteriosus (PDA)
patent foramen ovale
patent trifurcation
patent urachus
patent urethra
patent, widely
Paterson-Parker rules
Pathfinder catheter

pathognomonic findings
pathognomonic sign
pathological uptake
pathologic confirmation
pathologic correlation
pathologic diagnosis
pathologic dislocation
pathologic fracture
pathologic reflux
pathology, radiographic
pathophysiologic changes in airways
  obstruction
pathophysiology
pathway
  absorptive
  neural
  optic
  retrovestibular neural
patient motion artifact
pattern
  abdominal wall venous
  A fib (atrial fibrillation)
  air-space
  air-space filling
  alveolar
  AM (associative memory)
  anhaustral colonic gas
  anomalous topographic
  arterial deficiency
  bigeminal
  blood flow
  bone marrow edema pattern on
    MR imaging
  bowel
  bowel gas
  branching
  butterfly
  cobblestone
  cobweb
  contractile
  corduroy cloth (on myelogram)
  crazy-paving
  diffuse

pattern *(cont.)*
  dP/dt upstroke
  ductal
  early repolarization
  echo
  electron and x-ray diffraction
  enhancement
  extended
  fibrotic cavitating
  filigree
  fine reticular
  fold
  gas
  gastric mucosal
  haustral
  helical
  hemodynamic
  heterogeneous perfusion
  hierarchical scanning
  hole
  homogeneous
  honeycomb
  hourglass
  infiltration
  interstitial
  juvenile T wave
  lacy trabecular
  Laue
  left ventricular contraction
  left ventricular strain
  lobular
  M (on right atrial waveform)
  miliary
  macronodular
  marrow edema
  micronodular
  mosaic
  mosaic attenuation
  mosaic duodenal mucosal
  moth-eaten
  movement
  MR enhancement
  M-shaped mitral valve

pattern *(cont.)*
    mucosal
    nodular
    nonspecific gas
    parallel
    pin
    P pulmonale
    pseudoinfarct
    pulmonary flow
    pulmonary vascular
    recurrence
    reticular
    rheologic
    right ventricular strain
    rugal
    sclerosing
    sigmoid hair (on spine)
    signet ring
    small bowel mucosal
    SMPTE test
    speckled
    spectral
    spiral flow
    star
    stellate
    strain
    subtle abnormal perfusion
    sulcal
    surface convexity
    task-rest
    temporal sawtooth
    thermal convection
    tree-in-bud (TIB)
    trigeminal
    ventricular contraction
    vesicular
Patton laparoscopic catheter
patulous hiatus
pauciarticular
paucity of bowel gas
pause
    asystolic
    compensatory

pause *(cont.)*
    noncompensatory
    pauses
    postextrasystolic
    sinus
Pauwels angle of femoral neck
    fracture
Pauwels classification of femoral neck
    fracture
Pawlik trigone
Pawlow method (swimmer's view)
PAWP (pulmonary artery wedge
    pressure)
Payr disease
Payr sign
Pb (lead) (an element)
    Pb 212-labeled monoclonal anti-
        body imaging agent
PBC (primary biliary cirrhosis)
PBF (pulmonary blood flow)
PBN hysterosalpingography catheter
PBPI (penile-brachial pressure index)
    to assess cardiac disease
PBT Technologies PACS
PBVI (pulmonary blood volume index)
PC (phase contrast) imaging
PC (posterior commissure)
PCA (posterior cerebral artery)
PCA (posterior communicating artery)
PCL (posterior cruciate ligament)
PCoA (posterior communicating
    artery)
PCFP (postcatheterization false
    aneurysm)
PCP (pulmonary capillary pressure)
PCS (proximal coronary sinus)
PCVD (pulmonary collagen vascular
    disease)
PCWP (pulmonary capillary wedge
    pressure)
Pd (palladium)
PDA (patent ductus arteriosus)
PDA (personal digital assistant)

PDA (posterior descending artery)
P.D. Access over the needle catheter
PDI (power Doppler imaging)
PDR (pulsed brachytherapy)
PE (pericardial effusion)
PE (pulmonary embolism)
peak
    airway pressure
    diffraction
    juxtaphrenic
    main glow
    pressure
    single
peak airway pressure
peak count density
peak dP/dt
peak early diastolic filling velocities
peak enhancement
peak expiratory flow (PEF)
peak expiratory flow rate (PEFR)
peak filling rate (PFR)
peak fitting
peak flow
peak flow of urinary bladder
peak flow variability
peak flow velocity
peak identification
peak inflation pressures
peak inspiratory pressure (PIP)
peak late diastolic filling velocities
peak parenchymal activity
peak profile
peak regurgitant flow velocity
peak regurgitant wave pressure
peak systolic and diastolic ICA/CCA
    ratios
peak systolic pressure
peak systolic velocity (cm/sec)
peak tidal expiratory flow
peak to peak pressure gradient
peak velocity of blood flow on
    Doppler echocardiogram
pear-shaped bladder

pear-shaped defect
pear-shaped heart
pear-shaped uterus
Pearson bilateral AP projection of the
    acromoclavicular joints
pectoral
pectoralis major muscle
pectoralis major syndrome
pectoralis minor muscle
pectus carinatum
pectus excavatum deformity
pedal artery opacification
pedestal sign
pediatric biplane TEE (transesophageal
    echocardiography) probe
pediatric neuroradiology
pedicle
    IMA (internal mammary artery)
    musculofascial
    phrenic
    spinal
    vascular
pedicle bone grafts
pedicle erosion
pedicle of vertebra
pedicle sclerosis
peduncle
    cerebellar
    cerebral
    inferior cerebellar
peduncular segment of superior
    cerebellar artery
pedunculated myxoma
pedunculated polyp
pedunculated subserous myoma
pedunculated thrombus
pedunculated tumor
pedunculated uterine myoma
pedunculated vesical tumor
pedunculation
PEG (pneumoencephalogram)
Pel-Ebstein disease
Pellegrini-Stieda disease

pellet
  alanine-silicone
  radiopaque
pellet artifact (shotgun pellets)
pellucidum
pelviabdominal (or pelvi-abdominal)
pelvic abscess
pelvicaliceal changes
pelvicaliceal distention
pelvic bone
pelvic brim
pelvic cavity
pelvic collateral vessel
pelvic diameter
pelvic floor
pelvic floor laceration
pelvic fracture frame
pelvic girdle
pelvic inflammatory disease (PID)
pelvic inlet
pelvic inlet and outlet views
pelvic kidney
pelvic lymphadenectomy
pelvic node
pelvic notching
pelvic obliquity
pelvic outlet
pelvic rim fracture
pelvic ring fracture
pelvic tilt, bent knee
pelvic traction
pelvic ultrasound
pelvic ultrasound CT scan
pelvic venous plexuses, exaggeration
  of
pelvic view
pelviectasis
pelvimetry
  Mengert index in
  modified Ball
  Thoms

pelvis (pl. pelves)
  android
  anthropoid
  assimilation
  beaked
  bifid
  bony
  borderline
  brachypellic
  champagne glass
  contracted
  cordate
  cordiform
  Deventer
  dolichopellic
  dwarf
  elephant
  extrarenal
  false
  female
  flat
  frozen
  funnel-shaped
  greater
  gynecoid
  hardened
  heart-shaped
  infantile
  inlet contraction of
  inverted
  juvenile
  Kilian
  kyphoscoliotic
  kyphotic
  lesser
  longitudinal oval
  lordotic
  male
  masculine
  mesatipellic
  maternal
  Nägele
  osteomalacic

pelvis *(cont.)*
  Otto
  outlet contraction of
  platypelloid
  portable film of
  Prague
  pseudo-osteomalacic
  rachitic
  relaxation of
  reniform
  renal
  Rokitansky
  round
  scoliotic
  simple flat
  small
  spider
  spondylolisthetic
  transverse oval
  true
  ureteral
  ureteric
pelviureteral junction
pelviureteric junction
pelvocaliceal effacement
pencil beam approach
pencil beam navigator echoes
pencil in cup deformity
penciling of ribs
Pendred syndrome
pendulous urethra
pendulum movement
penetrating aortic ulceration
penetrating atherosclerotic ulceration
penetrating trauma
penetrating injury
penetrating injury to aortic arch
penetrating injury to innominate artery
penetrating injury to superior vena
  cava
penetrating lung injury
penetrating trauma to heart
penetrating ulceration

penetrating wound of descending
  thoracic aorta
penetration
  inadvertent
  3D
  x-ray
penetration rate
penetration syndrome
penile abscess
penile fibrosis
penile hypertrophy
penile malignancy
penile trauma
penile urethra
penis
  bulb of
  bulbospongiosus muscle of
  clubbed
  concealed
  corpora cavernosa
  corpus spongiosum
  crura of
  deep fascia of
  dorsal artery of
  dorsal nerve of
  dorsum of
  double
  glans
  ischiospongiosus muscle of
  root of
  suspensory ligament of
  webbed
penis hematoma
Pennal and Tile pelvic girdle injury
  classification
Pennal classification of pelvic ring
  fractures
Pennal views of pelvic inlet and outlet
penoscrotal junction
PenRad mammography clinical
  reporting system
Penrose drain
pentagastrin imaging agent

pentavalent DMSA(dimercaptosuccinic
acid)
Pentax EUP-EC124 ultrasound
gastroscope
Pentax-Hitachi FG32UA endosono-
graphic system
pentetreotide indium 111 (^{111}In)
penumbra, dosimetric
penumbra zone
PEP (pre-ejection period)
PE Plus II balloon dilatation catheter
peppermint oil (used with barium
enema)
peptic ulcer
acute
chronic
peptic ulcer disease (PUD)
peptide imaging agent
percentage signal intensity loss (PSIL)
perception, depth
Perception 5000 PC-based ultrasound
scanner
perceptual linearization
Perchloracap imaging agent
perchlorate washout test
Percor DL balloon catheter
Percor DL-II (dual lumen) intra-aortic
balloon catheter
Percor-Stat-DL catheter
Percuflex APD all-purpose catheter
with Fader Tip
Percuflex Plus flexible ureteral stent
Percuflex stent
PercuGuide
percussion wave of carotid arterial
pulse
PercuSurge GuardWire system
percutaneous antegrade biliary
drainage
percutaneous aortic balloon
valvuloplasty
percutaneous automated diskectomy
under fluoroscopy

percutaneous endoluminal placement
of stent-graft
percutaneous endomyocardial biopsy
percutaneous fibrin glue
percutaneous gastrostomy (PG), radiologic
percutaneous insertion via femoral
vein
percutaneous implantation of endovascular stent
percutaneous interventional radiology
percutaneous intracoronary angioscopy
percutaneously cannulated
percutaneous nephrolithotripsy (PNL)
percutaneous nephrostomy
percutaneous pericardial biopsy
percutaneous pericardioscopy
percutaneous pyelogram
percutaneous radiofrequency catheter
ablation
percutaneous radiofrequency ablation
percutaneous retrograde transfemoral
technique
percutaneous revascularization
percutaneous sclerotherapy
percutaneous thoracoscopy
percutaneous transcatheter ductal
closure (PTDC)
percutaneous transhepatic biliary
drainage with contrast monitoring
percutaneous transhepatic cholangiogram (PTC, PTHC)
percutaneous transhepatic liver biopsy
percutaneous transhepatic portography
with hemodynamic evaluation
percutaneous transluminal angioplasty
(PTA)
percutaneous transluminal coronary
angioplasty (PTCA)
percutaneous transluminal renal
angioplasty (PTRA)
percutaneous transluminal septal
myocardial ablation

percutaneous transmyocardial revascularization (PMR)
percutaneous transperineal seed implantation
percutaneous transvenous embolization
percutaneous ureteral occlusion
percutaneous ureteral stent
PerDUCER pericardial access device
perflenapent imaging agent
perflexane imaging agent
perflisopent imaging agent
perflubron contrast
perfluorocarbon F-19 (^{19}F) imaging agent
perfluoroctylbromide (PFOB) imaging agent
perflutren imaging agent
perforated diverticulum
perforating aneurysm
perforating arteries
perforating fracture
perforation
  bladder
  cardiac
  duodenal ulcer (DUP)
  transseptal
  ulcer
  walled-off esophageal
perforator vessel
Performa angiographic catheter
Performr (RF-Performr) electrophysiology catheter (*not* Performer)
perfusate
perfuse
perfusion
  adequate coronary
  antegrade
  coronary
  diminished systemic
  homogeneous
  hypothermic
  intraperitoneal hyperthermic (IPHP)

perfusion *(cont.)*
  luxury
  misery
  mosaic
  myocardial
  peripheral
  poor
  pulsatile
  quantitative cardiac
  regional (by mixed venous blood)
  regional cerebral
  renal
  retrograde cardiac (RCP)
  tissue
perfusion abnormality
perfusion agent
perfusion and ventilation lung scan
perfusion catheter
perfusion defect
perfusion deficit
perfusion gradient
perfusion lung scan
perfusion magnetic resonance imaging
perfusion-metabolism mismatch
perfusion pressure
perfusion scan
perfusion scintigraphy
perfusion-weighted imaging
perfusion-weighted MRI
perialveolar fibrosis
periampullary diverticulum
periampullary duodenal tumor
periaortic area
periaortic fibrosis
periapical granuloma
periapical lesion
periappendiceal abscess
periaqueductal gray matter
periaqueductal region
periarticular calcification
periarticular fracture
periarticular heterotopic ossification (PHO)

periarticular periostitis
periarticular tissues
peribronchial alveolar spaces
peribronchial connective tissue
peribronchial cuffing
peribronchial distribution
peribronchial fibrosis
peribronchial infiltrate
peribronchial lymph nodes
peribronchial markings
peribronchial thickening
peribronchiolar hemorrhage
pericallosal artery
pericardiacophrenic vein
pericardial absence
  congenital
  partial
pericardial cavity
pericardial constriction, occult
pericardial cyst
pericardial diaphragmatic adhesions
pericardial effusion
pericardial fat pad
pericardial fluid
pericardial fold
pericardial hematoma
pericardial infusion
pericardial reflection
pericardial sac
pericardial sinus
pericardial space
pericardiocentesis, ultrasonic guidance
  for
pericardioscopy, percutaneous
pericardium
  adherent
  autologous
  bread-and-butter
  calcified
  congenitally absent
  diaphragmatic
  empyema
  fibrous

pericardium *(cont.)*
  inelastic
  inflamed
  nondistensible
  parietal
  serous
  shaggy
  soldier's patches of
  tenting of
  thickened
  veins of
  visceral
pericardium calcareous deposits
pericardium exposed
pericardium fibrosum
pericatheter thrombus (pl. thrombi)
pericecal abscess
pericholecystic edema
pericholecystic fluid
pericicatricial emphysema
pericolonic fat
pericystic edema
periductal calcification
periductal fibrosis
peridural fibrosis
Periflow peripheral balloon catheter
perigastric deformity
perigraft hematoma
Peri-Guard patch
perihilar density
perihilar edema
perihilar edema haze
perihilar fat
perihilar fibrosis
perihilar infiltrate
perihilar markings
perihilar region
peri-ileal
peri-infarction ischemia
peri-infarctional defect
perilesional bone
perilunate carpal dislocation
perilunate fracture dislocation (PLFD)

perimalleolar pain
perimedullary
perimembranous ventricular septal
  defect
Perimount Plus heart valve
perimuscular plexus
perimylolysis
perinatal respiratory distress syndrome
perineal descent
perineal fibrosis
perineal hematoma
perineal hernia
perineal laceration
perineal muscle laceration
perineogram
perineoplastic edema
perinephric abscess
perinephric fat
perinephric hematoma
perinephric space
perineural invasion
perineural tumor
perineural fibroblastoma tumor
period
  diastolic filling
  noninteger
  raster
  rapid filling (RFP)
  reduced ventricular filling
periodic intermittent catheterization
periodic packing
periodontal ligament
perioperative myocardial infarction
periosteum, onion skin
periorbital Doppler study
periosteal bone formation
periosteal creep
periosteal fibroma
periosteal new bone formation
periosteal osteosarcoma
periosteal reaction
periosteal sarcoma

periostitis
  periarticular
  shaft
peripancreatic adenopathy
peripancreatic arteries
peripancreatic fluid collection
peripartal vaginal hemorrhage
peripelvic
peripelvic collateral vessel
peripheral adenopathy
peripheral air-space disease
peripheral angiography
peripheral arterial cannula
peripheral blood flow
peripheral circulatory vasoconstriction
peripheral consolidation
peripheral cutaneous vasoconstriction
peripheral embolus
peripheral equalization
peripheral fracture
peripheral gating technique
peripheral infiltrate
peripheral laser angioplasty (PLA)
peripheral lesion
peripherally inserted central (PICC)
  catheter
peripheral loading
peripheral lung disease
peripherally inserted central catheter
  (PICC)
peripheral MR angiography
peripheral nerve
peripheral nodule
peripheral ossification
peripheral parenchymal atelectasis
peripheral percutaneous interventions
  (PPI)
peripheral pulmonary artery stenosis
peripheral pulmonic stenosis
peripheral quantitative computed
  tomography technology (pQCT)
peripheral resistance

peripheral small airways study
peripheral vascular disease,
  arteriosclerotic
peripheral vascular resistance,
  decreased
peripheral veins, absent
peripheral vessels
peripheral washout sign
periphery, echogenic
periphery of the lung
periportal adenopathy
periportal area
periportal low attenuation
periportal tracking of blood
periprosthetic bone resorption
periprosthetic leak (leakage)
periradicular nerve
periradicular sheath
perirectal abscess
perirenal abscess
perirenal fat
perirenal hematoma
perirenal hemorrhage
perirenal mass
perirenal septum
perirenal space
perirolandic cortex
perisigmoid colon
perisinusoidal space
peristalsing bowel
peristalsis
  absent
  accelerated
  decreased
  increased
  reversed
  uterine
  visible
peristaltic contraction
peristaltic rush
peristaltic wave
peristriate cortex

peritoneal cavity
  greater sac of
  lesser sac of
peritoneal cavity abscess
peritoneal catheter
peritoneal ectopic pregnancy locations
peritoneal endometriosis
peritoneal enhancement
peritoneal effusion
peritoneal mouse (free body)
peritoneal-venous shunt patency test
peritoneogram
peritoneography, CT
peritoneovenous shunt (PVS)
peritoneum
  parietal
  pelvic
  visceral
peritonitis, bile
peritonsillar abscess
peritumoral injection
periureteral fibrosis
periureteric fibrosis
periurethral abscess
periurethral laceration
perivalvular dehiscence
perivalvular disruption
perivalvular dehiscence
perivalvular disruption
perivalvular leak
perivascular canal
perivascular distribution
perivascular edema
perivascular fibrosis
perivascular plane
perivascular space of Virchow-Robin
periventricular density
periventricular gray (PVG) matter
periventricular halo
periventricular leukomalacia (PVL)
periventricular white matter
perivenular nodularity

perivesical inflammation
perivitelline space
Perkins line
PermaCath dual lumen catheter
permanent brachytherapy
permeability
  capillary
  membrane
  tumor capillary
permeability-type pulmonary edema
permeative lesion
peroneal area
peroneal artery
peroneal muscles
peroneal obliterative thrombus
peroneal-tibial trunk
peroneal vein
peroneus tertius
perpetuation of atelectasis
perrenal hemorrhage
Persantine thallium scanning
Persantine thallium stress test
persistent bronchopleural fistula
persistent common atrioventricular
  canal
persistent fetal circulation
persistent occipitoposterior position
persistent splenomegaly
persistent truncus arteriosus
personal digital assistant (PDA)
perspective volume rendering (PVR)
Pertechnegas
pertechnetate sodium
Perthes-Bankart lesion
Perthes disease
Perthes epiphysis
pertrochanteric fracture
pertubation
  absorptive
  radiation dose
pertussoid eosinophilic pneumonia
perusal
pervenous catheter

pes abductus
pes adductus
pes anserinus
pes arcuatus
pes calcaneocavus
pes calcaneovalgus
pes calcaneus
pes cavovalgus
pes cavovarus
pes cavus
pes contortus
pes equinovalgus
pes equinovarus
pes equinus
pes excavatus
pes malleus valgus
pes planovalgus
pes plantigrade planus
pes planus
pes pronation
pes pronatus
pes supinatus
pes valgus
pes varus
pessary
PET (positron emission tomography)
  PET balloon, USCI
  PET balloon with window and
    extended collection chamber
  PET metabolic imaging
  PET myocardial fatty acid imaging
  PET perfusion imaging
  PET radioligands
  PET radiopharmaceuticals
  PET target material
petal-fugal flow on angiography
Petit disease
petroclinoid ligament
petroclival region
petromastoid
petro-occipital synchondrosis
petrosal bone
petrosal nerve

petrosal sinus
petrosphenoid
petrosquamosal
petrous bone
petrous carotid canal stenosis
petrous pyramid
petrous ridge
petrous segment of carotid artery
Peutz-Jeghers gastrointestinal
 polyposis
Peyer patch
Pezzer catheter
Pfeiffer-Comberg method
Pfeiffer syndrome
PFFD (proximal focal femoral
 deficiency)
P53-mediated radioresistance
PFOB imaging agent
PF-PACS system
PFR (peak filling rate)
PFR (proximal fragment ratio)
 measurement
PFWT (pain-free walking time) on
 treadmill
PG (percutaneous gastrostomy)
PGK (Panos G. Koutrouvelis, M.D.)
 stereotactic device
phagedenic ulcer
phagocytosis, MR imaging of
phakomatoses
phalangeal bones
phalangeal glenoidal ligament of hand
phalangeal herniation
phalanx (pl. phalanges)
 base of
 waist of
Phalen position
Phalen stress test
Phantom cardiac guidewire
pharmacodynamic study
pharyngoesophageal junction
pharyngoesophageal sphincter
pharmacologic intervention

pharmacologic stress dual isotope
 myocardial perfusion SPECT
pharmacologic stress echocardiography
pharmacoradiologic disimpaction of
 esophageal foreign body
PharmaSeed iodine-125 seeds
PharmaSeed palladium-103 seeds
pharyngeal area
pharyngoesophageal diverticulum
pharyngoesophageal function
pharynx
 laryngeal part of
 nasal part of
 oral part of
phase (see also *period*)
 corticomedullary (CP)
 delayed
 diastolic depolarization
 equilibrium
 expiratory
 hepatic arterial (HAP)
 inspiratory
 late
 NCP (noncontrast)
 NP (nephrographic)
 parenchymatous
 plateau (in cardiac action
  potentials)
 portal venous (PVP)
 prolonged expiratory
 prolonged inspiratory
 PVP (portal venous)
 rapid filling
 thin-section excretory
 vascular
 ventilation
 wash-in
 washout
phase analysis
phase angle
phase cycling
phase contrast angiography
phase contrast imaging

phase contrast MRE
phased-array surface coil
phased-array, symmetrical
phase delay
phase difference
phase-encoded motion artifact
phase encode pulse
phase encode time-reduced acquisition
   sequence
phase identification
phase image (imaging)
phase relation
phase sensitive detector
phase shift
phase shifting interferometry
phase shift velocity mapping
phase-unwrapping method
phase velocity image
phasic contractions
phenobarbital
phenomenological effective surface
   potential
phenomenon (pl. phenomena)
   A
   aberrant micturition
   aliasing
   anniversary
   Aschner
   Ashman
   Austin Flint
   baked brain
   Bancaud
   Bell
   booster
   Bowditch staircase
   combined-flexion
   coronary steal
   crus
   Cushing
   dip
   dip and plateau
   Doppler
   embolic
   extinction

phenomenon *(cont.)*
   flare
   flip-flop
   freezing
   Friedreich
   Gaertner (Gärtner)
   Gallavardin
   gap conduction
   Gibbs
   Goldblatt
   Gordon knee
   Gowers
   Hering
   Jod-Basedow
   Kasabach-Merritt
   Katz-Wachtle
   Kernohan notch
   kindling
   Litten diaphragm
   Marin-Amat
   no-reflow
   nonspecific
   on-off
   Piltz-Westphal
   Robin Hood (steal syndrome)
   R on T
   Schellong-Strisower
   Schiff-Sherrington
   Schramm
   staircase
   steal
   steal syndrome
   stone heart
   treppe
   Uhthoff
   unilateral Raynaud
   V
   vacuum
   vacuum joint
   vertebral steal
   Wenckebach
   zone
pheochromocytoma
Philips catheter

Philips CT scanner
Philips DVI 1 system
Philips Gyroscan ACS scanner
Philips Gyroscan Intera scanner
Philips Gyroscan NT; NT5; NT15
  scanner
Philips Gyroscan S5 scanner
Philips Gyroscan T5 scanner
Philips linear accelerator (LINAC)
Philips 1.5T NT MR scanner
Philips Tomoscan 350 CT scanner
Philips Tomoscan SR 6000 CT scanner
Philips ultrasound with endovaginal
  transducer
phlebogram (phlebography), MR
  ascending
  ascending contrast
  direct puncture
  impedance
phleboid
phlebolith
phleborheography (PRG)
phlebosclerosis
phlebostasis
phlebostenosis
phlebothrombosis
phlegmon
  Holz
  pancreatic
  periurethral
phlegmonous
phoenix abscess
PhorMax CR (computed radiography)
  system
Phosphocol P 32 (chromic phosphate
  P 32) radiotherapy agent
phosphoric acid imaging agent
phosphorus (P) (an element)
  ^{32}P chromic phosphate radiotherapy
    agent
  ^{32}P sodium phosphate
phosphorus, hand bone
phosphorus metabolites

phosphorus nuclear magnetic
  resonance spectroscopy (P-MRS)
phosphorus PMT (pyridoxyl-5-methyl
  tryptophan)
phosphorus-32 intracavitary irradiation
phosphorus-32 sodium phosphate
Phospho-Soda (Fleet) enema
photoabsorption
photo-plotter film
photoacoustic ultrasonography
photocell plethysmography
photodeficient region
photodetectors, CCD
photodiode
photodisruption
photoelasticity
photographic technique
  Debye-Scherrer
  Laue
photography, CT bone window
photolabel, long wavelength
photon
  annihilation
  soft
photon attenuation measurement
photon deficiency
photon deficient lesion
photon densitometry
photon interaction depth
photon-neutron mixed-beam
  radiotherapy
photon therapy beam line
photonic medicine
photopeak
photopenia
photopenic area on film or scan
photopenic defect
photopenic region
Photopic Imaging ultrasound system
photoplethysmographic digit
photoplethysmographic monitoring
photoplethysmography (PPG)
photoreceptor fractional velocity error

photoreceptor motion
photostimulable luminescence intensity
photostimulable phosphor dental
   radiography (PSP)
phrenic artery
phrenic pedicle
phrenoesophageal ligament
phrenogastric gastric
phrenovertebral junction
phrygian cap deformity
phthinoid chest
phthisis, aneurysmal
PHTN (pulmonary hypertension)
Phylax implantable cardioverter-
   defibrillator (Biotronik)
phyllodes tumor
physeal bar
physeal cartilage
physeal closure
physeal damage
physeal distraction
physeal fracture
physeal injury
physeal plate fracture
physicochemical speciation
physiological uptake
physiologic flow
physiologic regurgitation
physiologic shunt flow
physis (pl. physes)
   distal tibial
   fibular
   fused
   medial
   unfused
phytobezoar
PI (pulmonic insufficiency)
pia arachnoid
pia mater
pial vessels
PIBC (percutaneous intra-aortic
   balloon counterpulsation)
pica artifact

PICA (posterior inferior cerebellar
   artery)
PICA (posterior inferior communica-
   ting artery)
Pick body
Pick bundle
Pick disease
Picker camera
Picker CT scanner
Picker Magnascanner
Picker MR scanner
Picker PQ 5000 helical CT scanner
Picker PQ-2000 spiral CT scanner
Picker SPECT attenuation correction
Picket Fence fiducial localization
   stereotactic system
Pico-ST II low profile balloon catheter
picture archive and communication
   system (PACs) for imaging
picture archiving and communications
   systems in radiation oncology
   (PACSRO)
picture element (pixel)
picture frame pattern of vertebral
   bodies
PID (pelvic inflammatory disease)
PID (portal imaging device)
PIE (pulmonary interstitial
   emphysema)
piece, chin-occiput
Piedmont fracture
pigeon-breeder's lung
pigeon-breeder's pneumonitis
pigeon chest
pigeon-fancier's lung
Pigg-O-Stat x-ray chair for child
piggybacking
pigmented villonodular synovitis
pigtail catheter
pillar
   anterior cervical
   posterior cervical
pillar fracture (cervical spine)

pillar view
PillCam video capsule
pillion fracture
pillow fracture
pilonidal cyst
pilonidal sinus
pin pattern
PIN (posterior interosseous nerve)
    entrapment
pinchcock mechanism at esophago-
    gastric junction
pinched nerve
pincushion distortion, radiographic
pineal apoplexy
pineal body, calcified
pineal calcification displaced from
    midline
pineal gland, calcified
pineal gland tumor
pinealoma tumor
pineal region
pineoblastoma
pineocytoma
ping-pong fracture
pinhole, bone
pinhole collimator
pinhole image
Pinnacle 3 radiation therapy planning
    system
PION (posterior interosseous nerve)
PIP (peak inspiratory pressure)
PIP (proximal interphalangeal)
    PIP articulation
    PIP joint
Pipelle endometrial suction catheter
pipestem arteries
pipe-stemming of ankle-brachial index
PIPIDA (P-isopropylacetanilide-
    iminodiacetic acid)
    99mTcPIPIDA hepatobiliary scan
PIPJ (proximal interphalangeal joint)
Pipkin classification of femoral
    fracture

Pirie bone
Pirie sinus view
piriform muscle
pisiform bone of wrist
pisotriquetral joint
pistoning
piston sign
pit
    anal
    articular
    auditory
    central
    colonic
    costal
    cutaneous
    gastric
    postanal
pitch
    scan
    spiral CT
pitch ratio
Pittsburgh pneumonia
pituitary abscess
pituitary adamantinoma
pituitary flush
pituitary fossa
pituitary gland
pituitary microadenoma
pituitary stalk distortion (PSD)
pituitary tumor
pivoting table
pixel (picture element)
    edge-region
    maximum-intensity (MIP)
    normal-region
pixel block, 8 x 8
pixel noise
pixel-oriented algorithms
pixel projection
pixel values
    bright
    dark
Pixsys FlashPoint camera

placement
  annular
  catheter
  central venous line
  intracoronary stent
  intrapericardial patch lead
  percutaneous endoluminal
  poststent
  radiotherapy field
  shim
  shunt
  subannular
  subject
placement of radiation therapy fields,
  ultrasonic guidance for
placenta
  abnormal adherence of
  accessory
  adherent
  annular
  battledore
  bilobate
  chorioallantoic
  chorioamniotic
  cirsoid
  deciduate
  Duncan
  fetal
  first trimester
  fundal
  horseshoe
  incarcerated
  kidney-shaped
  marginal
  maternal
  nondeciduate
  panduriform
  retained
  Schultze
  second trimester
  third trimester
  velamentous
  villous

placental site trophoblastic tumor
placenta previa
  central
  complete
  incomplete
  lateral
  marginal
  partial
  total
placental abruption (abruptio
  placentae)
placental localization
placental polyp
placental souffle
placentography
plafond fracture
plafond, tibial
plagiocephalic
plagiocephaly
plague pneumonia
plain film
plain film radiography
plain-paper image
plain tomogram
planar exercise thallium-201
  scintigraphy
planar (2D) imaging
planar LAO image
planar spin imaging
planar thallium scan
planar thallium with quantitative
  analysis
planar view
Planck constant
plane (anatomical area)
  anatomic
  areolar
  auriculoinfraorbital
  axial
  axiolabiolingual
  axiomesiodistal
  bite
  buccolingual

plane *(cont.)*
  capsular
  circular
  coronal
  coronary oblique
  E
  eye-ear
  facial
  fat
  first parallel pelvic
  flexion-extension
  four-chamber
  fourth parallel pelvic
  Frankfort horizontal
  frontal
  gonion-gnathion
  Hensen
  Hodge
  horizontal
  imaging
  internervous
  interspinous
  intertubercular
  Ludwig
  median
  median sagittal
  mesiodistal
  midsagittal
  occlusal
  optimal imaging
  parallel tag
  paramedian sagittal
  pelvic
  perivascular
  sagittal
  sella-nasion
  semicoronal
  short axis
  slicing
  spinous
  sternoxiphoid
  subadventitial
  subcostal (SCP)

plane *(cont.)*
  supracristal (SCP)
  subintimal cleavage
  suprasternal
  tag
  thoracic
  transaxial
  transmedial
  transpyloric
  transtrabecular (TTP)
  transumbilical (TUP)
  transverse
  tumor cleavage
  valve
  varus-valgus
  vertical
  XY
  ZY
plane of cleavage of tumor
planigram
planigraphy
planimeter
planimetric analysis
planimetry
planogram
planography
planovalgus foot deformity
plantar aponeurosis
plantar axial view
plantar calcaneal spur
plantar compartment
plantar flexion-inversion deformity
plantar hyperplasia
plantar spur
plantar vault
plantaris muscle
plantaris rupture
plantarward
plantodorsal, axial
plaque (also plaquing)
  arterial
  arteriosclerotic
  atheromatous

plaque *(cont.)*
  atherosclerotic
  calcific
  calcified
  concentric atherosclerotic
  coral reef
  disrupted
  eccentric
  eccentric atherosclerotic
  echogenic
  echolucent
  endocardial
  fatty
  fibrofatty
  fibrotic
  fibrous
  fissured atheromatous
  gastrointestinal
  Hollenhorst
  Hutchinson
  iliac
  infiltrating
  intimal
  intraluminal
  Lichtheim
  lipid-laden
  luminal
  multiple sclerosis (MS)
  neuritic senile
  noncompliant
  obstructive
  pleural
  pulverized
  Randall
  residual
  sclerotic
  senile
  sessile
  stenotic
  talc
  ulcerated
  uncalcified
plaque cleaving

plaque compression
plaque-containing artery
plaque constituents
plaque erosion
plaque fracture (or fracturing)
plaquelike linear defect
plaque regression
plaque remodeling
plaque rupture
plaque splitting
plaque tearing
plaque vaporization
plaquing (see *plaque*)
plasma cell pneumonia
plasma cell pneumonitis (PCP)
plasma radioiron disappearance rate
plasma radioiron turnover rate
plasma volume
plastica, linitis
plastic clot
plastic retractor
plate
  acetabular reconstruction
  alar
  anal
  auditory
  axial
  basal
  bone
  bone flap fixation
  bony
  budding
  cap-and-anchor
  cardiogenic
  cartilaginous growth
  chorionic
  clinoid
  cloacal
  cloverleaf
  coaptation
  compression
  condylar
  connecting

plate *(cont.)*
    cortical
    cranial bone fixation
    cribriform
    dorsal
    dual
    dynamic compression (DCP)
    end
    epiphyseal cartilage
    ethmovomerine
    femoral
    fibrocartilaginous
    flat
    flexor palmar
    foot
    frontal
    fusion
    growth
    hilar
    interfragmentary
    intertrochanteric
    localization-compression grid
    meningioma of cribriform
    microfixation
    nail
    neutralization
    occipitocervical
    orbital
    orthotic
    overlay
    palmar
    pedicle
    planar
    plantar
    pterygoid
    skull
    stabilization
    stainless steel
    stem base
    subchondral bone
    supracondylar
    tarsal
    tectal

plate *(cont.)*
    tendon
    3-D or 3D (three-dimensional)
    titanium
    trapezoidal shaped sandwich
    vertebral body
    volar
plate and screw system, MRI-
    compatible
plateau
    multiple sclerosis
    tibial
plateau fracture
platelet-activating factor inhibitor
platelet-rich thrombus
platelet survival study
platelike atelectasis
platelike fibrous scar in lungs
platform, Cemax PACS
platinum coil
platinum coil used in interventional
    neuroradiology
platinum radiopaque catheter marker
    patterns
platybasia
platycephaly
platypellic pelvis
platypelloid pelvis
platypodia
platyspondylosis
platyspondyly
PLC (posterolateral corner) of knee
pleating of ligamentum flavum
pleating of small bowel
pledget(s)
pleomorphic adenoma
pleomorphic lymphoma
pleomorphic xanthoastrocytoma
pleomorphism, nuclear
plesiography (brachytherapy)
plethora of findings
plethoric
plethysmogram

plethysmograph, Medgraphics body
plethysmography
  air
  body box
  digital
  Doppler ultrasonic velocity
    detector segmental
  exercise strain gauge venous
  impedance (IPG)
  Medsonic
  photocell
  strain gauge
  venous
pleura (pl. pleurae)
  cervical
  congested
  costal
  costodiaphragmatic recess of
  diaphragmatic
  edematous
  mediastinal
  parietal
  pericardiac
  pulmonary
  silicotic visceral
  visceral
  wrinkled
pleural adhesions, fibrous
pleural apical hematoma cap
pleural-based area of increased
  opacity
pleural cap
pleural cavity
pleural cupula (pl. cupulae)
pleural effusion
  ipsilateral
  liquid
  loculated
pleural empyema
pleural exudate
pleural fibrosis, asbestos-induced
pleural fistula
pleural flap

pleural fluid
pleural implants, malignant
pleural involvement
pleural line
pleural margins
pleural plaque
pleural pressure
pleural reflection
  costal
  mediastinodiaphragmatic
  sternal
  vertebral
pleural rind
pleural sac
pleural space
pleural thickening
pleural trauma
pleurisy
  acute
  acute fibrinous
  adhesive
  blocked
  cholesterol
  chronic
  chyliform
  chyloid
  chylous
  circumscribed
  costal
  diaphragmatic
  diffuse
  double
  dry
  encysted
  exudative
  fibrinous
  hemorrhagic
  ichorous
  indurative
  interlobular
  latent
  mediastinal
  metapneumonic

pleurisy *(cont.)*
   plastic
   pneumococcal
   primary
   proliferating
   pulmonary
   pulsating
   purulent
   sacculated
   secondary
   septic
   serofibrinous
   serofibrous
   seropurulent
   serous
   single
   staphylococcal
   streptococcal
   suppurative
   typhoid
   visceral
   wet
pleurisy with effusion
pleuritic pneumonia
pleurocutaneous fistula
pleurogenic pneumonia
pleuroparenchymal plaque
pleuroperitoneal canal
pleuropulmonary adhesion
plexiform
plexiform neurofibromatosis
plexus
   abdominal aortic
   anterior coronary
   anterior pulmonary
   aortic
   Auerbach mesenteric
   autonomic
   axillary
   basilar
   Batson
   biliary
   brachial

plexus *(cont.)*
   calcification of choroid
   cardiac
   carotid
   cavernous
   celiac
   cervical
   choroid
   ciliary ganglionic
   coccygeal
   colic
   colonic myenteric
   common carotid
   coronary
   cystic
   deep cardiac
   deferential
   enteric
   esophageal
   Exner
   extradural vertebral
   facial
   femoral
   gastric
   gastroesophageal variceal
   great cardiac
   hemorrhoidal
   hepatic nerve
   hypogastric
   ileocolic
   inferior mesenteric
   intermesenteric
   lumbar
   lumbosacral
   lymph
   Meissner
   myenteric
   nerve
   pampiniform
   paravertebral nerve
   paravertebral venous
   pelvic
   perimuscular

plexus *(cont.)*
  pharyngeal
  presacral
  prostatic venous
  pulmonary
  rectal
  right coronary
  sacral
  sciatic
  solar
  spinal nerve
  submucosal venous
  superficial
  superior hypogastric
  superior mesenteric
  uterovaginal
  vaginal
  vascular
  venous
  vertebral
  vertebral venous
  vesical
  vesical venous
plexus injury
plica (pl. plicae)
  medial
  parapatellar
  suprapatellar
  synovial
plication defect
P-LINK software
PLL (posterior longitudinal ligament)
ploidy, DNA
P loop (on vectorcardiography)
plots, cluster
PLSA (posterolateral spinal artery)
plug
  meconium
  mucus
plugged liver biopsy
PMR (percutaneous transmyocardial
  revascularization)
Plummer disease

Plummer-Vinson syndrome
plump vessel
plurality of slices
plutonium, environmental
PM (posterior mitral)
PMD (papillary muscle dysfunction)
PML (posterior mitral leaflet)
pmol (picomole)
P-MRS (phosphorus magnetic resonance spectroscopy)
PMT (pyridoxyl-5-methyl tryptophan)
  imaging agent
PMT robotic fulcrumless tomographic
  system
PMV (percutaneous mitral balloon
  valvuloplasty)
PMV (prolapsed mitral valve)
PMVL (posterior mitral valve leaflet)
PNC (premature nodal contraction)
PNET (primitive neuroectodermal
  tumor)
pneumatic bone
pneumatization
pneumatocele
pneumencephalography, lumbar
pneumatocyst, cervical spine intraosseous
pneumoarthrogram
pneumoarthrogram sign
pneumocele
pneumocephalus
pneumococcal pleurisy
pneumoconiosis
pneumoconstriction
pneumocystic infection
pneumocystis
Pneumocystis carinii pneumonia
Pneumocystis pneumonia (PCP)
pneumocystography
pneumocystotomography
pneumoencephalogram (PEG)
pneumoencephalographic pattern
pneumoencephalography

pneumoencephalomyelogram
pneumoencephalomyelography
pneumogastrography
pneumogram
pneumography
  cerebral
  retroperitoneal
pneumogynogram
pneumohemothorax
pneumointestinalis
pneumolith
pneumomediastinography
pneumomediastinum
  postoperative
  radiolucent
pneumomyelography
pneumonia (see also *pneumonitis*)
  acute
  alcoholic
  allergic
  amebic
  anthrax
  apex
  apical
  Aspergillus bacterial
  aspiration
  asthmatic
  atypical bronchial
  atypical interstitial
  bacterial
  bilious
  bronchial
  bronchiolitis obliterans with
    organizing (BOOP)
  Buhl desquamative
  capillary
  caseous
  catarrhal
  central
  cerebral
  chelonian
  chemical
  chickenpox

pneumonia *(cont.)*
  chronic eosinophilic
  classic interstitial
  community-acquired (bacterial)
    (CAP)
  consolidative
  contusion
  Corrigan
  cryptogenic organizing
  cryptogenic organizing bacterial
  deglutition
  delayed resolution of
  desquamative interstitial (DIP)
  diffuse
  double
  Eaton agent
  Escherichia coli bacterial
  embolic
  exogenous lipoid
  eosinophilic
  ephemeral
  exogenous
  fibrinous
  fibrous
  Francisella tularensis bacterial
  Friedländer
  fungal
  gangrenous
  giant cell
  giant cell interstitial (GIP)
  gram-negative bacilli
  granulomatous
  gray hepatization stage of
  Group A hemolytic streptococci
  Haemophilus influenzae
  Hecht
  hypersensitivity
  hypostatic
  incomplete resolution of
  indurative
  infantile
  inhalation
  interstitial plasma cell

pneumonia *(cont.)*
    irradiation
    Klebsiella pneumoniae
    lingular
    lipoid
    lobar
    lobular
    Loeffler bacterial
    lymphoid interstitial
    massive
    metastatic
    migratory
    mycoplasmal
    necrotizing
    nonbacterial
    nosocomial
    obstructive
    oil-aspiration
    opportunistic fungal
    parenchymatous
    passive
    pertussoid eosinophilic
    Pittsburgh
    plague
    plasma cell
    pleuritic
    pleurogenic
    Pneumocystis
    Pneumocystis carinii
    postobstructive
    postoperative
    post-traumatic
    primary atypical
    protozoal
    purulent
    radiation
    red hepatization stage of
    resolving
    respiratory syncytial viral
    rheumatic
    rickettsial
    right-sided
    secondary

pneumonia *(cont.)*
    segmental
    septic
    staphylococcal
    streptococcal
    Staphylococcus aureus bacterial
    subacute allergic
    superficial
    suppurative
    terminal
    toxic
    toxemic
    traumatic
    tubercle bacillus
    tuberculous
    tularemic
    typhoid
    unresolved
    varicella
    ventilator-associated (VAP)
    viral
    walking
    wandering
    white
    woolsorter's
pneumonic infiltrate
pneumonitis (see also *pneumonia*)
    acid aspiration
    acute interstitial
    aspiration
    bacterial
    basilar
    chemical
    cholesterol
    chronic
    congenital rubella
    cytomegalovirus
    early
    granulomatous
    hypersensitivity
    interstitial
    lipoid
    lymphocytic interstitial

pneumonitis *(cont.)*
  malarial
  manganese
  Mycoplasma (mycoplasmal)
  pigeon-breeder's
  plasma cell (PCP)
  radiation
  staphylococcal
  trimellitic anhydritic
  uremic
  ventilation
pneumonocirrhosis
pneumonography
pneumopericardium
pneumoperitoneum
pneumopreperitoneum
pneumopyelography
pneumoradiography
pneumoroentgenogram
pneumoscrotum
pneumothorax
  artificial
  basilar
  blowing
  clicking
  closed
  congenital
  diagnostic
  extrapleural
  induced
  life-threatening
  open
  positive-pressure
  pressure
  simultaneous bilateral spontaneous
    (SBSP)
  spontaneous tension
  sucking
  tension
  therapeutic
  traumatic
  tuberculous
  uncomplicated
  valvular

pneumoventriculography
PNL (percutaneous nephrolithotripsy)
PO$_2$ imaging
pocket (see also *pouch*)
  air
  endocardial
  infraclavicular
  rectus sheath
  regurgitant
  subpectoral
  Zahn
pocket Doppler
pockets of Zahn
point (pl. points)
  Addison
  alveolar
  apophysary
  apophyseal
  auricular
  bleeding
  Cannon
  Cannon-Boehm
  cardinal
  Chauffard
  Clado
  congruent
  Cope
  coplanar contour
  craniometric
  dorsal
  end
  entry
  equilibrium
  frontopolar
  glenoid
  Hartmann
  lead
  Mackenzie
  midinguinal
  nodal
  output
  Pauly
  preauricular

point *(cont.)*
  random
  reentry
  saddle
  sample
  seed
  Sudek
  target
  white
point imaging
point in space stereotactic biopsies
point localization
point scanning
point spread functions
point to point protocol (PPP)
Poisson-distributed activity
  concentrations
POL (posterior oblique ligament)
Poland classification of epiphyseal
  fracture
polar coordinate system
polarity-altered spectral-selective
  acquisition (PASTA) imaging
polarization, chemically induced
  dynamic nuclear
polarized
polarographic needle electrode
  measurement
pole
  abapical
  cephalic
  fetal
  frontal
  germinal
  inferior
  kidney
  lower
  middle
  patellar
  pole
  scaphoid
  superior
  temporal
  upper

pole figure texture analysis
pole of kidney
Polhemus 3 digitizer
Politano-Leadbetter procedure
Pollack open-end Flexi-Tip ureteral
  catheter
pollex pedis
polyarticular symmetric tophaceous
  joint inflammation
polyclonal IgG
polycystic kidney disease
polycystic ovary (or ovarian) syndrome
polydactyly
PolyFlo catheter
PolyFlo peripherally inserted central
  catheter
polygelin colloid imaging agent
polygon mirror
polygyria
polyhydramnios
polymer
  friction-reducing
  PLA (polyactic acid)
polymer-coated drug-eluting stent
polymeric endoluminal paving stent
polynomial stepwise multiple-linear
  regression
polyorchidism
polyostotic bone lesion
polyostotic fibrous dysplasia
polyp
  adenomatous
  benign
  bleeding
  broad-based
  bronchial
  cardiac
  cervical
  choanal
  colon
  colonic
  colorectal
  cystic

polyp *(cont.)*
dental
duodenal
endometrial
fibrinous
fibroepithelial
fibrovascular
gastric
hamartomatous gastric
Hopmann
hydatid
hyperplastic gastric
inflammatory fibroid
juvenile
laryngeal
lipomatous
lymphoid
malignant
metaplastic
metastatic
mucous
multiple
myomatous
nasal
neoplastic
osseous
pedunculated
Peutz-Jeghers
placental
postinflammatory
rectal
regenerative
retention
sessile
sigmoid
single
stalk of
tubular
tubulovillous
urethral
uterine
vascular
villous

polyp of ureter
polyp of urethra
polypoid adenomyoma
polypoid calcified irregular mass
polypoid filling defect
polypoid lesion
polypoid lymphoid hyperplasia
polyposis
adenomatous
diffuse mucosal
familial adenomatous (FAP)
familial colorectal
familial gastrointestinal
familial intestinal
FAP (familial adenomatous)
filiform
gastric
hamartomatous
intestinal
juvenile
multiple
Peutz-Jeghers gastrointestinal
polyp stalk
polysplenia
Polystan venous return catheter
polystyrene, cross-linked
polytomographic radiology
polytomography
polytrauma
polyurethane foam embolus
polyurethane pail-handle coiled-tip
peritoneal dialysis catheter
polyurethane stent
polyvinyl alcohol (PVA) cryogel
polyvinyl alcohol particle size
Pompe disease
pond fracture
P1-P4 segments of posterior cerebral
artery (PCA)
pons (pl. pontes)
caudal
infarction of
pons and midbrain, tegmentum of

pontine angle
pontine contusion
pontine glioma tumor
pontine hemorrhage
pontine infarction
pontine-medullary levels
pontocerebellar fibers
pontocerebellar glioma
pontomedullary junction
pontomesencephalic junction
pool
  blood
  focal
  vascular blood
pooling of blood in extremities
pooling, venous
poorly differentiated tumor
poorly mobile leaflet
poor shimming of MRI magnet
poor uptake
popcorn calcification
popliteal aneurysm
popliteal artery entrapment syndrome
popliteal artery occlusive disease
popliteal bypass
popliteal fossa
popliteal in situ bypass
popliteal recess
popliteal space
popliteal to distal in situ bypass
popliteal trifurcation
popliteal vein
porcelain gallbladder
Porcher-Porot oblique transmaxillary
  view of the foramen jugulare
porencephalic cyst
porencephalous
porencephaly
porosis, cerebral
porous ingrowth
porous metallic stent
porous polyethylene dialysis catheter

port
  Aeon vascular access
  BardPort implantable
  BodyFlex
  B-port implant infusion
  injection
  noncoplanar multiple static
  parallel opposed unmodified
  Quinton vascular access
  RadPICC
  Rosenblatt implan table vascular
    access
  side entry access (SEA)
  single
  SlimPort implantable vascular
    access
  tangential
  Thora-Port
  treatment
  Triumph-I vascular
  vent
  Vital-Port vascular access
  Xtent vascular access
portable C-arm image intensifier
  fluoroscopy
portable x-ray
portable film
Port-A-Cath catheter
portacaval anastomosis, end to side
portacaval shunt
portal imaging device (PID)
portal-systemic shunt (or portosystemic)
portal to portal bridging
portal triad
portal vein cavernous transformation
portal venous-dominant phase (PVP)
  images (CT scan)
portal vein thrombosis
portal venography
portal venous phase (PVP)
PortalVision radiation oncology
  system

Portnoy ventricular catheter
porto-azygos collaterals
portogram
portography
  arterial
  CT arterial
  double spiral CT arterial
  percutaneous transhepatic
  splenic
portopulmonary shunt
portosystemic (or portal-systemic)
Posicam HZ PET scanner
Posicam PET (positron emission
  tomography) medical imaging
position (see also *projection*; *view*)
  ABER (abduction and external
    rotation)
  anatomic
  anatomical
  anterior oblique
  antero-oblique
  axial calcaneal
  axial sesamoid
  barber chair
  bayonet fracture
  beach chair
  Bertel
  Blackett-Healy (for teres minor or
    subscapularis insertion visualiza-
    tion)
  catheter tip
  curled-up
  decubitus
  dorsal
  dorsal lithotomy
  dorsal recumbent
  dorsal supine
  dorsosacral
  eccentric (of structure)
  erect
  feet-first
  Feist-Mankin
  fetal

position *(cont.)*
  flank
  Fowler
  frogleg or frog-leg
  frontoanterior
  frontoposterior
  frontotransverse
  full lateral
  genupectoral
  Harris and Beath
  head-first
  Holly
  horizontal
  infragenicular
  infrapulmonary
  Jones
  knee-chest
  kneeling
  LAO (left anterior oblique)
  lateral
  left anterior oblique (LAO)
  lateral decubitus
  lateral recumbent
  leapfrog
  left flank
  left frontoanterior (LFA)
  left frontoposterior (LFP)
  left frontotransverse (LFT)
  left lateral decubitus
  left mentotransverse (LMT)
  left occipitoposterior (LOP)
  left occipitotransverse (LOT)
  left sacroposterior (LSP)
  left side down decubitus
  lithotomy
  lordotic
  lotus
  LPO (left posterior oblique)
  mentoanterior (MA)
  mentoposterior (MP)
  mentotransverse
  modified dorsal lithotomy
  near anatomic

position *(cont.)*
  Nefertiti sniff
  neutral hip
  noncoaxial catheter tip
  normal anatomic
  occipitoanterior (OA)
  occipitoposterior (OP)
  occiput-anterior (OA)
  occiput left anterior (OLA)
  occiput-posterior (OP)
  orthopnea
  paramedian
  park bench
  partial flexion
  persistent occipitoposterior
  Phalen
  prayer
  prone
  pulmonary capillary wedge
  RAO (right anterior oblique)
  rectus
  recumbent
  reverse Trendelenburg
  right anterior oblique (RAO)
  right frontoanterior (RFA)
  right frontoposterior (RFP)
  right frontotransverse (RFT)
  right lateral decubitus
  right mentoanterior (RMA)
  right mentotransverse (RMT)
  right occipitoanterior (ROA)
  right occipitoposterior (ROP)
  right occipitotransverse (ROT)
  right sacroanterior (RSA)
  right sacroposterior (RSP)
  right sacrotransverse (RST)
  right posterior oblique (RPO)
  right-side-down decubitus
  sacroposterior (SP) breech
  sacrotransverse (ST)
  sacrum right posterior (SRP)
  semi-Fowler
  semilateral

position *(cont.)*
  semiprone
  side-lying
  Sims
  spiral
  squatting
  standing
  steep Trendelenburg
  stooped-over
  suboptimal
  supine
  swimmer's
  three-quarters prone
  tibial sesamoid
  Titterington
  transthoracic lateral
  Trendelenburg
  upright
  wedge
position confirmed by fluoroscopy
  with aid of radiopaque marking
positioning error
position of joint, near anatomic
positive GI contrast agent
positive predictive value
positive-pressure pneumothorax
positive tilt test
Positrol II catheter
positron emission computed
  tomography (PET) scan
positron emission tomography (PET)
positron emitters
positron imaging
positron scanning (see *PET scan*)
possible involvement
postablation
postangioplasty aortogram
postangioplasty mural thrombosis
postangioplasty stenosis
post beat filtration
postbiopsy mammogram
postcapillary venules

postcardiotomy lymphocytic splenomegaly
postcatheterization false aneurysm
(PCFP)
postcatheterization femoral (artery)
pseudoaneurysm
postcatheterization injury
postcatheterization urethral stricture
postcentral (sensory) gyrus
postcentral sulcus
postcontrast MR imaging
postcricoid area
postcubital
postdilatation arteriogram
postdrainage cystogram
postdrainage projection
postductal type of coarctation
posterior-anterior (PA)
posterior-aorta transposition of great
vessels
posterior apical segment
posterior axillary line
posterior border of lung
posterior bronchi
posterior cervical pillar (facet joints)
posterior cervical triangle
posterior circulation
posterior colliculus
posterior column deficits (of spine)
posterior commissure
posterior communicating artery (PCA)
posterior compartment lesion
posterior coronary plexus (of heart)
posterior cusp
posterior descending artery (PDA)
posterior fossa
posterior fracture-dislocation
posterior free wall
posterior gray column of cord
posterior gray horns of the spinal
canal
posterior inferior cerebellar artery
(PICA)

posterior inferior communicating
artery (PICA)
posterior intercostal artery
posterior interventricular groove
posterior interventricular vein
posterior joint syndrome
posterior-lateral (posterolateral)
posterior leaflet prolapse
posterior lip
posterior lumbar interbody fusion
(PLIF)
posterior mediastinum
posterior mitral leaflet (PML)
posterior mitral valve leaflet
posterior neck surface coil
posterior oblique position
posterior pericardial well
posterior olive in brain
posterior papillary muscle
posterior pulmonary plexus
posterior root entry zone (PREZ)
posterior root ganglia
posterior segment
posterior semilunar valve
posterior skull view
posterior spine fusion (PSF)
posterior spinocerebellar tract
posterior sulcus
posterior tibial artery
posterior tibial artery pseudoaneurysm
posterior tibiofibular ligament
posterior tibiotalar ligament
posterior tricuspid leaflet (PTL)
posterior wall myocardial infarction
posterior wall of urinary bladder
posterior wall thickness
posteroanterior (PA)
posterobasal wall myocardial
infarction
posteroinferior myocardial infarction
posterolateral aspect
posterolateral spinal artery (PLSA)

posterolateral wall myocardial
  infarction
posteromedial
posteroseptal myocardial infarction
postevacuation film
postganglionic gray fibers
postglomerular arteriolar constriction
postglucose loading exam
postictal cerebral blood flow scan
postinfarction course
postinfarction failure
postinfarction ventricular aneurysm
postinfarction ventriculoseptal defect
postinflammatory pulmonary fibrosis
postinjection image
postirradiation vascular insufficiency
postischemic recovery
postlymphangiography
postmastectomy lymphedema
  syndrome
postmetrizamide CT scan
post mortem orthopantomography
postmyocardiotomy infarction
postnatal ultrasound
postobstetric urethral stricture
postobstructive pneumonia
postoperative acute massive collapse
postoperative bronchopneumonia
postoperative chylothorax
postoperative hemorrhage
postoperative pelvic hematoma
postoperative pneumomediastinum
postoperative pneumonia
postoperative urethral stricture
postorchiectomy para-aortic
  radiotherapy
postpartum hemorrhage
postpartum pituitary apoplexy
postperfusion lung syndrome
postphlebitic incompetence
postprimary tuberculosis
postprocedure nephrostogram
postprocessing (of data)

post-PTCA residual stenosis
postpyelonephritis cortical scarring
postradiation fibrosis
postreduction x-ray
postsphenoidal bone
poststenotic dilatation
poststent placement
poststress ankle/arm Doppler index
poststress images
postsurgical
post-thrombolytic coronary reocclusion
post-tourniquet occlusion angiography
post-transplant acute renal failure
  (ARF)
post-transplantation complication
post-transplant coronary artery disease
post-transplant lymphoproliferative
  disorder (PTLD)
post-traumatic
post-traumatic angulation
post-traumatic cavus
post-traumatic fibrosis
post-traumatic hemophilia
post-traumatic neuroma
post-traumatic osteoporosis
post-traumatic pneumonia
post-traumatic pseudoaneurysm
post-ulnar bone
postvenography phlebitis
postvoid residual (PVR)
postvoid residual urine volume
postvoid(ing) film
potassium (^{43}K) (an element)
  potassium-43 (^{43}K) imaging agent
    (myocardial perfusion imaging)
potassium perchlorate imaging agent
potassium-perchlorate
potential
  electrostatic
  phenomenological effective surface
  sorption
potentiometer
potter's asthma

Pott fracture
Pott puffy tumor
Potts shunt
pouce flottant (floating thumb)
pouch
  antral
  apophyseal
  blind
  blind upper esophageal
  branchial
  Broca pudendal
  celomic
  deep perineal
  Douglas rectouterine
  dural root
  endodermal
  gastric
  Hartmann
  haustral
  Heidenhain
  hepatorenal
  hypophysial
  ileoanal
  ileocecal
  jejunal
  Kock
  Morison
  paracystic
  pararectal
  paravesical
  pendulous
  pharyngeal
  Physick
  Prussak
  Rathke
  rectal
  rectouterine
  rectovaginal
  rectovaginouterine
  rectovesical
  renal
  Seessel
  superficial inguinal

pouch *(cont.)*
  superficial perineal
  suprapatellar
  ultimobranchial
  uterovesical
  vesicouterine
  Zenker
pouching defect
pouch of Douglas abscess
pouchogram
pouchography, evacuation
Poupart inguinal ligament
power
  scanning
  stopping
power Doppler imaging (PDI)
power Doppler sonography
power injection
power injector
Powerline catheter
power-mode color Doppler imaging
PowerPICC catheter
PowerVision ultrasound system
PPAS (peripheral pulmonary artery
  stenosis)
PPH (primary pulmonary hypertension)
PPI (peripheral percutaneous interventions)
PPLO (pleuropneumonia-like
  organisms)
PPM (posterior papillary muscle)
PPP (point to point protocol)
PPRF (paramedian pontine reticular
  formation)
pQCT (peripheral quantitative computed tomography)
pQCT micro-scanner
prayer position
preablation
preacinar arterial wall thickness
preampullary portion of bile duct
preangioplasty stenosis

preaortic space, retropancreatic
preauricular point
precatheterization
precentral gyrus
precentral sulcus
precessing protons
precessional frequency
precharred fiber
precirrhosis
precision, test-retest
precluding catheter passage, tortuosity
preclusionary cue
precocious pseudopuberty
precommunicating segment of anterior
   cerebral artery
precontrast scan
precontrast T1 relaxation time
precordium
   active
   anterior
   bulging
   lateral
precursor sign to rupture of aneurysm
Predator angioplasty balloon catheter
predicted target heart rate
prediction, LSC background
predictive assay
predictive value
predictor
predominance
   anterior
   posterior
   predominant
   temporal
predominant flow loads
preductal coarctation of aorta
pre-ejection interval
pre-ejection period (PEP)
preferential shunting
preformed clot
preformed guidewire
prefrontal bone of von Bardeleben

pregnancy
   abdominal
   ampullar
   bigeminal
   broad ligament
   cervical
   combined
   compound
   cornual
   ectopic
   extrauterine
   fallopian
   false
   heterotopic
   hydatid
   gemellary
   heterotopic
   interstitial
   intraligamentary
   intraperitoneal
   intrauterine
   membranous
   mesenteric
   molar
   multiple
   mural
   ovarian
   ovarioabdominal
   oviductal
   parietal
   phantom
   plural
   post-term
   prolonged
   pseudointraligamentary
   sarcofetal
   sarcohysteric
   spurious
   stump
   toxemia of
   tubal
   tuboabdominal
   tuboligamentary

pregnancy *(cont.)*
  tubo-ovarian
  tubouterine
  twin
  uteroabdominal
  uterotubal
pregnancy tumor
preinvasive lesion
Preiser disease
preliminary film
Prelude vascular introducer
Prelude vascular introducer sheath
premalignant lesion
premammary abscess
premasking, interactive
premature atherosclerosis
premature closure of ductus arteriosus
premature mid-diastolic closure of
  mitral valve
premature rupture of membranes
premature valve closure
premedullary arteriovenous fistula
prenatal hydronephrosis
preoperative bronchoscopy
preoperative renal angiography
preoperative resting MUGA scan
prep (preparation)
  bowel
  kit
  on-column
  touch
prepared and draped (prepped and
  draped)
prepatellar bursa
Prepcat (barium sulfate) imaging agent
prepectorally
preponderance
preponderant
prepontine cistern
prepped and draped
prepulse, spin lock
prepyloric antrum
prepyloric atresia

prepyloric fold
prereduction x-ray
prerenal
presacral mass
presaturation
  fat-selective
  projection
  spatial
presbyesophagus
presbyophrenia
prescan, MRI
prescapula
presentation of fetus
  breech
  brow
  cephalic
  compound
  face
  footling
  frank breech
  parietal
  shoulder
  transverse
  vertex
presenting part
pre-slip changes on x-ray
presphenoidal bone
PRESS sequence
PRESS spectroscopy
pressure
  airway opening
  alveolar
  ambulant venous (AVP)
  ankle-arm
  ankle systolic
  AO or Ao (aorta)
  aortic
  aortic root
  arterial (ART or Art.)
  arterial peak systolic
  atmospheres of
  A wave (left or right atrial
    catheterization)

pressure *(cont.)*
  bile duct
  blood (BP)
  brachial artery
  brachial artery cuff
  brachial artery end diastolic
  brachial artery peak systolic
  C wave (right atrial catheterization)
  capillary
  capillary wedge
  cardiac filling
  central aortic
  central venous (CVP)
  cerebral perfusion
  collapse of jugular venous
  continuous descending (CDP)
  coronary artery perfusion (CPP)
  coronary wedge
  cuff blood
  diastolic blood (DBP)
  diastolic filling (DFP)
  diastolic perfusion
  diastolic pulmonary artery
  distal coronary perfusion
  Doppler ankle systolic
  Doppler blood
  Doppler calf systolic
  Doppler thigh systolic
  elevated
  end diastolic
  end systolic (ESP)
  endocardial
  equalized diastolic
  esophageal peristaltic
  extravascular
  femoral artery (FAP)
  filling
  hepatic wedge
  high blood (HBP)
  high filling
  high interstitial
  high wedge
  increased pulmonary arterial

pressure *(cont.)*
  interstitial fluid hydrostatic
  intracardiac
  intraluminal esophageal
  intrapericardial
  intrapleural
  intrapulmonary
  intrathoracic
  intrathoracic airway
  intraventricular
  intrinsic positive end expiratory
  in vivo balloon
  jugular venous
  LA (left atrium)
  left atrial (LAP)
  left atrial end diastolic
  left-sided heart
  left subclavian central venous
    (LSCVP)
  left ventricular (LV)
  left ventricular cavity
  left ventricular end diastolic
    (LVEDP)
  left ventricular filling
  left ventricular peak systolic
  left ventricular systolic (LVS)
  LES (lower esophageal sphincter)
  low wedge
  maximal respiratory
  maximum inflation
  mean
  mean aortic
  mean arterial (MAP)
  mean atrial
  mean blood
  mean brachial artery
  mean circulatory filling
  mean left atrial
  mean pulmonary artery (MPAP)
  mean pulmonary artery wedge
  mean right atrial
  minimum blood
  PA (pulmonary artery) systolic

pressure *(cont.)*
PAD (pulmonary artery diastolic)
PAS (pulmonary artery systolic)
passage
peak
peak-inflation
peak inspiratory (PIP)
peak regurgitant wave
peak systolic
peak systolic aortic (PSAP)
perfusion
phasic
pleural
portal venous (PVP)
pressure-controlled intermittent
    coronary occlusion
pressure-induced distortion
prevesicle space
primary atypical pneumonia
primary biliary cirrhosis (PBC)
primary diffuse large B-cell
    lymphoma
primary hypertrophic osteo-
    arthropathy (HOA)
primary lung neoplasm
primary vesical calculus
primordial duct
pulmonary arterial wedge (PAWP)
pulmonary artery (PAP)
pulmonary artery diastolic (PAD)
pulmonary artery end diastolic
    (PAEDP)
pulmonary artery mean (PAM)
pulmonary artery peak systolic
pulmonary artery/pulmonary
    capillary wedge
pulmonary artery systolic (PAS)
pulmonary artery wedge (PAWP)
pulmonary capillary (PCP)
pulmonary capillary wedge
    (PCWP)
pulmonary venous capillary (PVC)
pulmonary venous wedge

pressure *(cont.)*
pulmonary wedge
pulse
PV (pulmonary vein)
PVC (pulmonary venous capillary)
RA (right atrial)
recoil
regional cerebral perfusion (rCPP)
right atrial (RAP)
right-sided heart
right subclavian central venous
    (RSCVP)
right ventricular (RVP)
right ventricular diastolic (RVD)
right ventricular end diastolic
right ventricular peak systolic
right ventricular systolic (RVS)
right ventricular volume
RV (right ventricular)
RVD (right ventricular diastolic)
RVS (right ventricular systolic)
segmental lower extremity Doppler
stump
subatmospheric
supersystemic pulmonary artery
SVC (superior vena cava)
systemic
systolic
systolic blood (SBP)
toe systolic
transmyocardial perfusion
transpulmonary (PTP)
V wave (left or right atrial
    catheterization)
venous
ventricular
wedge
wedged hepatic venous (WHVP)
withdrawal
X' (prime) wave (right atrial
    catheterization)
Y wave
Z point

pressure catheter
pressure cuff
pressure difference, aortic-left
pressure equalization
pressure flow gradient
pressure fracture
pressure gradient on pullback
pressure injector
pressure measurement
pressure overload
pressure perfusion study
pressure pneumothorax
pressure pullback
pressure readings
pressure study
pressure waveform
Pressurometer
pretectal lesion
pretectal nucleus (region of midbrain)
pretectal region
pretendinous bands (of hand)
pretendinous cord
pretherapy imaging
pretibial region
prevertebral fascia
prevertebral soft tissue
PREZ (posterior root entry zone)
PRG (phleborheography)
Prima laser guidewire
primarily pulmonary hypertension
  (PPH)
primary atypical pneumonia
primary bronchi, right and left
primary, cancer of unknown (CUP)
primary complex
primary megaloureter
primary motor strip
primary neoplasm
primary pulmonary hypertension
primary pulmonary plasmacytoma
primary rhabdomyosarcoma
primary sarcoma
primary thrombus

primary tuberculosis
primary vesical calculus (pl. calculi)
primary visual cortex
primitive dislocation
primitive neuroectodermal tumor
  (PNET)
Primopac diagnostic catheter
primordial follicle
principal bronchus
principal eigenvector
principle, uncertainty
print reflectance modulation
printer
  Codonics color
  raster scanning
  Winprint laser
prism interpolation
prism method for ventricular volume
Privet coaxial catheter
Probe cardiac device
probability
  absolute emission
  emission
probe
  AngeLase combined mapping-laser
  balloon-expandable esophageal
  blood flow
  cardiac
  Chandler V-pacing
  Doppler flow
  echocardiographic
  eFlexTrial Probe2000
  electromagnetic flow
  gamma
  Hagar
  handheld
  handheld exploring electrode
  handheld mapping
  high frequency miniature
  laparoscopic Doppler
  magnetometer
  Medrad MRInnervu endorectal
  colon

probe *(cont.)*
NRM magnetometer
nuclear
oligonucleotide
Parsonnet
pediatric biplane TEE
Robicsek vascular (RVP)
sapphire contact
shear elasticity
side-hole cannulated
Siemens-Elema AB pulse transducer
Spectraprobe-Max
Teflon
transesophageal
USCI
truncated NMR
ultrasound
Verbatim balloon
Xtent
Probe balloon-on-a-wire dilatation
probehead, MRI
PROBE-SV spectrometer
probing catheter, USCI
procedure
process (pl. processes)
accessory
acromial
alar
alveolar consolidative
aortic root reconstruction
aortobifemoral reconstruction
apical
articular
ascending
auditory
basilar
bony
calcaneal
caudate
chainbead cystourethrogram
clinoid
cochleariform
condyloid

process *(cont.)*
conoid
consolidative
coracoid
coronoid
costal
dacrocystrography
digital image fusion (DIF)
endovascular coil embolization
energy transfer
ensiform
ethmoidal
falciform
fibroplastic
frontal
frontonasal
frontosphenoidal
glenoid
inflammatory
jugular
knobby
left ventricular posterior superior
lumbar transverse
neoplastic
neuroendovascular interventional
odontoid
olecranon
osseous destructive
percutaneous localization of
pulmonary nodules using
suture ligated microcoils
Politano-Leadbetter
pterygoid
radiation synovectomy
radiosynoviorthesis
sacral
sonographically guided human
thrombin injection
spinous
styloid
three-dimensional-connect
transverse
trochlear

process *(cont.)*
  ultrasound scan-guided compres-
    sion (to obliterate false aneu-
    rysm)
  ultrasound-guided percutaneous
    thrombin injection
  uncinate
  vermiform
  vertebrospinous (or vertebral
    spinous)
  vertebral
  xiphoid
  zygomatic
processing, Trex
processor, sequence
ProCross Rely over the wire balloon
  catheter
proctitis, radiation
proctogram
  balloon
  video
proctographic features
proctosigmoidoscopy
procurvature deformity
Prodigy bone densitometer
Prodigy bone densitometry
product cipher
product, daughter
production
  fast routine
  one-step
  pair
  remote controlled
  secondary electron
profile
  asymmetric metabolic
  excitation
  nonlinear excitation
  peak
  rectangular section
  section-sensitivity
  slice
  slice sensitivity
  three-dimensional dose

Profile Mammography System
Profile Plus dilatation catheter, USCI
Proflex 5 dilatation catheter
Pro-Flo XT catheter
profunda femoris artery
profuse uterine hemorrhage
progeny
progesterone-receptor-positive tumor
prognathic dilatation
prognostic importance
program
  Analyze software
  daemon
  ESOLAN
  Microsoft Access
  surveillance
progressive diaphyseal dysplasia
progressive hydrocephalus
progressive interstitial pulmonary
  fibrosis
progressive nodular pulmonary fibrosis
ProHance (gadoteridol) nonionic
  gadolinium contrast agent (MRI)
project
projection (see also *position*; *view*)
  anterior
  AP (anterior-posterior)
  average pixel (APP)
  Bigliani
  cartographic
  caudad
  caudal
  caudal-cranial angulation
  Cleaves axial hip
  Cleaves axial shoulder
  Colcher Sussman (AP and lateral)
  cone-beam
  craniocaudad
  cylindrical map
  Dunlap, Swanson, and Penner
  Eraso
  fan-beam
  filtered-back

projection *(cont.)*
  fingerlike
  frondlike papillary
  Fuchs
  Gaynor-Hart inferosuperior carpal
    tunnel
  Grashey
  half axial
  Harris
  Harris and Beath
  Hirtz submentovertex (SMV)
  Hough
  Hsieh PA oblique (of the hip)
  Isherwood
  Jaroschy
  Johnson axiolateral (femoral head
    and neck)
  Kandel (to demonstrate clubfoot)
  Kasabach oblique (of the odontoid
    process)
  Kemp-Harper submentovertex
    (SMV) (of the jugular foramina)
  kite
  Kuchendorf
  Kurzbauer unobstructed lateral (of
    the sternoclavicular articulation)
  Lambert
  Laquerriere and Pierquin ulnar
    groove
  LAO (left anterior oblique)
  lateral
  lateral oblique
  Lauenstein
  Lauenstein and Hickey lateral hip
  Law (facial bones)
  left lateral
  left posterior oblique
  Lilienfeld
  Lodge Moor (no hyphen)
  Low-Beers
  Low-Beers parietotemporal
    maximum intensity (MIP)
  medial oblique

projection *(cont.)*
  Miller
  minimum intensity
  modified Fuchs
  Nolke
  Norgaard
  oblique
  oblique foot
  Oppenheim cephaloscapular
    projection (for glenohumeral
    joint subluxation)
  Oppenheim cephaloscapular
  PA (posterior-anterior)
  Pearson
  posterior
  presaturation
  RAO (right anterior oblique)
  ray-sum
  right posterior oblique
  rotating tomographic
  saturation inversion (SIP)
  sliding thin-slab, maximum intensity
  sliding thin-slab, minimum intensity
  Staunig
  steep left anterior oblique
  stereographic
  stereotaxic surface (SSP)
  Taylor inferosuperior
  Taylor SMV
  thin-slab maximum intensity
  three dimensional stereotaxic
    surface
  Titterington half axial
  Towne
  Vogt bone-free
  Waters
  Wigby-Taylor open-mouth oblique
  Williams
  Zanelli
projection binning
projector, white light pattern
prolactinoma
prolactin-producing adenoma

prolapse
  anal
  anterior leaflet
  bladder
  cord
  genital
  gravid uterus
  holosystolic mitral valve
  intestinal
  intracranial fat
  massive genital
  mitral valve (MVP)
  mitral valve leaflet systolic
  neovaginal
  posterior leaflet
  rectal
  systolic
  tricuspid valve
  urethral
  urethral meatus
  uterine
  uterovaginal
  vaginal
  vaginal vault
  vaginal wall
  valve
prolapsed leaflet
prolapsed mitral valve leaflets
prolapsed tumor through mitral valve
  orifice
prolapse of leaflet
prolapsing scallop
proliferation
  alveoli
  angiofibroblastic
  bile duct
  bony
  collagen tissue
  connective tissue
  ductular
  fibroblastic
  fibrofatty mesenteric
  fibrous tissue

proliferation *(cont.)*
  glandular
  intimal
  myointimal
  myxomatous
  neointimal
  nodular
  osteophytic
  papillary
  synovial
  villous
proliferative bronchiolitis
prolonged ejection time
prolonged interval
prolonged left ventricular impulse
prominence
  aortic
  bony (spur)
  hilar
  mediastinal
  tibial tubercle
prominent rim of radiolucency
  surrounding ulcer
prominent septal lymphatics
prominent xiphoid process
promontory, sacral
prompt-gamma neutron activation
pronation
pronator quadratus
pronator sign
pronatory sign
prone lateral view
pronephric duct
prone position
prone view
Propac diagnostic catheter
propagation of dissection
properitoneal flank stripe
property (pl. properties)
  CTA dosimetric
  ferromagnetic
  ionic
prophylaxis, antibiotic

proportional counter
propria
  lamina
  substantia
  tunica
propulsive mechanism
propyliodone imaging agent
prospective analysis
ProSpeed CT scanner
ProstaCoil self-expanding urethral
  stent
ProstaScint (CYT-356 radiolabeled
  with indium [III]In) imaging agent
ProstaScint diagnostic imaging agent
ProstaScint monoclonal antibody
  imaging agent
ProstaSeed I 125 seeds
prostate
  apex of
  carcinoma of
  inferolateral surfaces of
  lateral lobe of
  lymph vessels of
  median lobe of
  posterior surface of
prostate carcinoma metastatic to heart
prostatectomy
  radical perineal
  radical retropubic
prostate implant
prostate seeding
prostatic abscess
prostatic adenoma
prostatic calculus
prostatic capsule
prostatic catheter
prostatic fossa
prostatic hemorrhage
prostatic lobe
prostatic malignancy
prostatic necrosis
prostatic obstruction
prostatic stone

prostatic stricture
prostatic urethra
prostatomembranous urethra
prosthesis (pl. prostheses)
  acetabular
  aortic valve
  aortofemoral
  ball and cage valve
  ball-cage
  ball valve
  bifurcated aortofemoral
  bileaflet valve
  bilioduodenal
  closure
  collar
  convexo-concave valve
  disk valve
  esophageal
  femoral
  femorofemoral crossover
  intraluminal sutureless
  intravascular
  iridium
  monostrut cardiac valve
  outflow tract
  tilting-disk aortic valve
  total hip replacement
  total knee replacement
prosthesis cup
prosthesis dehiscence
prosthetic femorodistal graft
prosthetic heart valve
protection
  myocardial
  radiation
protein kinase C localization (brain)
proteinosis, alveolar
protein synthesis rate
Proteus syndrome
protocol
  CT PE (computed tomography
    pulmonary embolus)
  dual phase

protocol *(cont.)*
  McHenry treadmill exercise
  MNP10
  MPRAGE
  neon particle
  RTOG
  2D GRE dynamic
  UCLA imaging
  urokinase
protodensity MRI image
protodiastolic gallop rhythm
protodiastolic reversal of blood flow
proton density
proton density images (MRI)
proton density-weighted images
proton irradiation
proton magnetic resonance
  spectroscopy
proton MRI
proton MR spectroscopy
protons
  methyl
  91-41 MeV
  precessing
protozoal pneumonia
protrude
protruding atheroma
protrusion
  disk
  spicular
  spoonlike (of leaflets)
  subtle nodular
  vascular
protrusion of navicular
protuberance, occipital
proximal anastomosis
proximal and distal portion of vessel
proximal anterior tibial artery
proximal articular set angle (PASA)
proximal carpal row
proximal circumflex artery
proximal coil

proximal focal femoral deficiency
  (PFFD)
proximal fragment ratio (PFR)
  measurement
proximal interphalangeal (PIP) joint
proximally
proximal part of prostatic urethra
proximal popliteal artery
proximal segment
proximal urethra
Pruitt-Inahara balloon-tipped perfusion
  catheter
pruned appearance of pulmonary
  vasculature
PS (pulmonary sequestration)
PS (pulmonic stenosis)
PSA (power spectral analysis)
PsA (psoriatic arthritis)
psammoma body
psammoma, Virchow
psammomatous meningiomas
pseudarthrosis
pseudoaneurysm (see also *aneurysm*)
  anastomotic
  aortic
  asymptomatic
  chronic
  exploration of
  femoral artery
  giant aortic
  hepatic artery
  iatrogenic
  infected
  left ventricular
  pancreatic
  postcatheterization femoral (artery)
  posterior tibial artery
  post-traumatic
  pulmonary
  ruptured
  superficial
  traumatic
  tuberculous

pseudoaneurysm cavity
pseudoaneurysm of arteriovenous
   fistula
pseudoangiomatous stromal hyperplasia
pseudocapsule
pseudocirrhosis, cholangiodysplastic
pseudocoarctation of aorta
pseudocolor B-mode display
pseudocyst
   adrenal
   lung
   mature pancreatic
   nonpancreatic
   pancreatic
   pulmonary
pseudodextrocardia
pseudodislocation
pseudodiverticulum
pseudodynamic MR imaging of the
   temporomandibular joints
pseudoemboli
pseudoendoleak
pseudoepiphysis
pseudoextrophy
pseudofracture artifact
pseudogestational sac
pseudohaustration
pseudojoints
pseudoleak
pseudolesion
pseudolipoma of Glisson capsule
pseudoluxation
pseudolymphoma, gastric
pseudomembrane
pseudomeningocele
pseudomitral leaflet
pseudomyxoma retroperitonei
pseudoneuroma
pseudo-obstruction
   bowel
   chronic idiopathic intestinal (CIIP)
   colonic

pseudo-obstruction *(cont.)*
   familial intestinal
   idiopathic intestinal
   nonfamilial intestinal
pseudopolyp
pseudopolyposis
pseudopregnancy
pseudopuberty, precocious
pseudosac
pseudosacculation
pseudosclerosis, spastic
pseudosheath
pseudostenosis
pseudostone
pseudothrombosis
pseudotumor
   fibrosing inflammatory
   orbital
pseudotumor cerebri (PTC)
PSF (posterior spine fusion)
PSG (peak systolic gradient)
PSIL (percentage signal intensity loss)
P623-Gd (gadolinium) imaging agent
psoas abscess
psoas muscle shadow, obliteration of
psoriatic arthritis (PsA)
PSP (photostimulable phosphor dental
   radiography)
PSS (Palmaz-Schatz stent)
P, substance
pTa-T2 tumor
PTA (percutaneous transluminal angioplasty)
PTBD (percutaneous transhepatic
   biliary drainage) catheter
PTBD (percutaneous transluminal
   balloon dilatation)
PTC (percutaneous transhepatic
   cholangiography)
PTC (pseudotumor cerebri)
PTCA (percutaneous transluminal
   coronary angioplasty)
PTCA catheterization

PTCA coronary angiogram
PTD (percutaneous transhepatic
drainage)
PTDC (percutaneous transcatheter
ductal closure)
pterion
pterygoid bone
pterygoid chest
pterygoideus hamulus
PTF (posterior talofibular) ligament
PTHC (percutaneous transhepatic
cholangiogram)
P-31 MR spectroscopy
PTL (posterior tricuspid leaflet)
PTLD (post-transplant lymphoproliferative disorder)
ptosis
ptotic
PTRA (percutaneous transluminal
renal angioplasty)
PTT (pulmonary transit time)
pT3 tumor
pT4 tumor
PTV (posterior terminal vein)
pubic bone
pubic ramus (pl. rami)
inferior
superior
pubic symphysis
pubic tubercle
pubis
mons
pecten
ramus of
symphysis
pubococcygeal line
pubococcygeus muscle
puboischial area
puborectalis loop
PUD (peptic ulcer disease)
puddle sign
puddling of contrast
puddling on barium enema

pudendal blood supply
pudendal hernia
puff of smoke (moyamoya) on angiography
Pugh Child grading system for
bleeding esophageal varices
Pugh classification of Child liver
criteria
Pulec and Freedman classification
of congenital aural atresia
pullback across aortic valve
pullback arterial markings
pullback from ventricle
pullback pressure recording
pullback study
pulmoaortic canal
pulmogram
pulmolith
pulmolithiasis
pulmonale, cor (c. pulmonale)
pulmonary abscess
pulmonary acinus
pulmonary agenesis
pulmonary alveolar microlithiasis
pulmonary alveolus (pl. alveoli)
pulmonary angiogram (angiography)
balloon occlusion
digital subtraction
pulmonary arterial circulation
pulmonary arterial input impedance
pulmonary arterial markings
pulmonary arterial occlusion
pulmonary arterial pressure, increased
pulmonary arterial vent
pulmonary arterial wedge pressure
pulmonary arteriolar vasoconstriction
pulmonary arteriosclerosis
pulmonary arteriovenous aneurysm
pulmonary arteriovenous fistula
pulmonary artery
aberrant left
anomalous
dilated

pulmonary artery agenesis
pulmonary artery apoplexy
pulmonary artery bifidity
pulmonary artery catheter, balloon-
    tipped flow-directed
pulmonary artery catheter-associated
    endocarditis
pulmonary artery catheter-related
    bacteremia
pulmonary artery compression
    ascending aorta aneurysm
pulmonary artery end diastolic
    pressure (PAEDP)
pulmonary artery engorgement
pulmonary artery pressure (PAP)
pulmonary artery stenosis, peripheral
pulmonary artery wedge pressure
    (PAWP)
pulmonary atresia
pulmonary AV O_2 difference
pulmonary barotrauma
pulmonary bed
pulmonary blood flow redistribution
pulmonary capillary endothelium
pulmonary capillary hemangiomatosis
pulmonary capillary permeability
    using Tc-DTPA
pulmonary capillary pressure (PCP)
pulmonary capillary venous wedge
    pressure
pulmonary capillary wedge position
pulmonary capillary wedge pressure
    (PCWP)
pulmonary capillary wedge tracing
pulmonary cartilage
pulmonary cavitation
pulmonary cavity
pulmonary circulation
pulmonary cirrhosis
pulmonary compliance, reduced
pulmonary compression by pleural
    fluid or gas
pulmonary confluence

pulmonary congestion
pulmonary consolidation
pulmonary contusion
pulmonary cyanosis
pulmonary cystic lymphangiectasis
pulmonary edema
    acute
    cardiogenic
    frank
    fulminant
    high altitude
    interstitial
    negative image
    neurogenic
    noncardiac
    noncardiogenic
    permeability-type
    postoperative
    reexpansion
pulmonary embolism (embolus,
    pl. emboli) (PE)
pulmonary emphysema
pulmonary eosinophilic infiltrates
pulmonary failure
pulmonary fibrosis (see *fibrosis*)
pulmonary fistula, congenital
pulmonary flotation catheter
pulmonary gangrene
pulmonary gas exchange
pulmonary hemorrhage
pulmonary hilus
pulmonary histoplasmosis
pulmonary incompetence
pulmonary infarction
pulmonary infiltrate
pulmonary insufficiency
pulmonary interstitial emphysema
    (PIE)
pulmonary interstitial idiopathic
    fibrosis
pulmonary interstitium
pulmonary ligament
pulmonary microcirculation

pulmonary microvasculature
pulmonary nodule enhancement
pulmonary orifice
pulmonary outflow tract
pulmonary overdistention
pulmonary parenchymal changes
pulmonary parenchymal infiltrates
pulmonary parenchymal window
pulmonary perfusion and ventilation
pulmonary perfusion imaging
pulmonary pleura
pulmonary plexus
pulmonary pseudoaneurysm
pulmonary quantitative differential
 function study
pulmonary regurgitant fraction
pulmonary regurgitation
pulmonary sarcoidosis
pulmonary scars
pulmonary scintigraphy
pulmonary sequestration (PS)
pulmonary stenosis
pulmonary sulcus tumor
pulmonary/systemic flow ratio
pulmonary TB (tuberculosis)
pulmonary thromboembolism (PTE)
pulmonary thrombosis
pulmonary time activity curve
pulmonary trunk idiopathic dilatation
pulmonary tuberculosis (TB)
pulmonary valve anulus
pulmonary valve atresia
pulmonary valve deformity
pulmonary valve insufficiency
pulmonary valve stenosis
pulmonary vascular bed impedance
pulmonary vascular congestion
pulmonary vascular markings
pulmonary vascular obstruction
pulmonary vascular pattern
pulmonary vascular redistribution
pulmonary vascular reserve

pulmonary vascular resistance (PVR)
pulmonary vascular resistance index
 (PVRI)
pulmonary vasculature
pulmonary vasoconstriction, hypoxic
pulmonary vein apoplexy
pulmonary vein atresia
pulmonary vein, congenital stenosis of
pulmonary vein diameter
pulmonary vein fibrosis
pulmonary vein stenosis
pulmonary vein wedge angiography
pulmonary veno-occlusive disease
pulmonary venous anomalous drainage
pulmonary venous anomalous drainage
 to right atrium
pulmonary venous congestion
pulmonary venous drainage
pulmonary venous hypertension
pulmonary venous obstruction
pulmonary venous system
pulmonary venous-systemic air emboli
pulmonary venous wedge pressure
pulmonary ventilation imaging
pulmonary vesicles
pulmonary vessels
pulmonary wedge angiography
pulmonary wedge pressure (PWP)
pulmonic atresia with intact
 ventricular septum
pulmonic infiltrate
pulmonic regurgitation
pulmonic stenosis-ventricular septal
 defect
pulmonic valve stenosis
pulposus, nucleus
pulsate
pulsatile flow, dampened
pulsatile perfusion
pulsatile tinnitus
pulsatility index (PI)
pulsation balloon

pulse (pl. pulses)
  adiabatic slice-selective rf (RF)
    (radiofrequency)
  DANTE-selective
  fat suppression
  narrow-band spectral-selective
  90 RF
  navigator
  phase-encode
  radiofrequency (RF)
  section-select
  spatially selective inversion
  2D spatially selective RF
pulsed brachytherapy (PDR)
pulsed Doppler transesophageal
  echocardiography
pulsed Doppler ultrasound
pulse deficit
pulsed electron paramagnetic NMR
pulsed gradient
pulsed infrared laser
pulsed L-band ESR spectrometer
pulse Doppler interrogation
pulsed magnetization transfer contrast
  MRI
pulsed ultrasound
pulse duration
pulsed-wave Doppler echocardiography
pulse height spectral analysis
pulse indicator, xylol
pulse inversion harmonic imaging
  ultrasound technique
pulse length
pulse reappearance time
pulse sequence, single shot adiabatic
  localization
pulse sequencing
PulseSpray injector
PulseSpray pulsed infusion system
pulse voltage
pulse volume recording (PVR)
pulse volume waveforms
pulse wave

pulse width
pulsion
pulverized plaque particulate matter
pulvinar region
pump
  angle port
  balloon
  cardiac balloon
  intra-aortic balloon (IABP)
  ion
  KAAT II Plus intra-aortic balloon
  pulmonary artery balloon (PABP)
punctate area
puncture
  fine-needle
  stereotactic
  venous
puncture fracture
puncture wound (types I-IV)
purification, one-line anion exchange
purified water contrast
purity, radionuclide
purulent mediastinitis
purulent pneumonia
putamen
putaminal hemorrhage, nondominant
putty kidney
PV (pulmonic valve)
PVD (peripheral vascular disease)
PVG (periventricular gray) matter
PVL (periventricular leukomalacia)
PVP (portal venous pressure)
PVP (portal venous-dominant phase)
  CT images
PVR (peripheral vascular resistance)
PVR (perspective volume rendering)
PVR (postvoiding residual)
PVR (pulmonary vascular resistance)
PVR (pulse volume recorder)
PVR fly-through viewing
PVRI (pulmonary vascular resistance
  index)
PW (posterior wall)

PW (pulse width)
PWT (posterior wall thickness)
pyelectasia
pyelectasis
pyelocaliceal
pyelocaliectasis
pyelocaliceal
pyelofluoroscopy
pyelogram
   antegrade
   excretory intravenous
   intravenous (IVP)
   percutaneous
   rapid-sequence intravenous
   retrograde
pyelographic appearance time
pyelography
pyelonephritic kidney
pyelonephritis, emphysematous
pyeloplasty, dismembered
pyelotubular backflow
pyeloureterography
pyeloureterostomy
pyemia
   cryptogenic
   portal
pyknomorphous
pyloric channel
pyloric hypertrophy
pyloric insufficiency
pyloric outlet obstruction
pyloric ring

pyloric stenosis
pyloric string sign
pyloric ulcer
pyloric valve
pyloroduodenal junction
pylorospasm, persistent
pylorus, hypertrophic
pyocephalus
pyogenic granuloma
pyomyositis
pyonephrosis
pyopneumothorax
pyothorax
pyoventricle
PYP (pyrophosphate) technetium
   myocardial scan
pyramid, petrous
pyramidal bone
pyramidal fracture (of maxilla)
pyramidal hemorrhagic zone
pyramidal layer of cerebral cortex
pyramidal lobe
pyramidal neurons
pyramidal tract
pyribenzamine
pyriform (piriform) sinus
pyriform cortex
pyriform sinus
pyrophosphate (PYP) myocardial scan
pyrophosphate crystals
pyruvate dehydrogenase complex
   deficiency

Q, q

Q (cardiac output)
Q (quotient, as in V-Q, ventilation perfusion scan)
QCA (quantitative coronary arteriography)
Q-cath catheterization recording system
Q space
QCT (quantitative computed tomography) test for bone loss
QDR-1500 bone densitometer
QDR-2000 bone densitometer
QHS (quantitative hepatobiliary scintigraphy)
QM (quantization matrix)
QO_2 (oxygen consumption)
Qp (pulmonary blood flow)
QPD (quadrature phase detector)
QR pattern
QRS interval
QRS loop, counterclockwise superiorly oriented frontal
QRS score
QRS-ST junction
QRS synchronized shock
QRS vector
QRS vertical axis

QRS-T angle, wide
Qs (systemic blood flow)
Qs/Qp ratio
Quad-Lumen drain with radiopaque stripe
Quadramet (samarium Sm 153 lexidronam) radiotherapy agent
QuadraPulse radiofrequency catheter
quadrangle cartilage
quadrangulation of Frouin
quadrant
    left lower (LLQ)
    left upper (LUQ)
    left upper outer
    right lower (RLQ)
    right upper (RUQ)
    right upper outer
quadrant of death (anterosuperior quadrant of hip)
quadrate lobe of liver
quadrature phase detector (QPD) artifact
quadrature RF receiver coil
quadrature setting
quadrature surface coil system
quadrature T/L surface coil
quadratus femoris muscle

543

quadratus, pronator
quad resonance NMR probe circuit
quadriceps muscle
quadrigeminal plate
quadrigeminy
quadrilateral brim
quadripolar catheter
quadripolar electrode catheter
QUAD 7000 high field, whole body,
    open MRI scanners
QUAD 12000 high field, whole body,
    open MRI scanners
Quain fatty degeneration of the heart
qualitative study
quality factor
Quanticor catheter
quantification
    automated
    flow
quantify
Quantison (human serum albumin
    microcapsule)
quantitative analysis
quantitative cardiac perfusion
quantitative computed tomography
    (QCT)
quantitative coronary arteriography
    (QCA)
quantitative CT during expiration
quantitative Doppler assessment
quantitative electroencephalography
    (QEEG)
quantitative exercise thallium-201
    variables
quantitative fluorescence imaging
quantitative gated SPECT (QGS)
quantitative hepatobiliary scintigraphy
    (QHS)
quantitative magnetization transfer

quantitative regional myocardial flow
    measurement
quantitative scan
quantitative spirometrically controlled
    CT
quantitative ultrasound sonometry
    (QUS)
quantity, spectrophotometric
quantization
    sequent scalar (SSQ)
    wavelet scalar (WSQ)
quantization matrix (QM) scaling
quantizer-design algorithms
Quantum Maverick coronary balloon
    dilatation catheter
quantum number
Quantum PTCA catheter
quench
quenching, sonoluminescence
Quénu-Muret sign
Quervain (de Quervain) fracture
Quesada method
questionable calcification
QuickFlash radial artery catheter
quiescence
Quik-Prep, Quinton
Quincke angioedema disease
Quinton catheter
Quinton Mahurkar dual lumen hemo-
    dialysis catheter
Quinton PermCath
Quinton PermCath vascular access
    catheter
Quinton Quik-Prep
Quinton vascular access port
quotient, Rayleigh
QUS (quantitative ultrasound sonom-
    etry)
Qwikstart catheter

R, r

Raaf Cath (vascular catheter)
RAAPI (resting ankle-arm pressure
  index)
RA (rheumatoid arthritis) factor
RA (rotational angiography),
  Integris 3-D
RA (right atrial) pressure
RA (right atrium) oxygen saturation
RAB (remote afterloading brachytherapy)
"rab'do-my-oly'sis"—see *rhabdomyolysis*
RACAT (rapid acquisition computed
  axial tomography)
rachioscoliosis
rachitic rosary sign
radiability
radial artery catheter
radial artery to cephalic vein fistula
radial bone
radial collateral ligament
radial deviation
radial drift
radial epiphyseal displacement
radial facing of metacarpal heads
radial forearm flap

radial fossa
radial head fracture
radial head subluxation (RHS)
radialized
radial ray defect
radial styloid process fracture
radial tuberosity
radial vascular thermal injury
radiate ligament
radiation (see also *irradiation; radiation therapy; radiotherapeutic
  agent*)
  acoustic
  adjuvant
  alpha
  cardiac
  Cerenkov
  diagnostic
  external beam
  fatal dose of
  intracavitary
  intrastitial
  ionizing
  monochromatic
  monochromatic synchrotron
  pseudomembranous (gastritis)

radiation *(cont.)*
  synchrotron
  therapeutic
  ultraviolet
radiation-absorbed dose (rad)
radiation changes
radiation colitis
radiation dosages
radiation dose pertubation
radiation dosimetry calculation
radiation fibrosis
radiation fistula
radiation-induced change
radiation-induced colitis
radiation-induced fibrosis
radiation-induced lung disease (RILD)
radiation-induced skin injury
radiation-induced ulceration
radiation-induced up-regulation
radiation intensity
radiation interrogation
radiation monitor
radiation necrosis
radiation osteonecrosis
radiation pericardial disease
radiation pneumonia
radiation pneumonitis
radiation port
radiation proctitis
radiation protection
radiation scatter
radiation source
  intracavitary
  intrastitial
radiation synovectomy
radiation therapy (see also *radiation;*
  radiotherapy; radiotherapy
  agents)
  accelerated hyperfractionated
  adjuvant
  adjuvant hypofractionated confor-
    mal
  chemoradiation therapy

radiation *(cont.)*
  combined-modality
  CT guidance for placement of
  concomitant boost
  concurrent (with chemotherapy)
  conformal
  conformal neutron and photon
  conventionally fractionated
    stereotactic
  craniospinal axis
  Cs 131 (cesium 131) Seed
  dynamic
  echography for placement of
  external beam (EBRT)
  eye-view 3D-CRT
  fractionated
  fractionated external beam
  fractionated stereotaxic
  hyperfractionated
  hypofractionated
  I-B1 radiolabeled antibody
    injection
  ICRU 50
  intensity-modulated (IMRT)
  interstitial
  intracavitary
  intraoperative (IORT)
  isotope
  large field
  MammoSite RTS (radiation therapy
    system)
  megavoltaFge
  neuroaxis
  orthovoltage
  palliative
  partial brain
  photon-neutron mixed-beam
  Pinnacle 3
  placement of
  PortalVision
  postorchiectomy para-aortic
  rotational
  RTP (radiation therapy planning)

radiation *(cont.)*
  short distance (brachytherapy)
  single field hyperthermia combined
    with ultrasound and
  split course accelerated
  split course hyperfractionated
  split hyperfractionated accelerated
  stereotactic or stereotaxic
  three-dimensional conformal
  3D-CRT
  upper mantle
  whole brain
radiation therapy planning (RTP)
  system
radiation toxicity syndrome
radical mastectomy
radical perineal prostatectomy
radical retropubic prostatectomy
radical trachelectomy
radicle, biliary
radicular arteries
radicular compression
radicular cyst
radicular vessels to spinal cord
radiculomedullary artery
radiculospinal artery
radioactive aerosol
radioactive bolus
radioactive cancer-specific targeting
  agent
radioactive cobalt
radioactive emissions from heart
radioactive fibrinogen scan
radioactive iodinated serum albumin
  (RISA) imaging agent
radioactive iodine uptake test (RAIU)
radioactive iodinated serum albumin
  (RISA)
radioactive isotope (see *imaging agent*)
radioactive label (labeling)
radioactively tagged
radioactive marker
radioactive material

radioactive source
radioactive string markers
radioactive thallium
radioactive tracer
radioactive xenon clearance
radioactive xenon gas inhalation
radioactivity, area of high
radioactivity detector, Neoprobe
radioactivity detention
radioaerosol clearance
radioaerosol imaging studies
radioallergosorbent test (RAST)
radioccipital
radiobiological
radiobiology
radiocalcium
radiocapitellar joint
radiocarcinogenesis
radiocardiogram
radiocardiography
radiocarpal angle
radiocarpal dislocation
radiocarpal joint
radiocarpal portal
radiochemical study
radiochemistry
radiochromic film
radiocolloid leakage
radiocolloid lymphoscintigraphy
radiocolloids
radiocontrast-induced nephropathy
radiocurable
radiode
radiodiagnosis
radiodiagnostics
radiodigital
radioelement application
  interstitial
  intracavitary
  surface
radioelement solution
radiofluorinated
Radiofocus Glidewire for angiography

radiofrequency (RF)
  RF ablation (RFA) therapy
  RF catheter ablation (RFCA)
  RF coil
  RF electrocautery
  RF energy
  RF field
  RF-generated thermal balloon
    catheter
  RF hyperthermia
  RF magnetic shield
  RF overflow artifact
  RF period
  RF-PMR (radiofrequency percuta-
    neous myocardial revasculariza-
    tion)
  RF pulse
  RF saturation bands
  RF screen
  RF modification transcatheter
  RF spatial distribution problem
  RF spatial distribution problem
    reconstruction artifact
  RF thermal ablation (RTA)
  RF transmitter
radiofrequency power amplifier
radiogenic leukopenia
radiogold
radiogram (radiograph) (see *imaging*)
radiographically firm synostosis
radiographic control
radiographic hallmark
radiographic imaging system,
  intensified (IRIS)
radioimmunoluminography
radioimmunoguided surgery (RIGs)
radiographic pelvimetry
radiographic pincushion distortion
radiographic urodynamic assessment
radiography (see *imaging*)
radiohumeral articulation
radioimmunity
radioimmunoassay (RIA)

radioimmunoassay, scintillation
  proximity
radioimmunodetection (RAID)
radioimmunodiffusion
radioimmunoelectrophoresis
radioimmunoimaging
radioimmunoscintigraphy
radioimmunoscintimetry
radioimmunosorbent
radioimmunotherapy
radioiodinated serum albumin (RISA)
radioiodination
  direct
  electrophilic
radioiodine
radioiron oral absorption
radioiron red cell utilization
radioisotope (isotope) (see *imaging
  agent*)
radioisotope assay, thyroxine (T_4RIA)
radioisotope bone imaging
radioisotope bone scan
radioisotope cisternography
radioisotope clearance assay
radioisotope-labeled antibody
radioisotope-labeled antigen
radioisotope labeling
radioisotope lung scan
radioisotope renal excretion test
radioisotope scan
radioisotope (static) scanning
radioisotope scanning of the thyroid
radioisotope scintigraphy
radioisotope stent
radioisotope uptake
radioisotope voiding cystography
radiolabeled anti-D-dimer antibodies
radiolabeled antifibrin antibody
radiolabeled compound
radiolabeled estrogen analog F-18
  ([18F]) estradiol (FES)
radiolabeled fibrinogen
radiolabeled MoAb

radiolabeled peptide alpha-M2
    imaging agent
radiolabeled platelets
radiolabeled RBC scan
radiolabeled water study
radiolabeled WBCs
radiolesion
radioligand
radiologically proven arthritis
radiologic-anatomic correlation
radiologic gastrostomy
radiologic guidance
radiologic-histopathologic study
radiologic-pathologic correlation
radiologic percutaneous gastrostomy
radiologic protection
Radiologic Society of North America
    (RSNA)
radiologist
radiology
    computed (CR)
    diagnostic
    interventional
    neurointerventional
    percutaneous interventional
    polytomographic
    skeletal
    storage phosphor
    therapeutic
radiology outcomes data
radiolucency, soap-bubble
radiolucent area
radiolucent center
radiolucent cleft
radiolucent filling defect
radiolucent focus (pl. foci)
radiolucent plastic occluder
radiolucent pneumomediastinum
radiolucent spine frame
radiolucent stone
radiolunotriquetral ligament
radiolymphoscintigraphy, intra-
    operative

radiomuscular
radionecrosis, cerebral
Radionics CRW stereotactic head
    frame
radionitrogen
radionuclear venography
radionuclide (see *imaging agent*)
    absorption of
    concentration of
    inhalation of
    inhaled
    injection of
    uptake of
radionuclide angiocardiogram
radionuclide angiogram (RNA)
radionuclide angioscintigraphy
radionuclide bladder scan
radionuclide blood flow (dynamic)
    studies
radionuclide carrier system
radionuclide cineangiography
radionuclide cisternography
radionuclide cystography (RNC)
radionuclide esophageal emptying time
radionuclide esophageal transit test
    (RETT)
radionuclide flow scan
radionuclide gated blood pool
    scanning
radionuclide injection
radionuclide label (labeling)
radionuclide-labeled leukocytes
radionuclide-labeled platelets
radionuclide liver scan
radionuclide mammography
radionuclide milk scan
radionuclide purity
radionuclide renal imaging
radionuclide renography
radionuclide scan (scanning)
radionuclide shuntogram
radionuclide shunt scintigram
radionuclide signals

radionuclide study, blood pool
radionuclide testicular scintigraphy
radionuclide uptake
radionuclide ventriculogram
radionuclide voiding study
radiopacity
radiopaque calculus
radiopaque catheter tip
radiopaque imaging agent
radiopaque density
radiopaque distal tip for location on
fluoroscopy
radiopaque FEP sheath
radiopaque fluid extravasation
radiopaque marker
radiopaque medium
radiopaque nanoparticulate
radiopaque pellet
radiopaque stone
radiopaque suture
radiopaque urine
radiopaque vesical calculus
radiopaque wire of counteroccluder
buttonhole
radiopaque xenon gas
radiopathology
radiopharmaceutical (see *imaging*
agent)
radiopharmaceutical ablation
radiopharmaceutical dacryocystography
radiopharmaceutical localization
radiopharmaceutical therapy
radiopharmaceutical voiding
cystogram
radiopharmaceutical volume-dilution
technique
radiophobia
radiophotography
radiophylaxis
radiopotassium
radiopulmonography
radioreaction
radioresistance

radioscaphocapitate ligament
radioscaphoid joint
radioscaphoid ligament
radioscapholunate ligament
radioscintigraphy
radioscopically tagged antihuman
antibody
radiosensibility
radiosensitive
radiosensitivity, fibroblast
radiosensitizer
carbogen
halogenated thymidine analogue
nicotinamide
radiostereometry
radiostereoscopy
radiostyloid process
radiosulfur
radiosurgery
Bragg-peak
charged-particle
CyberKnife
dynamic stereotactic
gamma knife
heavy-charged particle Bragg peak
image-guided
interstitial
LINAC or Linac (linear
accelerator)
multiarc LINAC
stereotactic or stereotaxic
radiosurgically
radiosynoviorthesis
radiotherapeutic agent
radiotherapist
radiotherapy (see *radiation; radiation*
therapy; radiotherapy agent)
radiotherapy agent (see also *imaging*
agent; *implant*)
Bexxar Dosimetric Package (iodine
I 131 tositumomab)
Bexxar Therapeutic Package
(iodine I 131 tositumomab)

radiotherapy *(cont.)*
    BrachySeed I-125 (iodine ^{125}I)
        implant
    BrachySeed Pd-103 (palladium
        ^{103}Pd) implant
    chromic phosphate P 32 (^{32}P)
    indium
        OctreoScan (^{111}In pentetreotide)
    iodine
        ^{125}I interstitial radiation implant
    Iodotope (sodium iodide ^{131}I)
    Metastron (strontium chloride
        Sr 89)
    octreotide acetate
    palladium 103 (^{103}Pd) radioactive
    Phosphocol P 32 (^{32}P chromic
        phosphate)
    Quadramet (samarium Sm 153
        lexidronam)
    samarium Sm 153 lexidronam
    sodium iodide (^{131}I); sodium
        iodide I 131
    strontium
        ^{89}Sr (strontium-89)
    Theraseed (palladium Pd 103)
radiotherapy with hyperthermia
radiotherapy without hyperthermia
radiotherapy field placement
radiotoxemia
radiotoxicity
radiotracer activity
radiotracer foil method
radiotracer foil method for sorption
    studies
radiotracer technique
radiotracer uptake
radiotransparency
radiotropic
radioulnar joint
radioulnar subluxation
radioulnar surface
radium radioactive source
radium seeds

radius
Radius coronary stent delivery
    catheter
RadNet radiology information system
radon seeds radioactive source
RadPICC catheter
RadPICC port
RADstation radiology workstation
radwaste radioactivity detection
RAE (right atrial enlargement)
Raeder-Arbitz syndrome
Raeder paratrigeminal syndrome
ragpicker's disease
RAID (radioimmunodetection)
railroad track pattern on x-ray in
    Sturge-Weber syndrome
railroad track sign
Raimiste sign
Raimondi ventricular catheter
raised intracranial pressure
RAIU (radioactive iodine uptake test)
rake retractor
rake ulcer
Raman spectroscopy
Ramesh and Pramod algorithms
rami (see *ramus*)
Ramirez shunt
ramp, folded step
Ramsay Hunt cerebellar myoclonic
    dyssynergia
ramus (pl. rami)
    dorsal
    dorsal primary
    inferior
    inferior pubic
    ischiopubic
    pubic
    superior
    ventral
    ventral primary
ramus intermedius artery branch
ramus medialis artery branch
R&F camera

Rand microballoon
random field, Gibbs
randomly distributed cortical perfusion
  defects
Ranfac LAP-013 cholangiographic
  catheter
Ranfac ORC-B cholangiographic
  catheter
Ranfac XL-11 cholangiographic
  catheter
range
  absorbed dose
  gray scale
  normal
  reference
  therapeutic
range-gated Doppler spectral flow
  analysis
Ranger PTCA catheter
Ranke angle
Ranke complex
Ranvier groove
Ranvier node
RAO (right anterior oblique)
  RAO breathing technique (on chest
    x-ray)
  RAO expiration technique
  RAO position for cardiac
    catheterization
  RAO projection
  RAO view
RAP (right atrial pressure)
raphe
  abdominal
  amniotic
  anococcygeal
  anogenital
  longitudinal
  median
  palpebral
  penile
  pterygomandibular
  scrotal
  tendinous

rapid acquisition computed axial
  tomography (RACAT)
rapid acquisition with relaxation
  enhancement (RARE)
rapid axial MRI
rapid contrast washout
rapid deceleration injury
rapid dephasing
rapid early repolarization phase
rapid exchange PTCA balloon angioplasty catheter
Rapid Exchange vein graft stent
  delivery system
rapid filling phase
rapid filling wave
rapid image transfer
rapid inspiratory flow rates
rapid oscillatory motion
rapid repolarization phase
rapid sequence intravenous pyelogram
  (IVP)
rapid sequential CT scan
rapid thoracic compression technique
Rapid-Trak balloon
Rapid-Trak catheter
Rapid-Trak guidewire
Rapid-Trak stent
Rapid-Trak stent delivery system
rapid uptake
rapid ventricular filling phase
rapid ventricular rate
rapid ventricular response
RapiSeal patch
Rappaport classification of gastric
  lymphoma
Rappaport disability rating scale
Raptor PTCA balloon
RaptorRail PTCA dilatation catheter
raptus of attention
RARE (rapid acquisition with relaxa-
  tion enhancement) MRI
RARE-derived pulse sequence
rarefaction of cortex

rarefied area
Rashkind double disk occluder
Rashkind double umbrella device
Rashkind occluder
Rashkind septostomy balloon catheter
Rasmussen mycotic aneurysm
Rastelli atrioventricular canal defect
    (type A, B, or C)
raster frequency
raster lines
raster period
raster scanning printer
raster spacing error
rate
    complication
    decay
    deposition
    instantaneous enhancement
    patency
    penetration
    protein synthesis
    shear
    slew
    transverse relaxation
    valley to peak
rate meter
Rathke pouch
Rathke duct
Rathke pouch (in the brain)
rating scale
ratio
    AH:HA
    ankle-brachial pressure
    AO:AC (aortic valve opening to
        aortic valve closing)
    aortic root
    artery/aortic velocity
    brain to background
    C/N (contrast to noise)
    cardiothoracic (CT, CTR)
    CBV/CBF
    cerebral blood volume/cerebral
        blood flow

ratio (cont.)
    chemical-shift
    CK:AST
    compression
    conduction (number of P waves to
        number of QRS)
    contrast to noise (C/N)
    E:A (on echocardiography)
    escape peak
    ESP-ESV
    ESWI-ESVI (end systolic wall
        stress index to end systolic
        volume)
    FL/AC (femur length to abdominal
        circumference)
    gray to white matter activity (also
        gray/white matter activity)
    gray to white matter utilization
    gyromagnetic
    HC/AC (head circumference to
        abdominal circumference)
    heart to background
    heart to lung
    Holdaway
    inferior-anterior (I-A) count
    Insall (in patella alta)
    Insall-Salvati
    inverse inspiratory–expiratory time
    isotopic
    I-E (inspiration to expiration, or
        inspiratory to expiratory)
    kidney to background
    LA–AR (left atrium/aortic root)
    L/A (liver/aorta) peak
    L/B
    left atrial to aortic (root) ratio
        (LA/Ao, LA-Ao)
    left ventricular systolic time
        interval
    lesion to background
    lesion to muscle
    lesion to nonlesion count
    liver/aorta (L/A) peak

ratio *(cont.)*
  liver/liver peak (L/LP)
  L/LP (liver/liver peak)
  magnetogyric
  maximum diameter to minimum
    diameter
  metatarsal length
  nasal to plasma radioactivity
  orifice to anulus
  P:A (peroneal to anterior
    compartment)
  PASP–SASP (pulmonary to
    systemic arterial systolic
    pressure)
  patellar ligament-patellar
  peak systolic and diastolic
  pitch
  Poisson
  P:QRS
  P–S flow (pulmonic–systemic)
  pulmonary–systemic blood flow
  pulmonary to systemic flow
  Qs/Qp
  R/S amplitude
  R/S wave
  risk–benefit
  RVP–LVP (right ventricular to left
    ventricular systolic pressure)
  RV6:RV5 voltage
  scatter to primary
  septal to free wall
  serum glucose:CSF glucose
  SI joint to sacrum
  signal to clutter
  signal to noise (S/N)
  spleen to liver
  stroke volume
  target to background
  thallium to scalp
  TME (trapezium-metacarpal
    eburnation)
  tumor to normal brain
  T–D (thickness to diameter of
    ventricle)

ratio *(cont.)*
  ventilation-perfusion (V-Q)
    (Q = quotient)
  VLDL-TG to HDL-C
rational drug design
Ratliff classification of avascular
  necrosis
rat-tail appearance on pancreatogram
Rau, apophysis of
Rauchfuss triangle
rauwolfia derivative
RAW (airway resistance)
ray (pl. rays)
  central
  digital
  grenz
  hypermobile first
  keV gamma
  long axis
  pollicized
ray amputation
ray-casting method
Rayleigh quotient
Rayleigh scattering law
Rayleigh-Tyndall scattering
Raymond-Cestan syndrome
Raynaud phenomenon
ray-sum projection
ray-sum views
Ray-Tec x-ray detectable surgical
  sponge
Ray TFC (threaded fusion cage)
Ray ventricular cannula
Razi cannula introducer
Rb (rubidium)
  ^{82}Rb-based cardiac imaging
RBBB (right bundle branch block)
RBC (red blood cell)
  labeled
  technetium-99m-labeled
RBG (red, blue, green)
RCA (retained cortical activity)
RCA (right coronary artery)

RCA (rotational coronary atherectomy)
rCBF (regional cerebral blood flow)
   PET scan
rCBV (regional cerebral blood
   volume) PET scan
RCC (renal cell carcinoma)
rCMRO$_2$ (regional cerebral metabolic
   rate for oxygen)
RCP (retrograde cerebral perfusion)
rCPP (regional cerebral perfusion
   pressure)
RCT (retinocortical time)
rd (rutherford) radioactive unit
RDG (retrograde duodenogastroscopy)
RDW (red cell diameter width)
RDX coronary radiation catheter
   delivery system
RE (reflux esophagitis)
RE (rehabilitation engineering)
Re (rhenium) (an element)
reabsorption, bony
reaccumulation
reaction
   endoergic
   exoergic
   hilar
   hypersensitivity
   lamellar
   layered periosteal
   onionskin periosteal
   periosteal
   pleural
   sarcoid-like
reactivation tuberculosis
reactive airways disease (RAD)
reactive airways dysfunction syndrome
reactive arterioles
reactive disease of smooth muscle
reactive hyperemia
reactivity, bronchial
reading
   batch-
   wet x-ray

readout wavelength
reagent, Wittig
real-time assessment
real-time biplanar needle tracking
real-time chirp Z transformer
real-time color flow Doppler imaging
   of blood flow
real-time CT fluoroscopy
real-time DAP (dose area product)
real-time display
real-time edge enhancement
real-time equipment
real-time format converter
real-time 4-D ultrasound
real-time images
real-time MR imaging tracking
real-time respiratory feedback
real-time scan ultrasound
real-time sonogram (sonography)
real-time two-dimensional (2D) blood
   flow imaging
real-time ultrasound (ultrasonography)
real-time volume rendering
realign
realignment, patellofemoral
reapproximating
reapproximation
Rebar microcatheter
rebleeding of aneurysm
rebreathing ventilation scan
rebypass
recalcitrant
recanalization technique
   angiographic
   argon laser
   laser
   percutaneous transluminal coronary
   peripheral laser (PLR)
recanalized artery
recanalized ductus
recanalizing
receiver coil
receiver operating characteristics
   (ROC)

receptor (pl. receptors)
  baro-
  benzodiazepine
  dopamine
  D2
  GABA
  serotonin
  S2
  transferrin
receptor antagonist
receptor binding
recess
  attic
  cecal
  cerebellopontine
  cochlear
  costodiaphragmatic
  costomediastinal
  duodenojejunal
  epitympanic
  hepatorenal
  ileocecal
  inferior duodenal
  infraglenoid
  intersigmoid
  optic
  popliteal
  paraduodenal
  peritoneal
  pleural
  prestyloid
  retrocecal
  retroduodenal
  sacciform
  sphenoethmoidal
  splenorenal
  sublabral
  subphrenic
  subscapularis
  superior duodenal
recessed balloon septostomy catheter
recession, nasion
recheck

recipient
  nonmyeloablative transplant
  syngeneic transplant
reciprocal changes
reciprocating conduction
recirculation peak
Recklinghausen disease of bone
recoarctation of aorta
recognition, high order curve
recoil
  arterial
  catheter
recoil pressure
recombinant human granulocyte
  colony stimulating factor
  (r-metHuG-CSF)
recon pitch
reconstituted via collaterals
reconstitution of blood flow in artery
reconstitution via profunda artery
reconstitution via collaterals
reconstructed with a 1:1 pitch at
  1 mm increments
reconstruction
  aortic
  Dor
  ECG-gated
  EKG-gated
  external gamma dose
  fan-beam
  gated 3D
  image
  multiplanar
  patch graft
  renovascular
  respiration gated 3D
  three-dimensional
  transannular patch
  zygomaticomalar
reconstruction algorithms
reconstruction artifact
reconstruction of aorta
reconstruction study

recording
    color Doppler
    continuous-wave Doppler
    evoked-potential
    pullback pressure
    pulsed-wave Doppler
    simultaneous
recovery
    fluid-attenuated inversion
    saturation
    shape
    uneventful
recovery period of myocardium
recovery time, corrected sinus node
recrudescence
recruitment potential
rectal endometriosis
rectal endoscopic ultrasonography
    (REU)
rectal fold
    inferior transverse
    superior transverse
rectal imaging agent
rectal multiplane transducer
rectal polyp
rectal pressure catheter
rectal prolapse
rectal shelf
rectal stricture
rectal stump
rectal trauma
rectal vault
rectangular non-single harmonic wave
rectangular section profile
rectilinear bone scan
rectilinear thyroid scan
rectolabial fistula
rectosigmoid function
rectourethral fistula
rectovaginal fistula
rectovaginal nodules of endometriosis
rectovaginal pouch

rectovaginal septum
rectovesical pouch
rectovesicovaginal fistula
rectovestibular fistula
rectovulvar fistula
rectum, blind-ending
rectus abdominis muscle
rectus muscle flap
rectus position
rectus sheath
rectus sheath pocket
recumbency
recumbent position
recumbent view
recur
recurred
recurrence
    local
    locoregional
    nodal
    pattern
    regional
    tumor
recurrent artery of Heubner
recurrent bladder neck obstruction
recurrent dislocation
recurrent laryngeal nerve
recurrent meningeal nerve
recurvatum deformity
recurvatum during gait
red/blue anaglyph glasses
red blood cell angioscintigraphy
red, blue, green (RBG)
red cell diameter width (RDW)
Reddick cystic duct cholangiogram
    catheter
red hepatization stage of pneumonia
Redifocus guidewire
RediFurl TaperSeal IAB catheter
RediGuard flexible IAB catheter
redirection of inferior vena cava
redistributed thallium scan

redistribution
  blood flow
  flow
  myocardial image
  pulmonary blood flow
  pulmonary vascular
redistribution image
redistribution study
Redi-Vu teleradiology system
red Robinson catheter
red rubber catheter
REDS (remote endoscopic digital
  spectroscopy)
reduced cardiac output
reduced circulation
reduced compliance of chamber
reduced plasma volume
reduced prominence of pulmonary
  vessels
reduced pulmonary compliance
reduced signal intensity
reduced stroke volume
reducible hernia
reduction
  afterload
  anatomic
  blood viscosity
  closed
  concentric
  congruent
  electrolytic
  fracture
  manual
  manual fracture
  open
  stable
  surgical
  thoracic volume
  trial
redundancy of interposed colon
  segment
redundant aortic leaflet
redundant aortic valve leaflets

redundant carotid artery
redundant mitral valve leaflets
redundant scallop of posterior anulus
redundant sigmoid colon
reefing, capsular
reefing of medial retinaculum of knee
reentry point
reexpansion of lung
reexpansion pulmonary edema
reexploration
reference coordinate system
reference line
reference site
reference standards, Wilmad
reference, sternospinal
referred pain
REFI (regional ejection fraction
  image)
refill, capillary
reflectance spectroscopy
reflectant
reflected edge of Poupart ligament
reflection
  costopleural
  epicardial
  hepatoduodenal
  hepatoduodenoperitoneal
  mediastinal
  mediastinodiaphragmatic pleural
  pericardial
  peritoneal
  sternal pleural
  vertebral pleural
Reflection acetabular cup
  cemented
  uncemented
reflectivity, high
reflectometer tuning unit
reflex (pl. reflexes)
Reflex steerable guidewire from
  Cordis
Reflotron bedside theophylline test

reflux
  abdominojugular
  acid
  bile
  duodenobiliary
  duodenogastric (DGR)
  duodenopancreatic
  free
  gastric
  gastroesophageal (GE, GER)
  hepatojugular (HJ)
  intra-renal
  left-sided
  nasopharyngeal
  nocturnal gastric
  vaginal
  vesicoureteral
reflux atrophy
reflux esophagitis
reflux gastritis
reflux grades I through V
refluxing megaureters
refluxing spastic neurogenic bladder
reflux of activity
reflux regurgitation
reformation, multiplanar
reformatted planar "Christmas tree"
  MR appearance of endolymphatic
  sac
reformatting, multiplanar
refractoriness, ventricular
refractory congestive heart failure
refractory hypertension
refractory hypoxemia
refractory period of myocardium (see
  period)
refractory to treatment
refracture
region
  anesthesic
  Broca
  dark
  insular

region *(cont.)*
  interseptal
  midfrontal
  periaqueductal
  photodeficient
  photopenic
  septal
  subfrontal
  task-activated brain
  temporal
  Wernicke
regional brain parenchymal fraction
  (RBPF)
regional brain parenchymal volume
  (RBPV)
regional cerebral blood flow (rCBF)
  PET tomography
regional cerebral blood volume
  (rCBV) PET scan
regional cerebral metabolic rate for
  oxygen (rCMRO$_2$)
regional cerebral oxygen saturation
regional cerebral perfusion pressure
  (rCPP)
regional ejection fraction image
  (REFI)
regional left ventricular function
regional lymph nodes
regional myocardial uptake of thallium
regional oxygen extraction fraction
  (rOEF)
regional perfusion by mixed venous
  blood
regional pulmonary perfusion
regional recurrence
regional tracer uptake
regional ventilation
regional ventricular function
regional wall motion abnormality, left
  ventricular
regional washout measurements
region of interest (ROI)
region of interest fluoroscopy

region of interest imaging technique
registration
  landmark
  robust
  spatial
  surface
  two-dimensional portal image
registration and alignment of 3D
  images
registry, STAR
Regnauld degeneration of MTP joint
regress
regression
  plaque
  polynomial stepwise multiple-
    linear
  spontaneous
  stepwise
regression analysis
regrowth delay
regular in outline fundus
regular wedge
regulation, defective volume
regurgitant flow
regurgitant jet
regurgitant lesion
regurgitant pandiastolic flow
regurgitant pocket
regurgitant stream
regurgitant velocity
regurgitant volume
regurgitation
  aortic (AR)
  aortic valve
  congenital
  congenital aortic
  congenital mitral (CMR)
  Dexter-Grossman classification of
    mitral
  Grossman scale for
  ischemically mediated mitral
  massive aortic
  mitral

regurgitation *(cont.)*
  mitral valve
  pansystolic mitral
  paravalvular
  physiologic
  pulmonary
  pulmonic (PR)
  pulmonic valve
  silent
  sour fluid
  transient tricuspid (of infancy)
  tricuspid (TR)
  tricuspid orifice
  tricuspid valve
  trivial mitral
  valvular (VR)
regurgitation index
rehabilitation (rehab), cardiac
rehydrated
Reichek method of calculating end
  systolic wall stress
Reichert flexible sigmoidoscope
Reichert-Mundinger-Fischer
  stereotactic frame
Reid baseline
Reil, island of
Reimer migration index
reimplantation technique
reimplant, common sheath
reinfarction
reinjection thallium stress exam
reinnervation, motor
reinsertion
reintimalization
reintubation
reirradiation
reirrigation
Reiter disease
rejection
  accelerated acute
  acute
  acute renal
  allograft

rejection *(cont.)*
    bordcrline severe
    chronic
    chronic humoral
    end stage
    first set
    focal moderate
    hyperacute
    low moderate
    resolved
    resolving
    second set
    severe acute
    transplant
    vasculitic
rejection crisis
relapsing course
relation
    end diastolic pressure-volume
    end systolic pressure-volume
    force-frequency
    force-length
    force-velocity
    Frank-Starling (of heart)
relationship
    dentoskeletal
    dose-response
    dose-volume
    globe-orbit
relative hypoxia
relative refractory period (RRP)
relative shunt flow
relativistic mass
relaxation
    ferromagnetic
    isovolumic
    longitudinal
    multiexponential
    multispin
    nuclear
    nuclear electric quadrupole
    paramagnetic
    reciprocal agonist-antagonist

rclaxation *(cont.)*
    spin spin
    spin lattice
    spin spin
    tissue-based T2
    T1
    transverse
    T2 star
relaxation atelectasis
relaxation effect, water
relaxation of pelvis
relaxation rate
relaxation techniques
relaxation time
    lattice
    longitudinal
    short T1
    spin lattice
    spin lattice proton
    spin spin
    T1
    T2
relaxivity
relaxometer
    Bruker PC-10
    IBM Field-Cycling Research
Release-NF (nitrofurazone Foley)
    catheter
Reliance urinary control insert catheter
Reliance urinary control stent
relief, mucosal
relief pattern
reloading, anode tube
remineralization
remitting course
remnant
    ductal
    heart
remodeling
    bone
    craniofacial
    para-articular bone
    regressive
    thrombus

remote afterloader
remote afterloading brachytherapy
(RAB)
remote afterloading high intensity
brachytherapy
remote control afterloading high dose
rate intracavitary brachytherapy
remote control afterloading machines
remote-controlled implantation of
radioactive source
remote-controlled production
remote diagnosis
remote endoscopic digital spectroscopy
(REDS)
remote history
remote lower motor neuron lesion
removal of urinary bladder
remyelination
renal adenoma
renal agenesis
renal angiogram
renal angiography
renal angiomyolipoma
renal angioscintigraphy
renal arteriography
renal artery, accessory
renal artery aneurysm
renal artery hemorrhage
renal artery obstruction
renal artery occlusion
renal artery stenosis
renal atrophy
renal axis
renal calculus
renal capsule
fatty
fibrous
renal cell carcinoma (RCC)
renal cell tumor
renal circulation imaging
renal cocktail
renal compromise
renal cortex, patchy atrophy of

renal cortical adenoma
renal cortical isotope scanning agent
renal cortical necrosis
renal cross-fused ectopia
renal cyst study
renal duct
renal duplex imaging
renal duplex scan
renal dysplasia
renal ectopia
renal failure
renal fibrosis
renal flow curve
renal fossa
renal function
renal function impairment
renal helical CT (RHCT)
renal hemorrhage
renal hemangiopericytoma
renal hypertension
renal hypertrophy
renal imaging
renal impression on liver
renal injury
renal isthmus
renal lithiasis (renolithiasis)
renal lobe
renal lymphangiectasia
renal malignancy
renal mass lesion
renal medulla
renal osteodystrophy
renal parenchymal disease
renal parenchyma
renal pelvic urothelial carcinoma
renal pelvis
renal perfusion
renal perfusion imaging
renal pyramids
renal resistive index
renal scan, diuretic
renal scarring
renal scintigraphy

renal sclerosis
renal shadow
renal shutdown
renal sinus echo
renal sinus echocardiogram
renal sinus fat
renal stent
renal transit time (RTT)
renal transplant
renal trauma
renal tubular ectasia
renal tubular function
renal tubular necrosis
renal tubular osteomalacia
renal tubules
renal ultrasound
renal vascular damage
renal vascular hypertension (RVH)
renal vein
renal vein thrombosis
rendering
    BabyFace 3-D surface rendering
        ultrasound
    perspective volume (PVR)
    quantitative spirometrically con-
        trolled CT angiography with
        volume rendering
    real-time volume rendering
    spiral CT with multiplanar
        reformatting and 3D rendering
    surface projection
    3D
    transparent
    volume
    voxel gradient
Rendu-Osler-Weber disease or syn-
    drome (also Weber-Osler-Rendu)
reniform contour
renin-angiotensin dependent outer
    cortex
renin-angiotensin mechanism
renin-secreting tumor

Renkin model
RenoCal-76 (diatrizoate meglumine
    66% and diatrizoate sodium 10%)
    imaging agent
Reno-Dip imaging agent
Reno-30, Reno-60 (diatrizoate meglu-
    mine) imaging agent
renogram curve
Renografin-60 imaging agent
renography
    captopril
    DTPA
    radionuclide
renolithiasis (renal lithiasis)
renovascular hypertension
renovascular reconstruction
renovascular stent
Renshaw cell
rent (tear or rupture)
Rentrop infusion catheter
reocclusion, post-thrombolytic
    coronary
reorganization, subtle neuronal
reoxygenation
repeatability
repeated FID (free induction decay)
repeated microtraumas
reperfuse
reperfusion
    acute myocardial infarction
    controlled aortic root
    coronary
    normokalemic
reperfusion edema after lung trans-
    plantation
reperfusion injury of postischemic
    lungs
reperfusion therapy
repetition time (TR)
repetitive seizures
repetitive strain (or stress) injury (RSI)
rephasing gradient

replacement
  aortic root
  aortic valve (AVR)
  ascending aneurysm
  bone
  fatty
  mitral valve (MVR)
  orthotopic total heart
replantation of amputated digit or
  extremity
repletion
reproducibility
reproducible baseline state
reproduction, colorimetric color
rerotation, varus
reroute, rerouted
rerouting
  intraventricular
  tendon
rerupture of aneurysm
resampling, volumetric
rescue defibrillation
rescue PTCA
rescue shock
resected, surgically
resecting fracture
resection, video-assisted thoracoscopic
  wedge
reserve
  cardiac
  contractile
  coronary flow (CFR)
  diastolic
  left ventricular systolic functional
  myocardial perfusion (MPR)
  preload
  pulmonary vascular
  regional contractile
  stenotic flow (SFR)
  systolic
  vascular
  ventricular
reserve force

reserve mechanism, heart rate
reservoir (also pouch)
  Accu-Flo CSF
  Braden flushing
  continent ileal
  Cordis implantable drug
  CSF (cerebrospinal fluid)
  double bubble flushing
  double barrel
  double J-shaped
  fecal
  flush
  flushing
  Foltz flushing
  ileal
  ileoanal
  intra-abdominal ileal
  J-shaped
  J-Vac suction
  Kock ileal
  lateral internal pelvic
  McKenzie
  Ommaya ventriculostomy
  Parks ileoanal
  peripheral venous
  Rickham intraventricular
  Salmon Rickham ventriculostomy
  Secor implantable drug
  S-shaped
  ventricular catheter
  W-stapled urinary
reservoir effect
residual
  fibrocalcific
  fibrocystic
  fibrotic
  gastric
  postvoid
  postvoiding (PVR)
residual cement
residual contrast material
residual deficit, significant
residual distortion

residual fraction (RF)
residual gradient
residual hemiparesis
residual interstitial changes
residual limb shape change
residual plaque
residual pulmonary dysfunction
residual renal function
residual stress analysis
residual urine
residual urine accumulation
residual volume (RV)
residual volume/total lung capacity
    (RV/TLC)
residue, fecal
residuum morphology
resilient artery
resistance
    airway (RAW)
    arteriolar
    calculated
    coronary vascular
    decreased peripheral vascular
    decreased systemic
    expiratory
    fixed pulmonary valvular
    increased airways
    increased cerebral vascular
    increased outflow
    increased peripheral
    increased pulmonary vascular
    index of runoff
    nasal airway
    peripheral vascular (PVR)
    pulmonary arteriolar
    pulmonary vascular (PVR)
    systemic vascular (SVR)
    total peripheral (TPR)
    total pulmonary (TPR)
    vascular
    vascular systemic
    Wood units index of
resistance blood flow

resistive exercise table
resistive index (RI)
resistive magnet
resolution
    contrast
    high temporal
    interval
    spatial
resolution stage
Resolve drainage catheter
resolving pneumonia
resolved (or resolving) rejection
resolving pneumonia
resolving time
resonance
    bandbox
    bubble
    cough
    cracked-pot
    nuclear magnetic (NMR)
    skodaic
    tympanic
    vesicular
    vesiculotympanic
    vocal
    whispering
    wooden
resonance line
resonant frequency
resonant percussion note
resonator
    bridged loop gap
    multicoupled loop gap
resorbable pin
resorbable plate
resorbable rod
resorbable screw
resorption
    bone
    bony
    dependent edema fluid
    fluid
    osteoclastic

resorption phase of healing
respiration gated three-dimensional
(3D) reconstruction
respiratory atrium
respiratory bronchiolitis
respiratory compensation
respiratory complications
respiratory compromise
respiratory decompensation
respiratory disturbance of acid base
respiratory embarrassment
respiratory excursions full and equal
respiratory frequency
respiratory gating technique
respiratory insufficiency
respiratory modulation of vascular
   impedance
respiratory motion artifacts
respiratory muscle weakness
respiratory ordered phase encoding
   (ROPE)
respiratory spasm
respiratory status, compromised
respiratory stridor
respiratory syncytial viral pneumonia
respiratory tract obstruction,
   mechanical
respiratory triggering
response
   abnormal ejection fraction
   blood oxygenation level-dependent
      (BOLD)
   cardioinhibitory
   controlled ventricular
   hemodynamic
   metabolic
   rapid ventricular
   regional cerebral blood flow
   slow ventricular
   therapeutic
   vagal
   vasoactive

response *(cont.)*
   vasoconstrictor
   vasodepressor
   vasodilatory
   ventricular
responsive to TSH manipulation
responsiveness, airway
restenosis after angioplasty
restiform body
resting electrocardiogram
resting end systolic wall stress
resting heart
resting imaging
resting MUGA scan, preoperative
resting perfusion
resting phase of cardiac action
   potentials
resting pulse
resting redistribution thallium-201
   scintigraphy
resting regional myocardial blood flow
resting regional myocardial
   hypoperfusion
rest injection
rest LV (left ventricular) function
rest-redistribution exam
rest RV (right ventricular) function
rest thallium-201 myocardial imaging
restoration algorithm
restoration of sinus rhythm
restriction, unilateral flow
restrictive abnormality
restrictive bulbo-ventricular foramen
restrictive cardiac syndrome
restrictive defect
restrictive hemodynamic syndrome
restrictive lung disease
restrictive myocardial disease
restrictive-obstructive lung disease,
   mixed
restrictive pattern
restrictive ventilatory defect

result (pl. results)
    concordant
    false-positive
    false-negative
    suboptimal
resurrection bone
retained bladder syndrome
retained cortical activity (RCA)
retained foreign body
retained secretions
retained urine
retard premature rewarming
rete (pl. retia)
rete pegs
rete ridges
retention cyst
retention of barium
retention of stool
reticular activating formation (RAF)
reticular activating substance
reticular activating system (RAS)
reticular formation of brain stem
reticular infiltrate
reticular opacity
reticular pattern
reticulation artifact
reticulocortical pathway
reticuloendothelial contrast agent
reticuloendothelial system
reticulogranular appearance
reticulogranular pattern
reticulonodular infiltrate
reticulospinal tract
reticulum
    hematopoietic (of marrow)
    arcoplasmic
reticulum cell sarcoma
retina, angiomatosis of
retinacular disruption
retinacular ligaments
retinaculum
    avulsed
    extensor

retinaculum *(cont.)*
    flexor
    patellar
    superior peroneal (SPR)
retinal exudate
retinoblastoma
retraction (pl. retractions)
    chest wall
    clot
    costal
    inspiratory
    intercostal
    late systolic
    leaflet
    midsystolic
    mild subcostal
    nipple
    postrheumatic cusp
    sternocleidomastoid
    sternum
    substernal
    suprasternal
    systolic
retractor, plastic
re-treating
retrieval
    microvascular
    transvaginal oocyte
retroappendiceal fossa
retroareolar dysplasia
retrobulbar hemorrhage
retrocalcaneal bursa
retrocalcaneal exostosis
retrocalcaneal spur
retrocardiac density
retrocardiac infiltrate
retrocardiac space
retrocecal appendix
retroclavicular
retrocrural lymph nodes
retroesophageal subclavian artery
retroflexed scope
retroflexed view

retroflexion
retrograde angiography
retrograde aortogram
retrograde arterial catheterization
retrograde atherectomy
retrograde atrial activation mapping
retrograde blood flow across valve
retrograde blood velocity
retrograde cerebral perfusion (RCP)
retrograde colonic washout
retrograde conduction
retrograde coronary sinus infusion
retrograde duodenogastroscopy (RDG)
retrograde fashion
   advanced in a
   catheter advanced in a
retrograde femoral arterial approach
retrograde filling
retrograde filling of vessels
retrograde flow on barium enema
retrograde imaging
retrograde index (RI)
retrograde injection
retrogradely (backward)
retrograde metastasis
retrograde percutaneous femoral artery
   approach for cardiac catheterization
retrograde perfusion
retrograde peristalsis
retrograde pyelogram
retrograde pyelography
retrograde refractory period
retrograde transfemoral aortography
retrograde ureteral catheterization
retrograde ureteral stent
retrograde ureterogram
retrograde urethrogram catheter
retrograde ureterography
retrograde ureteropyelogram
retrograde ventriculoatrial conduction
retrohepatic vena cava
retroileal appendix
retrolisthesis

retromammary space view in
   mammography
retromedullary arteriovenous
   malformation
retronuchal muscle
retroorbital space
retropancreatic preaortic space
retropancreatic tunnel
retropectoral mammary implant
retroperfusion
   coronary sinus
   synchronized
retroperitoneal actinomycosis
retroperitoneal adenopathy
retroperitoneal approach
retroperitoneal area
retroperitoneal bleeding
retroperitoneal fibrosis
retroperitoneal hematoma
retroperitoneal hemorrhage
retroperitoneal region
retroperitoneal space
retroperitoneal tumor
retroperitoneal tunnel
retroperitoneally
retroperitoneum
retropharyngeal abscess
retropubic space
retropulsion of bone fragment into
   spinal canal
retrosellar region
retrosomatic cleft
retrosternal chest pain
retrosternal thyroid
retrotorsion, femoral
retroversion, femoral
retrovestibular neural pathway
retrusion, midface
RETT (radionuclide esophageal transit
   test)
return
   anomalous
   anomalous pulmonary venous

return *(cont.)*
    central arterial
    infracardiac-type total anomalous
        venous
    paracardiac-type total anomalous
        venous
    pulmonary venous
    supracardiac-type total anomalous
        venous
    systemic venous
    total anomalous pulmonary venous
    total anomalous venous
    venous
return to baseline
Retzius
    ligament of
    line of
    space of
    system of
    vein of
REU (rectal endoscopic ultrasonog-
    raphy)
revascularization
    cerebral
    coronary
    coronary ostial
    endosteal
    foot
    graft
    heart
    infrainguinal
    intraoperative transmyocardial
        (ITMR)
    myocardial
    off-pump beating heart
    percutaneous
    radiofrequency percutaneous
        myocardial
    surgical
revascularized tissue
Reveal XVI PET/CT imaging
Revelation microcatheter
reverberation echoes

reversal of blood flow
reversal of cervical lordosis
reversal, shunt
reversal sign
reverse Barton fracture
reverse Berman angiographic balloon
    catheter
reverse Colles fracture
reversed coarctation
reversed differential cyanosis
reverse distribution
reversed greater saphenous vein
reversed Mercedes-Benz sign
reversed peristalsis
reversed-3 sign
reverse immunoassay
reverse redistribution
reverse Towne view
reverse transport
reverse Waters view
reversible (or resolving) ischemic
    neurologic deficit (RIND)
reversible airways disease (RAD)
reversible atrial pacing
reversible defect
reversible ischemia
reversible obstructive airway disease
    (ROAD)
reversible organic brain syndrome
reversible perfusion defects
revolving Ge-68 pins as transmission
    sources
Reye syndrome
Reynolds number
REZ (root exit zone)
RF (rapid filling)
RF (radiofrequency) (see *radiofre-
    quency*)
RF (residual fraction)
RFA (radiofrequency ablation)
RFCA (radiofrequency catheter
    ablation)
RFP (rapid filling period)

RF-PMR (radiofrequency percutaneous
   myocardial revascularization)
RFW (rapid filling wave)
Rh (rhodium) isoimmunization
rhabdoid suture
rhabdoid tumor
rhabdomyolysis
rhabdomyoma of heart
rhabdomyosarcoma
   alveolar
   cardiac
   childhood
   primary
   vaginal
RHCT (renal helical CT)
rhebosis
rhenium (Re) (an element)
   ^{186}Re hydroxyethylidene diphos-
      phonate (^{186}Re HEDP)
   ^{188}Re-labeled antibodies
rheologic pattern
rheography, light reflection
Rhese view of optic foramen
Rhese view of orbits
rheumatic adherent pericardium
rheumatic aortic insufficiency
rheumatic aortic stenosis
rheumatic chorea
rheumatic fever (RF)
rheumatic heart disease (RHD)
rheumatic lesion
rheumatic mitral stenosis
rheumatic nodule
rheumatic pneumonia
rheumatic valvular disease
rheumatoid arthritis (RA) factor
rheumatoid arthritis-associated
   interstitial lung disease
rheumatoid nodule
rheumatoid spondylitis
rheumatologist
rhinocerebral mucormycosis
rhodium (Rh)

rhomboid fossa
rhomboid ligament
rhomboid major muscle
rhomboideus muscle
rhonchus (pl. rhonchi)
RHS (radial head subluxation)
RHV (right hepatic vein)
rhythm disorder
rhythmic segmentation
rhythm, protodiastolic gallop
RI (resistive index) angiography
RI (retrograde index)
RIA (radioimmunoassay) test
rib (pl. ribs)
   angle of
   bed of
   bicipital
   bifid
   cervical
   facet for head of
   false
   first
   floating
   fused
   head of
   hypoplastic horizontal
   inferior border of
   inferior margin of superior
   intrathoracic
   lumbar
   minced
   neck of
   notching of
   penciling of
   periosteum of
   retracted
   rudimentary
   shaft of
   slipping
   sternal
   Stiller
   superior
   superior margin of inferior

rib *(cont.)*
  true
  tubercle of
  vertebral
  vertebrocostal
  vertebrosternal
ribbon application
rib contusion
rib fracture from cough
rib guillotine
rib notching
rib recession
rib spaces, narrowed
rib view
rice grain calcification
Richet, tibio-astragalocalcaneal canal
  of
Richter hernia
Richter-Monroe line
rickets, familial hypophosphatemic
rickettsial pneumonia
Rickham reservoir
rider's bone
ridge
  alveolar
  alveodental
  apical ectodermal (AER)
  basal
  bicipital
  bisagittal
  broad maxillary
  buccocervical
  buccogingival
  bulbar
  cerebral
  cranial
  cutaneous
  dental
  dorsal
  epicondylar
  epidermal
  epipericardial
  fibrocartilaginous

ridge *(cont.)*
  fibromuscular
  ganglion
  gastrocnemial
  genital
  gluteal
  greater multangular
  humeral
  interarticular
  interosseous
  intertrochanteric
  interureteric
  longitudinal
  marginal
  mesonephric
  mylohyoid
  oblique
  Outerbridge
  palatine
  pectoral
  petrous
  radial
  ridging
  sagittal
  semicircular
  septal
  sphenoid
  supra-aortic
  supracondylar
  supracoronary
  supraorbital
  tentorial
  transverse
  triangular
  ulnar
  urethral
  urogenital
  vastus lateralis
  wolffian
riding embolus
Ridley sinus
Ridley syndrome
Riechert-Mundinger (RM) head frame

Riechert-Mundinger (RM) technique
Riedel thyroiditis
Riedel lobe
Riedel struma
Rieux hernia
RIF-1 tumor
right and left atrial phasic volumetric
  function
right and retrograde left heart
  catheterization
right angle chest tube
right-angled telescopic lens
right anterior oblique (RAO) position
right aortic arch with mirror image
  branching
right atrial enlargement
right atrial extension of uterine
  leiomyosarcoma
right atrial patch positioned over the
  right atrioventricular sulcus
right atrial pressure (RAP)
right atrium
right border of heart
right bundle branch block (RBBB)
right bundle branch block with left
  anterior (or posterior) hemiblock
right coronary artery, dominant
right frontoanterior (RFA) position
right frontoposterior (RFP) position
right frontotransverse (RFT) position
right heart catheter
right heart failure
right heart pressure
right inferior epigastric artery
right internal iliac artery
right internal jugular artery
right internal mammary anastomosis
right Judkins catheter
right lateral decubitus position
right lateral decubitus view
right-left disorientation
right lower lobe (RLL) of lung
right main stem bronchus

right mentoanterior (RMA) position
right mentotransverse (RMT) position
right middle lobe
right middle lobe (RML) of lung
right middle lobe lingula
right occipitoanterior (ROA) position
right occipitotransverse (ROT) position
right posterior oblique (RPO) position
right sacroanterior (RSA) position
right sacroposterior (RSP) position
right sacrotransverse (RST) position
right-side-down decubitus position
right-sided empyema
right-sided heart failure
right-sided pneumonia
right subclavian artery, retroesophageal
right to left shift
right to left shunt with pulmonic
  stenosis
right to left shunting
right to left shunt of blood
right upper lobe (RUL)
right upper lobe consolidation
right upper quadrant (RUQ)
right ureter
right ventricle
  augmented filling of
  double outlet
  parchment
right ventricle adherent to posterior
  table of sternum
right ventricle outflow tract
right ventricle pulmonary artery
  conduit
right ventricular assist device (RVAD)
right ventricular coil
right ventricular conduction defect
right ventricular ejection fraction
  (RVEF)
right ventricular end diastolic volume
  (RVEDV)
right ventricular end systolic volume
  (RVESV)

right ventricular failure
right ventricular hypertrophy (RVH)
right ventricular impulse, hyperdynamic
right ventricular obstruction,
intraventricular
right ventricular outflow obstruction
right ventricular outflow tract
right ventricular overload
right ventricular pressure (RVP)
right ventricular stroke volume
right ventricular stroke work (RVSW)
right ventricular stroke work index
(RVSWI)
right ventricular systolic time interval
rigid ureter
Rigiflex TTS balloon catheter
Rigler sign
RIGS (radioimmunoguided surgery)
RILD (radiation-induced lung disease)
rim
acetabular
dark signal intensity
glenoid
high density
low density
sclerotic
signal intensity
rimlike calcium distribution
rim sign
RIND (reversible or resolving
ischemic neurologic deficit)
Rindfleisch, fold of
ring (pl. rings)
abdominal
Ace-Colles half
amnion
annular
anorectal
aortic subvalvular
apex of external
arc
atrial

ring *(cont.)*
atrioventricular
Bickel
Cannon
Carpentier
cartilaginous
CBI stereotactic
centering
Charnley centering
choroidal
ciliary
common tendinous
congenital (of aortic arch)
constriction
Crawford suture
crural
distal esophageal
double-flanged valve sewing
doughnut
drop-lock
esophageal A
esophageal B
esophageal contractile
esophageal mucosal
esophageal muscular
external
external inguinal
femoral
fibrocartilaginous
fibrous
fracture
fracture encircling foramen
magnum
half
halo
ilioinguinal
iliopsoas
Ilizarov
inguinal
internal abdominal
internal inguinal
intrahaustral contraction
ischial weightbearing

ring *(cont.)*
  Kayser-Fleischer
  lymphoid
  mitral
  mitral valve
  Mose concentric
  Ochsner
  olive
  orthosis drop-lock
  pelvic
  perichondral
  periosteal bone
  pleural
  prosthetic valve sewing
  prosthetic valve suture
  proximal to distal
  pyloric
  retraction
  Schatzki
  sewing
  Silastic
  silicone elastomer
  sizing
  sodium iodide
  sphincter contraction
  stereotactic or stereotaxic
  superficial inguinal
  supra-annular suture
  supravalvar
  tricuspid valve
  tubal
  valve
  vascular
  vertebral
  Vieussens
  Waldeyer
  Zinn
ring apophysis
ring blush on cerebral arteriography
Ring catheter
ring enhancement
ring-enhancing lesion
Ringer irrigation

Ringer solution (now Ringer irrigation)
ringlike configuration
ringlike contractions
Ring-McLean catheter
ring shadows with air-fluid levels
ring-sparing fracture
ring-sparing injury
ring-type imaging system
Riolan, arch of
Riolan bone (ossicle)
Riordan finger pollicization
Rippstein goniometer
Rippstein leg support
Rippstein method to view femoral neck
RISA (radioactive iodinated serum albumin)
Riseborough-Radin classification of intercondylar fracture
rise times
risk analysis
risk/benefit ratio
Risser-Ferguson method to measure scoliosis
Risser plaster corset
Risser scoliosis scale
Risser technique
Ritchie index
Riva-Rocci manometer
Riviere sign
RLE (right lower extremity)
RLL (right lower lobe) of lung
RLQ (right lower quadrant)
r-metHuG-CSF (recombinant human granulocyte colony stimulating factor)
RML (right middle lobe) of lung
RNA (radionuclide angiogram), gated
RNS terminal
RNV (radionuclide ventriculogram)
R/O (rule out)
ROA (regurgitant orifice area)

ROAD (reversible obstructive airway disease)
road-mapping for interventional radiography
road-mapping mode
Robert hyperpronated view of the thumb base
Robertson sign
Robicsek vascular probe (RVP)
robin's egg-blue gallbladder
Robin Hood phenomenon (steal syndrome)
Robinson catheter, red rubber
Robinson-Chung-Farahvar clavicular morcellation
Robinson straight urethral catheter
robotics-controlled stereotactic frame
robust registration technique
ROC (receiver operating characteristics)
Rocher view (skull)
rocking curve measurement
rocking precordial motion
Rockwood classification of acromioclavicular injury
Rockwood serendipity view
rod, TLD (thermoluminescent dosimeter)
RODEO (rotating delivery of excitation off-resonance), 3D
Rodriguez-Alvarez catheter
Roederer obliquity
rOEF (regional oxygen extraction fraction)
roentgen (R)
roentgen knife
roentgen stereophotogrammetric analysis (RSA)
roentgenkymography
roentgenogram
roentgenographic control
roentgenographic silhouette
roentgenography

roentgenologist
roentogenographically occult
Rogan teleradiology system
Roger syndrome
Roger ventricular septal defect
ROI (region of interest)
Rokitansky-Aschoff sinus
Rokitansky-Cushing ulcer
Rokitansky diverticulum
Rokitansky pelvis
Rolando angle
Rolando area
Rolando fissure
Rolando fracture
Rolando line
Rolando point
Rolando tubercle
Rolleston rule for systolic blood pressure
roll, radiolucent
Romano-Ward syndrome
Romberg-Wood syndrome
Romhilt-Estes score for left ventricular hypertrophy
ROMI (rule out myocardial infarction)
ROMIed (past tense verb for ruled out myocardial infarction)
roof
    acetabular
    intercondylar
root
    anatomical
    cochlear
    coronary sinus
    cranial
    dental
    dilated aortic
    facial
    insula
    lingual
    lung
    motor

root *(cont.)*
  nerve
  palatine
  retained
  sensory
  spinal
  ventral
  ventricle
rootlets of nerve
root-mean-squared gradient measure
ROPE (respiratory ordered phase
  encoding)
ropelike cord (in thrombophlebitis)
ropy
Roques syndrome
Rosch catheter
Rosch-Thurmond fallopian tube
  catheter
Rosch-Uchida transjugular liver access
  needle-catheter
rose bengal sodium ^{131}I radioactive
  biliary agent
Rosenbach syndrome
Rosenberg weightbearing view of knee
Rosenblatt implantable vascular access
  port
Rosen-Castleman-Liebow syndrome
Rosenmüller (Rosenmueller) fossa
Rosenthal, basal vein of (BVR)
rose thorn sign
rosette appearance of anus
rostral brain stem ischemia
rostral cervical nerve
rostral connection
rostral hypothalamus
rostral medulla
rostral pons
rostral spinal cord
rostral terminus
rostrally
rostrum of corpus callosum
rostrum sphenoidale
rotary instability

rotary scoliosis
rotary subluxation
rotary thoracolumbar scoliosis
rotatable pigtail catheter
rotating bur (or burr)
rotating delivery of excitation off-
  resonance), 3D (RODEO)
rotating frame imaging
rotating frame of reference
rotating gamma camera
rotating tomographic projection
rotating tourniquets for pulmonary
  edema
rotation
  360°
  tube position
rotation therapy
rotational alignment
rotational atherectomy system (RAS)
rotational coronary atherectomy (RCA)
rotational flaps
rotational force
rotational radiotherapy
rotator cuff tear
rotatory loads on spine
Rotch sign in pericardial effusion
Rotograph Plus panoramic dental
  tomography imaging system
Roubin-Gianturco flexible coil stent
rough zone
roughened state of pericardium
roughened surface
rouleaux formation
round cell tumors
round catheter tip
rounded border of lung
rounded convex borders
round pelvis
round pronator (pronator radii teres)
routine magnification view
routine view
Rouviere, ligament of
Roux-en-Y anastomosis

Roux-en-Y limb
row, carpal
Rowe calcaneal fracture classification
Rowe-Lowell fracture-dislocation
  classification system
row mode sinogram images
Royal Flush angiographic flush
  catheter
Royal women's coaxial catheter
Royer-Wilson syndrome
RPA (right pulmonary artery)
rpm (rotations per minute)
RPO (right posterior oblique) position
RPO 30° voiding cystogram
RPO and LPO 30° intravenous urog-
  raphy
RPT (rapid pull-through) technique
RPV (right pulmonary vein)
RSA (roentgen stereophotogrammetric
  analysis)
RSCVP (right subclavian central
  venous pressure)
RSI (repetitive stress injury)
RSNA (Radiologic Society of North
  America)
RT (repetition time)
RTA (radiofrequency thermal ablation)
RTT (renal transit time)
RT 3200 Advantage ultrasound
  scanner
RT 6800 ultrasound scanner
RTL cassette
RTOG protocol
RTP (radiation therapy planning)
  system
RTV cassette
rubidium (Rb) (an element)
  ^{82}Rb-based cardiac imaging
  ^{82}Rb-35S-33P
Rubin test
Rubratope-57 (cyanocobalamin Co-57)
  radioactive agent
rubrospinal tract

rubrous
rudimentary bone
rudimentary ribs
rudimentary sinus
rudimentary ventricular chamber
RUE (right upper extremity)
Ruedi-Allgower tibial plafond fracture
  classification
ruga (pl. rugae)
rugal folds
rugal pattern
rugger-jersey spine
RUL (right upper lobe) of lung
rule
  buccal object
  Clarke
rule-based scheme
rule out (R/O)
rule out myocardial infarction (ROMI)
rules, Paterson-Parker
Rumel catheter
runoff
  absent
  aortic
  aortofemoral
  arterial
  digital
  distal
  inadequate
  peripheral
  single vessel
  suboptimal
  three-vessel
  two-vessel
  vessel
runoff arteriogram
runoff resistance, index of
runoff vessel
runoff views, aortofemoral arteriography with
rupture
  abdominal aortic aneurysm
  aneurysmal

rupture *(cont.)*
  appendix
  Achilles tendon
  arch
  arterial
  buttonhole
  cardiac
  chordae tendineae
  chordal
  complete Achilles tendon
  contained aneurysmal
  forniceal
  interventricular septal
  large bladder
  myocardial
  nodal
  papillary muscle
  plantaris (tennis leg)
  plaque
  silicone implant
  ventricular free wall
  ventricular septal
  vessel
rupture of membranes (ROM),
  acoustically induced
rupture of uterus
ruptured capillaries
ruptured chordae tendineae
ruptured colonic wall
ruptured disk
ruptured pseudoaneurysm
ruptured urethra
ruptured emphysematous bleb
ruptured follicle
ruptured intracranial aneurysm
ruptured thoracic duct
RUQ (right upper quadrant)

Russell-Rubinstein classification of
  cerebrovascular malformation
Russell-Silver syndrome
Russian roulette (referring to a mix-
  ture of MR imaging techniques)
rutherford (rd) radioactive unit
Rutner percutaneous suprapubic
  balloon catheter
Ruysch disease
RV (residual volume)
RVA (right ventricular apical)
  electrogram
RVBF (reversed vertebral blood flow)
RVD (right ventricular diastolic)
  pressure
RVD (right ventricular dimension)
RVE (right ventricular enlargement)
RVFW (right ventricular free wall)
RVH (renal vascular hypertension)
RVH (right ventricular hypertrophy)
RVID (right ventricular internal
  diameter)
RVM (right ventricular mass)
RVOT (right ventricular outflow tract)
RVP (right ventricular pressure)
RVP–LVP (right ventricular to left
  ventricular systolic pressure) ratio
RV (right ventricle) pressure
RVS (right ventricular systolic)
  pressure
RVSTI (right ventricular systolic time
  interval)
RVSW (right ventricular stroke work)
RVSWI (right ventricular stroke work
  index)
RV/TLC (residual volume/total lung
  capacity)

S, s

SAA protein
SAB (sinoatrial block)
Sabathie sign
saber shin
sac
    abdominal
    abnormal gestational
    air
    alveolar
    amniotic
    aneurysmal
    aortic
    bursal
    chorionic
    common dural
    cystic
    decidual
    dental
    double decidual
    dural
    effacement of dural
    embryonic
    endolymphatic
    enterocele
    false
    fluid-filled
    gestational

sac *(cont.)*
    greater peritoneal
    heart
    hernia
    indirect hernia
    intrauterine
    lesser peritoneal
    narrowing of thecal
    pericardial
    peritoneal
    pleural
    spinal
    terminal air
    thecal
    tight dural
    widemouth
    wrapped aneurysmal
    yolk
sacciform kidney
sacciform recess
saccular aneurysm
saccular appearance, lobulated
saccular bronchiectasis
saccular collection
saccular formation
saccular mass
sacculated pleurisy

sacculation
saccule
sacculus ventricularis
Sack-Barabas syndrome
saclike spaces
sacral ala
sacral cyst
sacral dermatomes
sacral gutter
sacral insufficiency fracture (SIF)
sacralization of vertebrae
sacralized transverse process
sacral plexus
sacral promontory
sacroabdominoperineal pull-through
sacrococcygeal chordoma
sacrococcygeal joint
sacrococcygeal remnant tumor
sacrococcygeal teratoma
sacrococcyx
sacroiliac (SI)
sacroiliac articulation
sacroiliac disease
sacroiliac joint
sacroiliac sprain
sacroiliac subluxation
sacroposterior (SP) breech position
sacrotransverse (ST) position
sacropubic diameter
sacrosciatic foramen
sacrosciatic notch
sacrospinalis muscle
sacrotuberous ligament
sacrouterine
sacrovertebral angle
sacrum (sacral spine)
   alae of
   assimilation
   cornua of
   promontory of
   scimitar
   tilted
sacrum right posterior (SRP) position

SACT (sinoatrial conduction time)
saddle-area anesthesia
saddle coil
saddle embolism or embolus
saddle joint
saddle points
SADIA (small angle double incidence
   angiograms)
Sadowsky breast marking system
SaECG (signal-averaged electrocardiogram)
SAFER (saphenous [vein graft] angioplasty free of emboli randomized)
SAFHS (sonic-accelerated fracture-
   healing system)
SAFT (Synthetic Aperture Focusing
   Technique) in intravascular ultrasound imaging
Sage-Salvatore classification of
   acromioclavicular joint injury
sagging rope sign
sagittal 3D T1w-gradient echo
   sequence
sagittal image
sagittal gradient echo image
sagittal groove
sagittal image
sagittal oblique images
sagittal orientation
sagittal plane
sagittal plane faults
sagittal plane loop
sagittal roll spondylolisthesis
sagittal section
sagittal sinus
sagittal slice
sagittal suture
sagittal T-1 image
sagittal tomogram
sagittal transabdominal image
sagittal ultrasound
SAH (subarachnoid hemorrhage)
Sahara densitometry

sail-like anterior leaflet
sail sign (of fat pad in elbow joint)
Sakellarides classification of calcaneal
    fracture
saline
    heparinized
    hypertonic
    sterile
saline-enhanced MR arthrography
saline-enhanced RF tissue ablation
saline loading
saline solution
saline torch
salivagram
salivary gland function study
Salkowski test
salpingitis
    chronic interstitial
    follicular
    gonococcal
    hemorrhagic
    interstitial
    pseudofollicular
    purulent
    tuberculous
salpingogram
salpingography
    selective
    selective osteal
salpinx (pl. salpinges)
salt and pepper calvaria
salt and pepper duodenal erosion
Salter-Harris classification of fracture
    (I through VI, or 1-6)
Salter-Harris-Rang classification of
    fracture
salt wasting, cerebral
salvage, interventional limb
salvage of myocardium
salvage surgery
salvage therapy
salvo of echoes

salvo of premature ventricular
    complexes
SAM (scanning acoustic microscope)
SAM (systolic anterior motion) on
    2-D echocardiogram
samarium (Sm) (an element)
    ^{153}Sm EDTMP (ethylene diamine
        tetramethylene phosporic acid
        imaging agent
    ^{153}Sm lexidronam radiotherapy
        agent
same-day microsurgical arthroscopic
    lateral-approach laser-assisted
    (SMALL) fluoroscopic diskectomy
SampleMaster biopsy needle
sample points
sampling
    adrenal vein
    tissue
    zonal
sampling of mammographic lesion
Samuels Micro-Scler catheter
SAN (sinoatrial node)
Sanchez-Perez automatic film changer
sandbag hazard
sandbagging fracture of long bones
Sandhoff disease
Sandrock test for thrombosis
sandwiched infundibulum
sandwich patch closure, anterior
sandwich sign
Sanfilippo syndrome
SA (sinoatrial)
SA nodal reentry tachycardia
SA node (also called sinus)
Sansom sign in pericardial effusion
Sansregret modification of Chausse III
    method to view middle ear
Santiani-Stone classification of
    pancreatitis
Santorini
    duct of
    papilla of

saphenofemoral junction
saphenous [vein graft] angioplasty free
    of emboli randomized (SAFER)
saphenous vein fistula
saphenous varices
saphenous vein
    greater
    reversed greater
saphenous vein bypass graft
saphenous vein graft (SVG)
saphenous vein incompetence
sarcoid-like reaction
sarcoid of Boeck
sarcoidosis
    hepatic
    spinal cord
sarcoma (see also *carcinoma*, *tumor*)
    Abernethy
    alveolar soft-part (ASPS)
    ameloblastic
    angiolithic
    botryoid
    cardiac
    clear cell
    endobronchial Kaposi
    endometrial stromal
    epithelioid
    Ewing
    gastric Kaposi
    giant cell monstrocellular
    granulocytic
    hemangioendothelial
    high grade surface osteogenic
    immunoblastic
    intracolonic Kaposi
    intracortical osteogenic
    intrathoracic Kaposi
    Ito cell
    Jensen
    juxtacortical osteogenic
    Kaposi epicardial
    Kupffer cell
    leukocytic

sarcoma *(cont.)*
    lipoblastic
    low grade central osteogenic
    lymphatic
    malignant myeloid
    medullary
    mixed cell
    multicentric osteogenic
    multiple idiopathic hemorrhagic
    myelogenic
    myeloid
    myocardial infiltration by Kaposi
    neurogenic
    osteogenic
    Paget associated osteogenic
    parosteal osteogenic
    periosteal
    postirradiation osteogenic
    primary
    pulmonary Kaposi
    reticulum cell
    right atrial
    small cell osteogenic
    spindle cell
    synovial
    telangiectatic osteogenic
    vasoablative endothelial (VABES)
sarcoma botryoides
Sarns occluder
Sarns wire-reinforced catheter
SAS (supravalvular aortic stenosis)
Sassone score of appearance in
    transvaginal ultrasound
satellite lesion
satellite nodule
satumomab pendetide (OncoScint
    CR/OV) imaging agent
saturation
    jugular venous oxygen
    MT (magnetization transfer)
    oxygen
    regional cerebral oxygen
    spectroscopic fat

saturation inversion projection (SIP)
saturation recovery sequence
saturation recovery technique
saturation stripe
saturation transfer
saucerization of vertebra
saucer-shaped acetabulum
saucer-shaped excavation
sausage digit
sausage finger, in syringomyelia
sausaging of vein
SAVANT (Surgical Anatomy Visuali-
    zation and Navigation Tools)
sawtooth (also saw-toothed)
sawtooth appearance
sawtooth irregularity of bowel contour
SBDX (scanning-beam digital x-ray)
SBE (small bowel enteroscopy)
SBF (systemic blood flow)
SBFT (small bowel follow-through)
SBO (small bowel obstruction)
SBO (spina bifida occulta)
SBP (systolic blood pressure)
SBSL (single bubble sonolumines-
    cence)
SBSP (simultaneous bilateral
    spontaneous pneumothorax)
SCA (superior cerebellar artery)
SCAD (spontaneous coronary artery
    dissection)
SCA-EX ShortCutter catheter with
    rotating blades
scalar quantization, wavelet (WSQ)
scale
    AIS (Abbreviated Injury Scale)
    false color
    fish
    gray
    Moss staging for gastric adeno-
        carcinoma
    Risser scoliosis
scalene fat pad
scalene musculature

scalenus anterior muscle
scalenus anticus muscle hypertrophy
scalenus anticus syndrome
scalenus minimus
scallop of posterior anulus, redundant
scallop, prolapsing
scalloped bowel lumen
scalloped commissure
scalloped luminal configuration
scalloping contour
scalloping of margin of vertebral body
scalloping of vertebrae
scalloping osteolysis
scalloping, vertebral
scalpel, ultrasonic-driven
scan (scintiscan) (see *imaging;*
    scanner)
    abdominopelvic CT
    BladderScan
    bone
    C-11 palmitate uptake on PET
    colloid shift on liver-spleen
    computerized tomographic (CT)
    contrast-enhanced
    contrast-enhanced CT
    contrast material-enhanced MRI
    coronal CT scan of sinuses
    coronary artery scan (CAS) by
        Ultrafast CT
    DEXA (dual energy x-ray absorp-
        tiometry)
    DEXAscan
    diuretic renal
    fan-beam DEXA
    four-slice coronal CT scan of
        sinuses
    F-scan
    isotropic lung
    Jedmed/DGH A-scan
    MAG 3 dynamic renal
    milk
    noncontrast-enhanced
    radioisotope bone

scan *(cont.)*
  radionuclide
  radionuclide bladder
  Scan-O-Grams of lower extremities
  sequential
  serial
  tagged red blood cell nuclear
scan decrement
scan defect
Scanditronix PET scanner
Scanmaster DX scanner
Scanmaster DX x-ray film digitizer
scanned projection radiography (SPR)
scanned-slot detector system
scanner (also *digitizer*; see *imaging*)
  Acoma
  Acuson 128EP
  Acuson ultrasound
  Advanced NMR systems
  Agfa IMPAX PACS
  Agfa Medical
  Agfa RIS/PACS (Radiology Infor-
    mation System/Picture Archiv-
    ing and Communications
    System)
  All-Tronics
  Aloka ultrasound linear
  Aloka ultrasound sector
  American Shared-CuraCare
  ANMR Insta-scan MR
  Artoscan MRI
  ATL duplex
  ATL Mark 600 real-time sector
  ATL real-time Neurosector
  Aurora MR breast imaging system
  Biospec MR imaging system
  BI-RADS (Breast Imaging Report-
    ing and Data System)
  Bruel-Kjaer ultrasound
  Bruker
  Canon
  Cemax/Icon
  Cencit surface

scanner *(cont.)*
  charge-coupled device
  cine CT (computed tomography)
  Compuscan Hittman computerized
    electrocardioscanner
  CT Max 640
  CT9000
  CTI 933/04 ECAT
  CTI PET
  Delarnette
  Diasonics ultrasound
  DOBI (dynamic optical breast
    imaging system)
  Dornier
  DuPont
  Dynamic Spatial Reconstructor
    (DSR)
  Eastman Kodak
  ECG-triggered multidetector
  electron beam CT
  Elscint CT
  Elscint Gyrex Prestige 2.0T MR
    imaging
  Elscint MR
  Elscint Privilege 0.5T MR imaging
  Elscint Twin CT
  EMED
  EMI CT
  Evolution XP ultrafast CT
  Fonar
  Fonar-360 MRI
  4096 Plus PET
  4D Cardio-View
  4-row
  fused PET-CT
  Galen Scan
  Gammex RMI
  GE (General Electric)
  GE Advance PET
  GE CT Max
  GE Discovery LS CT/PET
  GE 9800 CT
  GE 8800 CT/T

scanner *(cont.)*
GE Genesis CT
GE GN 500 MHz
GE HiSpeed Advantage helical CT
GE Max MR
GE 9800 high resolution CT
GE Omega 500 MHz
GE 1.5 tesla Signa
GE Pace CT
GE QE 300 MHz
GE Signa 1.5 tesla
GE Signa 4.7 MRI
GE Signa 5.2 with SR-230 3-axis
   EPI gradient upgrade
GE single axis SR-230 echo-planar
GE Vectra MR
Gyroscan ACS NT MRI
Gyroscan S15
Heartscan heart attack prediction
   test using ultrafast CT
helical CT
Hewlett-Packard
high field open MRI
high field strength
Hilight Advantage System
Hispeed CT
Hitachi CT
Hitachi MR
Hitachi 0.3T unit
Hitachi Open MRI System
Hologic 2000
Howtek Scanmaster DX
IDSI
Imatron C-100 ultrafast CT
Imatron C-100XL CT
Imatron C-150L EBCT
Imatron Fastrac C-100 cine x-ray
   CT
Imatron Ultrafast CT
Innervision MR
InstaScan
Integris 3000

scanner *(cont.)*
intensified radiographic imaging
   system (IRIS)
Irex Exemplar ultrasound
Konica
large bore 0.6T imaging system
large bore 1.5T imaging system
Lumiscan 150
Lunar
LymphoScan nuclear imaging
   system
Magna-SL
Magnetom 1.5T
Magnetom SP63
Magnes 2500 WH (whole blood)
Magnex MR
Mallinckrodt
Marconi Infinion
Max Plus MR
MedImage
Medison
Medspec MR imaging system
midget MRI
Miraluma nuclear breast imaging
modified electron-beam CT
mPower PET scanner by Positron
MR catheter imaging and
   spectroscopy system
multiple jointed digitizer
multisensor structured light range
   digitizer
NeuroSector
Nishimoto Sangyo
Norlan pQCT XCT2000
1.5 tesla
Olympus endoscopic ultrasound
Open Sky MRI (trademarked)
Oxford 2T large bore imaging
   system
Pace Plus System
Park Medical Systems
Perception

scanner *(cont.)*
PETite
Philips CT
Philips 1.5T NT MR
Philips 4.7 T small bore system
Philips Gyroscan ACS
Philips Gyroscan Intera
Philips Gyroscan NT; NT5; NT15
Philips Gyroscan S5
Philips Gyroscan T5
Philips tomoscan 350 CT
Picker CT
Picker Magnascanner
Picker MR
Picker PQ 5000 helical CT
Picker PQ-2000 spiral CT
Polhemus 3 digitizer
Posicam HZ PET
PQCT micro-scanner
ProSpeed CT
Quad MRI
QUAD 12000 high field, whole
  body, open MRI
QUAD 7000 high field, whole
  body, open MRI
Quick CT9800
rectilinear
RT 3200 Advantage ultrasound
RT 6800 ultrasound
Scanditronix PET
Scanmaster DX x-ray film digitizer
Scan 2000 TransSpectral imped-
  ance
scintillation (scintiscanner)
sector
Sensation 16 MDCT
Shimadzu CT
Shimadzu MR
Siemens CT
Siemens DRH CT
Siemens Magnetom GBS II
Siemens Magnetom Impact
Siemens Magnetom 1.5 T

scanner *(cont.)*
Siemans Magnetom SP 4000
Siemens Magnetom Vision
Siemens One tesla
Siemens Somaform 512 CT
Siemens Somatom DR2 whole-
  body; also DR3
Siemens Somatom PLUS-S
Siemens Somatom Sensation 40
Siemens Somatom Sensation
  Cardiac 64
Siemens Sonoline Elegra ultra-
  sound
Siemens SP 4000
SieScape ultrasound
Signa 1.5T
Signa Horizon
Signa I.S.T. MRI
single field hyperthermia combined
  with radiation therapy and ultra-
  sound
16-row
Smart Prep
Somatom DR CT
Somatom Plus-S CT
Sonopsy 3-D ultrasound breast
  biopsy system
spiral CT
spiral XCT
Swissray
TCT900S helical CT
Tecmag Libra-S16 system
3D surface digitizer
3M
3 tesla
Toshiba CT
Toshiba Excelart Planissimo
Toshiba helical CT
Toshiba MR
Toshiba 900S helical CT
Toshiba 900S/XII
Toshiba TCT-80 CT
Toshiba Xpress SX helical CT

scanner *(cont.)*
   TransScan TS2000 electrical
     impedance breast scanning
     system
   Trex digital mammography system
     (TDMS)
   Trionix
   T-Scan 2000 TransSpectral imped-
     ance
   ultrafast computed tomography
   Ultramark
   UM 4 real-time sector
   Vidar
   Vision MRI
   Vision 1.5-T Siemens MRI
   Vision Ten V-scan
   whole-body 1.5T Siemens Vision
   whole-body 3T MRI system
   Xpress/SX helical CT
scanning (see *imaging*)
scanning acoustic microscope (SAM)
scanning-beam digital x-ray (SBDX)
scanning laser ophthalmoscopy
scanning locus
scanogram (see *imaging*)
Scan-O-Grams of lower extremities
scanography (see *imaging*)
scan pacing
scan parameters
scan pitch
scan time
scan volume
scan with contrast enhancement
scan without contrast enhancement
scaphocapitate joint
scaphocephalic head shape
scaphocephaly
scaphoid abdomen
scaphoid bone (navicular)
   pole of
   waist of
scaphoid nonunion advanced collapse
   (SNAC) grades I-III

scapholunate (SL)
scapholunate arthritic collapse (SLAC)
   wrist
scapholunate dissociation
scapholunate joint
scapholunate ligament (LSS)
scapholunate space
scapholunate widening
scapho-trapezium-trapezoid (STT)
   joint
scaphotrapezoid joint
scapula
   body of
   high-riding
   inferior tip of
   margin of
   winged
scapular bone
scapular flap
scapular notch
scapular winging
scapular Y view
scapuloclavicular
scapulocostal syndrome
scapuloperoneal muscular atrophy
scapulothoracic motion
scapulovertebral border
scar (see also *scarring*)
   dense
   infarcted
   linear (in lungs)
   myocardial
   nonviable
   pulmonary
   well-demarcated
   zipper
scar contracture
scar formation
scar tissue
scar tissue reaction
scarification of pleura
scarified duodenum

Scarpa
  canal of
  fascia of
  ganglion of
  ligament of
  method of
  triangle of
scarred duodenum
scarred fibrotic media
scarring
  apical
  basilar pleural
  interstitial
  narrowing of the lumen due to
  parenchymal
  pleural
  postnecrotic
  selective
  valve
  valvular
scar tissue in ureter
scatoma (stercoroma)
scatter
  collimator
  soft tissue
scatter compensation
scattered air bronchogram
scattered fat
scattering
  coherent
  Compton
  low angle
  small angle multiple
  Rayleigh-Tyndall
scattering angle
scattering foil compensator
scattering system
scatter to primary ratio
SCFE (slipped capital femoral
  epiphysis)
Schatzker fracture classification
  system
Schatzki ring

Schatzki view
Schaumann body
scheme
  CISS
  computer-aided diagnosis
  encryption
  rule-based
Scheuer histologic staging
Scheuermann juvenile kyphosis
Schick sign of tuberculosis
Schiefferdecker disk
schistosomiasis
Schlatter-Osgood disease
Schlesinger, vein of
Schmidt optics system
Schmitt disease
Schmorl disease
Schmorl node
Schneider method to view femoral
  head
Schneider PTCA instruments
Schneider-Shiley catheter
Schneider Wallstent
Schonander film changer
Schönlein purpura
Schoonmaker multipurpose catheter
Schüller (Schueller)
Schüller duct
Schüller view
Schwann tumor
schwannoma
  facial
  orbital
  vestibular
Schwarten balloon dilatation catheter
Schwartz test for patency of deep
  saphenous veins
SCI (spinal cord injury)
sciatic artery, persistent
sciatic endometriosis
sciatic foramen
  greater
  lesser

sciatic nerve irritation
sciatic notch
  greater
  lesser
sciatic plexus
sciatica
SciMed Express balloon
SciMed Express Monorail balloon
SciMed NC Ranger PTCA catheter
SciMed SSC "Skinny" catheter
scimitar deformity
scimitar-shaped flap
scimitar-shaped shadow
scimitar sign on chest radiograph
scimitar vein
Scinticore multicrystal scintillation
  camera
scintigram (see *scintigraphy*)
scintigraphic balloon
scintigraphic imaging
scintigraphic study
scintigraphy
  ACE inhibition
  AMA-Fab (antimyosin monoclonal
    antibody with Fab fragment)
  antifibrin
  bone
  bone marrow
  brain perfusion
  cortical
  dipyridamole thallium-201
  dual intracoronary
  exercise stress-redistribution
  exercise thallium
  gallium
  gated blood pool
  hepatobiliary
  HIDA ("high-dah")-CCK
  indium (In)
  ^{111}In-WBC (indium with white
    blood cells)
  infarct-avid hot-spot

scintigraphy *(cont.)*
  iodine (I)
    ^{131}I-19-iodocholesterol
    ^{131}I MIBG
  isotope
  labeled FFA (free fatty acid)
  lacrimal
  MIBG (metaiodobenzylguanidine)
  microsphere perfusion
  myocardial cold-spot perfusion
  NEFA (nonesterified fatty acid)
  NP-59
  perfusion
  planar thallium
  pulmonary
  pyrophosphate
  quantitative hepatobiliary (QHS)
  radioistope
  radionuclide shunt
  radionuclide testicular
  renal
  resting-redistribution thallium-201
  single photon planar (SPPS)
  somatostatin receptor (SRS)
  SPECT brain perfusion
  SPECT thallium
  stress perfusion
  technetium ^{99m}Tc-PYP (pyrophos-
    phate)
  thallium
  thallium perfusion
  thallium-201 myocardial
  three-phase bone (TPBS)
  vesicoureteral
  white blood cell (WBCS) with
    indium-111 (^{111}In)
  whole body bone
scintillating scotoma (pl. scotomata)
scintillation camera
scintillation counter
scintillation crystal
scintillation detector

scintillation, migrainous-like
scintillation proximity radioimmuno-
    assay
scintillation scan
scintillation spectrometry
scintillator
    aqueous
    benzene
    CeI
    cyclohexane
    organic liquid
    toluene
scintimammography (SMM)
scintiphotograph
scintirenography
scintiscan (see *imaging*)
scintiscanner (see *scanner*)
scintiscanning
Scintiview nuclear computer system
Scintron IV nuclear computer system
scirrhous carcinoma
scirrhous lesion
scissor gait
scissoring of legs
SCL (sinus cycle length)
SCLC (small cell lung cancer)
scleroderma of esophagus
sclerosing nonsuppurative osteo-
    myelitis
sclerosing adenosis
sclerosing mesenteritis
sclerosing pattern
sclerosis
    Ammon horn (mesial temporal)
    aortic
    arterial
    arteriocapillary
    arteriolar
    Baló
    calcified
    congenital hippocampal
    coronary
    diffuse

sclerosis *(cont.)*
    disseminated
    endocardial
    esophageal variceal
    familial amyotrophic lateral
    gastric
    hepatic
    hepatoportal
    hippocampal
    incisural
    Krabbe diffuse
    laser
    lobar
    medial calcific
    mesenteric
    mesial temporal
    Mönckeberg
    multiple (MS)
    pedicle
    posterolateral (of the spinal cord)
    progressive systemic
    pulmonary and cardiac
    renal
    segmental vein
    subchondral
    subendocardial
    tuberous
    valvular
    variceal
    vascular
    venous
sclerotherapy
    alcohol
    percutaneous
    variceal
sclerotic area
sclerotic coronary arteries
sclerotic degeneration
sclerotic plaque (plaquing)
sclerotic rims in gout
scoliosis
    adolescent idiopathic (AIS)
    Aussies-Isseis unstable

scoliosis *(cont.)*
    Cobb measurement of
    dextrorotary
    dextro-
    Dwyer correction of
    Fergusson method for measuring
    fixation of a
    functional
    idiopathic
    King classification of thoracic
    King-Moe
    levorotary
    levo-
    lumbar
    lumbar component of
    Moe and Kettleson distribution of
        curves in
    nonstructural
    rotary
    S-shaped
    structural
    thoracic
    thoracolumbar
    uncompensated rotary
    Winter-King-Moe
scoliotic spine
SCOOP 1 transtracheal oxygen
    catheter
SCOOP 2 catheter with distal and
    side openings
scorbutic white line
score
    late effects toxicity
    LENT (late effects of normal
        tissues)
    mean wall motion
    thallium SPECT
    wall motion
scorings on bone on x-ray
scotoma (pl. scotomata)
    absolute
    bilateral
    cecocentral

scotoma *(cont.)*
    central
    dense
    fortification
    homonymous scintillating
    paracentral
    relative
    scintillating
scotometry
scotomization
scotty dog sign
scout film
scout image
scout negative film
ScoutView targeting
scrambled image
screen
    guilt
    Lanex Medium
    RF (radiofrequency)
screen craze artifact
screen-film mammogram
screening-detected abnormality
screening mammography
screw
    cancellous
    metallic
    transfixing
screw and plate (screw-plate)
screw fixation
screw-in ceramic acetabular cup
scrotal abscess
scrotal hematoma
scrotal hernia
scrotal-testicular trauma
scrotal ultrasound
SCT (star-cancellation test)
SCTA (spiral CT angiography)
scybalum (pl. scybala)
scyphoid
SDBP (systemic diastolic blood
    pressure)
SDH (subdural hemorrhage)

S distortion
SDRI (small, deep, recent infarct)
SE (spin echo) image
SE 1500/40 MR images
SE 300/17 MR images
SEA (spinal epidural abscess)
seal and suction
seat belt fracture
seat belt injury
seat belt sign
sebaceum, adenoma (in tuberous
    sclerosis)
second cranial nerve (optic)
second portion of duodenum
secondary cartilaginous joint
secondary electron production
secondary extravasation of
    intravascular contents
secondary fracture
secondary hypertension
secondary pneumonia
secondary renal calculus
secondary sonographic findings
secondary stricture formation
secretory duct
secondary venous insufficiency
secretin
secretion-filled medium-sized bronchi
secretory capacity of the ACTH
    dependent inner adrenal cortex
secretory duct of Bartholin gland
    obstruction
section
    axial
    cesarean
    Compton scattering cross-
    coronal
    cross-
    elastic cross-
    flood
    sagittal
    serial

section *(cont.)*
    serpiginous
    step
    transverse
section-select flow compensation
section-select pulse
section-sensitivity profiles
sector
    lower field visual
    Sommer (of the hippocampus)
sector echocardiography
sector probe, biplane
sector scan echocardiography
sector scanning
secundum atrial septal defect (ASD)
Seddon classification of nerve injuries
seeding, seeds
    BrachySeed iodine-125
    BrachySeed palladium-103
    EchoSeed (iodine-125) brachy-
        therapy
    gold marker
    intracranial
    IoGold radioactive
    I-Plant radioactive iodine-125
    metastatic
    PharmaSeed iodine-125
    PharmaSeed palladium-103
    ProstaSeed I-125
    prostate
    radioactive
        radium
    Symmetra ^{125}I brachytherapy
    TheraSeed (palladium-103) active
        isotope in titanium capsule
    tumor
seeding of tumor
seed points
seeds (see *brachytherapy*; *seeding*)
seed voxel
SEE IT substernal epicardial echocar-
    diography segment

segment
  akinetic
  angulated
  anterior
  anterior basal
  anterobasal
  anterolateral
  apex
  apical
  apicoposterior
  arterial
  atretic
  bronchopulmonary
  cardiac
  coarcted
  contiguous
  diaphragmatic
  distal
  endarterectomized
  expansile aortic
  globus pallidus internal (GPi)
  hypokinetic
  infarcted lung
  inferior
  inferior basal
  inferoapical
  inferoposterior
  interleaved inversion-readout
  liver
  meatal
  nonassessable
  nonfilling venous
  noninfarcted
  posterior
  posterior apical
  posterobasal
  posterolateral
  proximal
  pulmonary
  septal wall
  septum
  superior
  Ta

segment *(cont.)*
  vaterian
  venous
segment distraction
segmental atelectasis
segmental bile duct
segmental bone loss
segmental bowel infarction
segmental branch of artery
segmental bronchus (pl. bronchi)
  cardiac
  lateral
  lateral basal
  medial
  medial basal
  posterior
  posterior basal
  superior
segmental consolidation
segmental defect
segmental distribution of syringomyelia
segmental fracture
segmental high intensity (SHI)
segmental infiltrating tumor
segmental ischemia
segmental lesion
segmental limb pressure
segmental lower extremity Doppler
  pressures
segmental misty mesentery (SSM)
segmental narrowing
segmental orifice
segmental perfusion abnormality
segmental plethysmography
segmental pneumonia
segmental renal artery waveform
segmental sign
segmental symptoms
segmental wall motion abnormality
  akinetic
  dyskinetic
  hyperkinetic
  hypokinetic

segmentation
  automatic lumen edge
  Cannon
  lung
  MR imaging
  rhythmic
  vascular
segmentation in coronal reoriented
  slices
segmentation method for real-time
  display
segmented k-space cardiac tagging
segmented k-space time of flight MR
  angiography
segmented k-space turbo gradient echo
  breath-hold sequence
segmented true fast imaging
segmented volume acquisition
segmenting dual echo MR head scan
Segond fracture
SEH (spinal epidural hemorrhage)
SeHCAT (selenium-labeled homo-
  cholic acid conjugated with
  taurine) test
SEI (subendocardial infarction)
Seikosha video printer for scans
Seinsheimer classification of femoral
  fracture
seizure
  generalized
  grand mal
  partial
  petit mal
seizure focus
seizure localization
seizure manifestations
seizure pattern
seizure phenomenon
seizure propagation
seizure threshold
Seldinger catheter
Seldinder technique angiography
selective adenosine A24 antagonist

selective angiography
selective arterial injection
selective arteriogram
selective cannulization
selective catheterization of vessels
selective cerebral arteriography
selective coronary arteriography
selective coronary cineangiography
selective excitation
selective excitation method
selective hole burning
selective injection
selective irradiation
selective line acquisition mode
selective nerve root block
selective osteal salpingography
selective ovarian vein angiography
selective partial inversion-recovery
  (SPIR)
selective percutaneous transhepatic
  embolization
selective presaturation MR
  angiography
selective reduction
selective renal artery angiography
selective renal artery embolization
selective salpingography
selective saturation method
selective scarring of posterobasal
  portion of left ventricle
selective separation
selective vascular ligation
selective venography
selective visceral arteriography
selective visualization
Select Performance balloon dilatation
  catheter
selenium (Se) (an element)
  Se detector
  ^{77}Se MRI spectroscopy
  ^{75}Se selenomethionine radioactive
    agent
self-aspirating cut-biopsy needle

self-articulating femoral (SAF) hip
  replacement
self-catheterization
self-expanding stent
self-expanding tulip sheath
self-limiting adult small bowel
  intussusception
self-organizing mapping (SOM)
self-positioning balloon
self-reinforced polyglycolide
self-retaining catheter
sella (pl. sellae)
  atrophy of dorsum
  ballooned
  ballooning of
  decalcified dorsum
  dorsum
  empty
  pressure
  tuberculum
sella-nasion plane
sellar tomography
sella turcica
semiautonomous nodule
semicircular canal
semicoronal plane
semidynamic splint
semiflexed, anteroposterior (SF-AP)
  view
semi-Fowler position
semilateral position
semilunar aortic valve regurgitation
semilunar bone
semilunar bony formation
semilunar cartilages
semilunar indentations
semilunar pulmonic valve
  regurgitation
semilunar-shaped fold
semilunar valve cusp
seminal duct
seminal vesicle fistula
seminoma testicular tumor

semiprone position
semiquantitative measurement
senescent aortic stenosis
senile ankylosing hyperostosis of spine
senile arteriosclerosis
senile dementia, Alzheimer type
  (SDAT)
senile emphysema
senile nevus
senile osteoporosis
senile subcapital fracture
Senographe 500 T mammography
Senographe 2000D digital mammography system
SenoScan full-field digital mammography system
SenoScan mammography
Sens-A-Ray digital dental imaging
  system
Sensation 16 MDCT scanner
SENSE (SENSitivity Encoding)
SENsitivity Encoding
sensing coil
sensitive plane projection reconstruction imaging
sensitive point scanning
sensitive volume
sensitivity
  line-shape
  percussion
  uniform
sensitize
sensitization
sentinel clot
sentinel fold
sentinel loop
sentinel node
sentinel pile (hemorrhoid)
sentinel transoral hemorrhage
separation
  AC (acromioclavicular)
  aortic cusp
  atlantoaxial

separation *(cont.)*
  atlanto-occipital
  carrier-free
  chromatographic
  costochondral junction
  fracture fragment
  leaflet
  selective
  shoulder
sepsis, intra-abdominal (IAS)
septal accessory pathway
septal amplitude
septal arcade
septal area
septal asymmetry
septal band
septal cardiac defect
septal collateral
septal cusp of valve
septal defect
  atrial
  atrioventricular
  interventricular
septal dip
septal hypertrophy, asymmetric
septal hypokinesis
septal hypoperfusion on thallium scan
septal infarction
septal leaflet
septal necrosis
septal papillary muscle
septal pathway
septal perforation
septal perforator branch
septal perforators
septal region
septal ridge
septal separation
septal thickness
septal wall thickness
septation
septic arthritis
septic embolism

septic embolus (pl. emboli)
septic lung syndrome
septic necrosis
septic pleurisy
septic pneumonia
septic pulmonary emboli
septic pulmonary infarction
septic shock
septic thrombosis
septicemia
septomarginal trabecula
septum (pl. septa)
  alveolar
  anal intermuscular
  anteroapical trabecular
  aortic
  aortopulmonary
  asymmetric hypertrophy of
  atrial
  atrioventricular
  bronchial
  bulbar
  canal
  cartilaginous
  conal
  conus
  crural
  distal bulbar
  dyskinetic
  femoral
  gingival
  infundibular
  intact ventricular
  interatrial (IAS)
  interhaustral
  interlobar
  interlobular
  intermuscular
  internal intermuscular
  interventricular (IVS)
  mediastinal
  membranous
  muscular atrioventricular

septum *(cont.)*
  nasal
  perirenal
  posterior median (of cord)
  rectovaginal
  rectovesical
  sinus
  thickened
  urorectal
  ventricular
sequela (pl. sequelae)
  clinical
  late normal tissue
  neuroendocrinological
  significant
sequence (pl. sequences)
  automated bolus detection
    three-dimensional fast gradient
    recalled echo
  auto-triggered elliptic centric-
    ordered
  breath-hold GRE
  Carr-Purcell
  Carr-Purcell-Meiboom-Gill
  conventional pulse
  CPMG
  DANTE
  diffusion pulse
  diffusion-weighted pulse
  dual echo
  dual GRE pulse
  echo planar
  echo planar pulse sequence
  FFE
  FLAIR
  FISP
  FLASH 3D
  flow-compensated gradient-echo
  FMPSRGR
  gradient echo
  gradient echo imaging
  gradient echo pulse
  GRASS pulse

sequence *(cont.)*
  in-phase
  interleaved GRE
  inversion recovery
  Klippel-Feil
  long echo train fast spin echo
  magnetization-prepared rapid
    acquisition gradient echo
  MP-RAGE (magnetization
    prepared 3D gradient echo)
  multiecho
  multislice spin echo
  opposed-phase
  partial saturation
  PRESS
  pulsed
  reduced MR imaging
  sagittal 3D T1 gradient echo
  saturation recovery
  short T1 inversion recovery (STIR)
  single breath-hold
  single slab three-dimensional pulse
  single shot adiabatic localization
    pulse
  single slice fast dynamic in vivo
  SPAMM
  spin echo
  spin echo pulse
  spin echo imaging
  spiral pulse
  susceptibility-sensitive
  3DFT-CISS
  3D GRE (gradient-recalled echo)
  3D-PSIF
  3D spoiled GRE
  3D time of flight MR angiographic
  TONE (tilted optimized nonsaturat-
    ing excitation)
  Turbo-FLASH
  turbo spin echo
  turbo spin echo T2-weighted
  turbo SE
  voiding

sequence processor
sequence time
sequential balloon inflation
sequential bypass graft
sequential dilatations
sequential extraction-radiotracer
  technique
sequential graft
sequential image acquisition
sequential in situ bypass
sequential monophasic shocks
sequential obstruction
sequential pacing
sequential plane imaging
sequential point imaging
sequential quantitative MR imaging
sequential scalar quantization (SSQ)
sequential compression device,
  Kendall
sequential CT imaging
sequential olfactory stimulation
sequential scans
sequestered lobe of lung
sequestration
  fluid
  third space
sequestrum (pl. sequestra)
  associated
  bony
  dorsolaterally organized
  necrotic
  primary
  secondary
  tertiary
Sequoia ultrasound system
serendipity view
SER-IV (supination, external
  rotation-type IV) fracture
serial CT slice
serial changes
serial contrast MR
serial cut film technique
serial duplex scan

serial images
serial lesions
serialography
serial scans
serial splinting
serial static image
series
  abdominal
  acute abdominal
  dynamic
  sinus
  small bowel
  upper GI (gastrointestinal)
Series-II humeral head
seriography
serofibrinous pleurisy
Seroma-Cath wound drainage catheter
seropurulent pleurisy
seromuscular layer
serosa
serosal surface
serosa of uterus
serosanguineous fluid
serotonin (5-HIAA)
serotonin (S2) receptors
serous cystadenoma
serous membrane
serous pericardium
serous pleurisy
serpiginous course
serpiginous ulceration
serrated catheter
serration, marginal
serratus anterior muscle
Sertoli-Leydig cell ovarian tumor
Sertoli-Leydig cell tumor
Sertoli stromal cell ovarian tumor
serum hepatitis (hepatitis B)
serum tumor marker
sesamoid bones of foot
  accessory
  bipartite
  entrapped plantar

sesamoid *(cont.)*
  fibular
  great toe
  hallux
  lateral
  medial
  quadripartite
  symptomatic bipartite
  tibial
  tripartite
sesamoid complex
sesamoid ligament
sesamoid migration
sesamoidometatarsal joint
sesamophalangeal ligament
sessile filling defect
sessile plaque
sessile polyp
sessile tumor
sestamibi polar map (CEQUAL)
sestamibi stress test
sestamibi technetium 99mTc SPECT
  with dipyridamole stress test
sestamibi technetium 99mTc stress test
set angle of toes
S.E.T. hemodialysis catheter
7E3 monoclonal antiplatelet antibody
Settegast method to view patella
setting
  quadrature
  wide window
setting-sun phenomenon
7-methoxy 11C methoxystaurosporine
  imaging agent
seven-pinhole tomography
seventh cranial nerve (facial nerve)
severe acute respiratory syndrome
  (SARS)
severe distortion
Severin classification
Severin grade
SFA (superficial femoral artery)

SF-AP (semiflexed, anteroposterior)
  view
SGA (small for gestational age)
shaded-surface display (SSD)
  algorithm
shaded-surface display CT angiography
shading sign
shadow (also shadowing)
  acoustic
  bandlike
  bat's wing
  breast
  butterfly breast
  cardiac
  centrilobular
  clean
  dirty
  discoid
  effusion
  fusiform
  hilar
  large thymus (obscuring cardiac
    silhouette)
  line
  linear
  paraspinal soft tissue
  Ponfick
  ring
  iliopsoas muscle
  renal
  snowstorm
  spindle-shaped
  toothpaste
  tramlines
  tumorlike
  widened heart
shadowing focus
shadowing, miliary
shadowing stone
Shadow over the wire balloon catheter

shaft
  bone
  distal third
  femoral
  French
  middle third
  ministem
  proximal third
shaft fracture
shaft periostitis
shag, aortic
shagging of cardiac borders
shaggy aorta syndrome
shagreen patches in tuberous sclerosis
Shames model
shape (shaped)
  barrel-
  boat
  brachycephalic head
  dumbbell-
  half-moon
  head
  horseshoe
  hourglass
  mesocephalic head
  oval
  ovoid-
  S-
  scaphocephalic head
  scaphoid
  sickle
  spherical
  spheroid-
shape distortion
Shape Maker system
shape recovery
Shapiro intrauterine insemination
  catheter
Sharp's angle
sharp border of lung
sharp carina
sharp dissection
sharp lateral margin

Sharp-Purser test
shaver catheter
shaving
  femoral condylar
  patellar
shavings, residual metal fragment
Shaw catheter
SHC (sclerosing hepatic carcinoma)
shear elasticity probe
shear fracture
shearing forces (on sacroiliac joints in
  runners)
shearing of white matter (in head
  injury)
shearing stress
shear stiffness
shear stress
shear wave motion
shear rate
shear stress
sheath
  Ancure EZ Path catheter
  angioplasty
  anterior rectus
  arterial
  carotid
  catheter
  caudal
  check-valve
  common synovial flexor
  Cordis
  crural
  dentinal
  dural
  extensor carpi ulnaris
  fascial
  femoral artery
  fenestrated
  fibrous
  flexor tendon
  ganglionic cyst in synovial tendon
  GlideCath
  Guidant

sheath *(cont.)*
  guiding
  Hemaquet
  Henle
  InnerVasc
  Innovante
  intratendon
  introducer
  Mullins
  muscle
  myelin
  nerve
  nerve root
  neural
  Passager introducing
  peel-away
  periradicular
  pilar
  plicated dural
  posterior rectus
  Prelude vascular introducer
  radiopaque FEP
  rectus
  Schwann cell of myelin
  self-expanding tulip
  Shuttle flexor
  Silastic
  Spectranetics (SLS)
  synovial
  tearaway
  tendon
  transseptal
  tulip
  unplicated
  USCI angioplasty guiding
  vascular
  venous
  X-Sept
sheath and side-arm
Shebele physician reporting
  workstation
sheetlike

Sheffield modification of Bruce
  treadmill protocol
Sheffield treadmill exercise protocol
Sheldon catheter
shelf
  Blumer rectal
  buccal
  dental
  lateral
  medial
  mesocolic
  palatine
  patellar
  rectal
shell, acetabular
shelling off of cartilage
shell osteochondral autograft
Shelton femur fracture classification
shelving edge of Poupart ligament
Shenton line
Shepard intrauterine insemination
  catheter
Shepherd fracture
shepherd's crook area of the right
  coronary artery
shepherd's crook deformity
Sherpa guiding catheter
SHG (sonohysterography)
SHI (segmental high intensity)
shield
  apron
  Faraday
  lead apron
  lead eye
  RF magnetic
  tungsten eye
shield apron
shielding, lead
shift
  anterior capsular
  chemical
  Doppler frequency

shift *(cont.)*
  intracranial
  lanthanide-induced
  left to right
  mediastinal
  midline
  navigator
  paradigm
  paramagnetic
  phase
  pineal gland
  pivot
  plantar
  reverse pivot (RPS)
  right to left
  ST segment
  superior frontal axis
  tracheal
  ventricular
  weight
shift of mediastinal structures
shift of midline structures (of the mid-brain)
shift to the left (white blood cells)
shift to the right (white blood cells)
Shiley guiding catheter
Shiley-Ionescu catheter
shill, protrusio
shim coil
shim magnet
shimming
shim placement
Shimadzu scanner
Shimazaki area-length method
shimmering, visual
shimming of MRI magnet, poor
shin bone
Shinobi Plus guidewire
Shinobi steerable guidewire
shin, saber
SHJR4s (side-hole Judkins right, curve 4 French, short)
shock-monitoring method

Sholkoff balloon hysterosalpingography catheter
Shone anomaly
short arm Grollman catheter
short axis acquisition
short axis images
short axis parasternal view
short axis plane on echocardiography
short axis slice
short bone
short bore magnet
short distance radiotherapy (brachytherapy)
short echo time
short echo time proton spectroscopy
shortening
  Achilles tendon
  fractional myocardial
  leg
  mean rate of circumferential
  phalangeal
  skeleton
  suboccipital
  tendon
  T2 (second thoracic vertebra)
shortening of carpus
shortening of tarsus
shortening of urethra
short half-life
short head of biceps
short inversion time inversion recovery (STIR)
short peroneal muscle tendon
short pulse
short rib-polydactyly syndrome
short scale contrast
short TE, long TR
short term patency
short T1 inversion recovery (STIR) sequence
short T1 relaxation time
short TR/TE (repetition time/echo time) (T1-weighted image)

shotty lymph node
shoulder
  baseball
  drop
  flail
  frozen
  knocked-down
  Little Leaguer
  loose
  Neviaser classification of frozen
  ring man (in gymnasts)
  sprained
  swimmer's
  tennis
shoulder compression test
shoulder depression test
shoulder-hand-finger syndrome
shoulder immobilizer
shoulder of heart
shoulder pointer
shoulder prosthesis
shoulder rock test
shoulder separation
shoulder-upper extremity-thoracic
  outlet syndrome
shower of echoes
shrinkage, graft
shrinkage of ganglion cells
shrugging sign
shrunken gallbladder
shudder of carotid arterial pulse
shunt (also shunting)
  Allen-Brown vascular access
  aorta to pulmonary artery
  aorticopulmonary
  aortopulmonary
  apicoaortic
  arterioportal
  arteriovenous (A-V, AV)
  arteriovenous bovine
  ascending aorta to pulmonary
    artery
  atrial right to left

shunt *(cont.)*
  barium-sulfate impregnated
  bidirectional
  biliopancreatic
  Blalock
  Blalock-Taussig
  Brescia-Cimino
  Buselmeier
  cardiac
  cardiovascular
  central aortopulmonary
  Cimino
  Cordis-Hakim
  CSF (cerebrospinal fluid)
  cysto-atrial
  Davidson
  Denver hydrocephalus
  Denver peritoneal venous
  descending aorta-pulmonary artery
  descending thoracic aorta to
    pulmonary artery
  dialysis
  distal splenorenal (DSR)
  DVP flush
  end to side portacaval
  esophageal
  extracardiac right to left
  gastric venacaval
  Glenn
  Gore-Tex
  Gott
  Hakim-Cordis ventriculoperitoneal
  hemodialysis access
  hermetic external
  Heyer-Schulte neurosurgical
  high pressure
  Holter
  Hyde
  infant
  intracardiac right to left
  intrapericardial aorticopulmonary
  intrapulmonary
  ISCI

shunt *(cont.)*
Javid endarterectomy
left to right
left to right cardiac
LeVeen peritoneal
Linton
low pressure
lumbar arachnoid peritoneal
lumboperitoneal (LP)
medium pressure
mesocaval H-graft
mesocaval interposition
migration of
modified Blalock-Taussig
net
Ommaya ventriculoperitoneal
one-piece
peritoneal-atrial
peritoneocaval
peritoneovenous (PVS)
portacaval
portopulmonary
portosystemic vascular
posterior fossa-atrial
Potts
preferential
proximal splenorenal
Pruitt-Inahara carotid
Pudenz
Quinton-Scribner
Ramirez
reversed (right to left)
right to left (reversed)
side to side portacaval
small bowel
Spetzler lumboperitoneal
splenorenal
subclavian artery to pulmonary
artery
subclavian-pulmonary
subdural to peritoneal
Sundt loop
supracardiac

shunt *(cont.)*
systemic-pulmonary artery
thecoperitoneal
Thomas vascular access
transjugular intrahepatic portosystemic
transvenous extrahepatic portacaval
T-tube
UNI-SHUNT hydrocephalus
vena cava to pulmonary artery
venoarterial
ventriculoatrial (VA)
ventriculojugular (VJ)
ventriculoperitoneal (VP)
ventriculopleural
ventriculovenous
vesicoamniotic
Wakabaushi
Warren splenorenal
Waterston
Waterston-Cooley
Winter
shunted blood
shunted tracer
shunt flow
anatomic
physiologic
relative
shunt function, cerebrospinal fluid
shunting of blood
left to right
marked
right to left
shuntogram
shunt placement
shunt quantification
shunt reservoir
shunt reversal
shunt scintigram
shunt syndrome, lumbar thecoperitoneal
shunt valve
shutdown, renal

Shuttle flexor sheath
SI (sacroiliac) joint
  SI joint to sacrum ratio
SI (saturation index) of bile
SI (signal intensity)
SI (sinus irregularity)
SI (stroke index)
Si(Li) x-ray detector
sialography CT
sialography MRI
Sibson fascia
sickle cell trait
sick sinus node
sick sinus syndrome (SSS)
  extrinsic
  intrinsic
sickle cell disease
sickle-shaped fold
SICOR (computer-assisted cardiac
  catheter recording system)
SID (source-image distance)
side-bending x-ray
side branch occlusion
side-by-side transposition of great
  vessels
side entry access (SEA) port
side-hole catheter
side to side anastomosis
siderosis
siderotic nodules
siderotic nodules in the spleen
siderotic splenomegaly
sideswipe elbow fracture
sidewall, pelvic
sidewinder catheter
Siemens AG system
Siemens DRH CT scanners
Siemens gamma camera
Siemens LINAC (linear accelerator)
Siemans Magnetom 1.5 T
Siemans Magnetom SP 4000 scanner
Siemens Mevatron 74 linear
  accelerator

Siemens one tesla scanner
Siemens Satellite CT Evaluation
  Console
Siemens Sensation 16 MDCT scanner
Siemens Somaform 512 CT scanner
Siemens Somatom DR2 whole-body
  scanner (also DR3)
Siemens Somatom PLUS-S imager
  (scanner)
Siemens Somatom Sensation 40
  scanner
Siemens Somatom Sensation Cardiac
  64 scanner
Siemens SP 4000 scanner
SieScape ultrasound imaging technology
sievert (Sv)
sigmoid cavity of radius
sigmoid cavity of ulna
sigmoid colon volvulus
sigmoid curve
sigmoid notch
sigmoid omentum
sigmoidovaginal fistula
sigmoidovesical fistula
sigmoid sinus
sigmoid valve
sign (see also *appearance*)
  Aaron
  Abrahams
  absent bow-tie
  accordion (on CT scan of colon)
  ace of spades (on angiogram)
  Achilles bulge
  Adson
  air bronchogram
  air crescent
  air meniscus
  Allen
  Allis
  Amoss
  amputation
  angel wing

sign *(cont.)*
Anghelescu
angiographic string
antecedent
anterior tibial
antler
antral pad
anvil
aortic arch aneurysm
aortic nipple
apical cap
Apley
applesauce
Ashhurst
Auenbrugger
"Aunt Minnie"
Babinski
Baccelli (of pleural effusion)
bagpipe
ball-bearing eye
Ballance
Bamberger
banana
Bancroft
barber pole
Barlow
Battle
bayonet
beading
Becker
Beevor
Bethea
beveled edge
Biermer
bilateral pyramidal
Biot
Bird
blade of grass
Blumberg
Bouillaud
bow-tie
bowler hat
bowstring

sign *(cont.)*
Boyce
Bozzolo
Bragard
brain stem
Branham arteriovenous fistula
Braunwald
brim
Broadbent inverted
Brockenbrough-Braunwald
Brudzinski
Bryant
Burton
buttock
C
camelback
Cantelli
Cardarelli
cardinal
cardiorespiratory
Carnett
carotid string
Carvallo
Castellino
Cegka
cerebral
Chaddock
chain of lakes
Chilaiditi
choppy sea
Christmas tree
Chvostek-Weiss
Claybrook
Cleeman
clockwise whirlpool
cobblestoning
cobra head
Codman
coffee bean
Cogan lid twitch
cogwheel
Cole
Collier

sign *(cont.)*
colon cutoff
comet tail
commemorative
Comolli
contralateral
Coopernail
cord
Corrigan
cortical
cortical ring
corticospinal tract
cottage loaf
coughing
Courvoisier
cranial nerve
crazy-paving
crescent
crescent-in-doughnut (for
    intussusception)
cross-chest impingement
crossed sciatica
crowded carpal
Cruveilhier
CT angiogram
CT arrowhead
cuff
Cullen
cushion
dagger
D'Amato
Dance
Dawbarn
deep lateral femoral notch
deep sulcus
Dejerine
de la Camp
de Musset (aortic aneurysm)
de Mussey (pleurisy)
Delbet
Delmege
delta
Demianoff

sign *(cont.)*
dense metaphyseal band
dense sigmoid sinus
dense vein
Desault
Deyerle
dirty fat
displaced fat pad
dog leg
doll's eye
dome
doorbell
Dorendorf
dorsal column
double bubble
double bubble duodenal
double camelback
double halo
double line
double PCL (posterior cruciate
    ligament)
double stripe
double wall
drooping lily
Drummond
Duchenne
duct-penetrating
duodenal wind sock
Dupuytren
dural tail
Duroziez
d'Espine
E
Ebstein
Egawa
elbow fat pad
Ellis
empty delta
Erb
Erichsen
Ewart
extrapyramidal tract
eye-of-the-tiger

sign *(cont.)*
Fajersztajn crossed sciatic
false localizing
fan
fat-blood interface (FBI)
fat C2
fat pad
FBI (fat-blood interface)
Federici
figure-3
fingertip
Finkelstein
fissure
flapping tremor
Fleck
Fleischner
flow void
focal neurologic
football
Forestier bowstring
Frank
Fränkel (Fraenkel)
Franz
Friedreich
Froment paper
frontal lobe
Fürbringer
Gaenslen
Gage
Galant
Galeazzi
Gerhardt
Gilbert
Glasgow
gloved finger
goblet
Goldthwait
gooseneck
Gordon
Gowers
Grancher
Green-Joynt
Greene

sign *(cont.)*
Grey Turner
Griesinger
Grocco
Grossman
guarding
Guilland
Gunn crossing
hair on end
Hall
halo
hamburger
Hamman pneumopericardium
harlequin eye
Hart
Hawkins
heel pad
Heim-Kreysig
Helbing
Henning
hide-bound bowel
Hill
Hill-Sachs
Hirschberg
Hoffmann
Homans
Honda
Hoover
Hope
Horn
hot cross bun skull
hot nose
Howship-Romberg
Huchard
Hueter fracture
Huntington
hyperattenuating ring
hyperdense middle cerebral artery
hyperintensive ring
iliopsoas
incomplete border
intervertebral vacuum cleft
intradecidual

sign *(cont.)*
ivory phalanx
ivory vertebra
ivy
inverted V
J
Jaccoud
Jackson
Jenet
jugular
jump
Jürgensen
Kanavel
Kantor
Kaplan
Karplus
Katz-Wachtel
Keen
Kehr
Kellgren
Kellock
Kernig
Kerr
Klemm
knuckle
Kocher-Cushing
Korányi-Grocco
Kussmaul venous
Lachman
Laënnec
Lancisi
Landolfi
Langoria
Lasègue
lateral femoral notch
lateralizing
Laugier
Lazarus
Leichtenstern
lemon
Lennhoff
leptomeningeal ivy
Leri

sign *(cont.)*
Leser-Trelat
Levine
Lhermitte
Linder
linguine (in breast)
liver flap
liver-jugular
Livierato abdominocardiac
localizing neurological
lollipop tree
long tract
Lorenz
Lowenberg
lower motor neuron
lower soft tissue attenuation of the
accordion
Ludloff
Macewen
Mahler
Maisonneuve
Mannkopf
Marie-Foix
McBurney
McCort
McGinn-White
McMurray
Meltzer
Mendel-Bekhterev
meningoencephalitic
meniscus
Mennell
Mercedes-Benz
milk of calcium
Minor
Morquio
Morton-Horwitz nerve cross-over
Moschcowitz (of arterial occlusive
disease)
motor
moulage
movie
Mulder

sign *(cont.)*
Müller (Mueller) aortic regurgitation
Murphy
musculoskeletal crescent
Musset (de Musset)
mute toe
Myerson
Naffziger
naked facet
Neer impingement
negative delta (on CT)
Negro
Nelson
Neri bowing
neurologic soft
Nicoladoni-Branham
nubbin
obturator
oculomotor
Oliver-Cardarelli
ominous
Oppenheim
optic nerve tram-track
orbicularis
organic (of brain damage)
Ortolani
Osler
pad
panda
parallel track
parietal lobe
Parrot
patent bronchus
pathognomonic
pathologic lid retraction
Paul
Payr
pearl necklace
pedestal
percussion
Perez
peripheral washout

sign *(cont.)*
peritoneal
peroneal
Pfuhl-Jaffé
Phalen
phonatory
piano key
pillow
Pins
Piotrowski
piston
pivot-shift
plane
plumb-line
Plummer
pneumoarthrogram
positive bottle
postural motor
Potain
Pott
Pottenger
precursor
premonitory
Prevel
Prévost
pronation
pronator
pronatory
proximal and distal hyperattentuating middle cerebral artery
pruning
Prussian helmet
pseudo-Babinski
pseudobulbar
pseudocalculus
pseudokidney
pseudo-Foster-Kennedy
pseudo-Romberg
psoas
puddle
pupillary
pyloric string
pyramidal

sign *(cont.)*
Queckenstedt
Quénu-Muret
Quincke
rabbit ear
raccoon eyes
rachitic rosary
radial bands
radialis
railroad track
Raimiste
rat-tail
rebound
Renee creak
reversal
reversed 3
reversed Mercedes Benz
Rigler
rim
ring of cribriform plate fracture
Riordan
Risser
Rivero-Carvallo
Riviere
Robertson
Romberg
Rosenbach
rose thorn
Rotch
Rothschild
Rovighi
Rovsing
Rust
Sabathie
sagging rope
sail
Sanders
sandwich
Sansom
Sarbo
sawtooth appearance
Schepelmann
Schick

sign *(cont.)*
Schlesinger
Schoeber
scimitar
scotty dog
seat belt
segmental
Seguin
Seitz
setting-sun
shading
Shapiro
Shibley
shrugging
signet ring
silhouette
Sister Mary Joseph
Skoda
small bowel feces
Smith
soft neurologic
soft tissue rim
somatic
sonographic Murphy
Soto-Hall
Spalding
Speed
spinal
spread suture
Spurling
square-root
squeeze
stairs
steeple
Steinberg thumb
Steinmann
Sterles
Sterling-Okuniewski
Sternberg
Stewart-Holmes
Stierlin
Strauss
string

sign *(cont.)*
string of pearls
stripe
Strümpell (Struempell)
Strunsky
subtle
supinatory
swirl
Sumner
tandem Romberg
target
target
tattoo
tau
teardrop
Terry fingernail
Terry-Thomas
tethered-bowel
theater
Thomas
thorn
thumbprinting
Thurston-Holland
tibialis (of Strümpell)
Tinel percussion
toe spread
tooth
track
tram-track
trapezius ridge
Traube aortic regurgitation
tree-in-bud
triangular cord
Trimadeau
tripod
Troisier
trolley-track
Trömner (Troemner)
Trousseau
tumbling bullet
Turner
turtle

sign *(cont.)*
Turyn
twin peak
Uhthoff
unilateral Babinski
upper motor neuron
VAD (voluntary anterior drawer)
Vanzetti
vein
versive motor
vital
voluntary posterior drawer (VPD)
Voshell
VPD (voluntary posterior drawer)
Waddell
wall echo shadow (WES)
Walter-Murdoch wrist
Wartenberg
washout
Weill
Weiss
WES (wall echo shadow)
Westermark
wet leather
whirl
whirlpool
white cerebellum
white matter
Williams
Williamson
Wilson
wind sock (echocardiogram)
windshield wiper
winking owl spinal
Wintrich
Yergason
Signa GEMS MR imaging system
Signa Horizon scanner
Signa I.S.T. MRI scanner
Signa 1.5 tesla MR scanner
Signa Special Procedures (SP) system
Signa SP/i 0.5T MR imaging unit

signal
  blood oxygenation level-dependent
    (BOLD)
  color Doppler
  D
  differential
  disk water
  Doppler flow
  flow
  hyperintense
  hypointense
  lipid
  magnetic resonance
  mosaic-jet
  NAA metabolite
  stimulus-correlated
  water
signal acquisitions
signal amplification
signal blooming
signal dephasing
signal fallout
signal intensity (SI)
signal intensity curve
signal intensity time curves
signal loss
signal magnification
signal mass
signal time-course
signal to clutter ratio
signal to noise ratio (SNR or S/N
  ratio)
signal void
signature, echo
signet ring appearance
signet ring carcinoma
signet ring pattern
signet ring sign
significant axis deviation
significant, clinically
significant distortion
significant residual deficit
significant sequelae

Silastic catheter
Silastic sheath
Silastic stent
Silber aspiration catheter
silence, electrocerebral (ECS)
silent areas of brain
silent gallstone
silent ischemia
silent mitral stenosis
silent myocardial infarction
silent myocardial ischemia
silent patent ductus arteriosus
silent regurgitation
silhouette
  cardiac (large thymus shadow
    obscuring)
  cardiovascular
  enlarged cardiac
  luminal
  roentgenographic
  widened cardiac
silhouette image
silhouette sign
silicone catheter
silicone Foley catheter
silicone Malecot catheter
silicone stent
Silicon Graphics Reality Engine
  system
silicone implant rupture (seen on
  MRI)
Silicore catheter
silicosis
silicotic fibrosis of lung
silicotic nodule with central necrosis
silicotic visceral pleura
silicotuberculosis
Silitek stent
silver-fork deformity
silver-fork fracture
SilverSpeed guidewire
SIM (small intestine mesentery)
Simmons 1, 2, and 3 catheter

Simmons-type sidewinder catheter
Simmons view to demonstrate talipes
equinovarus
Simon nitinol percutaneous IVC filter
simple dislocation
simple flat pelvis
simple fracture, complex
simple shift
simplex, xanthoma tuberosum
SimpliCT guidance system
Simplus PE/t dilatation catheter
Simpson atherectomy catheter
Simpson atherectomy device, PET
balloon
Simpson Coronary AtheroCath (SCA)
system
Simpson-Robert catheter
Simpson rule method for ventricular
volume
Simpson Ultra-Low Profile II balloon
catheter
Sims position
simulation-aided field setting
simulated annealing methods
simulated equilibrium factor study
simulation, laboratory
simulation of converging ports
simulation of tangential portals
simulation of treatment area
simulator
Maxwell 3D Field
MR
virtual reality
Ximatron
simultaneous balloon inflation
simultaneous bilateral spontaneous
pneumothorax (SBSP)
simultaneous fluoroscopy and
manometric evaluation of
pharyngeal swallowing and
dysphagia
simultaneous pacing and coronary
blood flow measurement

simultaneous volume imaging
simultaneous waveforms, exponential
sincalide (synthetic CCK)
sincalide cholescintigraphy
sincalide imaging agent
singer's node
Singh index of osteoporosis
single atrium
single breath-hold
single breath-hold sequence on CT
scan
single breath view
single bubble cavitation
single bubble sonoluminescence
(SBSL)
single contrast arthrography
single cuff dialysis catheter
single dose gadolinium imaging
single energy spectrum quantitative
computed tomography
single extrastimuli
single fill/void technique
single harmonic wave
single isocenter
single lumen femoral vein catheter
single lumen silicone breast implant
single lumen subclavian vein catheter
single lung transplantation
single outlet heart
single peak
single photon emission CT with MR
single photon absorptiometry (SPA)
single photon emission computed tomography (SPECT)
single photon planar scintigraphy
(SPPS)
single pleurisy
single port
single shot adiabatic localization pulse
sequence
single shot fast spin echo (SSFSE)
single shot fast spin echo and
gadolinium-enhanced fat-suppressed
spoiled gradient-echo MR imaging

single shot MR cholangiography
single slab three-dimensional pulse
  sequence
single slice fast dynamic in vivo
  sequence
single slice long axis tomograms
single stripe colitis (SSC)
single ventricle with pulmonic stenosis
single vessel disease
single vessel runoff
single voxel proton spectroscopy
sinistral portal hypertension
sink-trap malformation
sinoatrial (SA)
sinoatrial branch
sinoatrial node (SA or S-A node)
  Flack
  Koch
sinoatrial node artery
sinoatrial node dysfunction
sinoatrial node infarction
sinoauricular node
sinodural plate
Sinografin imaging agent
sinogram
sinotubular junction
sintering
sinus
  accessory
  aortic valve
  atlas articular
  barber's pilonidal
  basilar
  Breschet
  carotid
  cavernous
  cerebral venous
  cervical
  circular
  coccygeal
  coronary (of Valsalva)
  costomediastinal
  cranial

sinus *(cont.)*
  distal coronary (DCS)
  draining
  dura mater venous
  dural
  dural venous
  ethmoid
  frontal
  Guérin
  inferior sagittal (ISS)
  lateral
  left coronary
  lumbosacral dermal
  lymph node
  marginal
  mastoid
  maxillary
  medullary
  middle coronary (MCS)
  nasal
  noncoronary
  oblique pericardial
  osteomyelitic
  paranasal
  pericardial
  perineal
  Petit
  petrosal
  pilonidal
  piriform
  precoronal sagittal
  prostatic
  proximal coronary (PCS)
  pulmonary
  pyriform
  renal
  Ridley
  Rokitansky-Aschoff
  rudimentary
  sagittal
  sigmoid
  sphenoid
  sphenoparietal

sinus *(cont.)*
  subeustachian
  superior sagittal (SSS)
  tarsal
  thickened
  transverse pericardial
  UG (urogenital)
  Valsalva
  valve of coronary
  venous
  vertebral articular
sinus aneurysm, aortic
sinus irregularity (SI)
sinusitis, allergic fungal
sinus lesion, cavernous
sinus mechanism
sinus nodal reentry
sinus node automaticity
sinus node depression
sinus node dysfunction
sinus node recovery time, corrected
sinus node reentry
sinus of Morgagni
sinus of pulmonary trunk
sinus of Valsalva aneurysm
sinus of venae cavae
sinusoidal non-single harmonic wave
sinusoidal vascular spaces
sinusoid reference function
sinusoids, hepatic
sinus pause
sinus retroperfusion, coronary
sinus segment
sinus septum
sinus series
sinus slowing
sinus tarsi syndrome
sinus tract study
sinus venous defect
sinuvertebral nerve (of Luschka)
SIP (saturation inversion projection)
siphon, carotid
SIR angiogram

SISCOM (Subtraction Ictal SPECT
  co-registered to MRI)
Sister Mary Joseph node
site
  arterial access
  de-airing
  fracture
  ipsilateral antegrade
  reference
site of arterial puncture
site of maximal intensity
Site-Rite and Site-Rite II ultrasound
  system for vascular imaging
site-specific labeling
sitting-up view
situs ambiguus of atria
situs
  atrial
  D-loop ventricular
  L-loop ventricular situs
situs atrialis solitus
situs concordance
situs inversus
situs inversus totalis
situs inversus viscerum
situs perversus
situs solitus
  atrial
  visceral
situs transversus
situs viscerum inversus
Sitzmarks (polyvinyl chloride) imaging
  agent
6-[^{18}F] fluoro-DOPA
16–detector row computed tomography
16-row scanner
sixth compartment
sixth cranial nerve (abducens nerve)
sixth intercostal space
60° left anterior oblique projection
60 MHz Fourier Transform NMR
  spectrometer

60 MHz Rapid Scan spectrometer
size and caliber
size and configuration
size estimation error
size of uterus
size, particle
sizer, prosthetic valve
sizing, balloon
sizing ring
Sjögren syndrome
SJS (Schwartz-Jampel syndrome)
skeletal amyloidosis
skeletal angioscintigraphy
skeletal bed
skeletal disruption
skeletal emphysema
skeletal hyperostosis
skeletal hypoplasia
skeletally immature
skeletally mature
skeletal metastasis (pl. metastases)
skeletal radiology
skeletal survey, isotopic
skeletal traction
skeleton
  appendicular
  articulated
  axial
  bony
  cardiac
  fibrous
  gill arch
  osteoporotic
  spidering
  spiky
  sulcal
  visceral
skeleton shortening
skeletonizing
Skene duct
skier's fracture
skier's thumb

Skillern fracture
skin bridge
skin crease artifact
skin depth
skin fold artifact
skin lesion artifact
skin lines
Skinny over the wire balloon catheter
skin-rolling scapular tenderness
skin thickening
skip lesions of Crohn disease
Skoda sign
skull
  beaten silver appearance of
  cloverleaf
  foramen magnum of
  hammer-marked, secondary to
    thinning
  hot cross bun
  lytic lesion of the
  molding of
  sonolucent
skull asymmetry
skull base
skullcap
skull defect, postoperative
skull films
skull fracture
  basilar
  compound
  depressed
  depressed and compound
  linear
  simple
  stellate
  undepressed stellate
skull hyperostosis
skull plate
Skylight system
skyline view of patella
SL (sonoluminescence)
SL (scapholunate) joint

slab (pl. slabs)
  coronal
  interleaved axial
slab imaging
SLAC (scapholunate arthritic collapse)
  wrist
slant hole collimator
SLAP (superior labrum anterior
  posterior) lesion
slate-gray cyanosis
SLE (systemic lupus erythematosus)
slew rate
slice
  angled
  apical short axis
  axial
  basal short axis
  contiguous
  coronal
  coronal reoriented
  digitized CT
  horizontal long axis
  intermediate CT
  long axis
  midsagittal
  midventricular short axis
  plurality of
  sagittal
  serial CT
  short axis
  texture
  tissue
  tomographic
  transaxial
  transverse
  vertical long axis
slice format
slice fracture
slice orientation
slice-overlap artifact
slice profile
slice sensitivity profile (SSP)
slice thickness

slice volume
slicing planes
sliding hernia
sliding-type hiatal hernia
slightly retroflexed uterus
SlimPort implantable vascular access
  port
Slinky catheter
slip angle
slip-in connection
slippage, film
slipped capital femoral epiphysis
slipped disk
slipped tendon
slipped upper femoral epiphysis
  (SUFE)
slipping rib syndrome
slip-ring camera
slip-ring CT
slip-ring technology
SLJD (Sinding-Larsen-Johansson
  disease)
slope
  closing (on echo)
  D to E (of mitral valve)
  decreased E to F (E-F)
  disappearance
  E to F (of mitral valve)
  flat diastolic
  flattened E to F
  opening (on echo)
  ST/HR (ST segment/heart rate)
  valve opening
slot blot analysis
sloughed mucosa
sloughed papilla
sloughed urethra syndrome
slow channel blocking drugs
slow filling wave
slow flow lesions
slow flow vascular anomaly
slow flow vascular malformation
slow neutron

sludge
  biliary
  blood
  gallbladder
sluggish enterohepatic circulation
sluggishly flowing blood
slurp sound (on proper catheter
  positioning)
SLUScan for Your Heart
Sm (samarium) (an element)
SMA (smooth muscle antibody)
SMA (superior mesenteric artery)
SMALL (same-day microsurgical
  arthroscopic lateral-approach laser-
  assisted) fluoroscopic diskectomy
small airway dysfunction
small angle multiple scattering
small aorta syndrome
small atrophic kidney
small bore catheter
small bore catheter thoracostomy
small bowel feces sign
small bowel adenoma
small bowel enteroscopy (SBE)
small bowel contents
small bowel follow-through (SBFT)
small bowel infarct
small bowel series
small bowel transit time
small cardiac vein
small cell carcinoma of the lung
small cell lung cancer (SCLC)
small cuff syndrome
small defibrillating patch
small feminine aorta
small for gestational age (SGA)
small kidney
small-lunged emphysema
small saphenous vein
small vessel stroke
small volume disease
small water-hammer pulse
Smart Prep imaging agent

Smart Prep scanner
SmartScore (using high speed CT
  images)
SmartSpot high resolution digital
  imaging system
SMAS (superior mesenteric artery
  syndrome)
smear fragment
Smec balloon catheter
SMIS console
Smith fracture
SMM (scintimammography)
smokelike echoes
smoker's bronchiolitis
smoker's lung
smooth hyperplasia
smooth muscle tumor
SMPTE (Society of Motion Picture
  and Television Engineers) test
  pattern (teleradiology)
SMS coaxial catheter
SMV (submentovertex) view
SMV (superior mesenteric vein)
SNAC (scaphoid nonunion advanced
  collapse) grades I-III
S/N (signal to noise) ratio
snake graft
snapping hip syndrome
snapping triceps syndrome
snapshot, contrast-enhanced dynamic
snowboard (or snowboarding) injury
snowman appearance of heart
snowman deformity
snowman heart
snowplow occlusion
snowstorm shadow on chest x-ray
SNR (signal to noise ratio)
SNRT (sinus node recovery time)
snuffbox, anatomic
snufftaker's pituitary disease
soap bubble appearance of exudate
soap bubble radiolucency
soapsuds enema (SSE)

"SO-as"—phonetic for "psoas"
socket/residuum interface
socket-stump interface
sodium amidotrizoate imaging agent
sodium bicarbonate solution
sodium bicarbonate and tartaric acid
sodium chloride 0.9%
sodium diatrizoate imaging agent
sodium diatrizoate with menaquinon
   imaging agent
sodium iodide (^{131}I); sodium iodide
   I 131 radiotherapy agent
sodium iodide ring
sodium iodine (^{123}I); sodium iodide
   I 123
sodium iodipamide imaging agent
sodium iodohippurate contrast
   medium
sodium iodomethamate contrast
   medium
sodium iothalamate imaging agent
sodium ioxaglate
sodium ipodate (sodium iopodate)
   imaging agent
sodium methiodal imaging agent
sodium mitrizoate
sodium pertechnetate ^{99m}Tc
sodium tyropanoate imaging agent
Sof-Flex loop suprapubic catheter
Soft-Cell catheter
soft coaxial catheter
soft copy computed radiography
soft disk herniation
softening and swelling of cartilage
softening of brain
soft neurologic sign
soft palate
soft photon
Softip diagnostic catheter
Soft-Pass laparoscopic catheter
SoftScan laser mammography system
Softscan laser scanner
Soft Seal cervical catheter

Soft Seal transcervical balloon catheter
soft silicone rubber dialysis catheter
soft tissue abnormality
soft tissue abscess
soft tissue calcification
soft tissue contracture
soft tissue contusion
soft tissue defect
soft tissue density structure
soft tissue entrapment
soft tissue interposition
soft tissue mass
soft tissue necrosis
soft tissue ossification
soft tissue osteochondroma
soft tissue radiograph
soft tissue rim sign
soft tissue scatter
soft tissue, stippled
soft tissue swelling
soft tissue window
Soft Torque uterine catheter
Softouch guiding catheter
soft uterus
Soft-Vu angiographic catheter
Soft-Vu Omni flush catheter
software (see also *program*)
   DecThreads
   Kodak
   low acoustic pressure harmonic
   low mechanical index harmonic
   modified vessel image processor
   NeatMed radiology toolkit
   Neuro Echo
   Neuro Lobe
   Neuro SPGR
   P-LINK
   SPARC
   Starlink
   VERT
   Viewnex
   Voxel-Man
   VoxelView

Solayrès obliquity
soldier's heart syndrome
soldier's patches of pericardium
soldier's spot
soleal line
soleal vein
solenoid surface coil
Solera thrombectomy catheter
soleus muscle
solid bolus challenge
solid bone
solid edema of lung
solid lesion, echogenic
solid modeler
solid renal lesion
solid state manometry catheter
solid state nuclear track detector
solitary cold lesion
solitary functioning kidney
solitary kidney
solitary lung nodule
solitary mass
solitary pulmonary nodule (SPN)
solitus
  atrial situs
  situs
  visceral situs
Solo catheter with Pro/Pel coating
Solomon syndrome
SoloPass stent and catheter
SOMA scale
Somatom DR CT scanner
Somatom Plus-S CT Scanner
Somatom Sensation Cardiac 64
  scanner
Somatom Sensation 40 scanner
Somatom Volume Zoom computed
  tomography system
somatosensory cortex
somatostatin receptor
somatostatin receptor scintigraphy
  (SRS)
S1-S5 (five sacral vertebrae)

Sonablate 200 high intensity focused
  ultrasound system
Sonde enteroscope
Sones Cardio-Marker catheter
Sones Hi-Flow catheter
Sones selective coronary arteriography
sonicated albumin microbubbles
sonicated imaging agent
sonicated meglumine sodium
sonicated Renografin-76
sonications
Sonicator portable ultrasound
Sonifer sonicating system
Sonnenberg classification of erosive
  esophagitis
sonoangiogram
Sonoblate 200 ultrasound system
sonochemiluminescence
SonoCT real-time spatial compound
  imaging
Sonocut ultrasonic aspirator
sonogram (see *ultrasound*)
sonographically guided human
  thrombin injection
sonographic feature analysis
sonographic Murphy sign
sonographic parameter
sonography (see also *ultrasound*)
  Acuson computed
  Acuson transvaginal
  anal endosonography
  Biosound AU (Advanced Ultra-
    sonography)
  blooming artifacts in ultrasonog-
    raphy
  color-coded duplex
  color-coded real-time
  color duplex ultrasound
  color power transcranial Doppler
  compression ultrasonography
  continuous wave Doppler ultra-
    sonography
  Doppler ultrasonography

space
adnexal
alveolar dead
anatomical dead
antecubital
apical
apical air
axillary
Baros
Berger
Bogros
Bottcher
Bowman
Burns
capsular
cartilage
Chassaignac
Cloquet
Colles
Cotunnius
C-Y color
dead
disk
Disse
dorsal subaponeurotic
dorsal subcutaneous
echo-free
epicardial
epidural
episcleral
epitympanic
extradural
extraperitoneal
extrapleural
fifth intercostal
first intercostal
foraminal
fourth intercostal
free pericardial
gingival
Henke
His perivascular
Holzknecht

space *(cont.)*
hyperintense marrow
increased lateral joint
intercellular
intercondylar (ICS) joint
intercostal
intermetatarsal
interpeduncular
interpleural
interscalene
interstitial
intervertebral disk
intervillous
intrathecal
intravascular
joint
k-space
Kiernan
Kretschmann
Kuhnt
lateral joint
left intercostal (LICS)
Lesgaft
Lesshaft
lung air
Magendie
Malacarne
masticator
Meckel
medial joint
midpalmar
Mohrenheim
narrowing of joint
parapharyngeal
Parona (subtendinous)
patellofemoral joint
peribronchial alveolar
pericardial
perineal
perinephric
perirenal
perisinusoidal
peritoneal

space *(cont.)*
  perivitelline
  plane of intercostal
  pleural
  Poirier
  Poiseuille
  popliteal
  posterior septal
  presacral
  prevesicle
  Prussak
  pulp
  Q
  Reinke
  retrocardiac
  retromammary
  retro-orbital
  retropancreatic preaortic
  retroparotid
  retroperitoneal
    retropubic
  retrosphenoidal
  retrovesical
  Retzius
  scapholunate
  Schwalbe
  subarachnoid
  subdural
  subhepatic
  subperitoneal
  subtendinous
  subumbilical
  suprahepatic
  supralevator
  syndesmotic clear
  Talairach
  Tarin
  Tenon
  thenar
  tibiocalcaneal
  tissue
  Traube semilunar
  Trautmann triangular

space *(cont.)*
  ventricular
  vesicovaginal
  Virchow-Robin space of the brain
  Waldeyer
  web
  Westberg
  Zang
  zonular
space deficits
Spacemaker balloon dissector
space-occupying lesions
spacing error, raster
spacing, multiple beam interface
spade-shaped valvotome
Spalding sign
SPAMM sequence
span
  levator
  liver
SPARC software
spare
sparing, arytenoid
sparkling appearance of myocardium
spasm
  artery
  bowel
  bronchial
  catheter-induced coronary artery
  colonic
  coronary artery (CAS)
  coughing
  diffuse arteriolar
  diffuse esophageal (DES)
  hemifacial
  inspiratory
  muscle
  muscular
  postbypass
  respiratory
  vascular
  vein
  venous

spastic colon
spastic esophagus
spastic ileus
spatial and temporal resolution
spatial dose fractionation
spatial EPR imaging
spatially selective inversion pulse
spatial mapping
spatial modulation magnetization
spatial peak intensity
spatial presaturation
spatial registration
spatial resolution
specific activity
specificity
  high
  low
specimen, breast core biopsy
speckled pattern
SPECT (single photon emission
    computed tomography)
  acetazolamide-enhanced
  brain perfusion
  dual head
  dynamic volumetric
  electrocardiogram-gated
  FDG
  ictal
  interictal
  quantitative gated (QGS)
  Tc-99m red blood cell
  Trionix
SPECT brain perfusion scintigraphy
SPECT/MRI imaging system
SPECT technetium sestamibi scan
SPECT thallium scintigram
SPECT tomography
SPECT with ^{18}Fl-2-deoxy-D-glucose
  (FDG)
spectography, nuclear magnetic
  resonance (NMR)
spectra (pl. of spectrum)
spectral analysis

spectral diffusion
spectral Doppler
spectral noise distribution
spectral pattern
spectral US (ultrasound)
spectral wave analysis
Spectranetics excimer laser for
  coronary angioplasty
Spectranetics sheath (SLS)
Spectraprobe-Max probe
spectrofluorometry
spectrometer, SISCO (Spectroscopy
  Imaging Systems Corporation)
  4.7T/33 cm diameter imaging
spectrometry
  AMS (accelerator mass)
  Bruker NMR
  Compton suppression
  EDXRF (energy dispersive x-ray
    fluorescence)
  4.0T/31cm Surrey Medical Imaging
    Systems (SMIS) imaging
  GE NMR
  GN300 7.05T/89 mm bore multi-
    nuclear
  IBM NMR
  liquid scintillation
  Nicolet NMR
  NMR
  PROBE-SV
  pulsed L-band ESR
  scintillation
  60 MHz Fourier Transform NMR
  60 MHz Rapid Scan
  tandem mass
  360 MHz VT multinuclear
  270 MHz VT multinuclear
  Varian Associates 11.7T
    (500 MHz)/51 mm bore
  Varian NMR
spectrophotometer
  F-1200 Fluorescence
  F-2000 Fluorescence

spectrophotometer *(cont.)*
  F-4500 Fluorescence
  U-1100 UV-Vis
  U-2001 UV-Vis
  U-2020 UV-Vis
  U-3000 UV-Vis
  U-3010 UV-Vis
  U-3300 UV-Vis
  U-3310 UV-Vis
  UV-Visible
spectrophotometric calculation
spectrophotometric quantity
spectroscopic fat saturation technique
spectroscopic imaging
spectroscopy
  contrast-enhanced in vivo proton
    MR
  COSY H-1 MR
  CSI
  diffuse near-infrared
  double spin echo proton
  fluorescence
  Fourier transform infrared
  Fourier transform Raman
  glutamate
  H-1 MR
  hydrogen-1 (or 1H) magnetic
    resonance
  in vivo proton MR
  INVOS 2100 optical
  ISIS
  laser correlational (LCS)
  localized H1
  magnetic resonance (MRS)
  MR H-1 stimulated-echo
    acquisition mode
  near-infrared (NIRS)
  NMR (nuclear magnetic resonance)
  nonresonance Raman
  1H magnetic MR
  oxygen-17 NMR
  P-31 MR

spectroscopy *(cont.)*
  phosphorus nuclear magnetic
    resonance (P-MRS)
  PRESS
  proton magnetic resonance
  Raman
  remote endoscopic digital (REDS)
  selenium-77 NMR
  short echo time proton
  single voxel proton
  STEAM
  2D J-resolved 1H MR
Spectrum silicone Foley catheter
specular echo
Speedy balloon catheter
Spence, tail of
Spens syndrome
sperm abscess
spermatic cord
spermatic duct
spermatic fistula
spermatic vein
SP-501 Sonoprobe endoscopy system
SPGR (spoiled gradient-recalled) echo
  sequences
sphenocephaly
sphenoethmoidal encephalocele
sphenoethmoidal recess
sphenoethmoidal suture
sphenoid bone
sphenoid ridge tumors
sphenoid sinus
sphenoid wing
sphenoidal fissure syndrome
sphenoidal sinusitis
spheno-occipital suture
spheno-occipital synchondrosis
spheno-orbital suture
sphenopalatine ganglion
sphenopalatine neuralgia
sphenoparietal suture
sphenopetrosal suture

sphenopharyngeal meningoencephalocele
sphenosquamous suture
sphenotemporal suture
sphenoturbinal bone
sphenovomerine suture
spherical lesion
spherical map
spherical mass
spherocytosis, hereditary
spheroid-shaped
spheroids, tumor
sphincter
anal
antral
basal
bicanalicular
Boyden
canalicular
choledochal
colic
cricopharyngeal
duodenal
duodenojejunal
external anal
extrinsic
first duodenal
hypertensive lower esophageal
Hyrtl
inferior esophageal (IES)
Lutkens
Nélaton
O'Beirne
Oddi
pancreatic duct
pancreaticobiliary
pharyngoesophageal
prepyloric
pyloric
upper esophageal (UES)
sphincteric ureterocele
sphingolipidosis

sphingomyelin lipidosis
sphingomyelinase
Shprintzen velocardiofacial syndrome
sphygmography
sphygmomanometer cuff
SPI-Argent II peritoneal dialysis
catheter
spicular density
spicular protrusion
spiculated mass
spiculations on colon
spicule of bone
spicules in profile
SPIDER (steady state projection
imaging with dynamic echo train
readout)
spike-related functional MR imaging
spider angioma (pl. angiomata)
spidering skeleton
spider nevus (pl. nevi)
spiderweb appearance
spiderweb circulation on angiography
of glioblastomas
spider x-ray view
spike loading
spiky outgrowths of bone
spiky skeletons
spin (pl. spins)
flowing
J-coupled
stationary
uncoupled
spina bifida
spina bifida occulta (SBO)
spina bifida posterior
spinal abscess, epidural
spinal accessory nerve (eleventh
cranial nerve)
spinal angiogram
spinal angiolipoma
spinal arthritis
spinal axial loading

spinal axis
spinal block by cord compression
spinal canal narrowing
spinal column
spinal cord
    caliber of
    compression of
    decompression of
    hemisection of
    infarction of the
    laceration of the
    multiple focal lesions of (in
        multiple sclerosis)
    posterolateral sclerosis of
    size of
    tethered
    transection of
spinal cord ependymoma
spinal cord injury (SCI)
spinal cord lesion
spinal cord parenchyma
spinal cord stroke
spinal cord tumor
spinal dural arteriovenous fistula
spinal dysraphism
spinal elements, neoplastic destruction
    of
spinal ependymoma
spinal epidural abscess
spinal epidural hematoma
spinal fixation
spinal fusion
spinal hemiplegia
spinal hydatid cyst
spinal instability
spinal involvement
spinal lordosis
spinal myeloscopy
spinal roots
    C1-7 (cervical)
    Co. 1 (coccygeal)
    L1-5 (lumbar)
    S1-5 (sacral)
    T1-12 (thoracic)

spinal subarachnoid hemorrhage
spinal subdural hematoma
spinal tuberculosis
spinal videofluoroscopy
spin coupling
spin density
spindle
    aortic
    His
spindle-shaped shadow
spine
    alar
    angulation of
    anterior column of
    anterior maxillary
    anterior superior iliac
    anteroposterior iliac
    cervical (C)
    Charcot
    coccygeal (coccyx)
    dendritic
    dorsal (D)
    functional units of
    iliac
    ischial
    kinetic cervical
    kissing
    lateral bending views of the
    lumbar (L)
    lumbarized
    lumbosacral (LS)
    maxillary
    mental
    nasal
    poker
    posterior-inferior
    posterior column of
    posterior-inferior
    rotatory loads on
    rugger-jersey
    sacral (S)
    splinting of
    static cervical

spine *(cont.)*
   thoracic (T)
   thoracolumbar
   trochanteric
spin echo (SE)
   breath-hold fast-recovery optimized
     fast
   T2-weighted turbo
spin echo image
spin echo imaging sequence
spin echo pulse sequence
spin label method
spin lattice relaxation time
spin lock and magnetization transfer
   imaging
spin lock imaging
spin lock induced T1rho-weighted
   image
spin-locking, adiabatic off-resonance
spin lock prepulse
spinocerebellar ataxia
spinocerebellar degeneration
spinoglenoid notch
spinographic analysis
spinography, digitized
spinoreticular tract
spinotectal tract
spinothalamic tract
spinous process
spin spin relaxation time
spin warp imaging
SPIO (superparamagnetic iron oxide)
   oral contrast agent
SPIR (selective partial inversion-
   recovery)
spiral (also spiraling)
spiral appearance
spiral band of Gosset
spiral computed tomography
spiral CT (computed tomography)
   angiography (SCTA)
spiral CT pitch
spiral CT scanner

spiral CT with multiplanar
   reformatting and 3D rendering
spiral dissection
spiral fracture
spiral oblique fracture
spiral position
spiral pulse sequence
spiral scanning technique
SpiraStent ureteral stent
spiral-tip catheter
spiral XCT (x-ray computed
   tomography) scanner
SpiroFlo bioabsorbable prostate stent
spirometric gating (or guidance) in
   helical CT technology
spirometric acquisition
spirometrically controlled CT
Spirtos coaxial catheter
splanchnic arterial stenosis
splanchnic vascular imaging
splanchnic vasculature
splanchnic vessels
splash, succussion
splashing bruit
splayed
splayfoot deformity
splaying of pedicles
spleen
   accessory
   floating
   inflammatory
   long axis of
   tip of
   wandering
spleen to liver ratio
splenic artery
splenic enhancement pattern
splenic flexure
splenic lobule
splenic notch
splenic portography
splenic venography
splenium of corpus callosum

splenization
splenobronchial fistula
splenogonadal fusion
splenography
splenomegaly
  congenital
  congestive
  Egyptian
  fibrocongestive
  Gaucher
  hemolytic
  infectious
  myelophthisic
  Opitz thrombophlebitic
  persistent
  siderotic
splenoportography
splenorenal anastomosis
splenorenal arterial bypass graft
splenorenal recess
splenorenal shunt
splinter hemorrhage
splinting of the spine
split brain studies
split compression fracture
split course accelerated radiotherapy
split course hyperfractionated radiation
  therapy
split echo diffusion-weighted MR
  imaging
split function
split hyperfractionated accelerated
  radiation therapy
split liver transplantation
split renal function (SRF)
split renal function decrease
split sheath catheter
splitting
  directional bremsstrahlung (DBS)
  interaction
  uniform bremsstrahlung (UBS)
  zero-field
SPN (solitary pulmonary nodule)

SpO_2 (oxygen saturation)
spoke bone
spoiled gradient-recalled (SPGR) echo
  sequences
spoiler, Lucite beam
spoking, cortical
spondylitic change
spondylitis
  ankylosing
  rheumatoid
  tuberculous
spondylitis deformans
spondylolisthesis
  sagittal roll
  slip angle
  traumatic (grades 1-4)
spondylolisthetic pelvis
spondylolysis
spondylomalacia
spondylosis
  cervical
  degenerative
  diffuse
  Nurick classification of
spondylosyndesis
sponge
  gelatin
  Ivalon
  Ray-Tec x-ray detectable surgical
    sponge
  Vistec x-ray detectable
spongiocytoma
spongiosa of mitral valve
spongy appearance
spongy bone
spongy degeneration leukodystrophy
spongy urethra
spongy uterus
spontaneous cardioversion
spontaneous closure of defect
spontaneous coronary artery dissection
  (SCAD)
spontaneous deposition

spontaneous detorsion
spontaneous echo contrast
spontaneous fracture
spontaneous infantile ductal aneurysm
spontaneous involution
spontaneous passage of stone
spontaneous pneumothorax
spontaneous regression
spontaneous subsidence
spontaneous tension pneumothorax
spontaneous transient vasoconstriction
spoonlike protrusion of leaflets
sporadic subcortical arteriosclerotic
  encephalopathy
spot
  capitate soft
  hot
  pituitary bright
  z-flying focal (zFFS)

spot compression
spot film
spot film fluorography
spot images
S phase fraction
S pouch, ileal
SPP (superparamagnetic particle)
  imaging agent
SPPS (single photon planar
  scintigraphy)
SPR (scanned projection radiography)
SPR (superior peroneal retinaculum)
sprain
  acute
  chronic
  eversion
sprain fracture
sprain-strain
spread
  pattern of
  transfascial
Sprengel deformity
Spring catheter with Pro/Pel coating

Springer fracture
spring hookwire
spring-loaded vascular stent
sprinter's fracture
sprodiamide imaging agent
SP6 camera
spur (spurring)
  acromial
  anterior
  bone (or bony)
  calcaneal
  calcific
  degenerative
  heel
  hypertrophic marginal
  impingement
  inferior
  marginal
  Morand
  osteoarthritic
  plantar calcaneal
  posterior
  prominent
  retrocalcaneal
  traction
  uncovertebral
spur formation
spurring
Spyglass angiography catheter
squamocolumnar junction
squamous cell carcinoma in situ (CIS)
squamous intraepithelial lesion (SIL)
squaring-off (of bone after fracture)
squatting position
squeeze sign
Squibb catheter
Sr (strontium) (an element)
SRF (split renal function)
SRS (somatostatin receptor scintigraphy)
SSD (shaded surface display) algorithms
SSFP (steady state free precession)

SSFSE (single shot fast spin echo)
SSH (spinal subdural hemorrhage)
S-shaped pouch
S-shaped scoliosis
SSKI (saturated potassium iodide
    solution)
SSM (segmental misty mesentery)
SSP (slice sensitivity profile)
SSS (sick sinus syndrome)
SSS (subclavian steal syndrome)
SSQ (sequential scalar quantization)
SSS (subclavian steal syndrome)
stabilization, Bremer AirFlo Vest for
    thoracic
stabilizing bullet
stable fracture
stable isotope
stable-state tuberculosis
stab wound to kidney
Stack autoperfusion balloon
stacked foil technique
stacked metaphor workstation
stacked ovoid lesions
stacked scans
stacked tomograms
Stack perfusion coronary dilatation
    catheter
STAE (subsegmental transcatheter
    arterial embolization)
staghorn calculus
staghorn renal calculus
staging (see also *grading*)
    axillary lymph node
    Berndt-Harty talar lesion
    distraction-flexion (DFS)
    Ficat avascular necrosis
    Gottschalk
    Greulich and Pyle skeletal
        maturation
    Jackson
    neuroblastoma
    Outerbridge degenerative arthritis
    pre-slip

staging *(cont.)*
    Scheuer histologic
    whole-body
stagnant loop syndrome
stagnant urine
stain, tumor (on cerebral angiography)
stainless steel mesh stent
staircase phenomenon
stairstep air-fluid levels
stairstep artifact
stairstep fracture
stalk
    body
    infundibular
    pituitary
    polyp
    tumor
stalk-section effect
Stamey-Malecot catheter
standard-dose enhanced conventional
    MR imaging
standardized uptake value (SUV)
standards
    ACR teleradiology standard
    age-based
    Taveras
    Wilmad reference
standby rate
standing position
standing postvoid view
standoff
standstill
    atrial
    cardiac
    ventricular
Stand-Up MRI, Fonar
Stanford type B aortic dissection
stannous pyrophosphate
stannous sulfur colloid imaging agent
staphylococcal pleurisy
staphylococcal pneumonia
staphylococcal pneumonitis

Staphylococcus aureus bacterial
  pneumonia
STAR angiography
Starcam camera
star-cancellation test (SCT)
Stargate falloposcopy catheter
Starling curve
Starlink software
star pattern
STAR registry
STARRT Falloposcopy System
star-shaped vessel lumen
stasis, venous
stasis edema
stasis of blood flow
stasis ulcers
state, chronic constrictive
static 3D FLASH imaging
static image
status post (S/P)
Staunig inferosuperior projection of
  pelvic bones
steady state free precession (SSFP)
steady state MRE
steady state precession
steady state projection imaging with
  dynamic echo train readout
  (SPIDER)
steal
  arterial
  coronary artery
  subclavian
stealing of cerebral blood by
  subclavian artery
steal phenomenon
STEAM (stimulated echo acquisition
  mode)
STEAM spectroscopy
steatosis
Stecher method to view scaphoid bone
steep left anterior oblique (LAO) view
steeple sign on chest x-ray
steep Towne projection

steep Trendelenburg position
steerable catheter
steerable guidewire system
steering catheter
steering, electronic independent beam
Steerocath catheter
steganography
stellar nevus
stellate defect
stellate lesion
stellate pattern
stellate skull fracture
stem
  brain
  bronchus
  reticular formation of the brain
  roundback
  straight
stem cell transplantation
Stener lesion
stenocardia
steno-occlusive disease
stenosing lesion
stenosing ring of left atrium
stenosis
  acquired mitral
  American Heart Association
    classification of
  ampullary
  anal
  antral
  aortic (AS)
  aortic valve
  aortoiliac
  aqueductal
  arterial
  atypical aortic valve
  benign papillary
  bicuspid valvular aortic
  bilateral carotid
  bladder neck
  bowel
  branch pulmonary

stenosis *(cont.)*
   breast duct
   bronchial
   buttonhole mitral
   calcific aortic
   calcific bicuspid valvular
   calcific senile aortic valvular
   calcific valvular
   cardiac valvular
   carotid artery
   central canal
   central spinal
   cerebral artery
   cervical
   choledochoduodenal junctional
   common pulmonary vein
   concentric hourglass
   congenital esophageal
   congenital pyriform aperture
   coronary artery
   coronary luminal
   coronary ostial
   critical coronary
   critical valvular
   cross-sectional area
   culprit
   diffuse
   discrete subaortic
   discrete subvalvular aortic (DSAS)
   distal urethral
   dynamic subaortic
   eccentric
   esophageal
   external iliac
   femoropopliteal atheromatous
   fibromuscular subaortic
   fish-mouth mitral
   fixed-orifice aortic
   flow-limiting
   focal
   granulation
   hemodynamically significant
   high grade

stenosis *(cont.)*
   hypercalcemia supravalvular aortic
   hypertrophic infundibular
     subpulmonic
   hypertrophic pyloric
   hypertrophic subaortic
   idiopathic hypertrophic subaortic
     (IHSS)
   iliofemoral venous
   infrainguinal bypass
   infrarenal
   infrarenal aortic
   infundibular pulmonary
   infundibular subpulmonic
   innominate artery
   intrarenal
   juxta-anastomotic
   linear
   luminal
   meatal
   membranous subvalvular aortic
   mitral (MS)
   mitral valve
   multifocal short
   muscular subaortic
   napkin-ring
   neoplastic
   neovagina
   noncalcified coronary
   noncritical
   nonrheumatic valvular aortic
   ostial renal artery
   papillary
   peripheral arterial
   peripheral pulmonary artery
     (PPAS)
   petrous carotid canal
   post-PTCA
   postangioplasty
   preangioplasty
   pulmonary
   pulmonary artery
   pulmonary valve

stenosis *(cont.)*
    pulmonary vein
    pulmonic (PS)
    pyloric
    rectal
    relative mitral
    renal artery
    rheumatic aortic valvular
    rheumatic mitral
    rheumatic tricuspid
    saphenous vein
    segmental
    senescent aortic
    severe
    silent mitral
    spinal
    splanchnic arterial
    stomal
    subaortic
    subclavian artery
    subinfundibular pulmonary
    subpulmonic infundibular
    subvalvar aortic
    supra-aortic
    supraclavicular aortic stenosis
    suprarenal
    supravalvular aortic (SAS, SVAS)
    supravalvular pulmonic
    tapering
    tight
    tracheal
    tricuspid (TS)
    true mitral
    truncal renal artery
    tubal
    tubular
    tunnel subvalvular aortic
    unicuspid aortic valve
    unilateral carotid
    unilateral renal artery
    ureteral
    urethral
    vaginal

stenosis *(cont.)*
    valvar aortic
    valvular pulmonic
    vertebral artery
stenosis of breast duct
stenotic but patent tricuspid valve
stenotic isthmus
stenotic lesion
stenotic ureter
stenotic valve
Stensen duct
stent (stenting)
    ACS Multilink coronary
    ACS RX Multi-Link
    activated balloon expandable
        intravascular
    antegrade ureteral
    balloon expandable flexible coil
    balloon expandable intravascular
    balloon expandable metallic
    balloon uterine
    Beamer
    beStent balloon-expandable
    biliary
    biodegradable
    Bio divYsio stent
    BioSorb resorbable urologic
    Bridge X3 renal
    CardioCoil self-expanding coronary
    Circon
    coil vascular
    covered Gianturco
    covered retrievable, expandable
        nitinol
    Dacron-covered
    double J indwelling
    double J ureteral
    double pigtail
    drainage
    Endocare Horizon prostatic
    ENDOcare nitinol urinary
    EndoCoil biliary
    endoluminal

stent *(cont.)*
   EsophaCoil biliary stent
   esophageal
   Fader Tip ureteral
   gastroduodenal
   Gianturco-Rösch Z-stent
   Greene renal implant
   heat-expandable
   helical coil
   Horizon nitinol temporary
   Horizon temporary urinary
   hydrophilic-coated urologic
   iliac artery
   indwelling
   indwelling ureteral
   Innovante
   InStent CarotidCoil
   InStent self-expanding and balloon
      expandable
   interdigitating coil
   IntraCoil self-expanding nitinol
   intracoronary
   IntraStent DoubleStrut LD
   IntraStent DoubleStrut renal artery
   IntraStent DoubleStrut XS renal
      artery
   intravascular
   iridium-192 (^{192}Ir)-loaded
   Jocath
   Jography
   Joguide
   Kwart AQ Retro-Inject
   Kwart Retro-Inject
   lacrimal duct
   Litespeed
   LSe Kwart Retro-Inject
   Lubri-Flex urologic
   Magic Wallstent
   Mardis firm stent with HydroPlus
      coating
   Medinvent
   Medivent vascular
   Micro-Driver

stent *(cont.)*
   MicroStent II over the wire PTCA
   MINI Crown
   Mobius vascular
   Multi-Flex urologic
   Multilink Duet noncoated coronary
   Multilink Penta coronary
   Multilink Tetra coronary
   Multi-Link Vision RX and OTW
      (over the wire) coronary
   Navius
   Neuroform microdelivery
   NexStent carotid
   NIR ON
   NIR premounted
   NIR Prince (or NIR pRINce)
   NIR with SOX over the wire
      coronary
   NIRflex coronary
   NIRoyal Elite Monorail coronary
   nitinol
   nitinol thermal memory
   Omnir
   OmniStent
   ostiomeatal
   Outcomes by Design
   Palmaz balloon-expandable iliac
   Palmaz-Schatz (PSS)
   Palmaz-Schatz coronary
   pancreatic duct
   Paragon coronary
   patent
   Percuflex
   Percuflex Plus flexible ureteral
   percutaneous
   percutaneous implantation of endo-
      vascular
   percutaneous ureteral
   pigtail
   polymer-coated drug-eluting
   polyurethane
   porous metallic
   ProstaCoil self-expanding urethral

stent *(cont.)*
    radioisotope
    Rapid-Trak
    Reliance urinary control
    renal
    renovascular
    retrograde ureteral
    Roubin Gianturco flexible coil
    Schatz-Palmaz tubular mesh
    self-expanding
    Silastic
    silicone
    Silitek
    SpiraStent ureteral
    SpiroFlo bioabsorbable prostate
    spring-loaded vascular
    stainless steel mesh
    straight
    Strecker balloon-expandable
    Strecker tantalum
    Surgitek
    tantalum
    Tecoflex
    thermal memory
    transhepatic biliary
    T-tube
    U-tube
    Ultraflex self-expanding
    ureteral
    urethral
    UroCoil self-expanding
    UroLume endoprosthesis wire
    UroLume urethral
    UroLume urinary
    UroLume Wallstent
    Vistaflex biliary
    Wallstent spring-loaded
    Wiktor
    wire-mesh self-expandable
    XT radiopaque coronary
    zig-zag
stent deployment
stent embolization

stent expansion
stent-graft
    Dacron-covered
    endovascular
    Jocath
    Jography
    percutaneous endoluminal
        placement of
stent-guide, Joguide
stentless porcine aortic valve
stent migration
stent-mounted allograft valve
stent-mounted heterograft valve
stent recanalization
stent thrombosis
stent-vessel wall contact
Stenver view
stepdown deformity of shoulder
step-oblique mammography
stepoff between bone fracture frag-
    ments
stepoff, orbital rim
stepped-care antihypertensive regimen
stepping kinematic imaging platform
stepping-table gadolinium-enhanced
    digital subtraction MR angiography
stepup (or step-up)
stepwise regression analysis
stercoral ulcer
stercoroma
stereocinefluorography
stereofluoroscopy
stereographic projections
stereogram
stereolithography
stereologic method of volume
    estimation
stereoradiography
stereoscopic fly-through
stereoscopic view
stereoscopic vision
stereotactic (or stereotaxic)
stereotactic ablation

stereotactic add-on device
stereotactically guided
stereotactic biopsy
stereotactic CT scan
stereotactic data
stereotactic directional vacuum-assisted
breast biopsy
stereotactic localization
stereotactic method for intracranial
navigation
stereotactic neurosurgery
stereotactic procedure
stereotactic proton irradiation
stereotactic radiation therapy
stereotactic radiosurgery
stereotactic resection, computer-
assisted
stereotactic surface projection (SSP)
stereotactic vacuum-assisted breast
biopsy
stereotactic vacuum-assisted directional
biopsy
stereotaxis
computer-assisted volumetric
imaging-based
volumetric
stereotaxy
sterile
sternal angle of Louis
sternal border and apex
sternal cartilage
sternal edge
sternal joint
sternal lift
sternal marrow
sternal notch
sternal pleural reflection
sternal splitting
sternal view
Sternberg myocardial insufficiency
sternoclavicular angle
sternoclavicular joint

sternocleidomastoid muscle
sternocostal joint
sternocostal surface of heart
sternohyoid muscle
sternopericardial ligament
sternothyroid muscle
sternum
anterior bowing of
nonunion of operated
steroid cell ovarian tumor
Stertzer brachial guiding catheter
stethoscope
Littmann
ultrasound
Stieda fracture
Stierlin sign
stiffening
stiffness, shear
Still disease (juvenile rheumatoid
arthritis)
Stiller rib
stimulated echo acquisition mode
(STEAM)
stimulated echo artifact
stimulated echo-tagging technique
stimulation
odor
secretin
sequential olfactory
stimulus-correlated signal
stippled calcification
stippled epiphysis
stippled soft tissue
stippling of lung fields
STIR (short T1 inversion recovery)
scan
STIR (short tau inversion recovery)
sequence
Stockert/Shiley venous occluder
Stockholm C view of skull
stocking-glove distribution

stoma
  abdominal
  bowel
  diverting
  gastrointestinal
  permanent
  prolapsed
  retracted
  Silastic collar-reinforced
stomach
  aberrant umbilical
  antrum of
  bilocular
  canal of
  cardiac
  cascade
  convex border of
  coronary artery of
  cup-and-spill
  distal blind
  distended
  dumping
  greater curvature of
  Holzknecht
  hourglass
  intrathoracic
  leather bottle
  lesser curvature of
  miniature
  Pavlov
  pit of
  riding
  scaphoid
  sclerotic
  sour
  thoracic
  trifid
  upset
  upside-down
  water-trap
  waterfall
stomal bag

stone (see also *calculus*; *gallstone*)
  barrel-shaped
  bile duct
  biliary
  biliary tract
  bilirubinate
  black faceted
  bladder
  bosselated
  calcium bilirubinate
  CBD (common bile duct)
  common bile duct
  gall
  gallbladder
  high attenuation
  impacted urethral
  intrahepatic
  intraluminal
  intravesical
  kidney
  lung
  metabolic
  noncalcified
  nonopaque
  opaque
  passage of renal
  prostatic
  radiolucent
  radiopaque
  renal
  residual
  salivary
  spontaneous passage of
  staghorn
  shadowing
  ureteral
  ureteric
  urinary
  vein
  womb
stone differentiated from tumor
stone disintegration in ureter

stone formation, vesical
stonelike calculus
stone manipulation, percutaneous
stop action images
stopcock
stooped-over position
stopping power
storage phosphor radiology
storage-phosphor system
storiform pattern
stork method to view symphysis pubis
straddle fracture
straddle injury of urethra
straight AP pelvic injection
straight catheterization
straight chest tube
straight flush percutaneous catheter
straight-line HT (Hough transform)
   mapping
straight ureter
straight veins of kidney
strain
   ligamentous
   lumbosacral spine
   muscle
strain fracture
strain rate MR imaging
strain-sprain injury
stranding
   fascial
   mesenteric
   soft tissue
strands of increased density on chest
   x-ray
strandy pulmonic infiltrate
strangulated bowel
strangulated hernia
stratigraphy
Stratis II MRI system
stray neutron field
streak artifact
streaks of atelectasis on chest film
streaks of increased density

Strecker balloon-expandable stent
Strecker tantalum stent
streptococcal pleurisy
streptococcal pneumonia
stress
   adduction (to fingers)
   adenosine-induced
   biomechanical
   hydraulic shear
   mediolateral
   orthostatic
   shear
   shearing
   torque
   valgus
   varus
stress and rest images
stress cystogram
stress films
stress fracture
stress gated blood pool cardiac
   examination
stress images (imaging)
stress-induced left ventricular
   dilatation
stress-injected sestamibi-gated SPECT
   with echocardiography
stress management
stress Myoview noninvasive nuclear
   imaging technique
stress perfusion and rest function by
   sestamibi-gated SPECT
stress perfusion scintigraphy
stress radiography
stress redistribution exam
stress-rest-reinjection examination
stress test
   dipyridamole thallium
   Persantine thallium
stress thallium scan
stress thallium-201 myocardial
   imaging
stress ulcer

striations, subcallosal
stricture
    anal
    anastomotic
    annular esophageal
    antral
    benign biliary
    bile duct
    bulbar urethral
    bulbomembranous urethral
    cervical
    cicatricial
    congenital
    contractile
    esophageal
    irritable
    longitudinal esophageal
    male urethral
    peptic
    postcatheterization urethral
    postobstetric urethral
    postoperative urethral
    prostatic
    pyloric
    rectal
    recurrent
    spasmodic
    traumatic urethral
    ureteral
    urethral
    urinary meatal
    vaginal
    vulvar
stricture of ureter
string guideline
stringlike bands of fibrous tissue
string of beads appearance
string of pearls nuclear arrangement
string of pearls sign
string sign in terminal ileum
strip, primary motor

stripe
    Baillarger
    central intraluminal saturation
    flank
    Gennari
    paraspinal pleural
    paratracheal
    properitoneal flank
    Retzius
    saturation
    vertebral
    Vicq d'Azyr
stripe sign
striping, horizontal
stroke
    cerebrovascular
    hyperacute
    thromboembolic (TE)
stroke distance, Doppler-derived
stroke ejection rate
stroke force
stroke index (SI)
stroke power
stroke scale score
stroke volume (SV)
stroke volume image
stroke volume index (SVI)
stroke volume ratio
stroma
stromal endometriosis
strongyloidiasis
strontium (Sr) (an element)
    ^{82}Sr
    ^{85}Sr bracelet
    ^{89}Sr chloride (Metastron) radio-
        active drug
    ^{90}Sr-loaded eye applicator
structural epilepsy
structural scoliosis
structural weakness of bronchial wall
    supports

structure (pl. structures)
  adjacent
  angiographically overlapping
  anomalous
  biliary
  bony
  branching linear
  branching tubular
  calcified density
  central hilar
  cord
  denture-supporting
  elongated
  high density
  hollow
  hypoechoic tubular
  intratumoral
  KUB (kidneys, ureters, bladder)
  labyrinthine
  low contrast
  low density
  organoid
  osseous
  renal collecting
  ringlike
  satellite
  soft tissue density
  submillimeter
  subtle
  superior mediastinal
  supraglottic
  tubular
  vascular
structured coil electromagnet
Strümpell-Lorrain disease
Strümpell-Marie disease
strut
  corticocancellous
  optic
  tricuspid valve
  valve outflow
STT (scapho-trapezium-trapezoid)
  joint

Stryker notch view of humeral head
studded fissures
study (see also *imaging*)
  aerosol ventilation
  anisotropic 3-D or volume
  biplane pelvic oblique
  bladder contractility
  blood flow
  bone density
  bone length
  bone mineral content (BMC)
  bubble (contrast echocardiography)
  carotid duplex
  cerebrospinal fluid leak
  conventional
  cornflake esophageal motility
  defecographic
  Doppler blood flow
  Doppler flow probe
  dual contrast
  dynamic contrast-enhanced
    subtraction
  electromagnetic blood flow
  endovascular flow wire
  FibroSpect
  first pass
  fistula tract
  flow
  gallbladder (oral cholecystogram)
  gas ventilation
  gated blood (pool) cardiac wall
    motion
  ictal phase
  in vivo disposition
  inhalation
  interictal PET FDG
  interictal SPECT
  isotropic 3D or volume
  kidney function
  marker transit
  meniscus sign on upper GI
  minute sequence
  morphine-augmented

study *(cont.)*
 motility
 multibreath washout
 multitracer
 noncontrast
 noninvasive imaging
 nuclear-tagged red blood cell
  bleeding
 paleopathologic and radiologic
 periorbital Doppler
 peripheral small airways
 pharmacodynamic
 platelet survival
 pressure
 pressure perfusion
 pullback
 pulmonary quantitative differential
  function
 qualitative
 radiochemical
 radiolabeled water
 radiologic-histopathologic
 radionuclide blood pool
 radionuclide voiding
 reconstruction
 redistribution
 renal cyst
 rest-dobutamine stress myocardial
  perfusion
 salivary gland function
 scintigraphic
 simulated equilibrium factor
 sinus tract
 TECA (technetium albumin)
 ureteral reflux
 videofluoroscopy swallowing
  (VFSS)
 voiding
 wall motion
stump
 appendiceal
 cervical
 duodenal

stump *(cont.)*
 gastric
 rectal
Sturge-Weber telangiectasia
stuttering myocardial infarction
S2 (serotonin) receptor
styloid process
subacromial bursitis
subacromial impingement syndrome
subacute allergic pneumonia
subadventitial plane
subadventitial tissue
subannular region
subaortic curtain
subaortic glands
subaortic muscle
subaortic stenosis
subapical
subarachnoid cavity
subarachnoid hemorrhage (SAH)
subarachnoid instillation of contrast
  material
subarachnoid metastatic disease
subarachnoid phenol block (SAPB)
  with fluoroscopy
subarachnoid space
subareolar abscess
subarticular cyst
subastragalar dislocation
subatmospheric pressure
sub-band (or subband), wavelet
subcallosal gyrus
subcallosal striations
subcapital fracture
subcapsular hematoma
subcardinal vein
subcarina (pl. subcarinae)
subcarinal adenopathy
subcarinal angle
subcarinal node
subchondral bone cyst
subchondral bone plate
subchondral microfractures

subchorionic hemorrhage
subclavian aneurysm
subclavian approach for cardiac
   catheterization
subclavian artery occlusion
subclavian artery steal of cerebral
   blood
subclavian artery stenosis
subclavian catheter
subclavian junction
subclavian loop
subclavian-pulmonary shunt
subclavian steal phenomenon (SSP)
subclavian steal syndrome (SSS)
subclavian vein, blind percutaneous
   puncture of
subclavian vein catheterization
subclavicular approach
subcollateral gyrus
subcoracoid dislocation of shoulder
subcortical infarct
subcortical ischemic vascular dementia
subcortical intracerebral hemorrhage
subcortical intracranial lesion
subcortical lesion
subcortical tumor
subcostal approach
subcostal artery
subcostal branch
subcostal margin
subcostal nerve
subcostal window
subcu (subcutaneous)
subcutaneous air
subcutaneous array electrode
subcutaneous emphysema
subcutaneous fat line
subcutaneous fracture
subcutaneous granuloma annulare
subcutaneous hemangioma
subdural hemorrhage
subcutaneous injection of contrast
   artifact

subcutaneous patch
subcutaneous pocket
subcutaneous tissue
subcutaneous tissue gas
subcutaneous tunnel
subcutaneous veins
subcuticular layer
subdeltoid bursal adhesion
subdiaphragmatic abscess
subdural abscess
subdural blood
subdural cavity
subdural clot
subdural effusion
subdural empyema
subdural hematoma
subdural hemorrhage
subdural hygroma
subdural space
subdural window on CT scan
subendocardial infarction (SEI)
subendocardial injury
subendocardial ischemia
subendocardial myocardial infarction
subendocardial necrosis
subendothelial hyalinization
subependymal hemorrhage
subepithelial hematoma
subeustachian sinus
subfalcine (subfalcial) herniation
subfascial hematoma
subfascial transposition
subfascially
subfrontal meningioma tumor
subgaleal abscess
subgaleal hematoma
subglenoid dislocation of shoulder
subglottic area
subglottic edema
subhepatic area
subhepatic space
subinfundibular pulmonary stenosis
subintimal cleavage plane

subintimal dissection
sublabral foramen
sublabral recess
subligamentous disk herniation
sublingual varices
sublux
subluxated
subluxation
   atlanto-axial
   clement
   forward
   occult
   patellar
   posterior
   radial head (RHS)
   reduced
   rotary
   tendon
   Volkmann
submandibular ganglion
submandibular triangle
submammary abscess
submaxillary
submental vertex view
submentovertex [or submentovertical]
   (SMV) view
submillimeter structures
submucosal arterial malformation
submucosal edema in distal ileum
submucosal fat deposition
submucosal lesion
submucosal thickening
submucous myoma
suboccipital shortening
suboptimal film due to film quality;
   patient cooperation; positioning
suboptimal position
suboptimal results
suboptimal runoff
suboptimal visualization
suboptimally visualized
subparcellated
subpectoral pocket

subperiosteal abscess of frontal sinus
subperiosteal fracture
subperiosteally
subperiosteal new bone formation
subperiosteal orbital abscess
subphrenic abscess
subphrenic biloma
subpleural bleb
subpleural curvilinear lines
subpleural dots
subpleural lines
subpubic arch
subpulmonic fluid
subpulmonic infundibular stenosis
subpulmonic obstruction
subrectus placement
subsartorial tunnel
subscapular hematoma
subsegment of lung
subsegmental bibasilar atelectasis
subsegmental bronchus
subsegmental perfusion abnormality
subsegmental transcatheter arterial
   embolization (STAE)
subsegments, right middle lobe
subseptate uterus
subsequent hernia formation
subserosal fibrosis
subserosal layer
subspinous dislocation
substantia propria
substernal angle
substernal goiter
substernal thyroid
substitution bone
substrate, main energy
subtalar articulation
subtalar coalition on x-ray of the foot
subtalar joint space
subtendinous space
subtentorial lesion
subtle abnormalities

subtle cerebral and cerebellar morphologic anomalies
subtle change
subtle clue
subtle collapse
subtle deficits
subtle depression
subtle differences
subtle dispersion anomalies
subtle effects
subtle features
subtle inflammation
subtle injury
subtle lesion
subtle markers
subtle microcalcification
subtle mobile atlantoaxial dislocation
subtle mural abnormality
subtle myelin pallor
subtle neuroanatomical changes
subtle neuronal reorganization
subtle nodular protrusions
subtle signs
subtle structural alterations
subtle structural changes
subtle structure
subtle variations
subtle white matter changes
subtotal lesion
subtraction, Epistar
subtraction films
    digital
    manual
    serial
Subtraction Ictal SPECT co-registered
    to MRI (SISCOM)
subtraction, temporal
subtraction images
subtraction technique
subtrochanteric fracture
subvalvular aneurysm
subvalvular aortic obstruction
subvalvular aortic stenosis

subvesical duct
subxiphoid echocardiography view
subxiphoid implantation
subxiphoid view
sucking pneumothorax
Sucquet-Hoyer anastomosis
Sucquet-Hoyer canal
sucrose dosimeter
sucrose polyester contrast
suction line, aortic vent
Sudbury system
sudden blockage of coronary artery
Sudeck atrophy
Sudeck osteoporotic atrophy
SUFE (slipped upper femoral
    epiphysis)
suite, angiography
sulcal skeleton
sulcation
sulcus (pl. sulci)
    angularis
    basilar
    blunted posterior
    cortical
    costal
    Harrison
    atrioventricular
    calcarine
    callosal
    central
    cingulate
    collateral
    dilatation of the
    effacement of
    frontal
    hypothalamic
    lateral occipital
    lips of lateral
    occipitotemporal
    olfactory
    parieto-occipital
    pontomedullary
    postcentral

sulcus *(cont.)*
  posterior
  posterior interventricular
  precentral
  pulmonary
  rami of lateral
  rolandic
  superior frontal
  superior temporal
  supracallosal
  temporal
  ulnar
  widened (on scan)
sulesomab (technetium Tc 99m
  sulesomab)
sulfobromophthalein (BSP) imaging
  agent
sulfur colloid labeled with Tc 99m
  scan
sulfur colloid, technetium bound to
SULP II catheter
sum-peak method
summation shadow artifact
summing correction
Summit LoDose collimator
summit, ventricular septal
sump catheter
Sun SPARCstation system
Sun workstation
sunburst pattern
sunrise view of patella
sunset view
superabsorbent polymer (SAP) embolic material
super scan appearance
superciliary arch
superconducting magnet
superconductor
superdominant left anterior descending
  artery
superficial femoral artery
superficial external pudendal artery
superficial femoral arteries (SFAs)

superficial femoral artery occlusion
superficial femoral vein
superficial lesion
superficial palmar arterial arch
superficial pneumonia
superficial posterior compartment
superficial pseudoaneurysm
superficial vein
superimposed
superimposition artifact
superimposition of signals
superincumbent spinal curves
superior border of heart
superior border of rib
superior bronchus
superior caval defect
superior caval obstruction
superior colliculus
superior costotransverse ligament
superior epigastric artery
superior facet
superior frontal gyrus
superior frontal sulcus
superior genicular artery
superior intercostal artery
superior intercostal vein
superior lobe of lung
superior margin of inferior rib
superior marginal defect
superior mediastinal structures
superior mediastinum
superior mesenteric artery (SMA)
superior mesenteric vein (SMV)
superior parietal lobule gyrus
superior pubic ramus
superior pulmonary artery
superior pulmonary vein
superior retraction
superior sagittal sinus
superior segment
superior semicircular canal
superior temporal gyrus
superior temporal sulcus

superior thoracic aperture
superior thyroid artery
superior vena cava obstruction
supernormal conduction
supernormal excitation
supernumerary bone
supernumerary sesamoid bones
superoinferior heart
superolaterally
superomedial portal
superparamagnetic contrast agent
superparamagnetic iron oxide-
enhanced imaging
superparamagnetic iron oxide (SPIO)
oral contrast agent
superselective (*not* supraselective)
superselective adrenal arterial
embolization
superselective angio-CT
superselective angiography
superselective angioscintigraphy
superselective catheterization
superselective intra-arterial
chemotherapy
superselective transcatheter embolization
supination-adduction fracture
supination, degrees of
supination-eversion fracture
supinatory sign
supine film
supine position
supplemental beam filtration
Supple Peri-Guard patch
support, Rippstein leg
suppression
    Cytomel (thyroid hormone)
    double echo three-point Dixon
      method
    fat
    outer-volume
    paradoxical
    uniform fat

suppressor mesh
suppuration
suppurative pneumonia
supra-annular constriction
supra-aortic ridge
supra-aortic stenosis
supracallosal sulcus
supracardiac shunt
supracardiac-type total anomalous
venous return
supraceliac aorta
supraclavicular aortic stenosis
supraclavicular lymph node
supraclavicular node
supraclavicular region
supraclavicular triangle
supraclinoid internal carotid artery
supracolic compartment
supracollicular spike of cortical bone
supracondylar femoral fracture
supracondylar humerus fracture
supracoronary ridge
supracristal ventricular septal defect
supradiaphragmatic aorta
supraduodenal approach
supraepicondylar
supraepitrochlear
supraglottic larynx
supraglottic structures
suprahepatic caval cuff
suprahepatic space
suprahepatic vena cava
suprainterparietal bone
supralevator space
supraligamentous disk herniation
supramalleolar region
supramarginal gyrus
supranuclear lesion
supraoccipital bone
supraorbital fissure
supraorbital ridges
suprapatellar bursa
suprapatellar plica

suprapatellar pouch
suprapharyngeal bone
suprapubic area
suprapubic catheter
suprapubic catheterization
suprapubic tube
suprapubic urodynamic catheter
suprarenal aneurysm
suprarenal extension of aneurysm
suprarenal gland
suprarenal stenosis
suprascapular nerve entrapment
"supraselective" (see *superselective*)
suprasellar adenoma
suprasellar aneurysm
suprasellar cistern
suprasellar extension of tumor
suprasellar lesion
suprasellar mass
suprasellar region
suprasellar tumor
supraspinatus nerve
supraspinous ligaments
suprasternal bone
suprasternal bulging
suprasternal notch view on
    echocardiogram
suprasternal window
supraspinatus outlet view
suprasyndesmotic fixation
supratentorial brain tumor
supratentorial cerebral blood flow
supratentorial primitive neuro-
    ectodermal tumor (PNET)
suprathreshold
supratip nasal tip deformity
supratrochlear
supravalvular aortic stenosis (SAS,
    SVAS)
supravalvular aortogram
supravalvular mitral stenosis
supravalvular pulmonic stenosis
supraventricular crest (SVC)

supraventricular plane
supravesical fossa
supravesical obstruction
sural nerve
SureStart feature of Aspire continuous
    imaging
surface
    acromial articular
    anterolateral
    anteromedial
    apposing articular
    articular
    articulating
    arytenoidal articular
    auricular
    axial
    basal
    bone
    bosselated
    buccal
    calcaneal articular
    carpal articular
    cartilaginous joint
    cerebral
    colic
    contiguous articular
    costal
    cuboidal articular
    diaphragmatic
    distal
    endosteal
    endothelial
    fibular
    fibular articular
    gastric
    glenoid
    grooving of articular
    joint articular
    occlusal
    parallelism of articular
    posterior
    radioulnar
    roughened articular

surface *(cont.)*
  superomedial
  weightbearing
surface application of radioelement
surface coil localization
surface distance
surface matching technique
surface projection rendering
surface registration
surface tension of lungs
surface variable attenuation correction
surfer's knots
surgery
  cryoreductive
  IMR-image-guided general
  laparoscopic Roux-en-Y gastric
    bypass
  ligation reversal
  lung volume reduction
  salvage
  video-assisted thoracic (VATS)
Surgical Anatomy Visualization and
  Navigation Tools (SAVANT)
surgical cardiac tamponade
surgical emphysema
surgical intervention
surgically implanted hemodialysis
  catheter
surgical margin involvement
surgical neck fracture
surgical neck of humerus
surgical revascularization
Surgical Simplex P radiopaque bone
  cement
surgical simulation CT
surgical staples
surgical venous interruption
Surgilase 150 laser
Surgilase CO_2 laser
SurgiScope
Surgitek stent
Surgi-Vision Intercept urethral coil

Surgi-Vision prostate MRI microcoil
  imaging
survey
  anatomic
  bone
  four-view wrist
  joint
  metastatic bone
  metastatic skeletal
  osseous
survey-view images
susceptibility artifact
susceptibility, diamagnetic
susceptibility-sensitive sequence
susceptibility-weighted MR
suspended heart syndrome
suspension, barium
suspension characteristics
suspicious calcification
sustained anterior parasternal motion
sustained apical impulse
sustained left ventricular heave
sutural bone
sutural diastasis
suture
  apical
  basilar
  biparietal
  bregmatomastoid
  coronal
  cranial
  delayed closure of
  dentate
  diastasis of the
  ethmoidolacrimal
  ethmoidomaxillary
  frontal
  frontoethmoidal
  frontolacrimal
  frontomaxillary
  frontonasal
  frontoparietal

suture *(cont.)*
    frontosphenoid
    frontozygomatic
    Gillies
    Gruber
    interparietal
    jugal
    lambdoidal cranial
    mamillary
    metopic
    nonfusion of cranial
    occipital
    occipitomastoid
    occipitoparietal
    occipitosphenoid
    overlapping
    parietal
    parietomastoid
    parieto-occipital
    petrobasilar
    petrosphenobasilar
    petrospheno-occipital
    petrosquamous
    prematurely closed
    radiopaque
    rhabdoid
    sagittal
    sagittal cranial
    sphenoethmoidal
    spheno-occipital
    spheno-orbital
    sphenoparietal
    sphenopetrosal
    sphenosquamous
    sphenotemporal
    sphenovomerine
    splayed cranial
    spread (cranial sign)
    squamosomastoid
    squamosoparietal
    squamososphenoid
    squamous
    temporal

suture artifact
suture-ligated embolization microcoils
SUV (standardized uptake value)
SV (stroke volume)
SVAS (supravalvular aortic stenosis)
SVC (superior vena cava)
SVC (supraventricular crest)
SVI (stroke volume index)
SvO$_2$ (venous oxygen saturation)
SVR (systemic vascular resistance)
SVRI (systemic vascular resistance
    index)
swallow
    barium
    dry
    Gastrografin
    ice-water
    water-soluble contrast esophageal
    wet
swallowing artifact
swallowing center
swallowing dysfunction
swallowing function
swallowing mechanism, video-
    fluoroscopy of
swallow syncope
swamp-static artifact
Swan-Ganz balloon-flotation catheter
Swan-Ganz thermodilution catheter
swan-neck catheter
swan-neck deformity
swan neck shape of ventricular
    outflow
Swanson finger joint
Swanson method to view acetabula in
    profile
Swartz SL Series Fast-Cath introducer
Swediaur disease
sweep, duodenal
sweeper
Sweet method for localization of
    foreign bodies in the orbit
Sweet sternal punch

swelling, soft tissue
SWI (stroke work index)
swimmer's view
swinging flashlight test
swirling smokelike echoes
swirled appearance (on ultrasound)
swirl sign
Swiss cheese appearance
Swiss cheese ventricular septal defect
Swissray scanner
swiss roll technique
swivel dislocation (of midfoot)
swollen tissues
Swyer-James unilateral hyperlucency
   of lung
SXA (single energy x-ray) absorptiometer
SXCT (spiral x-ray computed
   tomography)
Sydenham chorea
Syed-Neblett brachytherapy method
Symmetra ^{125}I brachytherapy seeds
Symmetra ^{125}I seed brachytherapy
symmetrical uterus
sympathetic nerve block
symphalangia
symphalangism
sylvian aqueduct syndrome
sylvian candelabra
sylvian fissure
sylvian operculum
sylvian/rolandic junction
Sylvius
   aqueduct of
   cistern of
   fossa of
Syme amputation
symmetrical chest
symmetrical narrowing
symmetrical phased array
symmetric distribution
symmetric pulmonary congestion
symmetry

sympathetic chain
sympathetic denervation
sympathetic ganglia
sympathetic innervation
sympathetic nervous tissue
sympathetic vascular instability
symphysis, pubic
symphysis pubis
symptomatic metastatic spinal cord
   compression
symptomatology
symptom complex
synaptic cleft
synaptic dopamine concentration
synaptic pathways
synchronicity
synchronization device
synchronous carotid arterial pulse
synchrotron, monochromatic
synchrotron radiation
syndactylization of digits
syndactyly
syndesmosis, tibiofibular
syndrome
   acute compartment
   adrenogenital
   adult respiratory distress (ARDS)
   Aicardi
   air-block
   Alagille
   Albright-McCune-Sternberg
   amyostatic
   anomalous vein of scimitar
   anterior cerebellar artery
   anterior compartment
   antiphospholipid
   antiphospholipid antibody
   Anton
   aortic arch hypoplasia
   apple peel
   Archer
   arrhythmogenic right ventricular
      dysplasia (ARVD)

syndrome *(cont.)*
  Asherson
  atherosclerotic occlusive
  Avellis
  axonopathic neurogenic thoracic
    outlet
  Balint
  ballooning mitral valve prolapse
  Barré-Lieou
  Bartter
  basilar
  basilar artery
  beat knee
  Behr
  Bernard-Horner
  Beuren
  Bing-Horton
  Blackfan-Diamond
  blind loop
  blue rubber-bleb nevus
  Bouveret
  Bouveret-Hoffmann
  Bradbury-Eggleston
  Brett
  Brissaud
  Brock middle lobe
  bronchiectasis-bronchomalacia
  bubbly lung
  buckled innominate artery
  Budd-Chiari
  Bureau-Barriere
  Burke
  Cacchione
  Caplan
  carcinoid
  cardiac radiation
  cardiocutaneous
  cardiofacial
  Carney
  carotid blowout
  carotid sinus (CSS)
  carpal tunnel (CTS)
  Carpenter

syndrome *(cont.)*
  cauda equina (CES)
  cauda equina compression
  cavitating mesenteric lymph node
  Cayler
  Ceelen-Gellerstedt
  celiac artery compression
  celiac axis
  cerebellar
  cerebral steal
  cerebrohepatorenal
  cervical aorta
  cervical dorsal outlet
  Chédiak-Higashi
  Chiari-Budd
  chronic fatigue
  Churg-Strauss
  circulatory hyperkinetic
  Clarke-Hadfield
  Claude
  Clerc-Levy-Cristesco (CLC)
  clumsy-hand
  cobbler chest
  Cockayne
  Colinet-Caplan
  Collet-Sicard
  compartment
  compression
  congenital vascular–bone (CVBS)
  Conn
  Conradi-Hünermann
  constriction band
  Cornelia de Lange
  coronary artery steal
  coronary steal
  coronary-subclavian steal
  Corvisart
  costal margin
  costoclavicular
  Cotton-Berg
  craniomandibular
  Cronkhite-Canada
  cubital tunnel

syndrome *(cont.)*
Curracino-Silverman
Cushing
Cyriax
Dandy-Walker
Davies-Colley
de Lange
De Martini-Balestra
DeGimard
Demons-Meigs
Determann
DiGeorge
double outlet right ventricle (I–IV)
Down
Dressler postmyocardial infarction
Dubin-Johnson
dumping
Dusart
Eisenmenger
Elsner
empty sella
entrapment
Erdheim I
euthyroid sick
Evans
external carotid steal
extrinsic sick sinus
facet
facioauriculovertebral (FAV)
failed back surgery (FBSS)
Farber
fat embolism (FES)
Feldaker
Felty
fibrocystic breast
Fiessinger-Rendu
Foix-Alajouanine
Forney
Forrester
Foster-Kennedy
Fraley
Friedel Pick (Pick disease)
Gaisböck (Gaisboeck)

syndrome *(cont.)*
Garcin
Gardner-Diamond
gas-bloat
gastrocardiac
Goldenhar
Goodpasture
Gorlin
Gouley
Gowers
Graham-Burford-Mayer
Gsell-Erdheim
Guillain-Barré (GBS)
Haim-Munk
Hajdu-Cheney
Hale
Hallermann-Streiff-François
Hamman-Rich (idiopathic
  pulmonary fibrosis)
Harkavy
Hayem-Widal
Heerfordt
Hegglin
hepatopulmonary
hepatorenal (HRS)
heterotaxy
Hippel-Lindau
holiday heart
hollow chest
Holmes
Holt-Oram
Horner
Hughes-Stovin
Hunter
Hurler
Hutinel-Pick
hypogenetic lung
hypoplastic aorta
hypoplastic left heart (HLHS)
hypoplastic left ventricle
hyposensitive carotid sinus
iliocaval compression
ilioinguinal

syndrome *(cont.)*
iliotibial band friction
impingement
incomplete Kartagener
infantile
inferior vena cava
inflammatory response
inframammary
infrapatellar contracture (IPCS)
inguinal ligament
intercoronary steal
intermediate coronary
internal snapping hip
intestinal hypoperistalsis
intrinsic sick sinus
irritable bowel (IBS)
Ivemark
Janus
Jarcho-Levin
Jeune-Tommasi
Joubert
jugular foramen
Kartagener
Kast
Katayama
Kearns-Sayre
Kemp-Elliot-Gorlin
Kinsbourne
Klauder
Klein-Waardenburg
Klippel-Trénaunay-Weber
Koerber-Salus-Elschnig
Korsakoff
Laubry-Pezzi
Laurence-Moon-Biedl-Bardet
Leitner
LEOPARD
Leriche
Liddle
Löfgren
Looser-Milkman
low cardiac output
low flow

syndrome *(cont.)*
Lown-Ganong-Levine (LGL)
Lucey-Driscoll
lumbar thecoperitoneal shunt
Lutembacher
lymph node
Macleod
Maffucci
Mal de Meleda
Manson schistosomiasis-pulmonary
   artery obstruction
manubriosternal
Marable
Marfan
Marine-Lenhart
Maroteaux-Lamy
Martorell aortic arch
Martorell-Fabre
Master
Maugeri
McArdle
MEA IIa and IIb
Meadows
Meigs
Meigs-Cass
Menkes kinky-hair
midaortic
middle aortic
middle lobe
Mikulicz
Milkman (also Looser-Milkman)
Miller-Dieker
Millikan-Siekert
Minot–von Willebrand
mitral regurgitation-chordal
   elongation
Mohr
Morel
Morgagni-Adams-Stokes (MAS)
Morgagni-Stewart-Morel
Morquio
Mounier-Kuhn
Moynahan

syndrome *(cont.)*
mucocutaneous lymph node
(MCLS)
multiple hamartoma
multiple system atrophy (MSA)
myelodysplastic
nervous heart
Noonan
Nothnagel
oculosubcutaneous syndrome
of Yuge
Ogilvie (pseudo-obstruction
of colon)
organic brain (OBS)
Ortner
Osler-Libman-Sacks
osmotic demyelination
overuse
Paget-von Schroetter
Pancoast
pancreaticohepatic
Papillon-Lefevre
parchment heart
pectoralis major
Pendred
penetration
perinatal respiratory distress
Pfeiffer
Plummer-Vinson
polycystic ovary (or ovarian)
popliteal artery entrapment
posterior joint
postmastectomy lymphedema
postperfusion lung
Proteus
radiation toxicity
Raeder paratrigeminal
Raeder-Arbitz
railroad track pattern on x-ray
in Sturge-Weber
Raymond-Cestan
reactive airways dysfunction
Rendu-Osler-Weber

syndrome *(cont.)*
restrictive cardiac
restrictive hemodynamic
retained bladder
reversible organic brain
reversible posterior leukoencephalopathy
Reye
Ridley
Robin Hood steal
Roger
Romano-Ward
Romberg-Wood
Roques
Rosenbach
Rosen-Castleman-Liebow
Royer-Wilson
Russell-Silver
Sack-Barabas
Sanfilippo
scalenus anticus
scapulocostal
Schwartz-Jampel
septic lung
severe acute respiratory (SARS)
shaggy aorta
short rib-polydactyly
shoulder-hand-finger
shoulder-upper extremity-thoracic
outlet
Shprintzen velocardiofacial
shunt
sick sinus (SSS)
sinus tarsi
Sjögren
slipping rib
sloughed urethra
small aorta
small cuff
snapping hip
snapping triceps
soldier's heart
Solomon

syndrome *(cont.)*
    spastic bowel
    Spens
    sphenoidal fissure
    Sphrintzen velocardiofacial
    stagnant loop
    steal
    subacromial impingement
    subclavian steal (SSS)
    superior mesenteric artery (SMAS)
    suspended heart
    sylvian aqueduct
    systemic inflammatory response
    tarsal tunnel (TTS)
    Taussig-Snellen-Alberts
    temporomandibular joint (TMJ)
    terminal reservoir
    tethered cord (TCS)
    thoracic inlet (Pancoast)
    thoracic outlet (TOS)
    Tietze
    Tolosa-Hunt
    tram track pattern on x-ray in
        Sturge-Weber
    transient bone marrow edema
    Treacher Collins
    Turkish sabre
    twin to twin transfusion (TTTS)
    Uhl
    ulnar abutment
    uncal herniation
    unroofed coronary sinus
    upper-limb cardiovascular
    Upshaw-Schulman
    vanishing bile duct (VBDS)
    vanishing lung syndrome (on
        x-ray)
    vascular
    vena cava
    vertebral artery
    vertebral-basilar artery
    vestibular aqueduct (VAS)
    Villaret-Mackenzie

syndrome *(cont.)*
    visceral cholesterol embolization
    von Hippel-Lindau (VHL)
    von Recklinghausen
    Von Rokitansky
    VSD (ventricular septal defect) and
        absent pulmonary valve
    Wallenberg lateral medullary
    wasting
    Waterhouse-Friderichsen
    Weber-Osler-Rendu
    Weil
    Weinberg-Himelfarb
    Weingarten
    Weisenburg
    Weiss-Baker
    Werner
    Wernicke-Korsakoff
    wet lung
    white clot
    white lung
    Williams
    Williams-Beuren
    Williams-Campbell
    Wilson-Mikity
    Wiskott-Aldrich
    Wolff-Parkinson-White (WPW)
    Wolf-Hirschhorn
    xiphoid process
    Zeek
    Zellweger
    Ziegler
    Zollinger-Ellison (ZES)
Synergy ultrasound system
syngeneic transplant recipient
synkinesis (pl. synkineses)
synostosis
    cervical
    congenital radioulnar
    coronal
    lambdoid
    multiple suture
    nonsyndromic bicoronal

synostosis *(cont.)*
  nonsyndromic unicoronal
  premature suture
  radiographically firm
  sagittal
  single suture
  terminal
  tibiofibular
synovectomy, radiation
synovial cavity
synovial chondrosarcoma
synovial hemangioma
synovial membrane
synovial osteochondromatosis
synovial plica
synovial proliferation
synovial sarcoma of heart
synovial surface
synovial thickening
synoviogram
synovitis
  hand joint
  pigmented villonodular
  transient
synovium
  boggy
  exuberant
  hyperplastic
  opaque
synpneumonic empyema
synthesis
  automated
  facile
synthetase, nitrous oxide
Synthetic Aperture Focusing Technique (SAFT) in intravascular ultrasound imaging
synthetic interposition graft
syphilitic abscess
syringe, Ultraject pre-filled contrast media
syringobulbia
syringocele

syringocoele
syringoencephalia
syringoencephalomyelia
syringomeningocele
syringomyelia
syringopontia
syrinx cavity
syrinx, traumatic
system (see also *scanner*; *ultrasound*)
  ABBI (advanced breast biopsy instrumentation)
  Acolysis ultrasound intravascular thrombolysis
  Acuson 128XP ultrasound
  Add-On Bucky digital x-ray image acquisition
  Advantx LC+ cardiovascular imaging
  Agfa CR
  Agfa IMPAX PACS
  Agfa PACS
  Agfa RIS/PACS (Radiology Information System/Picture Archiving and Communications)
  AI 5200 diagnostic ultrasound
  Altaire high-field-performance open MR imaging
  ALT Ultrasound
  Angiomat 6000 contrast delivery
  AngioVista angiographic
  AquaSens FMS 1000 fluid monitoring
  Arcitumomab diagnostic imaging
  Artoscan MRI
  Aspen digital ultrasound
  Aspire continuous imaging (CI)
  Aurora dedicated breast MRI
  Aurora MR breast imaging
  automated angle encoder
  BAK-1 interbody fusion
  BAK Vista interbody fusion
  Bard percutaneous cardiopulmonary support (CPS)

system *(cont.)*
  Beamer injection stent
  biad SPECT imaging
  biliary
  Biosound AU
  Biospec MR imaging
  biphasic
  BI-RADS (breast imaging and
    reporting data system of the
    American College of Radiology)
  Bracco
  Bremer Halo Crown
  Bristol-Myers
  Bruker CSI MR
  CADstream
  caliceal
  Cartesian reference coordinate
  CathTrack catheter locator
  central nervous (CNS)
  CGR biplane angiographic
  Chemo-Port perivena catheter
  circumflex coronary
  collateral
  collecting
  Compass stereotactic frame
  Compton-suppression
  computerized phonoenterography
  computerized texture analysis of
    lung nodules and lung paren-
    chyma
  Concentric retriever (CRS)
  continuous wave high frequency
    Doppler ultrasound
  continuous wave laser
  Continuum MR-compatible
    infusion
  contoured tilting compression
    mammography
  Contour mammography
  Cordis endovascular
  COROSKOP C cardiac imaging
  CRYOguide ultrasound
  CT-MRI-compatible stereotactic
    head frame

system *(cont.)*
  Curix Capacity Plus film process-
    ing
  C-VEST ambulatory radionuclide
    monitoring
  Cyberware
  dedicated breast biopsy
  DELTAmanager MedImage
  Desilets introducer
  Diasonics
  DICOM
  Dictaphone Digital Express
    clinical reporting
  digital Add-On Bucky x-ray image
    acquisition
  digital holography
  Digital Equipment
  digital mammographic
  DIMAQ integrated ultrasound
  directly coupled sample changer
  Discovery LS imaging
  dominant left coronary artery
  dominant right coronary
  dual head gamma camera
  Dynarad portable imaging
  Eccocee compact ultrasound diag-
    nostic
  EchoEye 3-D ultrasound imaging
  Echovar Doppler
  Elscint
  Encompass cardiac network
  endocavitary applicator
  engorged collecting
  EnSite 3000 imaging system
  ExAblate 2000
  Excelart short bore MRI
  Exogen SAFHS (sonic accelerated
    fracture healing system)
  Explorer X 70 intraoral radiog-
    raphy
  external jugular
  extracranial carotid
  FlimFax teleradiology

system *(cont.)*
 FluoroNav virtual fluoroscopy
 FluoroPlus angiography
 FluoroTrak surgical navigation
 Fonar
 foreign body retrieval
 full-field digital mammography
 Galen teleradiology
 GE (General Electric)
 GE Senographe 2000D fully digital
  mammography
 Given diagnostic imaging
 greater saphenous
 Greenfield vena cava filter
 Haid Universal bone plate
 HDI (high definition imaging)
  3000 ultrasound
 hepatic ductal
 Hewlett Packard
 high field
 Hi-Star midfield MRI
 homonuclear spin
 House grading
 HyperPACS
 IBM Speech Server clinical
  reporting
 IDXrad radiology information
 IMAC
 image analysis
 Imagecast imaging management
 Imatron
 immunomedics
 Impax PACS
 Instrumentation Laboratory
 internal carotid
 intracaval endovascular ultrasonog-
  raphy (ICEUS)
 intrahepatic
 intraoperative navigation (iON)
 IRIS (Intensified Radiographic
  Imaging System)
 Isocam scintillation imaging
 Jackson staging

system *(cont.)*
 Lanier clinical reporting
 left biliary duct
 lesser saphenous
 Liebel-Flarsheim CT 9000 contrast
  delivery
 lipophilic sequestration
 Luma cervical imaging
 LymphoScan nuclear imaging
 Magnes biomagnetometer
 Magnetom Open
 Magnetom Vision MR
 Magnex Alpha MR
 Mammex TR computer-aided
  mammography diagnosis
 Mammomat Novation full-field
  digital mammography
 MammoReader imaging
 Marex MRI
 MEDDARS cardiac catheterization
  analysis
 Medspec MR imaging
 Medweb clinical reporting
 MicroLYSUS ultrasound-enhanced
  drug delivery
 multidetector
 Multi-Link Vision RX and OTW
  (over the wire) coronary stent
 Neuroform microdelivery stent
 nonduplex collecting
 Novacore left ventricular assist
  (LVAS)
 Octreoscan
 OEC Series 9600 cardiac
 1.5T Signa Advantage
 open architecture
 open-configuration MR
 OpenPACS
 Optical Tracking System
 OSCAR ultrasonic bone cement
  removal
 OsteoView x-ray
 Ovation Falloposcopy

system *(cont.)*
  Paris
  PenRad mammography clinical
    reporting
  Pentax-Hitachi FG32UA endosono-
    graphic
  PF-PACS
  Philips
  PhorMax CR (computed radiog-
    raphy)
  Photopic Imaging ultrasound
  Picker
  Pinnacle 3 radiation therapy
    planning
  PMT robotic fulcrumless
    tomographic
  polar coordinate
  PortalVision radiation oncology
  PowerVision Ultrasound
  Probe balloon-on-a-wire dilatation
  Profile Mammography
  ProstaScint
  pulmonary venous
  PulseSpray pulsed infusion
  Q-cath catheterization recording
  quadrature surface coil MRI
  radiation therapy planning (RTP)
  radionuclide carrier
  RadNet radiology information
  Rapid Exchange vein graft stent
    delivery
  Rapid-Trak stent delivery
  RDX coronary radiation catheter
    delivery
  Redi-Vu teleradiology
  reference coordinate
  renal collecting
  reticuloendothelial
  Retzius
  Reveal XVI PET/CT imaging
  ring-type imaging
  Rogan teleradiology
  RTP (radiation therapy planning)

system *(cont.)*
  saphenous
  Scanmaster DX
  scanned-slot detector
  scanning beam digital
  scattering
  Schmidt optics
  Scintiview nuclear computer
  Scintron IV (four) nuclear
    computer
  screen-film
  ScnoScan full-field digital mam-
    mography
  Sens-A-Ray digital dental imaging
  sequestration
  Sequoia ultrasound
  Shape Maker
  Shimadzu
  SICOR (computer-assisted cardiac
    catheter recording)
  Siemens AG
  Signa GEMS MR imaging
  Signal
  Silicon Graphics Reality Engine
  SimpliCT guidance
  SmartSpot high resolution digital
    imaging
  SoftScan laser mammography
  Somatom Volume Zoom computed
    tomography
  Sonablate 200 high intensity
    focused ultrasound
  SonoHeart handheld digital echo-
    cardiography
  Sonoline Elegra ultrasound
  Sonoline Sierra ultrasound
    imaging
  Sonoprobe SP-501 system for endo-
    scopic procedures
  SonoSite 180 hand-carried ultra-
    sound
  SP-501 Sonoprobe endoscopy
  SPECT/MRI imaging system

system *(cont.)*
  Squibb
  STARRT Falloposcopy
  steerable guidewire
  storage-phosphor
  Sudbury
  Summit LoDose collimator
  Sun SPARCstation
  SureStart imaging
  Synergy ultrasound
  Tesio twin catheter
  tesla imaging system
  thermal dosimetry
  TMS 3-dimensional radiation
    therapy planning
  transluminal lysing
  Triad SPECT imaging
  TRON 3 VACI cardiac imaging
  UltraPACS diagnostic imaging
  Ultraseed ultrasound-guided
    brachytherapy
  UltraSTAR computer-based ultra-
    sound reporting
  uPACS picture archiving system
  upper collecting
  USCI Probe balloon-on-a-wire
    dilatation
  Varian brachytherapy
  VARIS radiation oncology
  VasoView balloon dissection
  VAX 4100
  ventricular
  VentTrak monitoring system
  vertebral artery
  Vingmed Sound CFM ultrasound
  Virtuoso portable three-dimensional
    imaging
  Vitrea 3-D
  VIVENDI virtual endoscopy
  VoiceRAD clinical reporting
  Voluson ultrasound
  VoxelView
  Xillix LIFE-GI fluorescence
    endoscopy

system *(cont.)*
  XKnife stereotactic radiosurgery
  Xplorer filmless high resolution
    digital radiography imaging
  x-ray shadow projection
    microtomographic
  systematic ultrasound-guided biopsies
  systemic anticoagulation with heparin
  systemic arterial circulation
  systemic arterial oxygen desaturation
  systemic arterial vasoconstriction
  systemic AV O_2 difference
  systemic blood
  systemic carnitine deficiency
  systemic circulation
  systemic diastolic blood pressure
    (SDBP)
  systemic disorder affecting heart
    function
  systemic heparinization
  systemic hypoperfusion
  systemic inflammatory response
    syndrome
  systemic lupus erythematosus (SLE)
  systemic mean arterial pressure
    (SMAP)
  systemic mercury intoxication
  systemic oxygen saturation measured
    after balloon-occluding each
    collateral
  systemic perfusion, diminished
  systemic pressure
  systemic-pulmonary artery shunt
  systemic vascular resistance (SVR)
  systemic vascular resistance index
    (SVRI)
  systemic venous hypertension
  systemic venous return
  systolic acceleration time
  systolic and diagnostic gating
  systolic anterior motion (SAM) on
    2D echocardiogram
  systolic blood pressure (SBP)

systolic-diastolic blood pressure
systolic ejection period (SEP)
systolic fractional shortening
systolic gradient
systolic heart failure
systolic hypertension
systolic impulse
systolic mammary souffle
systolic pressure

systolic pressure determination (SLP)
systolic pressure-time index
systolic prolapse of mitral valve leaflet
systolic reserve
systolic retraction of apex
systolic S waves
systolic time interval (STI)
systolic upstroke time
systolic velocity-time integral

T, t

T (temporal)
T (tesla)
T (thoracic)
Ta (tantalum) (an element)
table
  continuously rolling platform
  dual lookup
  floating
  Hydradjust IV
  pivoting
  tilt
table feed
table movement
TAE (transcatheter arterial
  embolization)
Tagarno 3SD cine projector for
  angiography
tagged red blood cell nuclear scan
tagging, barium-based fecal
tagging, fecal
tag image file format (TIFF)
tag of cartilage
tag plane
tagged antibody, fluorescently
tagged atom
tagged, radioactively
tagging cine magnetic resonance

tailgut cyst
tail-like segment
tail of breast in mammography
tail of pancreas
tail of Spence in mammography
takeoff of vessel
takeup of radioactive material
Talairach space
talar avascular necrosis
talar declination angle
talar dome
talar impingement
talar neck view
talar osteochondral fracture
talar tilt angle
talcosis
talc plaque
talipes arcuatus
talocalcaneal angle
talocalcaneal articulation
talocalcaneal coalition
talocalcaneal index
talocalcaneal joint
talocalcaneal ligament
talocrural angle
talocrural fusion
talocrural joint

talofibular joint
talofibular ligament
talometatarsal angle
Talon balloon dilation catheter
talonavicular angle
talonavicular beaking
talonavicular capsule
talonavicular joint
talonavicular ligament
talus (ankle)
   congenital vertical
   flat top
   neck of
   sulcus
   vertical
tamponade
   balloon
   cardiac
   chronic
   esophagogastric
   ferromagnetic
   florid cardiac
   full-blown cardiac
   heart
   low pressure cardiac
   pericardial chyle with
   subacute cardiac
   surgical cardiac
tandem and ovoids
tandem, external beam with
tandem lesion
tandem mass spectrometry
tangential
tangentially
tangential breast fields
tangential constriction
tangential cut
tangential layer of hand
tangential ports
tangential scapular view
tangential view
tantalum bronchogram

tantalum (^{183}Ta) (an element) (see
   imaging agent)
tantalum marker
tantalum stent
tape, LeMaitre Glow 'N Tell
tapering occlusion
tapering off
tapering stenosis
tapers, fiberoptic
TAPVR (total anomalous pulmonary
   venous return)
target (targeting)
   angiographic
   gas
   internal cyclotron
   metal technetium
   ScoutView
   three-dimensional reconstructed
   tungsten
target appearance
target calcification
target lesion
targetlike appearance
target MIPcor
target organ
target sign
target sign on CT scan
target tissues
target to background ratio
target volume
Targis catheter
Tarrant axial view of the clavicle
tarsal-metatarsal (or tarsometatarsal)
   joint space
tarsal arch
tarsal bone
tarsal canal
tarsal coalition
tarsal navicular
tarsal sinus
tarsal tunnel syndrome
tarsometatarsal (or tarsal-metatarsal)
   joint space

tarsus shortening
Tar symptoms
T artifact
task-activated brain regions
task rest pattern
tattoo sign
tau sign
Taussig-Bing congenital malformation
of heart
Taussig-Snellen-Alberts syndrome
taut pericardial effusion
TAV (transcutaneous aortovelography)
Taveras, standards of
Tawara atrioventricular node
Taylor inferosuperior projection of
pubic and ischia rami
Taylor SMV projection to demonstrate
mastoid processes
TB (tuberculosis)
TBED (trabecular bone equivalent
density)
TBNA (transbronchial needle
aspiration)
TBT (transcervical balloon tuboplasty)
Tc (technetium) (an element)
99mTc, Tc 99m (see *imaging agent,
technetium*)
Tc 99m tetrofosmin (technetium
Tc 99m tetrofosmin)
TCA (transcondylar axis)
TCBF (total cerebral blood flow)
TCD (transcranial Doppler)
ultrasonography
TCCS (transcranial color-coded sonog-
raphy)
Tc HIDA ("tek-high-dah")
Tc HIDA (technetium hepatoiminodi-
acetic acid) scan
T condylar fracture
TCP/IP (transmission control protcol/
Internet protocol)
TCS (tethered cord syndrome)

TCT900S helical CT scanner
TDMS (Trex digital mammography
system)
TDoG (tissue Doppler gated)
T/D (thickness to diameter of
ventricle) ratio
TE (echo delay time)
TE (echo time)
TE (tracheoesophageal) fistula
tear (rupture)
attritional
bowstring
bucket-handle (of knee meniscus)
cleavage
dural
entry
fishtail
flap
full thickness
ligament
linear
Mallory-Weiss
micro
parrot-beak
partial-thickness
radial
rotator cuff
serosal
tendon (types I-IV)
tearaway sheath
teardrop figure
teardrop sign
teardrop-shaped density
teardrop-shaped flexion-compression
fracture
teboroxime cardiac scan for
myocardial infarction
teboroxime resting washout (TRW)
TEC (transluminal endarterectomy
catheter)
TEC (transluminal extraction catheter)
TECA (technetium albumin) study

Technegas
Technescan Gluceptate (technetium
  Tc 99m gluceptate)
TechneScan MAA (technetium ^{99m}Tc
  macroaggregated albumin) imaging
  agent
TechneScan MAG3 (^{99m}Tc mertiatide)
  renal diagnostic imaging
TechneScan PYP (technetium ^{99m}Tc
  pyrophosphate) imaging agent
technetated aggregated human albumin
  (technetium Tc 99m albumin aggregated)
technetium (Tc 99m or ^{99m}Tc) (see
  imaging agent)
technetium bound to DTPA
technetium bound to serum albumin
technetium bound to sulfur colloid
technetium-labeled sulfur colloid
  imaging
technetium 99m-labeled fibrinogen
technetium 99m venogram
technetium pyrophosphate scanning
Technicare camera
technique (see also *approach*; *method*)
  acquisition
  algebraic reconstruction (ART)
    bolus chase imaging
  Amplatz
  background subtraction
  bayesian
  blended
  bolus chase
  brain surface matching
  bread-loaf
  Brown-Roberts-Wells
  bull's-eye
  chase bolus imaging
  clearance
  contralateral subtraction
  coronal oblique
  counterstaining
  cross-correlation

technique *(cont.)*
  cuboid squeeze
  cuboid whip
  cut-film
  deblurring
  deconvolution
  double contrast
  double umbrella
  Dunn and Rippstein
  echo-tagging
  Egan
  endoscopic ultrasound-assisted
    band ligation
  EPISTAR perfusion
  equilibrium radionuclide
    angiocardiography
  esophageal balloon
  exclusion-HPLC
  Exorcist respiratory compensation
  fast-FLAIR
  fast spin echo acquisition
  FAT SAT (fat saturation)
  field-fitting
  first pass
  flow mapping
  fluoroscopic road-mapping
  full bladder
  gated
  gradient echo cine
  Gruentzig (Grüntzig) PTCA
  half-wedged field
  HARC-C wavelet compression
  in vivo
  inhalation
  integrated parallel acquisition
    (IPAT)
  intercomparison measurement
  intravascular MRI
  IR-guided pigtail catheter place-
    ment
  inverse radiotherapy
  inversion recovery
  isolation perfusion

technique *(cont.)*
  Judkins
  kissing atherectomy
  kissing balloon
  Leksell
  loading
  low-angle shot (flash)
  low dose film mammographic
  Markov chain
  MIDCAB (minimally invasive
    direct coronary artery bypass)
  ML/EM reconstruction
  Monte Carlo
  MRCP using HASTE with a
    phased array coil
  MR hydrography
  MR peritoneography
  multimodal image fusion
  multiphasic multislice MRI
  multiplanar
  multislice multiphase spin echo
    imaging
  multislice spin echo
  navigator echo motion correction
  NEUGAT (neutron/gamma
    transmission)
  neutron/gamma transmission
    (NEUGAT)
  no-gap
  noncoplanar arc
  noninvasive
  packing, extraction, and calculation
  partial saturation
  PASTA (polarity-altered spectral-
    selective acquisition)
  PCICO (pressure-controlled
    intermittent coronary occlusion)
  percutaneous transfemoral
  pharmokinetic
  pressure half-time
  pulse inversion harmonic imaging
    ultrasound
  radiotracer

technique *(cont.)*
  RAO breathing
  RAO expiration
  reduced radiation dose
  region of interest imaging
  Riechert-Mundinger
  Risser
  road-mapping
  robus registration
  scanning-beam digital x-ray
    (SBDX)
  scintillation counting
  Seldinger percutaneous
  sequential extraction-radiotracer
  serial cut film
  silhouette
  single field hyperthermia combined
    with radiation therapy and ultra-
    sound
  single fill/void
  sliding thin-slab, minimum
    intensity projection
  small bowel enteroscopy (SBE)
  Sones cineangiography
  spectroscopic fat saturation
  spin echo
  spin label
  stacked-foil
  stereotactic or stereotaxic
  stimulated echo-tagging
  stress Myoview noninvasive nuclear
    imaging
  subclavian turndown
  subtraction
  tandem mass spectrometry
  tetrahedral interpolation
  three-dimensional (3D, 3-D)
  THRIVE (T1 high resolution
    isotropic volume examination)
  timed imaging
  tissue characterization
  Todd-Wells
  transcatheter

technique *(cont.)*
  transgluteal CT-guided
  trephine
  triple dose gadolinium-enhanced
    MR imaging without MT
    (magnetization transfer)
  two-dimensional (2D, 2-D)
  ultrasound-guided compression
  upgated
  ureteral compression
  ureterorenoscopy
  ureteroscopy
  variance reduction
  Viehweger
  volumetric interpolated breathing-
    hold
  volumetric mapping
  whiplash
  xenon Xe 133-clearance
technology
  e-Touch
  slip-ring
Technos ultrasound
Tecmag Libra-S16 system
Tecoflex stent
tectal lesion
tectoral ligament
tectospinal tract
TED (thromboembolic disease)
Tedlar bags
TEE (transesophageal echocardiography) imaging with DTI
teeth
  Hutchinson
  incisor
  milk
  molar
  premolar
  primary
  secondary
  wisdom
TEF (tracheoesophageal fistula)
Tefcat intrauterine catheter

Teflon-coated guidewire
Teflon ERCP catheter
Teflon intracardiac patch
tegmental tract
tegmentum
  medullary
  midbrain
  pontine
tegmentum of pons
Teichholz ejection fraction in
  echocardiogram
Teichholz equation for left ventricular
  volume
"tek-high-dah" (Tc HIDA) scan
telangiectatic focal nodular hyperplasia
telangiectatic osteosarcoma
telangiectatic vessel
telecobalt
telecom integration
Telectronics defibrillator patch
Telepaque imaging agent
teleradiology videoconferencing
teletherapy, C-60
Telos radiographic stress device
temperature, firing
temperature sensors
template irradiation
Templeton and Zim carpal tunnel view
temporal aliasing
temporal artery
temporal bone fracture
temporal horn
temporal instability
temporal instability artifact
temporal lobe epilepsy
temporal lobe lesion
temporal lobe tumor
temporally
temporal-occipital junction
temporal phase delay
temporal subtraction
temporo-occipital region
temporomandibular joint (TMJ)

temporoparietal region
temporo-parieto-occipitopontine tract
temporopontine tract
temporozygomatic region
Tenacath HSG (hysterosalpingography)
  catheter
Tenckhoff peritoneal dialysis catheter
Tenckhoff silicone catheter
tenderness over kidney
tender uterus
tendinitis, calcific shoulder
tendinosis, patellar
tendo (pl. tendines)
tendo Achillis (Achilles tendon)
tendo calcaneus (Achilles tendon)
tendon
  Achilles
  calcaneal
  central (of diaphragm)
  central perineal
  collagen fibrils within
  common
  conjoined
  conjoint
  coronary
  cricoesophageal
  hamstring
  heel (tendo calcaneus)
  membranaceous
  patellar
  peroneal
  rider's
  slipped
  Todaro
  Zinn (common tendinous ring)
tendon loop procedure
tendon rerouting procedure
tendon rupture
tendon-sheath space infection
tendon, short peroneal muscle
tendon sling
tendon split and rerouting procedure
tendon tear (types I-IV)

tennis elbow
tennis leg (plantaris rupture)
Tennis Racquet angiography catheter
tennis shoulder
tennis toe
tension hydrocephalus
tension, left atrial
tension pneumothorax
tension time index (TTI)
tentative diagnosis
tented up
tenth cranial nerve (vagus nerve)
tenting of hemidiaphragm
tenting of pericardium
tenting of diaphragm
tentorial edge
tentorial herniation
tentorial meningioma
tentorial notch herniation
TER (therapeutic external radiation)
teratocarcinoma testicular tumor
teratoma
  cystic
  malignant
  malignant ovarian
  ovarian
  pineal
  sacrococcygeal
  solid
  suprasellar atypical
  testis
teratoma testicular tumor
terminal
  character cell
  dumb
  X-
terminal air sac
terminal air space
terminal bronchiole
terminal crest
terminal ileum
terminal inversion
terminal pneumonia

terminal reservoir syndrome
terminal thrombosis
termination
  early phase
  late phase
territorial infarction
Terry-Thomas sign
tertiary collimation
tertiary contractions
Tesio hemodialysis access catheter
Tesio twin catheter system
tesla (T)
tesla field
tesla imaging system
test (see also *imaging*)
  abduction stress
  acetazolamide (Diamox) challenge
  adjunctive
  antinuclear antibody (ANA)
  axial manual traction
  Balke protocol for cardiac exercise
    stress
  Barlow hip instability
  Bayes theorem in exercise stress
  bolus challenge
  bronchial provocation
  capillary resistance
  contraction stress (CST)
  costoclavicular
  Cytomel suppression
  Dehio
  dexamethasone suppression
  dipyridamole echocardiography
  dipyridamole handgrip
  dipyridamole infusion
  dipyridamole thallium stress
  dipyridamole tomographic thallium
    stress
  Doppler ultrasound segmental
    blood pressure
  drop test for pneumoperitoneum
  duplex screening
  ectopic

test *(cont.)*
  Ellestad protocol for treadmill
    stress
  ergonovine
  exercise thallium-201 stress
  exercise tolerance (ETT)
  flat-hand
  fluorescein dye disappearance
    (DDT)
  HDM bronchial provocation
  Heartscan heart attack prediction
  ^{125}I iothalamate GFR (glomerular
    filtration rate)
  injection test for pneumoperito-
    neum
  isometric exercise stress
  ^{131}I uptake (thyroid function)
  Korotkoff test for collateral circula-
    tion
  Kveim
  Mann-Whitney
  Master two-step exercise stress
  Mester test for rheumatic disease
  nonstress (NST)
  nuclear gated blood pool
  O'Connor finger dexterity
  Osteo-Gram bone density
  perchlorate washout
  peritoneal-venous shunt patency
  Persantine thallium stress
  Phalen stress
  positive tilt
  quantitative computed tomography
    (QCT) test for bone loss
  radioactive iodine uptake (RAIU)
  radioallergosorbent (RAST)
  radioimmunoassay (RIA)
  radioisotope renal excretion
  radionuclide esophageal transit
    (RETT)
  Reflotron bedside theophylline
  Rubin
  Salkowski

test *(cont.)*
    Sandrock test for thrombosis
    Schwartz test for patency of deep
        saphenous veins
    selenium-labeled homocholic acid
        conjugated with taurine
        (SeHCAT)
    sestamibi ^{99m}Tc SPECT with
        dipyridamole stress
    sestamibi ^{99m}Tc stress
    sestamibi stress
    Sharp-Purser
    shoulder compression
    shoulder depression
    shoulder rock
    SLUScan for Your Heart
    star-cancellation (SCT)
    swinging flashlight
    3-D CE (three-dimensional
        contrast-enhanced) magnetic
        resonance angiography (MRA)
    T3 resin uptake
    thyroid suppression
    thyrotropin releasing hormone
        (TRH) stimulation
    treadmill exercise (TET)
    treadmill exercise stress
    treadmill stress (TMST)
    Whitaker
    Wilcoxon signed-rank
    Yergason of shoulder subluxation
testicle
testicular abscess
testicular adenomatoid tumor
testicular adrenal rest tissue
testicular artery
testicular deformity
testicular duct
testicular hematoma
testicular infarction
testicular microlithiasis
testicular torsion

testicular tumor (see also *tumor*)
    choriocarcinoma
    embryonal cell
    functional interstitial cell
    nonseminomatous-type
    seminoma
    teratocarcinoma
    teratoma
testis (pl. testes)
    appendix
    descended
    ectopic
    efferent ductules of
    infarcted
    rete
    torsion of
    undescended
testis ectopia
test meal
test-retest precision
"tet" (tetralogy) of Fallot
tethered bowel sign
tethered cord
tethered spinal cord
tetrad, Fallot
tetrahedral interpolation technique
tetralogy of Fallot (TOF)
tetrapolar esophageal catheter
tetrofosmin (technetium Tc 99m tetro-
    fosmin)
texture, echo
texture mapping
texture slice
TFA (thigh-foot angle)
TFA (tibiofemoral angle)
TFC (triangular fibrocartilage)
TFCC (triangular fibrocartilaginous
    complex)
T fracture
TGA (transposition of great arteries)
thalamic fracture of the calcaneus
thalamic infarct
thalamic lesion

thalamocaudate artery
thalamoperforate artery
thalamostriate vein
thalamotegmental involvement
thalamus
thallium (Tl) (an element)
thallium 201 (^{201}Tl) (see *imaging agent*)
combined Myoscint/thallium imaging
combined thallium-Tc-HOMPAO imaging
dipyridamole thallium-201 scintigraphy
dipyridamole thallium ventriculography
dipyridamole tomographic thallium stress test
dipyridamole thallium stress test
dobutamine thallium angiography
doughnut configuration on thallium imaging
exercise thallium-201 stress test
exercise thallium-201 tomography
four-hour delayed thallium imaging
homogeneous thallium distribution
horseshoe configuration on thallium imaging
lung/heart ratio of thallium 201 activity
MI adenosine thallium imaging
myocardial uptake of thallium
Persantine thallium scanning
Persantine thallium stress test
planar exercise thallium-201 scintigraphy
planar thallium scan
planar thallium with quantitative analysis
planar thallium imaging
quantitative exercise thallium-201 variables
radioactive thallium

thallium *(cont.)*
redistributed thallium imaging
redistributed thallium scan
redistribution thallium-201
regional myocardial uptake of thallium
reinjection thallium stress exam
resting-redistribution thallium-201 scintigraphy
rest thallium-201 myocardial imaging
septal hypoperfusion on thallium scan
SPECT thallium imaging
SPECT thallium scintigram
stress thallium-201 myocardial imaging
thallium debris
thallium SPECT score
thallium-201 single photon emission
thallium to scalp ratio
whole body thallium imaging
thallium SPECT score
thallium to scalp ratio
thatched-roof worker's lung
THC (translepatic cholangiography)
THE (transhepatic embolization)
thebesian circulation
thebesian foramen
thebesian valve
thebesian vein
theca (pl. thecae)
theca externa
theca interna
theca lutein ovarian cyst
thecal sac
thecoma
thecoperitoneal shunt
thenar eminence
thenar muscle
thenar space abscess
theophylline attenuation

theory
  Beer-Bouguer
  density matrix
  fuzzy set
  hot spot
  Kubelka-Munk
  quantum
therapeutic application of radioactive
  source
therapeutic embolization
therapeutic external radiation (TER)
therapeutic pneumothorax
therapeutic radiation
therapeutic radiology
therapy (see also *radiation therapy*
  adjuvant hypofractionated confor-
    mal radiation
  adjunctive
  adjuvant radiation
  antineoplastic
  antitubercular
  arc
  boron neutron capture (BNCT)
  brachytherapy
  Bragg-peak photon-beam
  brisement
  chemo-
  chemoradiation
  combined-modality radiation
  concurrent radiation therapy and
    chemotherapy
  conformal radiation (CRT)
  conventionally fractionated
    stereotactic radiation
  craniospinal axis radiation
  electron arc
  electron beam
  endoscopic sclerosing
  endovascular
  ethanol
  external beam
  eye-view 3D-CRT radiation
  fast neutron

therapy *(cont.)*
  fibrinolytic
  fluoroscopy-guided subarachnoid
    phenol block (SAPB)
  four-fiber
  fractionated radiation
  fragmentation
  gadolinium neutron capture
  grid
  hyperfractionated radiation
  hypertonic glucose
  hypofractionated
  immunosuppressive
  indicator dilution
  indomethacin
  intensity-modulated radiation
  interstitial radioactive colloid
  intra-articular radiopharmaceutical
  intracavitary radioactive colloid
  intracoronary thrombolytic
  intraoperative radiation (IORT)
  intravascular radiopharmaceutical
  iodine ^{192}I high dose rate single
    catheter
  IORT (intraoperative radiation)
  laser
  laser-induced thermotherapy
  megavoltage grid
  megavoltage radiation
  megavoltage x-ray
  neoadjuvant hormonal
  neutron
  neutron capture
  neutron/gamma transmission
  nonballoon
  orthovoltage radiation
  palliative
  partial-brain radiation
  percutaneous microwave coagula-
    tion
  three-dimensional conformal
    radiation
  radiation

therapy *(cont.)*
  radiotherapy
  radiofrequency ablation
  radiopharmaceutical
  rotation
  salvage
  split hyperfractionated accelerated
    radiation
  split-course hyperfractionated
  stereotactic radiation
  supportive
  three-dimensional conformal
    radiation (3D-CRT)
  thrombolytic
  tiered
  total androgen suppression
  transcatheter
  ultraearly thrombolytic
  ultrasound-guided percutaneous
    microwave coagulation
  vascular gene
  updraft
  whole-brain radiation
therapy tomographs
therapy zones
TheraSeed (palladium Pd 103) active
  isotope in titanium capsule
thermal ablation
thermal convection patterns
thermal diffusion
thermal dosimetry system
thermal equilibrium
thermal memory stent
thermal neutron
thermal treatment parameters
therminoluminescent dosimetry
thermistor catheter
thermistor plethysmography
thermoacoustic CT with radio waves
thermoacoustics
thermochemotherapy
thermodilution balloon catheter
thermodilution cardiac output

thermodilution catheter
thermodilution ejection fraction
thermodilution method of cardiac
  output measurement
thermodilution Swan-Ganz catheter
thermogram, liquid crystal
thermography
  blood vessel
  laser-induced (LITT)
  liquid crystal contact (LCT)
thermoluminescence
thermoluminescent dosimeter
thermoradiotherapy, interstitial
thermotherapy
  laser-induced (LITT)
  MR imaging-guided laser-induced
    interstitial
thickening
  aortic valve
  beaded
  coarse
  diffuse
  fascial
  focal intimal
  interlobular septal
  intralobular interstitial
  irregular gallbladder wall
  intimal
  ligamentous
  mediastinal
  mottled
  myocardial
  partial
  peribronchial
  pleural
  submucosal
  synovial
  urothelial
  valve
  wall
thickened leaflet
thickening of the mesentery
thickening of the omentum

thickened pelvic brim
thickened pericardium
thickness
  full
  interleaf
  junctional zone
  myometrial zone
  nominal section
  section
thick slice image
thick-walled
Thiemann disease
thigh-foot angle
thin border
thin collimation images
thin collimation multidetector row
  spiral CT
thin cylindrical uniform field volumes
thin film analysis
thin fibrous cap
thin needle percutaneous cholangiography
thin plate spline
thin section (or slice) CT
thin section excretory phase CT
thin section multidetector row CT
  colonography
thin slab maximum intensity projection
thin slice (or section) CT
thin slice image
thin-walled
third cranial nerve (oculomotor nerve)
third intercondylar tubercle of Parsons
third intercostal space
third left interspace
third order chordae
third portion of duodenum
third space sequestration
third stage hemorrhage
third ventricle tumors
30° position
30° right anterior oblique projection

Thomas vascular access shunt
Thoms method (pelvimetry)
thoracentesis, ultrasonic guidance for
thoraces (see *thorax*)
thoracic aortic aneurysm
thoracic aortography
thoracic asymmetry
thoracic cage configuration
thoracic catheter
thoracic cavity
thoracic component of scoliosis
thoracic computed tomography
thoracic deformity
thoracic duct
thoracic empyema
thoracic esophagus
thoracic fistula
thoracic gas volumes
thoracic inlet
thoracic inlet (Pancoast) syndrome
thoracic kyphosis, loss of
thoracic outlet syndrome (TOS)
thoracic scoliosis
thoracic spine (T spine)
thoracic stomach
thoracic vertebrae (T1-T12)
thoracic wall
thoracoabdominal aorta
thoracoabdominal aortic aneurysm
thoracoabdominal wall
thoracoepigastric vein
thoracofemoral conversion
thoracolumbar scoliosis
thoracolumbar spine
Thoracoport
thoracoscopy, percutaneous
thoracostomy, small bore catheter
Thora-Port port
thorax (pl. thoraces, thoraxes)
  asymmetrical
  bony
  cylindrical
  squared off
  symmetrical

thorax view
Thorel bundle of muscle fibers in
heart
Thorel pathway
thorium (Th) (an element)
threatened vessel closure post-PTCA
30 sec./frame time
three-axis gradient coil
three-compartment wrist angiography
three-dimensional (3D or 3 D)
  3D anthropometry
  3D CE (3-D contrast-enhanced)
    magnetic resonance angiography
    (MRA)
  3DCE MRA technique
  3D CEMRA (3-D contrast-
    enhanced MR angiography)
  3D CISS MR imaging
  3D conformal radiation therapy
  3D connect operation
  3D CRT (conformal radiation
    therapy)
  3D CT densitometry
  3D data set
  3D dose profile
  3D echocardiography
  3D freehand ultrasound
  3DFT (3D Fourier transform)
  3DFT-CISS sequence
  3DFT GRASS MR imaging
  3DFT magnetic resonance
    angiography
  3DFT SPGR MR imaging
  3D gadolinium-enhanced sub-
    tracted MR angiography
  3D gadolinium-enhanced magnetic
    resonance angiography for
    aortoiliac inflow
  3D GRE (gradient-recalled-echo)
    MRI
  3D H-1 magnetic resonance
    spectroscopic imaging

three-dimensional *(cont.)*
  3D helical computerized tomo-
    graphic angiography (3D helical
    CTA)
  3D holography
  3D image reconstruction
  3D inflow MR angiography
  3-D IVUS (three-dimensional
    intravascular ultrasound)
  3D MRI data sets
  3D magnetic resonance microscopy
  3D magnetic source imaging (MSI)
  3D modeling
  3D MSI (magnetic source imaging)
  3D penetration
  3D phase-contrast magnetic
    resonance angiography
  3D portocholangiography
  3D processed ultrafast computer-
    ized imaging
  3D-PSIF sequence
  3D reformatted images
  3D spoiled gradient-recalled
    sequences
  3D stereotaxic surface projections
  3D surface anthropometry
  3D surface digitizer
  3D technique
  3D time of flight magnetic reso-
    nance (3D TOF MR) angio-
    graphic sequences
  3D time-resolved motion
  3D T1-gradient echo sequence,
    sagittal
  3D transesophageal echocardi-
    ography
  3D Turbo-FLAIR (fluid-attenuated
    inversion recovery)
  3D turbo SE imaging
  3D ultrasound
three-head camera
three-head scan

3M scanner
three-part fracture
three-phase bone scintigraphy (TPBS)
three-phase helical CT
3-Scape real-time 3-D imaging
3 tesla scanner
three time-point contrast-enhanced
  MR imaging
3:2 block ("three to two")
three-vessel coronary disease
three-vessel runoff
three-way catheter
three-way stopcock
thresher's lung
threshold, malignancy
thresholding method
THRIVE (T1 high resolution isotropic
  volume examination) technique
thrombi (pl. of thrombus)
thrombin, percutaneous
thromboatherosclerotic process
thromboembolus
thromboembolism
thromboembolization
  catheter-induced
  deep venous
  pulmonary
  venous
thrombolysis
  mechanical
  pharmacomechanical
  pulse-spray
thrombolytic therapy
thrombo-obliterative process
thromboresistance
thrombosed
thrombosed dialysis fistula
thrombosis
  acute basilar artery
  catheter-related upper extremity
    deep venous
  intentional reversible
  left atrial

thrombosis *(cont.)*
  nonpyogenic
  syndrome of impending
  therapeutic
thrombostasis
thrombosuction catheter
thrombotic infarct
thrombus
  calcified
  intramural
  mural
thrombus formation
through-and-through fracture
Thruflex PTCA balloon catheter
thumb, gamekeeper's
thumbprints (or thumbprinting) on
  surface of colon in barium enema
Thurston Holland sign
thymic cyst
thymic lesion
thymidine kinase
thymoma of heart
thymus gland
thyrocardiac disease
thyrocervical collateral veins
thyrocervical trunk of subclavian
  artery
thyroglossal duct cyst
thyroid
  lingual
  multinodular
  substernal
thyroid artery
thyroid cartilage
thyroid dysgenesis
thyroid follicle
thyroid gland
  accessory
  enlarged
thyroid imaging
thyroid isthmus
thyroid lobe
thyroid nodule

thyroid radioiodine uptake
thyroid scan
thyroid stunning
thyroid suppression test
thyroid uptake of radioactive iodine
thyroiditis
thyroxine radioisotope assay (T$_4$RIA)
TI (inversion time)
TIA (transient ischemic attack)
TIB (tree-in-bud) pattern
"tib-fib" (tibia-fibula)
tibial artery disease
tibial crest
tibial flare
tibial obliterative thrombi
tibial outflow tracts, blind
tibial plafond fracture
tibial plateau fracture
tibial sesamoid ligament
tibial sesamoid position
tibial tendon
tibial torsion
tibial tuberosity
tibial-peroneal trunk
tibioastragalocalcaneal canal of Richet
tibiocalcaneal fusion
tibiocalcaneal joint complex
tibiocalcaneal ligament
tibiocalcaneal space
tibiofibular diastasis
tibiofibular fracture
tibiofibular syndesmosis
tibionavicular ligament
tibioperoneal occlusive disease
tibiotalar angle
tibiotalocalcaneal fusion
tibiotarsal dislocation
TICA (traumatic intracranial
    aneurysm)
tidal wave of carotid arterial pulse
Tietze syndrome
TIFF (tag image file format)
tight lesion

Tile classification of pelvic ring
    fracture
Tile-Pennal classification system
Tile views of pelvic inlet and outlet
Tillaux-Kleiger fracture
tilt
    head-up
    palmar
tilted optimized nonsaturating
    excitation (TONE)
time
    abnormal intestinal transit
    acceleration
    acquisition
    asymmetric appearance
    atrial activation
    atrioventricular
    data acquisition
    decay
    deceleration
    diastolic perfusion
    dwell
    echo (TE)
    echo delay
    ejection (ET)
    emptying
    esophageal transit
    gastric transit
    image acquisition
    interpulse
    inversion (TI)
    isovolumic contraction
    isovolumic relaxation (IVRT)
    left ventricular ejection (LVET)
    maximum inflation
    maximum walking (MWT)
    mean
    mean tissue transit
    myocardial contrast appearance
    (MCAT)
    perfusion
    precontrast T1 relaxation
    prolonged ejection renal transit
    (RTT)

time *(cont.)*
  pulmonary transit (PTT)
  pulse reappearance
  pyelographic appearance
  radionuclide esophageal dead
  reaction recovery
  real-time
  recovery
  relaxation
  repetition (TR)
  resolving
  right ventricle to ear
  scan
  short echo
  sinoatrial conduction (SACT)
  sinus node recovery (SNRT)
  small bowel transit
  spin lattice proton relaxation
  systolic acceleration
  systolic upstroke
  T1 relaxation
  T2 relaxation
  transit
  venous filling (VFT)
  venous return (VRT)
  ventricular activation (VAT)
  ventricular isovolumic relaxation
time activity curve of contrast agent
time attenuation curve
time-averaged flow
timed bolus delivery
time density curve
timed imaging technique
time insensitive
time intensity curve
time lapse quantitative computed
  tomography lymphography
time of flight (TOF)
time of flight angiography
time of flight echoplanar imaging
time of flight (TOF) magnetic
  resonance angiography
time of flight measurement

time of flight (TOF) PET imaging
  systems
time-out, ventriculoatrial
time-resolved imaging by automatic
  data segmentation (TRIADS)
time sensitive
time to peak activity
time to peak contrast (TPC)
time to peak filling rate (TPFR)
TIMI (thrombolysis in myocardial
  infarction) classification
tip, basilar
tipped uterus
TIPS (transjugular intrahepatic
  portosystemic shunt)
tissue
  aberrant
  abnormal
  adventitial
  aerated
  areolar
  bony
  cartilaginous
  cavernous
  chondroid
  chorionic
  collagenous
  connective
  cortical
  crushed
  damaged
  dartoic
  dead
  degenerated
  dense
  destruction of
  ectopic
  exuberant
  fatty
  fibroadipose
  fibroareolar
  fibrocartilaginous
  fibrofatty

tissue *(cont.)*
  fibroglandular
  fibromuscular
  fibrosing
  fibrotic
  fibrous
  fibrous scar
  fibrovascular
  gangrenous
  gelatinous
  glandular
  granulation
  grumous
  hyperplastic
  hypertrophic
  interlobular
  isointense soft
  joint
  lipomatous-like
  lymph node
  lymphatic
  lymphoid
  lymphoreticular
  mesenchymal
  mesenteric
  muscle
  muscular
  necrotic
  neoplastic
  nodal
  noncritical soft
  nonviable
  osseous
  ossification of soft
  parenchymal
  periarticular
  proliferation of fibrous
  regeneration of
  scar
  soft
  subadventitial
  subcutaneous
  synovial

tissue *(cont.)*
  taenia
  tendon
  tuberculosis granulation
  underlying
tissue-based T2 relaxation
tissue-borne
tissue characterization technique
tissue contrast
tissue deficit compensator
tissue density
tissue Doppler gated (TDoG) dynamic
  three-dimensional ultrasound imaging
tissue Doppler imaging
tissue harmonic imaging
tissue inhomogeneity factors
tissue mass
tissue migration
tissue outflow valve
tissue perfusion
tissue sequelae
tissue slice
tissue veil
tissue viability
Tis-U-Trap endometrial suction
  catheter
titanium capsule
titanium plate
Titterington half axial projection
Titterington position
Tl (thallium)—see *thallium*
TLC (triple lumen catheter)
TLD (thermoluminescent dosimeter)
  rod
TLI (total lymphoid irradiation)
T loop (vectorcardiography)
TMA (true metatarsus adductus)
TME (trapezium-metacarpal
  eburnation)
TMJ (temporomandibular joint)
  syndrome

TMR CA PACS (triple modular
redundancy, continuous-availability,
picture archiving and communication system)
TMS three-dimensional radiation
therapy planning system
TMST (treadmill stress test)
TNM classification of carcinoma
Todaro, triangle of
Todd cirrhosis
TOF (tetralogy of Fallot)
TOF (time of flight) magnetic
resonance angiography
toit externe angle
Tolosa-Hunt syndrome
toluene scintillator
Tomocat (barium sulfate) imaging
agent
tomogram (see *imaging*)
tomographic cut
tomographic image
tomographic section
tomographic slice
tomography (see also *imaging*)
ACAT (automated computed
[computerized] axial
ante mortem orthopantomography
arthrotomography of shoulder,
double contrast
biplanar cardiac blood pool
cardiac positron emission (PET)
Cardiac Protect
cervical CT
computed tomography angiographic
portography (CTAP)
computed transmission
computerized axial (CAT)
dynamic computerized (CT)
dynamic single photon emission
electron beam computed (EBCT)
endoscopic optical coherence
(EOCT)
exercise thallium-201

tomography *(cont.)*
expiratory computed tomography
FACT (focused appendix computed)
GE SPECT (single photon emission computerized tomography,
multidetector computed
(MDCT)
helical biphasic computed (CT)
hemoglobin
high resolution computed (HRCT)
H_2 ^{15}O PET (positron emission
tomography)
hypocycloidal ankle tomography
indirect computed tomography
isotropic thin slice CT
kidney
lateral
linear
magnetic resonance (MRT)
mastoid polytomography
microtomography
MSCT (multislice computed
tomography)
multidetector computed (CT)
multidetector row spiral computed
multiphasic renal computerized
(CT)
myocardial perfusion
nephrotomography
PETT (positron emission transaxial tomography)
pneumocystotomography
polytomography
positron emission (PET)
pQCT (peripheral quantitative
computed tomography)
QCT (quantitative computed
tomography) (for bone loss)
quantitative hemoglobin
quantitative spirometrically
controlled CT
rapid acquisition computed axial
(RACAT)

tomography *(cont.)*
  regional cerebral blood flow
    (rCBF) PET
  renal computed (CT)
  Rotograph Plus panoramic dental
  sellar
  seven-pinhole
  single photon emission computed
    (SPECT)
  16-detector row computed
  spiral computed
  time-lapse quantitative computed
  TOF PET (time of flight positron
    emission tomography)
  tuned aperture computed (Delta 32
    TACT)
  ultrafast CT (UFCT) electron beam
  ultrasound diffraction
  view microtomography
  volumetric computed
  water-contrast computed
  XCT (x-ray computed tomography)
  XeCT (xenon computed tomog-
    raphy)
  Z-dependent computed
tomomyelography
tomoscanner, Philips T-60
tomoscintigraphy
tomosynthesis
  digital circular
  digital x-ray
T1 ("tee-one") (longitudinal or spin
    lattice relaxation time)
  T1 constant
  T1FS (T1-weighted fat-suppressed)
    images
  T1 high resolution isotropic volume
    examination (THRIVE) tech-
    nique
  T1 lesion load
  T1 pulse sequence
  T1 relaxation time
  T1-weighted coronal image

T1 *(cont.)*
  T1-weighted fat-suppressed images
    (T1FS)
  T1-weighted gadolinium-enhanced
    SE images
  T1-weighted image (short TR/TE)
  T1-weighted sagittal image
  TONE (tilted optimized nonsaturating
    excitation)
  T1-T12 (twelve thoracic vertebrae)
tongue and trough bone
tongue of tissue
tongue-type fracture
Tönnis (Toennis) hip dysplasia classifi-
    cation
Tonopaque (barium sulfate) imaging
    agent
tonsil, herniated cerebellar
tonus
toothpaste shadow
tooth sign
tophaceous gout
tophus (pl. tophi) formation
topical water-soluble contrast media
top normal limits in size
topodermatography
topogram
topograph
topographic identification
topographic measurement
topographic pattern, anomalous
topography (mapping) (do not confuse
    with *tomography*)
  arterial
  ocular globe
  vessel
Torcon NB selective angiographic
    catheter
Tornwaldt cyst in nasopharynx
torpid development
torr pressure
torsed appendage
torsion fracture

torsion of fracture fragment
torsional abnormalities
torsional alignment
torsional impaction force
torsional stress
torso phased-array coil (TPAC)
tortuosity and elongation
tortuosity precluding catheter passage
tortuous emptying
tortuous ureter
torus fracture
TOS (thoracic outlet syndrome)
Toshiba Aspire CI (continuous
　imaging)
Toshiba CT scanner
Toshiba EccoCee ultrasound system
Toshiba echocardiograph machine
Toshiba Excelart Planissimo scanner
Toshiba helical CT scanner
Toshiba MR scanner
Toshiba 900S helical CT scanner
Toshiba 900S/XII scanner
Toshiba TCT-80 CT scanner
Toshiba 270 ultrasound system
Toshiba Xpress scanner
Toshiba Xpress SX helical CT
　scanner
Toshiba Xvision scanner
tositumomab monoclonal antibody
　(iodine I 131 tositumomab)
total anomalous pulmonary venous
　drainage (TAPVD)
total atrial refractory period (TARP)
total body irradiation
total body scanning
Total-Cross PTA catheter
total fracture
total lymphoid irradiation (TLI)
Towne projection in skull x-rays
Towne view
toxemic pneumonia
toxic adenoma
toxic nodular goiter

toxic pneumonia
toxicity, flutamide-associated liver
TPAC (torso phased-array coil)
TPBS (three-phase bone scintigraphy)
TPC (time to peak contrast)
TPFR (time to peak filling rate)
Tpot (potential doubling time), flow
　cytometry
TPR (total peripheral resistance)
TPR (total pulmonary resistance)
TR (repetition time)
TR (tricuspid regurgitation)
TR/TE (repetition time/echo time),
　long (T2-weighted image)
　short (T1-weighted image)
trabecula (pl. trabeculae)
trabecular bone
trabecular bone equivalent density
　(TBED)
trabecular displacement
trabecular pattern
trabeculated atrium
trabeculated outline
trabeculation
　effaced
　endocardial
trace (see *imaging agent*)
trace amount of radiopharmaceutical
trace element distribution
tracer accumulation
tracer activity
tracer bolus
tracer dose
tracer
　neutron-rich biomedical
　radioactive
tracer uptake
trachea
　annular ligament of
　carina of
　scabbard
tracheal anastomosis
tracheal atresia

tracheal bifurcation
tracheal deviation
tracheal displacement
tracheal distortion
tracheal ring
tracheal shift
tracheal stenosis
trachelectomy, radical
tracheobronchial fistula
tracheobronchial foreign body
tracheobronchial tree
tracheoesophageal fistula (TEF)
tracheomalacia
tracing, vessel-
track cone length
Tracker catheter
track etching
tracking
  active
  bolus
  brain fiber
  magnetic resonance needle
  passive
  real-time biplanar needle
  real-time magnetic resonance
    imaging
tracking limit
track sign
tract
  alimentary
  ascending
  atriohisian
  Bekhterev
  biliary
  Bruce and Muir
  bulbar
  Burdach
  central tegmental
  cerebellorubral
  cerebellorubrospinal
  cerebellospinal
  cerebellotegmental
  cerebellothalamic

tract *(cont.)*
  comma tract of Schultze
  conariohypophyseal
  corticobulbar
  corticopontine
  corticorubral
  corticospinal
  corticotectal
  crossed pyramidal
  cuneocerebellar
  Deiters
  dentatothalamic
  descending
  digestive
  direct pyramidal
  dorsolateral
  extracorticospinal
  extrapyramidal
  fastigiobulbar
  fistulous
  Flechsig
  flow
  frontopontine
  frontotemporal
  gastrointestinal (GI)
  geniculocalcarine
  geniculostriate
  genital
  genitourinary
  GI (gastrointestinal)
  Goll
  Gombault-Philippe
  Gowers
  habenulopeduncular
  Helweg
  hepatic outflow
  hypothalamicohypophysial
  ileal inflow
  intermediolateral
  internodal
  intersegmental
  interstitiospinal
  intestinal

tract *(cont.)*
  intrahepatic biliary
  Lissauer
  long
  Lowenthal
  lower
  Maissiat
  mamillopeduncular
  mamillotegmental
  mamillothalamic
  Marchi
  mesencephalic
  Meynert
  Monakow
  motor
  Muir and Bruce
  nigrostriate
  occipitopontine
  pancreaticobiliary
  paraventriculohypophysial
  parietopontine
  patent needle
  peduncular
  Philippe-Gombault
  pilonidal
  posterior spinocerebellar
  pulmonary conduit outflow
  pulmonary outflow
  pyramidal
  respiratory
  reticulospinal
  rubrobulbar
  rubroreticular
  Schultze comma
  Schutz
  semilunar
  sensory
  septomarginal
  sinus
  spinal
  spinocerebellar
  spinocervical
  spinocervicothalamic

tract *(cont.)*
  spinothalamic
  Spitzka-Lissauer
  strionigral
  sulcomarginal
  tectobulbar
  tectocerebellar
  tegmental
  tegmentospinal
  temporopontine
  testobulbar
  thalamo-olivary
  transverse
  triangular
  trigeminal nerve
  trigeminothalamic
  tuberohypophysial
  upper
  upper gastrointestinal (UGI)
  urinary
  uveal
  ventral amygdalofugal
  vestibulocerebellar
  Vicq d'Azyr
  white matter
tract embolization
traction diverticulum
tragus
train, fast SE
trait, sickle cell
trajectory, bullet
trajectory of creatinine (Cr) rise
TrakBack ultrasound catheter
tramline cortical calcification
tramlines shadow
tram-track pattern on x-ray in
  Sturge-Weber syndrome
tram-track sign
transabdominal scanning
transabdominal ultrasound
transaortic radiofrequency ablation
transapical endocardial ablation
transarterial chemoembolization

transarterial embolization
transaxial CT scan
transaxial fat-saturated 3-D images
transaxial images
transaxial maximum-intensity
    projection (MIP)
transaxial slice
transaxillary lateral view
transbronchial lung biopsy
transbronchial needle aspiration
    (TBNA)
transcapitate fracture
transcatheter ablation
transcatheter arterial chemoemboliza-
    tion
transcatheter arterial embolization
    (TAE)
transcatheter filter placement
transcatheter introduction of
    intravascular stent
transcatheter oily chemoembolization
transcatheter therapy
    embolization
    infusion
transcatheter variceal embolization
transcervical balloon tuboplasty (TBT)
transcervical catheter
transcervical catheterization of fallop-
    ian tube
transcervical fracture
transcervical tubal access (T-TAC)
    catheter
transchondral talar fracture
transchoroidal approach
transclival approach
transcondylar axis (TCA)
transcondylar fracture
transcranial color-coded duplex
    sonography
transcranial color-coded real-time
    sonography
transcranial color-coded sonography
    (TCCS)

transcranial Doppler ultrasound
transcranial Doppler (TCD)
    ultrasound (sonography)
transcutaneous extraction catheter
    atherectomy
transcutaneous oxygen pressure
transducer
    Acuson linear array
    broadband
    catheter-borne
    curved-array
    epicardial Doppler flow
    linear
    Metricath catheter and transducer
    M-mode
    magnetic resonance imaging-guided
        focused ultrasound
    sector
    V5Ms shielded
transect, transected
transection
transependymal uptake of tracer
transepiphyseal fracture
transesophageal Doppler color flow
    imaging
transesophageal echocardiography
    (TEE)
transesophageal imaging
transesophageal multiplanar echocar-
    diography
transesophageal probe
transesophageal transducer
transfemoral arteriogram
transfer
    energy
    magnetization
    rapid image
    saturation
    ultrafast video
transfer mode, asynchronous (ATM)
transferrin receptor
transfontanellar ultrasound, high-
    resolution

transform
   cosine
   fast Fourier
   Fourier
   K-L
transformation, cavernous (of portal
   vein)
transformation matrix
transform-based skeletonization
transgluteal approach
transgluteal CT-guided technique
transhamate fracture
transhepatic cholangiography (THC)
transhepatic embolization (THE)
transhepatic cholangiography (THC)
transient bone marrow edema
   syndrome
transient elastography
transient ischemic attack (TIA)
transient shunt obstruction
transient synovitis
transiliac approach
transillumination
transit, bolus
transition zone
transitional rhythm
transitional vertebra
transit time, abnormal intestinal
transjugular cholangiogram
transjugular intrahepatic portosystemic
   shunt (TIPS)
transjugular intrahepatic portosystemic
   shunt with stent-graft
translation-invariant filter
translocation of coronary arteries
translucency
   first trimester nuchal
   nuchal (NT)
translucent depression in interatrial
   septum
translucent zone
translumbar aortogram
translumbar aortography

transluminal angioplasty, percutaneous
   (PTA)
transluminal atherectomy
transluminal balloon angioplasty
transluminal coronary angioplasty
transluminal coronary artery
   angioplasty complex
transluminal dilatation
transluminal endatherectomy catheter
   (TEC)
transluminal extraction catheter (TEC)
transluminally placed stented graft
transluminal lysing system
transluminal ultrasonic angioplasty
   (TUA)
transmalleolar axis (TMA)-thigh angle
transmedial plane
transmesenteric hernia
transmesenteric plication
transmetatarsal amputation (TMA)
transmission block
transmission control protocol/Internet
   protocol (TCP/IP)
transmission CT
transmission data
transmission dosimetry
transmission scan
transmitral flow
transmitral gradient
transmitted carotid artery pulsations
transmural cryoablation
transmural fibrosis
transmural infarct
transmural linear lesion
transmural match
transmural myocardial infarct
transmural myocardial infarction
transmural steal
transmutation
transmyocardial perfusion pressure
transnasal endoluminal ultrasonography
   of GI tract
transnasally

transoral
transorbital view
transorally
transparent rendering
transpedicular decompression
transphyseal
transplant (or transplantation)
transport
  forward
  reverse
transporter, dopamine
transposed aorta
transposition
  atrial
  carotid-subclavian
  congenitally corrected
  corrected great arteries
  gastric
  great vessel
  Jatene
transposition cipher
transposition of great arteries (TGA)
  (great vessels)
  complete
  corrected (CTGA)
  partial (of great vessels)
transosseous approach
transpedicular access
transperineal prostatic cryoablation
transperineal ultrasonography
transpharyngeal view of the head of
  the mandibular condyle
transplant
  nonmyeloablative
  syngeneic
transplantation
  hematopoietic stem cell
  percutaneous transhepatic
    pancreatic islet cell
  single lung
  split liver
  stem cell
transplanted kidney

transpulmonary echo ultrasound
  reflectors
transpulmonary pressure (PTP)
transpulmonic gradient
transradial styloid perilunate
  dislocation
transradiancy
transradiant air
transradiant zone
transrectal echography
transrectal ultrasound (TRUS)
transrenal arteriovenous dialysis graft
transsacral approach
TransScan 2000 breast mapping device
TransScan TS2000 electrical impedance breast scanning system
transscaphoid perilunate dislocation
transsection, spinal cord
transseptal angiocardiography
transseptal left heart catheterization
transseptal perforation
transseptal puncture
transseptal radiofrequency ablation
transsternal approach
transsyndesmotic screw fixation
transtentorial herniation
transtentorial
transtentorially
transthoracic echocardiography (TTE)
transthoracic imaging
transthoracic needle aspiration,
  ultrasound-guided
transthoracic needle biopsy (TNB)
transthoracic 3DE (three-dimensional
  echocardiography)
transthoracic imaging
transthoracic lateral position
transtriquetral fracture-dislocation
transtympanic iontophoresis
transudate
transudation
transudation of fluid
transudative pericardial fluid

transurethral ultrasound-guided laser-
induced prostatectomy (TULIP)
transurethral
transurethrally
transvaginal echography
transvaginal oocyte retrieval
transvaginal sonography
transvaginal ultrasound (TVS)
transvaginal uterine cervical dilation
with fluoroscopic guidance
transvalvular gradient
transvenous extrahepatic portacaval
shunt
transvenous implantation
transverse arch
transverse colon
transverse cord lesion
transverse diameter
transverse fracture
transverse heart
transverse hypoplasia
transverse ligaments of atlas
transverse magnetization
transverse orientation
transverse pelvic diameter
transverse plane
transverse plane forces
transverse presentation
transverse process
transverse relaxation rate
transverse section
transverse slice
transverse sinus
transverse ultrasound
trapeziometacarpal joint
trapezioscaphoid joint
trapeziotrapezoid joint
trapezium (greater multangular) bone
trapezius muscle
trapezoidal-shaped sandwich plate
trapezoid (lesser multangular) bone
trapezoid bone of Henle
trapezoid bone of Lyser

trapezoid ligament
Trapper catheter exchange
trapping, air
trapping of radioisotope
Traube aortic regurgitation sign
Traube semilunar space
trauma
  acoustic
  anal
  birth
  bladder
  blunt
  blunt abdominal
  iatrogenic
  kidney
  multiple
  nonpenetrating (to heart)
  obstetrical
  penetrating
  penile
  physical
  pleural
  rectal
  renal
  scrotal-testicular
  urethral
traumatic aneurysm
traumatic avulsion
traumatic brain injury (TBI)
traumatic dislocation
traumatic disruption
traumatic emphysema
traumatic infarct
traumatic intracranial aneurysm
traumatic meningeal hemorrhage
traumatic pneumonia
traumatic pneumothorax
traumatic pseudoaneurysm
traumatic rupture
traumatic spondylolisthesis (grades 1-4)
traumatic spondylolysis
traumatic thrombus
traumatic urethral stricture

traumatogenic occlusion
traversing the fracture
Treacher Collins syndrome
treadmill exercise stress test
treadmill exercise test (TET)
treadmill inclination, incremental
   increases in
treadmill slope
treadmill speed, incremental
   increases in
treadmill stress test (TMST)
treated premalignant lesion
treatment energy
treatment port
tree
   airway
   arterial
   biliary
   bronchial
   coronary artery
   hepatobiliary
   iliocaval
   intrahepatic biliary
   lower extremity arterial
   tracheobronchial
tree artifact
tree-in-bud (TIB)
tree-in-bud pattern
tree-in-bud sign
tree-in-winter appearance
tree-like airway structure
tree-shaped spot on radiograph
trefoil balloon catheter
Treitz hernia
Treitz ligament
trend-correction
Trendelenburg position
Trevor disease
Trex digital mammography system
   (TDMS)
Trex processing
TRH (thyrotropin releasing hormone)
   stimulation test

T_4RIA (thyroxine radioisotope assay)
triad
   acute compression
   Charcot
   Dieulafoy
   hepatic
   portal
   Saint
   Whipple
TRIADS (time-resolved imaging by
   automatic data segmentation)
Triad SPECT imaging system
triangle
   anal
   aponeurotic
   auricular
   axillary
   Burger scalene
   Calot
   cardiohepatic
   carotid
   cephalic
   cervical
   clavipectoral
   Codman
   crural
   cystohepatic
   deltoideopectoral
   digastric
   Einthoven
   facial
   femoral
   Garland
   Gerhardt
   Grynfeltt
   Henke
   Hesselbach
   iliofemoral
   inguinal
   insular
   internal jugular
   Koch
   Korányi-Grocco

triangle *(cont.)*
  Labbé
  Langenbeck
  Lesgaft
  Livingston
  lumbocostoabdominal
  mesenteric
  paramedian
  Pawlik
  posterior
  scalene
  Scarpa
  submandibular
  supraclavicular
  Todaro
  urogenital
  vertebrocostal
  Ward
triangular area of dullness
triangular bone
triangular cord sign
triangular defect
triangular external ankle fixation
triangular fibrocartilage (TFC)
triangular fibrocartilage complex
  (TFCC)
triangular ligament
triangular non-single harmonic wave
triangular uterus
triangulation of Carrel
tributary (pl. tributaries)
trichinous embolism
trichophytic granuloma
tricuspid aortic valve
tricuspid valve leaflet
trifid stomach
triflanged nail
trifoil balloon
trifurcation of artery
trigeminal cavernous fistula
trigeminal cavity
trigeminal hemangioma
trigeminal nerve (fifth cranial nerve)

trigeminal neuralgia
trigeminal pattern
trigeminy
trigger delay
triggering ventricular contraction
trigonal hypertrophy
trigone
  angles of
  collateral
  deltoideopectoral
  fibrous
  Henke
  hypertrophied
  hypoglossal
  inguinal
  lateral ventricle
  Lieutaud
  Müller (Mueller)
  Pawlik
  vertebrocostal
trigone of urinary bladder
Triguide guide catheter
triisocyanide ^{99m}Tc imaging agent
trilaminar appearance
trilayer appearance
trileaflet
trilinear interpolation
trileaflet
trilobar hypertrophy
Trilogy acetabular cup, uncemented
trimalleolar fracture
trimellitic anhydritic pneumonitis
Trionix camera
Trionix scanner
Trionix SPECT
triphasic spiral CT
triplane fracture
triple dose gadolinium-enhanced MR
  imaging without MT (magnetization transfer)
triple dose gadolinium imaging
triple head SPECT with FDG
triple label

triple lumen central venous catheter
triple lumen umbilical catheter
triple match
triple modular redundancy, continuous-availability, picture archiving and communication system (TMR CA PACS)
triple phase helical CT
triple resonance NMR probe circuit
triple ripple
triplet beat
triplication of ureter
tripod position
tri-point bullet
tripolar electrode catheter
triquetral bone
triquetral fracture
triquetrohamate joint
triquetrohamate ligament
triquetrolunate dislocation
triradiate cartilage
trisacryl gelatin microspheres
trisomy 21
tristimulus values
Triumph-I vascular port
trochanter
   greater
   lesser
trochlear nerve (fourth cranial nerve)
trochlear notch
trochlear process
Troisier node
trolley-track sign
TRON 3 VACI cardiac imaging system
trophedema
trophic fracture
trophoblastic material
trophoblastic neoplasm
trough line
Tru-Cut liver biopsy
true channel
true conjugate

true fast imaging
true lumen
true posterior wall myocardial infarction
truncal artery
truncal renal artery stenosis
truncal valve
truncated NMR probe
truncation band artifact
truncular venous malformation
truncus arteriosus
   embryonic
   persistent
trunk
   articulations of
   atrioventricular (AV)
   bifurcation of
   brachiocephalic
   bronchomediastinal
   bronchomediastinal lymph
   celiac
   celiac-bimesenteric
   cordlike
   costocervical
   joints of
   lumbosacral
   lymph
   nerve
   posterior vagal
   thyrocervical
   vagal
Trunkey fracture classification system
TRUS (transrectal ultrasound)
Tru-Scint AD (technetium Tc 99m MAb-170) imaging agent
Tru-Trac high pressure PTA balloon
TRW (teboroxime) resting washout
trypanosomiasis
TS (tricuspid stenosis)
T-shaped fracture
TSH (thyroid-stimulating hormone)
   TSH-dependent functioning nodule
   TSH stimulation test

T spine (thoracic spine)
TSPP (technetium stannous pyrophos-
    phate) rectilinear bone scan
TTC (T-tube cholangiogram)
TTE (transthoracic echocardiography)
T3 resin uptake test
T-Scan 2000 transpectral impedance
    scanner
T-score on bone densitometry
TS2000 (TransScan 2000)
T-TAC (transcervical tubal access)
    catheter
TTS (tarsal tunnel syndrome)
T-tube cholangiogram
T tubogram
T2 (transverse or spin spin relaxation
    time) constant
    T2-lesion load
    T2 pulse sequence
    T2 QMRI (T2 quantitative MRI)
    T2 relaxation time
    T2 shortening
    T2 star relaxation
    T2 time constant
    T2-weighted image (long TR/TE)
    T2-weighted spin echo image
    T2-weighted turbo SE images
    T2-weighted turbo spin echo
TUA (transluminal ultrasonic angio-
    plasty)
tubal insufflation
tubal obstruction
tubal pregnancy
tubal ring
tubal rugae abscess
tubal stenosis
tube
    anode
    auditory
    bilateral pleural
    blocked shunt
    bronchial
    calices (calyces)

tube *(cont.)*
    capillary
    cathode-ray
    Chaoul voltage x-ray
    chest
    collecting
    corneal
    cuffed endotracheal
    digestive
    double lumen endobronchial
    endobronchial
    endotracheal (ET)
    enterolysis
    Entristar skin-level gastrostomy
    Eppendorf
    ET (endotracheal)
    eustachian
    fallopian
    feeding
    fenestrated
    jejunostomy
    J-shaped
    large caliber
    Malecot
    Miser
    muscular
    nasogastric (NFG)
    nasotracheal
    neural
    NG (nasogastric)
    non-endhole nasojejunal feeding
    obstructed shunt
    oroendotracheal
    orogastric
    pharyngotympanic
    pickup
    pleural
    polyethylene
    right-angle chest
    separator
    Shiner radiopaque
    shunt
    solid-phase extraction

tube *(cont.)*
  stomach
  straight chest
  suction
  suprapubic
  T-
  T self-retaining drainage
  tracheal
  uterine
  water-seal chest
  x-ray
tube current
tube drainage
tube geometry module of VIDA
tube position rotation
tuber cinereum
tubercle
  accessory
  acoustic
  adductor
  amygdaloid
  articular
  auricular
  calcaneal
  carotid
  Chaput
  conoid
  corniculate
  costal
  crown
  cuneiform
  darwinian
  dental
  dissection
  epiglottic
  fibrous
  genial
  genital
  Gerdy
  Ghon
  greater
  iliac
  intercondylar

tubercle *(cont.)*
  lesser
  Lister
  Parsons
  prominent
  pubic
  rib
  scalene
  sella turcica
  tibial
tubercle bacillus
tubercle bacillus pneumonia
tubercular empyema
tuberculoma
tuberculosis (TB)
  bone
  colonic
  disseminated
  exudative
  fulminant
  genitourinary
  hematogenous
  inhalation
  mammary
  meningeal
  miliary
  postprimary
  primary
  pulmonary
  renal
tuberculosis of kidney
tuberculosis of ureter
tuberculous arthritis
tuberculous pneumonia
tuberculous pseudoaneurysm
tuberosity (pl. tuberosities)
  bicipital
  calcaneal
  coracoid
  costal
  deltoid
  femoral
  greater

tuberosity *(cont.)*
  iliac
  infraglenoid
  ischial
  lesser
  navicular
  omental
  radial
  tibial
  ulnar
tuberous sclerosis
tubogram
tubo-ovarian abscess
tuboplasty
  balloon
  ultrasound transcervical
  ultrasound-guided transcervical
tubular adenoma
tubular aneurysm
tubular bone
tubular cancer
tubular carcinoma
tubular cavity
tubular degeneration, renal
tubular dilation
tubular ectasia
tubular ectasia, renal
tubular lesion
tubular magnet
tubular mesh
tubular necrosis, acute
tubular obstruction
tubular polyp
tubular stenosis
tubular structure
tubular tumor
tubular ventricle
tubule
  collecting
  connecting
  convoluted
  dental
  dentinal

tubule *(cont.)*
  discharging
  distal convoluted
  mesonephric
  proximal convoluted
  renal
  seminiferous
  straight
  tortuous
tubulointerstitial inflammation
tubulointerstitial lesion
tuft fracture
tularemic pneumonia
tulip sheath
TULIP (transurethral ultrasound-
  guided laser-induced prostatectomy)
tumbling bullet sign
tumor
  adenomatoid
  adenomatoid oviduct
  aggressive angiomyxoma
  AML (angiomyolipoma) solid renal
  androgen-secreting
  aneuploid
  angiomyxoma
  apple core
  Askin
  benign
  bladder
  borderline ovarian
  Brenner
  bulky
  carcinoid
  cavernous
  chondrogenic
  chordoma
  chromophobe adenoma
  clivus meningioma
  CNS (central nervous system)
  colloid cyst
  craniopharyngioma
  cutaneous
  cystic

tumor *(cont.)*
　deep-seated
　desmoplastic small round cell
　diffuse infiltrating
　discrete
　dumbbell
　dysgerminoma
　cchogcnic
　embryonal
　endometrioid
　ependymoma
　epidermoid
　estrogen-producing ovarian
　estrogen receptor positive (ER+)
　estrogen receptor negative (ER-)
　estrogen-secreting testicular
　Ewing
　extension of
　extracompartmental
　extramedullary
　fatty
　fetal
　fibroadenoma
　fibrohistiocytic
　fibroid
　fibrous
　finger of
　focal
　focal infiltrating
　ganglion
　gastrointestinal stromal
　germ cell (GCT)
　globular
　glomus
　gross
　granulosa cell
　granulosa-theca cell
　hepatic adrenal rest
　highly vascular
　hourglass
　hypoechogenic
　inflammatory myofibroblastic
　invasive ductal

tumor *(cont.)*
　invasive lobular
　intra-axial brain
　intracompartmental
　intracranial
　intradural
　intramedullary
　invasive
　kidney
　Krukenberg
　lobulated
　locally invasivc
　lymphoid
　macroscopically evident
　main
　malignant
　malignant peripheral nerve sheath
　malignant teratoma
　medullary
　metastatic
　microadenoma
　mixed mesodermal
　mobile pedunculated left atrial
　MPNST (malignant peripheral
　　nerve sheath tumor)
　mucocutaneous
　napkin ring
　necrotic
　neuroendocrine
　neurogenic
　nonechogenic
　non-neoplastic
　non-neurogenic gastrointestinal
　　mesenchymal
　nonseminomatous germ cell
　ovarian
　ovarian granulosa cell
　Pancoast
　papillary
　papilloma
　pedunculated
　pedunculated vesical
　phyllodes

tumor *(cont.)*
  pilocytic
  pinealoma
  placental site trophoblastic
  pontine glioma
  poorly circumscribed
  poorly differentiated
  Pott puffy
  pregnancy
  primary
  progesterone-receptor-positive
  prolactin-secreting adenoma
  pseudomalignant
  pseudotumor
  pulmonary sulcus
  radiosensitive
  renal cell
  RIF-1
  scirrhous
  secondary
  seeding of
  segmental infiltrating
  Sertoli-Leydig cell
  Sertoli-Leydig cell ovarian
  Sertoli-stromal cell ovarian
  sessile
  smooth muscle
  solid
  spread of
  steroid cell ovarian
  stone differentiated from
  subcortical
  submucosal
  subserosal
  tubular
  urothelial
  uterine
  vascular
  virilizing
  vulvar
  Warthin (adenolymphoma)
  well-circumscribed

tumor *(cont.)*
  well-differentiated
  Wharton (cystadenoma)
  Wilms
tumor ablation, focused-heat
tumoral invasion
tumor base
tumor-bearing bone
tumor bed
tumor bed boost (of radiopharmaceutical)
tumor blush on cerebral angiography
tumor boundary
tumor capillary permeability
tumor cleavage plane
tumor embolism
tumor embolization
tumor erosion
tumor extirpation
tumor halo (on ultrasound image)
tumor-infiltrated lymph nodes
tumor involvement
tumorlike shadow
tumor marker
tumor mass
tumor matrix
tumor necrosis
tumor osteoid
tumor recurrence
tumor staining on cerebral
  angiography
tumor to normal brain ratio
tumor vascularity
tumor volume
tumor volume-based dose selection
tumor volumetry
tungsten eye shield
tungsten target
tunica adventitia
tunica intima
tunica media
tunica propria

tuning unit, reflectometer
tunnel
　carpal
　cross-trigonal
　cubital
　retropancreatic
　tarsal
tunneled hemodialysis catheter
tunnel view
turbid effusion
turbinate bone
Turbo-FLAIR imaging
Turbo-FLASH sequence
turbo SE sequences
turbo spin echo sequences
turbo spin echo T2-weighted sequence
turbo STIR images
turbulence
turbulent flow
turbulent signal
turcica, sella
turf-toe
Turkish sabre syndrome
Turner marginal gyrus
turning-point morphology (TPM)
turricephaly
turtle sign
TV (tricuspid valve)
TV-interlaced (TVI)
T vector
TVS (transvaginal ultrasound)
twelfth cranial nerve (hypoglossal
　nerve)
24-bit image
twig
　cutaneous
　muscular
twin (pl. twins)
　cephalothoracopagus
　conjoined
　dorsal union
　Janus
　monochorionic co-twin

twin (cont.)
　monozygotic
　ventral union
twinkling artifact
twin peak sign
twin to twin transfusion syndrome
　(TTTS)
twin trunk
twisting of the bowel around itself
two-channel phased array RF receiver
　coil system
two-dimensional (2D or 2-D)
　2D B-mode ultrasound machine
　2D color-coded imaging of blood
　　flow
　2D echocardiography (sector scan)
　2D format
　2D Fourier imaging
　2D Fourier transform (2DFT)
　2DFT (two-dimensional Fourier
　　transform)
　2D GRE dynamic protocol
　2-D IVUS (two-dimensional
　　intravascular ultrasound)
　2D J-resolved 1H MR spectros-
　　copy
　2D portal image registration
　2D pulsatility index mapping
　2D resistance index mapping
　2D sector scan
　2D spatially selective radio-
　　frequency (RF) pulses
two-frame gated imaging
two-part fracture
two-phase CT
two-phase computed tomographic
　imaging
two-phase helical computed tomog-
　raphy
2-nitroimidazole nucleoside analog
270 MHz VT multinuclear spec-
　trometer
two-vessel runoff

two-view chest x-ray
Tygon catheter
tympanic bone
typhoid pneumonia
tyropanoate sodium imaging agent
type A aortic dissection

type B aortic dissection
type I, II, and III dens fracture
typhoid pneumonia
tyropanoate (tyropanoate sodium)
  imaging agent

U, u

U (uranium) (an element)
UAE (uterine arterial embolization)
UAL (ultrasonic-assisted lipoplasty (or liposuction)
UBIS 5000 ultrasound bone sonometer
UBM (ultrasound backscatter microscopy)
UBM (ultrasound biomicroscopy)
UBOs (unidentified bright objects)
UBS (uniform bremsstrahlung splitting)
UC (ulcerative colitis)
UCAC (uterine cornual access catheter)
UCG (ultrasonic cardiography)
UCL (ulnar collateral ligament)
UCLA imaging protocol
UEs (upper extremities)
UES (upper esophageal sphincter)
UFCT (ultrafast computed tomography)
UGI (upper gastrointestinal) series
UGI SBF (upper GI series with small bowel follow-through)
UG (urogenital) sinus
Uhl syndrome
UHMM (ultra-high magnification mammography)

UJ (uncovertebral joint)
ulcer (ulceration)
  acid peptic
  active duodenal
  acute peptic
  amebic
  anastomotic
  anterior wall antral
  antral
  aortic
  arteriolar ischemic
  atheromatous
  atherosclerotic aortic
  Barrett
  bear claw
  benign
  bleeding
  bulbar peptic
  chronic
  chronic peptic
  collar button
  colonic mucosal
  craterlike
  Cruveilhier
  Curling
  Cushing
  Cushing-Rokitansky

ulcer *(cont.)*
    duodenal
    esophageal
    flask-shaped
    focal
    gastric
    gastrointestinal
    giant peptic
    greater curvature
    healing
    Hunner
    indolent
    intestinal
    intractable
    ischemic
    jejunal
    juxtapyloric
    kissing
    Kocher dilatation
    lesser curvature
    linear
    malignant
    marginal
    minute bleeding
    necrotic
    patchy colonic
    penetrating
    peptic
    perforated
    perforating
    postbulbar duodenal
    postsurgical recurrent
    prepyloric gastric
    punched-out
    punctate
    puncture
    pyloric channel
    radiation-induced
    rake
    recurrent
    Rokitansky-Cushing
    thorn
    round

ulcer *(cont.)*
    sea anemone
    secondary
    serpiginous
    stercoral
    stomach
    stomal
    stress
    trophic
    urinary
    V-shaped
ulcerated atheromatous plaque
ulcerated plaque
ulcerative colitis (UC)
ulcerative lesion
ulcer base
ulcer bed
ulcer crater
ulcerlike lesion of aorta
ulcer osteoma
ulcer with heaped-up edges
Uldall *(not* Udall) subclavian hemo-
    dialysis catheter
ulna
ulnar abutment syndrome
ulnar bone
ulnar bursa
ulnar collateral ligament
ulnar deviation
ulnar extensor
ulnar facing of metacarpal heads
ulnar hand
ulnar nerve dislocation
ulnar nerve entrapment
ulnar nerve lesion
ulnar notch
ulnar pulse
ulnar sesamoid bone
ulnar styloid process
ulnar tubercle
ulnarward
ulnocarpal ligament
ulnolunate ligament

ulnotriquetral ligament
ULP (ultra low profile) catheter
ultracardiography imaging
UltraCision ultrasonic knife
ultraearly thrombolytic therapy
ultrafast computed tomography
(UFCT) scanner
ultrafast CT electron beam tomography
ultrafast video transfer
ultra-high magnification mammography (UHMM)
Ultraject pre-filled contrast media syringe
UltraLite flow-directed microcatheter
ultra-low profile fixed-wire balloon dilatation catheter
Ultramark 4 ultrasound
Ultramark 8 transducer
Ultramark 9 scanner
UltraPACS diagnostic imaging system
Ultraseed ultrasound-guided brachytherapy system
ultrasmall superparamagnetic iron oxide (USPIO) imaging agent
ultrasonically activated scalpel
ultrasonic aortography
ultrasonic aspiration
ultrasonic assessment
ultrasonic-assisted lipoplasty (or liposuction) (UAL)
ultrasonic body contouring
ultrasonic cardiogram
ultrasonic cardiography (UCG)
ultrasonic-driven scalpel
ultrasonic elastography
ultrasonic guidance for interstitial radioelement application
ultrasonic guidance for intrauterine fetal transfusion
ultrasonic guidance for placement of radiation therapy fields
ultrasonic knife, UltraCision

ultrasonic lithotripsy
ultrasonic nebulizer (USN)
ultrasonic scalpel
ultrasonic tomographic image
ultrasonographic catheter
ultrasonographic images, crosssectional
ultrasonography (see also *sonography; ultrasound*)
ultrasonography-guided fine-needle aspiration biopsy
ultrasound (US), ultrasonography (see also *imaging; sonography*)
abdominal
Ablatherm HIFU (high intensity focused ultrasound) system
ACM (automated cardiac flow measurement)
Acuson
Acuson computed sonography
ADR
AI 5200 diagnostic
Aloka linear
Aloka scctor
A-mode
Aspen
Aspen digital
ATL real-time
BABE
BabyFace
BabyFace 3-D surface rendering
bilateral whole-breast
BladderManager
BladderScan
BladderScan BVI 2500
B-mode
breast
Bruel-Kjaer
CathScanner ultrasound imaging system
color-coded duplex
color-coded real-time
color Doppler

ultrasound *(cont.)*
   color duplex
   color flow Doppler (CDUS)
   color power transcranial Doppler
   compression
   contact B-scan
   continuous wave
   contrast echocardiography
   contrast-enhanced
   cranial
   CRYOguide ultrasound system
   CUSALap
   diagnostic
   diagnostic range
   Diasonics
   diathermy
   DIMAQ integrated
   Doppler
   double bubble appearance of fetus
     on
   duplex (DU)
   duplex B-mode
   duplex carotid
   duplex Doppler
   duplex pulsed-Doppler
   DUST (dynamic ultrasound of
     shoulder)
   echocolonoscope
   echo-enhanced transcranial color-
     coded
   EchoEye 3-D
   EchoFlow blood velocity meter
     system (BVM-1)
   echogastroscope
   Echo-Gen enhanced
   echogenic immunoliposomes
     (ELIPs)
   endoanal
   endorectal
   endoscopic (EUS)
   endovaginal (EVUS)
   endovascular
   EUS (endoscopic ultrasonography)

ultrasound *(cont.)*
   fatty meal (FMS)
   fetal
   5 MHz
   focused extracorporeal
   freehand interventional
   frequency domain imaging (FDI)
   full bladder
   gallbladder
   gastrointestinal endoscopic
   GI (gastrointestinal) endoscopic
   graded compression
   gray-scale
   harmonic power Doppler
   HDI 3000 ultrasound system
   Hewlett-Packard
   high frequency therapeutic
   high intensity focused (HFU,
     HIFU)
   high resolution
   high resolution transfontanellar
   high spatial resolution
   Hitachi
   hypoechoic
   immersion B-scan
   intracaval endovascular (ICEUS)
   intracavitary prostate
   intracoronary
   intraoperative (IOUS)
   intraportal endovascular (IPEUS)
   intrarectal
   intravascular (IVUS)
   Irex Exemplar
   laparoscopic (LUS)
   laparoscopic contact (LCU)
   laparoscopic intracorporeal (LICU)
   low intensity pulsed
   low mechanical index continuous-
     mode contrast-enhanced
   Mammotome
   M-mode
   MUSTPAC (medical ultrasound
     3D portable, with advanced
     communications)

ultrasound *(cont.)*
neonatal adrenal
NeuroSector
Nicolet Elite Doppler
noninvasive
obstetric
Olympus endoscopic
Olympus EU-M30S endoscopic
ultrasonography receiver
pancreaticobiliary (or pancreatic-
biliary)
pelvic
Pentax EUP-EC124 ultrasound
gastroscope
Pentax-Hitachi FG32UA endo-
sonographic system
Philips ultrasound with endovaginal
transducer
photoacoustic
Photopic Imaging
postnatal
power Doppler
PowerVision
pulsed
pulsed Doppler
pulse inversion
real-time
real-time 4-D
rectal endoscopic
renal
RT 3200 Advantage
RT 6800
sagittal
scrotal
Sequoia ultrasound system
Siemens Sonoline Elegral
SieScape
single field hyperthermia combined
with radiation therapy and
Site-Rite and Site-Rite II
Site-Rite and Site-Rite II ultrasound
systems for vascular imaging
Sonablate 200

ultrasound *(cont.)*
Sonablate 200 high intensity
focused ultrasound system
Sonicator portable
sonohysterography
Sonoline Sierra ultrasound imaging
system
Sonoprobe SP-501 system for
endoscopic procedures
SonoSite 180 hand-carried ultrasound system
SonoSite portable
sonourethrography
Synergy
TDOG (tissue Doppler gated)
dynamic three-dimensional
Technos
Technos ultrasound system
three-dimensional (3D) freehand
three-dimensional intravascular
(3-D IVUS)
tissue Doppler gated (TDoG)
dynamic three-dimensional
ultrasound imaging
transcranial color-coded duplex
transcranial Doppler (TCD)
transluminal ultrasonic angioplasty
(TUA)
transnasal endoluminal
transperineal ultrasonography
transrectal (TRUS)
transthoracic
transvaginal (TVS)
transverse
TRUS (transrectal ultrasound)
two-dimensional (2D) B-mode
transabdominal
two-dimensional intravascular (2-D
IVUS)
Ultramark 4
ultrasonic body contouring
vaginal
Versalab ultrasonic medical device

ultrasound *(cont.)*
  VingMed
  Voluson
ultrasound augmented mammography
ultrasound backscatter microscopy
  (UBM)
ultrasound biomicroscopy (UBM)
ultrasound biopsy needle
ultrasound diagnosis
ultrasound diathermy
ultrasound diffraction tomography
ultrasound disruption of stone
ultrasound echocardiography
ultrasound-enhanced stylet, INRAD
  HiLiter
ultrasound for foreign body detection
ultrasound gel
ultrasound guidance
ultrasound-guided anterior subcostal
  liver biopsy
ultrasound-guided compression
ultrasound-guided echo biopsy
ultrasound-guided hookwire
ultrasound-guided needle biopsy
ultrasound-guided percutaneous
  interstitial laser ablation
ultrasound-guided percutaneous
  microwave coagulation therapy
ultrasound-guided percutaneous
  thrombin injection
ultrasound-guided pneumatic reduction
  of intussusception
ultrasound-guided pseudoaneurysm
  compression
ultrasound-guided stereotactic biopsy
ultrasound-guided transcervical tuboplasty
ultrasound-guided transthoracic needle
  aspiration
ultrasound-guided transvaginal aspiration of eggs

ultrasound-guided TULIP (transurethral laser-induced prostatectomy)
ultrasound hyperthermia treatment
ultrasound imaging technology
ultrasound monitoring
ultrasound monitoring of ovarian
  follicle diameter
ultrasound needle guidance for amniocentesis
ultrasound needle guidance for fetal
  transfusion
ultrasound pad
ultrasound probe
  Olympus UM-1W transendoscopic
  Versadopp 10 Doppler
ultrasound scan
ultrasound scanning, high resolution
ultrasound stethoscope
ultrasound system (see *ultrasound*)
ultrasound transcervical tuboplasty
ultrasound velocity dilution
ultrasound venography
UltraSTAR computer-based ultrasound
  reporting system
ultrastructural abnormality
Ultravist (iopromide) imaging agent
UMB-E umbilical catheter
umbilical artery
umbilical artery (UAC) catheter
umbilical catheter
umbilical cord
  three-vessel
  two-vessel
umbilical cord compromise
umbilical cyst
umbilical duct
umbilical fistula
umbilical hemorrhage
umbilical hernia
umbilical vein catheterization

Umbili-Cath Tecoflex umbilical
  catheter
UM 4 real-time sector scanner
UMI catheter
unattached fractions
unbuttoning of device
uncalcified pleural plaque
uncal gyrus
uncal herniation syndrome
uncemented Reflection acetabular cup
uncemented Trilogy acetabular cup
uncertainty principle
unciform bone
uncinate aura
uncinate gyrus
uncinate process of pancreas
uncinate region of temporal lobe
uncoil
uncomplicated non-Q-wave myocardial
  infarction
uncomplicated Q-wave myocardial
  infarction
uncommitted metaphyseal lesion
uncommon pneumoconioses
uncomplicated myocardial infarction
uncontrolled bronchospasm
uncoupled spins
uncovertebral joint (UJ)
uncovertebral spurring
uncus, arachnoid of
uncus corporis
undepressed stellate fracture
undercorrection
underdetection
underdistention
underdrive termination
under fluoroscopic guidance
underinflation of lung
underloading, ventricular
underperfused
underperfusion
under-scan method/projection
undersurface

underventilation
undifferentiated nasopharyngeal
  carcinoma (UCNT)
undisplaced fracture
undulant impulse
undulating contour
undulating course
unenhanced helical CT
unenhanced imaging
unenhanced magnetic resonance
  imaging scan
unfundibular tubal ectopic pregnancy
  locations
unfused physis
unguicular tuberosity
unicameral bone cyst
unicameral brain
unicommissural aortic valve
unicommissural valve
unicompartmental knee prosthesis
unicorn
unicornuate uterus
unicoronal synostosis
unicortical screw
unicorn uterus
unidentified bright objects (UBOs)
unidirectional lead configuration
unifascicular block
unifocal
unifocalization uniform bremsstrahlung
  splitting (UBS)
uniform attenuation coefficient
uniform fat suppression
uniform loading
uniform resource locator (URL)
uniform sensitivity
uniform TR (repetition time)
  excitation
uniformly progressive deterioration
uniform uptake throughout
unigravida
unilateral cervical root avulsion injury
unilateral fragmentation

unilateral hypertrophy
unilateral involvement
unilateral renal artery stenosis
unilateral small kidney
unilateral transpedicular percutaneous
  vertebroplasty
unilocular macrocystic serous cystadenoma
union
  bony
  delayed fracture
  faulty
  fibrous
  osseous
  secondary
  vicious
union of fracture fragments
unipara
uniphasic imaging agent
unit
  BICAP
  EMI
  gamma
  Hounsfield (HU)
  HU (Hounsfield)
  Leksell gamma
  linear accelerator
  musculotendinous
  reflectometer tuning
  rutherford (rd)
  Sheffield gamma
  stepdown
  Wood (of pulmonary vascular
    resistance)
unit of measure
  becquerel (Bq)
  centigray (cGy)
  centimeter (cm)
  cubic centimeter (cc)
  deciliter (dl)
  electron volt (eV)
  femtoliter (fL)
  gauss (G)

unit *(cont.)*
  gigaelectron volt (GeV)
  gram (g)
  gray (Gy)
  international unit (IU)
  joule (J)
  kelvin (K)
  kiloelectron volt (keV or kev)
  kilogram (kg)
  kilohertz (kHz)
  kilometer (km)
  liter (L)
  megaelectron volt (MeV)
  megahertz (MHz)
  meter (m)
  milliampere (mA)
  milliequivalent (mEq)
  milligram (mg)
  milliliter (ml)
  millimeter (mm)
  millimeter of mercury (mm Hg
    or mmHg)
  millimole (mmol)
  milliunit (mU)
  tesla (T)
univentricular heart
University of Florida LINAC (linear
  accelerator)
Unix/X11 workstation
unleveling, pelvic
unmitigated (unrelieved)
unmodulated radiofrequency current
unmyelinated nerve fibers
unopacified
unopacification
unopposed images
unreliable marker
unresectable
unresolved pneumonia
unresponsive programming
unroofed coronary sinus syndrome
unroofing of nerve
unruptured follicle

unsharp masking
unshunted hydrocephalus
unstable angina
unstable fracture
unsuppressed exam
untether
untethered
ununited (nonunited) fracture
U-1100 UV-Vis spectrophotometer
   (also U-2001, U-2010, U-3000,
   U-3010, U-3300, U-3310)
UOAC (uterine ostial access catheter)
U1-NA cephalometric measurement
up-regulation, radiation-induced
uPACS picture archiving system
updraft therapy
UPJ (ureteropelvic junction)
UPJO (ureteropelvic junction obstruction)
upper airway obstruction, foreign body
upper collecting system
upper gastrointestinal series
upper GI (gastrointestinal) series
upper GI with small bowel follow-
   through
upper-limb cardiovascular syndrome
upper limits of normal
upper lobe vein prominence
upper lung field
upper mantle radiotherapy
upper pole collecting system
upper pole moiety
upper pole ureter
upper rate interval
upper respiratory tract disease
upper tract obstruction
upright chest film
upright chest, PA
upright PA (posteroanterior) film
upright postvoid view
upright view
upright weightbearing view
UP7 film

Upshaw-Schulman syndrome
upstairs-downstairs heart
upstream blood
upstroke, carotid pulse
upstroke phase of cardiac action
   potentials
uptake (of organ)
   contrast
   decreased
   decreased uptake with patchy
     distribution
   diffuse
   dye
   fluorescein
   focal
   heterogeneous
   iodine ^{131}I (thyroid function)
   localized
   observed maximal
   pathological
   physiological
   poor
   predicted maximal
   radioiodine
   radioisotope
   radionuclide
   rapid
   radiotracer
   thyroid (of radioactive iodine)
   tracer
   uniform
   variegated (of radioiodine)
uptake and excretion
uptake and retention
uptake in radionuclide scan
upward and backward dislocation
upward retraction
urachus, patent
uranium (U) (an element)
^{235}U (uranium-235)
Ureflex ureteral catheter
Ureflex ureteral catheter for intravenous pyelogram

Ureflex urethral catheter
uremia
uremic pneumonitis
ureter
  abdominal part of
  angulation of
  atonic
  bifid
  circumcaval
  construction of intestinal
  crushing of
  curlicue
  dilatation of
  dilated
  distal right
  ectatic
  ectopic
  extraperitoneal excision of lower
    one-third of
  fishhook appearance of
  fishhooking of
  hook-shaped
  ileal
  intramural portion of distal
  intravesical
  J-hook deformity of distal
  kinked
  kinking of
  left
  looped
  lower pole
  moderately dilated
  mucosa of
  muscular layer of
  native dilated
  occlusion of
  orthotopic
  partial obstruction of
  polyp of
  postcaval
  retrocaval
  retroiliac
  right

ureter *(cont.)*
  rigid
  scar tissue in
  stenotic
  stone disintegration in
  straight
  stricture of
  tenderness over
  tortuosity of
  tortuous
  tuberculosis of
  upper pole
ureteral achalasia
ureteral bud, accessory
ureteral calculus
ureteral catheter
ureteral catheter (with an olive-shaped
    tip)
ureteral catheter tip
ureteral clipping
ureteral compression technique
ureteral dilatation
ureteral dilation
ureteral distention
ureteral division
ureteral ectasia
ureteral ectopia
ureteral endometriosis
ureteral filling
ureteral filling defect
ureteral fistula
ureteral notching
ureteral occlusion
ureteral reflux imaging
ureteral reflux study
ureteral stasis
ureteral stenosis
ureteral stent
ureteral stricture
ureteral valve
ureteral vascular compromise
ureter and skin fistula
ureterectasis

ureteric compression on intravenous
  urolography, AP
ureteric dilation
ureteric obstruction
ureteric stone
ureterocele
  bilobed
  ectopic
  sphincteric
ureterocele disproportion
ureterocervical fistula
ureterocutaneous fistula
ureterogram, retrograde
ureterography
ureterohydronephrosis
ureterolithiasis
ureteropelvic junction (UPJ)
  obstruction (UPJO)
ureteropyelogram, retrograde
ureteropyelography
ureterorenoscopy
ureteroscopy
ureterostomy, high-loop
ureterovaginal fistula
ureterovesical junction (UVJ),
  competence of
ureterovesical obstruction
urethra
  angle of inclination of
  anterior
  blocked
  bulbous
  distal
  distal part of prostatic
  female
  hypermobile
  intermediate part of
  male
  membranous
  mucosa of
  muscular layer of
  muscular layer of spongy
  navicular fossa of

urethra *(cont.)*
  nontraumatic rupture of
  patent
  pendulous
  penile
  polyp of
  posterior
  prostatic
  prostatomembranous
  proximal
  proximal part of prostatic
  ruptured
  shortening of
  spongy
urethral abscess
urethral adenomatoid metaplasia
urethral adenomatous tumor
urethral calculus
urethral catheter
urethral dilation
urethral diverticulum
urethral fistula
urethral gland abscess
urethral meatus prolapse
urethral obstruction
urethral polyp
urethral prolapse
urethral stenosis
urethral stent
urethral trauma
urethral atresia
urethral fistula
urethral induration
urethral meatus prolapse
urethral prolapse
urethral stricture
urethral trauma
urethral valve
urethra and penile skin fistula
urethra and vagina fistula
urethrocutaneous fistula
urethrocystography
urethrocystogram

urethrocystography
  retrograde
  voiding (VCU)
urethrogram
urethrography
  retrograde
  voiding
urethroperineal fistula
urethroperineal fistula
urethrorectal fistula
urethroscrotal fistula
urethrovesical angle (UVA)
urethrovesical fistula
urethrovesical junction
urethrovesicovaginal fistula
urinary ascites
urinary bladder
  anterior wall of
  apex of
  dome of
  epithelium of
  fundus of
  lateral wall of
  peak flow of
  posterior wall of
  removal of
  trigone of
urinary extravasation
urinary fistula
urinary meatal stricture
urinary tract
urinary tract calculus
urinary tract fistula
urinary tract inflammation
urinary tract obstruction
urinary tumor
urine
  nonopaque
  postvoid residual
  radiopaque
  residual
  retained
  stagnant

urinoma
Urist view of acetabular rim in profile
URL (uniform resource locator)
UroCoil self-expanding stent
urodynamic loop catheter
urogenital diaphragm
urogenital duct
urogenital fistula
urogenital ridge
urogenital sinus
urogram
urography
  antegrade
  CT
  excretory (EU)
  intravenous
  magnetic resonance (MRU)
  retrograde
  RPO and LPO 30° intravenous
urokinase protocol
UroLume endoprosthesis wire stent
UroLume flow-directed catheter
UroLume flow-directed microcatheter
UroLume urethral stent
UroLume urinary stent
UroLume Wallstent
UroMax II urethral balloon catheter
UroQuest On-Command catheter
uroradiology
urorectal septum
urosepsis
urothelial carcinoma in situ (CIS)
urothelial striations
urothelial thickening
urothelial tumor
US (ultrasound, ultrasonography)
USCI angioplasty guiding sheath
USCI Mini-Profile balloon dilatation
  catheter
USCI probing catheter
US (under-scan) method/projection
USPIO (ultrasmall superparamagnetic
  iron oxide)

USPIO (ultrasmall superparamagnetic
   iron oxide) imaging agent
uterine adenomyosis
uterine adenosarcoma
uterine agenesis
uterine arterial embolization (UAE)
uterine calculus
uterine cirsoid aneurysm
uterine cornual access catheter
   (UCAC)
uterine didelphia
uterine endometriosis
uterine fibroid, pedunculated
uterine fistula
uterine hemorrhage
uterine laceration
uterine lipoma
uterine malignancy
uterine myoma (pl. myomata)
uterine myoma deformity
uterine ostial access catheter (UOAC)
uterine peristalsis
uterine prolapse
uterine tumor
uterine neck
uterocervical
uterogram
uterography
uteropelvic
uteroperitoneal fistula
uteroplacental
uterorectal fistula
uterosalpingography
uterotubography
uterotubal junction
uteroureteric fistula
uterovaginal anastomosis
uterovaginal fistula
uterovaginal prolapse
uterovesical fistula
uterus
   anomalous
   anteflexed

uterus *(cont.)*
   anterior lip of
   anteverted
   aplastic
   arcuate
   atonic
   atony of
   band of
   bicameral
   bicornis
   bicornuate
   bifid
   biforate
   bilocular
   bimanual abdominorectal palpation
      of
   bimanual abdominovaginal
      palpation of
   bipartite
   cervix of
   cochleate
   cornu of
   Couvelaire
   didelphic
   double
   double-mouthed
   duplex
   endometriosis
   external os of
   fetal
   fibroid
   firm
   fluid-filled mass in
   fundus of
   Gilliam suspension of
   gravid
   heart-shaped
   helicine artery of
   horn of
   hourglass
   hourglass contraction of
   incarcerated gravid
   incudiform

uterus *(cont.)*
  infantile
  isthmus of
  inverted pear-shaped
  involuted
  isthmus of
  lateral angle of
  malposition of
  masculine
  midposition
  miniature
  mobile
  mobility of
  multiparous
  myomatous
  neck of
  normal-size
  one-horned
  opening of
  orifice of
  outline of
  pear-shaped
  position of
  posterior lip of
  postpartum subinvoluted
  pregnant
  prolapse of
  prolapse of gravid
  prostatic
  pubescent
  retroflexed

uterus *(cont.)*
  retroverted
  ribbon
  round ligament of
  rupture of
  saddle-shaped
  septate
  serosa of
  size of
  slightly retroflexed
  soft
  spongy
  subseptate
  symmetrical
  unicornuate
  prostatic
  tender
  tipped
  triangular
  unicorn
  urethral
uterus to abdominal wall fistula
utricle
utricular
utriculus (utricle)
UV (ultraviolet)
UVA (urethrovesical angle)
uveal melanoma
uvula, cerebellar
uvula palatina

V, v

V (ventricular)
V (volume of lung)
VA (ventriculoatrial)
　VA conduction
　VA interval
V-angle, femoral torsion
VABES (vasoablative endothelial
　sarcoma)
vacuum-assisted breast biopsy
vacuum cleft
vacuum disk
vacuum, facet joint
vacuum joint phenomenon
vacuum phenomenon, spontaneous
vacuum ultraviolet light (VUV)
vagina
　anterior fornix of
　azygos artery of
　double
　fornix of
　vestibule of
vaginal agenesis
vaginal cavity
vaginal cone irradiation
vaginal endometriosis
vaginal fistula
vaginal hematoma

vaginal laceration
vaginal ligament of hand
vaginal neofornix
vaginal prolapse
vaginal reflux
vaginal rhabdomyosarcoma
vaginal stenosis
vaginal stricture
vaginal ultrasound
vaginal vault prolapse
vaginal wall prolapse
vaginogram
vaginoperineal fistula
vaginovesical fistula
vagus (tenth cranial) nerve
vagus trunk
Valdini method to demonstrate
　squamous portion of occipital bone
　and foramen magnum
valgus
　adolescent hallux
　Coldman Hakim programmable
　fulguration of
　hallux (HV)
　hindfoot
　insufficiency of aortic
　metatarsus

valgus *(cont.)*
   myxomatous degeneration of
   myxomatous degeneration of mitral
   Passage hemostasis
   Perimount Plus heart
   pes
   posterior semilunar
   talipes
   ureteral
valgus carrying angle
valgus deformity
valgus foot
valgus fracture, impacted
valgus heel
valgus stress
valgus tilt
vallecula cerebelli
Valle hysteroscope
valley to peak dose rate
Valsalva maneuver
value
   attenuation
   bright pixel
   comparative
   CT attenuation
   dark pixel
value flips
   negative predictive
   P
   positive predictive
   predictive
   tristimulus
valvar aortic stenosis
valve
   absent
   aortic (AV)
   Bauhin
   bicuspid
   bileaflet
   billowing mitral
   blunting of
   calcified
   capillary

valve *(cont.)*
   cardiac
   caval
   cleft
   competent
   conduit
   congenital absence of
   coronary
   coronary sinus
   disc-type
   doming of
   dysplastic
   early opening of
   echo-dense
   eustachian
   extirpation of
   failed
   fibrotic
   flail
   flexible
   floppy
   foramen ovale
   frenulum of
   globular
   hammocking of
   Heimlich
   Heister
   Houston
   hypoplastic
   ileocecal
   Kerckring
   leaky
   mitral (MV)
   monocusp
   narrowed
   native
   notching of
   parachute mitral
   premature closure of
   prosthetic heart
   pulmonic
   pulmonary (PV)
   pyloric

valve *(cont.)*
  quadricuspid pulmonary
  rectal
  regurgitation of
  rheumatic heart
  semilunar (aortic and pulmonary)
  sigmoid
  spiral
  stenotic
  synthetic
  thebesian
  tilting-disk valve
  track
  tricuspid (TV)
  tricuspid aortic
  trileaflet aortic
  truncal
  unicommissural
  urethral
  vegetation of
  venous
  Vieussens
  xenograft
valve attenuation
valve bladder
valve calcification
valve cusps
valved conduit
valve dehiscence
valve incompetence
valve leaflets
valve outflow strut
valve plane
valve pockets
valve replacement
valve scarring
valve strut
valve thickening and scarring
valve tip
valviform
valvular aortic insufficiency
valvular aortic stenosis
valvular apparatus

valvular atresia
valvular cardiac defect
valvular damage
valvular disease
valvular dysfunction
valvular heart disease
valvular incompetence
valvular opening
valvular orifice
valvular pneumothorax
valvular pulmonic stenosis
valvular regurgitant lesion
valvular regurgitation
valvular stenosis
VAN (vein, artery, nerve)
van Andel catheter
vanishing bile duct syndrome (VBDS)
vanishing lung syndrome (on x-ray)
VAP (ventilator-associated pneumonia)
Vaquez disease
variability
  anatomic
  beat to beat
  interacquisition
  interpretive
  peak flow
variable-angle uniform signal
  excitation (VUSE)
variable energy
variable flip angle excitation
variable murmur
variable response rate
Varian Associates 11.7T (500 MHz)/
  51 mm bore spectrometer
Varian brachytherapy system
variance reduction technique
Varian LINAC (linear accelerator)
Varian NMR spectrometer
variance images
variant
  anatomic
  labral
  ossification

variant angina pectoris
variation
  area/hemidiameter
  BO field
  diurnal
  exposure
  normal anatomic
  positional
  subtle
variation in density
variceal column
variceal hemorrhage
variceal sclerotherapy
varicella pneumonia
varices (pl. of varix)
varicocele, idiopathic
varicography
varicose aneurysm
varicose bronchiectasis
varicose vein
varicosity (pl. varicosities)
variegated uptake of radioiodine
Variflex catheter
VARIS radiation oncology system
varix (pl. varices)
varum, genu
varus
  metatarsus
  rearfoot
  subtalar
  talipes
  tibial
varus angle
varus deformity
varus heel
varus metatarsophalangeal (MTP)
  angle
varus tilt
VAS (vestibular aqueduct syndrome)
Vas-Cath catheter
Vas-Cath catheter for percutaneous
  thromboarterectomy
Vas-Cath Flexxicon II catheter

Vas-Cath Opti-Flow long term dual
  lumen hemodialysis catheter
Vas-Cath PTA balloon catheter
Vas-Cath Soft-Cell permanent dual
  lumen hemodialysis catheter
Vascu-Guard patch
vascular access
vascular accident
vascular anastomosis
vascular and airway modeling
vascular anomaly
vascular atrophy
vascular attachments
vascular bed, pulmonary
vascular blush (on carotid
  angiography)
vascular bud
vascular bundle
vascular catastrophe
vascular channels, aberrant
vascular cirrhosis
vascular compromise
vascular congestion
vascular cord damage
vascular disease, peripheral
vascular ectasia
vascular encasement
vascular engorgement
vascular enhancement
vascular flasks
vascular flow imaging
vascular gene therapy
vascular graft
vascular hamartoma
vascular hemangioma
vascular heterograft
vascular hydraulic conductivity
vascular impedance
vascular insult
vascular invasion
vascular involvement
vascularization

vascular jejunization of the ileum on
   CT scan
vascular lesion
vascular lumen
vascular malformation
vascular markings
vascular network
vascular obstruction
vascular occlusive disease
vascular patency
vascular pedicle
vascular permeability
vascular phase
vascular plexus
vascular protrusion
vascular redistribution
vascular reserve
vascular resistance
vascular ring
vascular segmentation and extraction
vascular sling
vascular spasm
vascular supply
vascular syndrome
vascular systemic resistance
vascular tone
vascular tuft
vascular wall
vascular xenograft
vascularity
vasculature
   crossing
   peripancreatic
   pruned appearance of pulmonary
vasculitic lesion
vasculopathy, cardiac
vasoconstriction
vasodepressive
vasodepressor reaction (VDR)
vasodilate
vasodilation
vasodilatation
vasography

vasopressor
vasoreactivity, pulmonary
vasospasm
vasospastic vessel
vasovagal phenomenon
VasoView balloon dissection system
vastus lateralis muscle
vastus medialis advancement (VMA)
vastus medialis muscle
vastus medialis obliquus (VMO)
VAT (vaso-occlusive angiotherapy)
VAT (ventricular activation time)
Vater
   ampulla of
   papilla of
VATER (acronym for vertebral or vascular defects, anorectal malformation, tracheoesophageal fistula, and
   radial, ray, or renal anomaly)
Vater diverticulum
vaterian segment
VATS (video-assisted thoracic surgery)
vault
   cranial
   plantar
   rectal
VAX 4100 system
VBDS (vanishing bile duct syndrome)
VBI (vertebrobasilar insufficiency)
VC (vital capacity)
VCB (ventricular capture beat)
VCF (ventricular contractility function)
VCG (vectorcardiogram)
VCO_2 (venous CO_2 production)
VCUG (vesicoureterogram)
VCUG (voiding cystourethrogram)
VD (valvular disease)
VD (videodensitometry)
VDI (venous distensibility index)
VDR (vasodepressor reaction)
VDS (ventral derotating spinal)
VEA (ventricular ectopic activity)
VEB (ventricular ectopic beat)

vector
  expression
  mean cardiac
vectorcardiogram, vectorcardiography
  (VCG)
  Frank
  frontal plane
  sagittal plane
  spatial
  transverse plane
Vector catheter
Vector X catheter
vector loop
vegetation of valve
vein (pl. veins)
  accessory cephalic
  accessory hemiazygos
  accessory saphenous
  accessory vertebral
  accompanying
  ALSVs (arm and lesser saphenous
    veins)
  anal
  anastomosing
  anastomotic
  aneurysmal
  angular
  anonymous
  antebrachial
  antecubital
  anterior cardiac
  anterior jugular
  anterior terminal (ATV)
  appendicular
  aqueous
  arciform
  arcuate
  arterial
  ascending lumbar
  auditory
  auricular
  autogenous
  axillary

vein *(cont.)*
  azygos
  basal
  basal vein of Rosenthal (BVR)
  basilic
  basivertebral
  Boyd perforating
  brachial
  brachiocephalic
  bronchial
  bulb of
  cannulated central
  capacious
  capillary
  cardiac
  cardinal
  cavernous
  central
  cephalic
  cerebral
  cervical
  choroid
  ciliary
  circumflex
  colic
  common basal
  common cardinal
  common facial
  communicating
  companion
  condylar emissary
  congenital stenosis of
  conjunctival
  coronary
  costoaxillary
  cutaneous
  cystic
  deep
  digital
  dilated (due to obstruction of the
    hepatic portal circulation)
  diploic
  distended

vein *(cont.)*
Dodd perforating group of
dorsispinal
duodenal
embryonic umbilical
emissary
engorged
epigastric
episcleral
esophageal
ethmoidal
external jugular
external pudendal
facial
familial varicose
feeder
femoral
fibular
flat neck
frontal
gastric
gastroepiploic
great cardiac
great cerebral vein of Galen
great saphenous
harvested
hemiazygos
hepatic
ileocolic
iliofemoral
inferior pulmonary
inferior rectal
inferior thyroid
infradiaphragmatic
innominate
intercostal
internal cerebral (ICV)
internal jugular
internal thoracic
intussusception of
jugular
Labbé
labial

vein *(cont.)*
leaking
left hepatic
lesser saphenous
limb of
lobe of azygos
marginal
Marshall
median antebrachial
medullary
meningeal
mesenteric
middle cardiac
middle rectal
nodularity
oblique
palmar cutaneous
pancreatic
paraumbilical
parent
pericardial
peroneal
portal
posterior auricular
posterior interventricular
posterior terminal (PTV)
prepyloric
pudendal
pulmonary
pulsating
renal
Retzius
reversed
Rosenthal basal
saphenous
sausaging of
Schlesinger
scimitar
scrotal
septal
small cardiac
small saphenous
soleal

vein *(cont.)*
  spermatic
  splenic
  subcardinal
  subclavian
  subcutaneous
  superficial
  superficial femoral
  superior intercostal
  superior mesenteric (SMV)
  superior pulmonary
  superior rectal
  systemic
  testicular
  thalamostriate
  thebesian
  thoracoepigastric
  thyrocervical collateral
  tortuous
  varicose
  vermian
  vertebral
vein graft
  blood flow patterns in
  color-flow duplex imaging of
  patency of
vein graft occlusion
vein graft stenosis
vein graft thrombosis
vein of Retzius
vein patch angioplasty
vein patency
vein sign
velocimetry, laser Doppler
velocity
  aortic wave
  blood flow
  closing
  coronary blood flow (CBFV)
  decreased closing
  diastolic regurgitant
  fiber-shortening
  forward

velocity *(cont.)*
  maximal transaortic jet
  mean aortic flow
  mean posterior wall
  mean pulmonary flow
  meter per second (m/sec)
  muzzle velocity in handgun injury
  peak aortic flow
  peak flow
  peak pulmonary flow
  peak systolic
  peak transmitted
  regurgitant
velocity-encoded cine MR (magnetic
  resonance) imaging
velocity encoding on brain magnetic
  resonance angiography
velocity mapping, phase
velocity-time integral of early diastole
velocity-time integral of late diastole
velocity waveforms (VWFs)
velopharyngeal closure
Velpeau axillary lateral view
velum
vena cava (pl. venae cavae)
  flat inferior
  inferior (IVC)
  infrahepatic
  superior (SVC)
  suprahepatic
vena cava (or caval) filter
vena cava syndrome
vena comitans (pl. venae comitantes)
venacavography
venetian blind artifact
venoarterial shunting
venodilators
venofibrosis
venogram
venography
  adrenal
  cerebral CT
  contrast

venography *(cont.)*
  conventional
  epidural
  free hepatic
  hepatic
  iliac
  intraosseous
  isotope
  lower limb
  MR
  portal
  radionuclear
  radionuclide
  selective
  splenic
  technetium Tc 99m
  venous enhanced subtracted peak
    arterial MR
  vertebral
  wedged hepatic
veno-occlusive disease (VOD)
venostasis
venous access
venous angiography
venous angioma
venous anomaly
venous backflow
venous blood, arterialization of
venous blood gas values
venous cannula
venous capillaries
venous catheter
venous channel, deep
venous circulation
venous congestion
venous decompensation
venous defects
venous distention
venous Doppler exam
venous embolus
venous engorgement

venous enhanced subtracted peak
  arterial MR venography
venous excursion
venous filling
  early
  late
venous gangrene
venous hyperemia
venous hypertension
venous injection
venous insufficiency
venous junction
venous lake
venous malformation (VM)
venous motion
venous obstruction
venous oxygen content
venous phase image
venovenous hemodialysis
venous plexus
venous pooling
venous pressure
venous pulse, trough of
venous refill time (VRT)
venous reflux
venous reservoir
venous return
  anomalous pulmonary
  total anomalous
venous scan
venous segment, nonfilling
venous segments of kidney
venous sinus
venous spasm
venous stasis
venous thromboembolic disease
  (VTED)
venous thromboembolism
venous thrombosis
venous ulcer
venous valve

venous vascular malformation
venous waveform
ventilation
   airway pressure release
   alveolar (VA)
   high minute
   maximal voluntary (MVV)
   mechanical
   minute
   partial liquid
   reduced alveolar
   uneven
   volume-controlled inverse ratio
   volume-cycled
ventilation defect
ventilation image
ventilation lung scan
ventilation-perfusion defect
ventilation-perfusion lung scan
ventilation-perfusion (V-Q, VQ) ratio
   [Q = quotient]
ventilation phase
ventilation pneumonitis
ventilation scan
ventilator-associated pneumonia (VAP)
ventilatory capacity-demand imbalance
ventilatory defect, restrictive
ventilatory dysfunction
ventilatory effort
ventilatory failure
vent port
ventral aorta
ventral branch
ventral cochlear nucleus
ventral dilation
ventral hernia
ventral spinocerebellar tracts
ventral spinothalamic tracts
ventral surface
ventral union twins
Ventra PTA catheter

ventricle (of brain, heart, larynx)
   absent
   akinetic left
   apex of left
   Arantius
   atrialized
   atrium of
   augmented filling of
   auxiliary
   ballooned floor of
   cephalic
   cerebral
   common
   compensatory enlargement of
   dilatation of
   dilated
   double inlet
   dual
   Duncan (fifth)
   dysfunctional
   effacement of
   elongation of
   enlargement of
   fifth
   floor of
   fourth
   frontal horn of lateral
   Galen
   hypokinetic
   hypoplastic
   laryngeal
   lateral
   left (LV)
   loculate
   Mary Allen Engle
   Morgagni
   outflow of
   papilloma of the fourth
   parchment right
   pineal
   primitive

ventricle *(cont.)*
  right (RV)
  roof of
  rudimentary
  shift of
  single
  sixth (Verga)
  slit
  Sylvius
  temporal horn of lateral
  terminal
  thick-walled
  third
  thrusting
  tiny
  trigone of
  tubular
  Verga
ventricles of brain
ventricular aberration
ventricular activation time (VAT)
ventricular actuation, direct mechanical
  (DMVA)
ventricular afterload
ventricular aneurysm
ventricular apex
ventricular assist device (VAD)
ventricular capture beat
ventricular catheter blockage
ventricular cavity
ventricular cineangiogram
ventricular contraction pattern
ventricular couplets
ventricular D-loop
ventricular decompensation
ventricular depolarization
ventricular depression
ventricular dilatation
ventricular disproportion
ventricular drainage
ventricular dysfunction
ventricular dysrhythmia
ventricular ectopy

ventricular effective refractory period
  (VERP)
ventricular ejection fraction
ventricular elastance, maximum
  (EMAX)
ventricular electrical instability
ventricular enlargement
ventricular escape mechanism
ventricular extrastimulation
ventricular failure
ventricular filling
ventricular free wall thickness
ventricular function, compromised
ventricular function curve
ventricular function parameters
ventricular gallop
ventricular gradient
ventricular hypertrophy
ventricular intracerebral hemorrhage
ventricular inversion
ventricular irritability
ventricular left-handedness
ventricular myocardium
ventricular myxoma
ventricular obstruction
ventricular outflow obstruction
ventricular outflow tract obstruction
ventricular overdrive pacing
ventricular paroxysmal tachycardia
ventricular perforation
ventricular pre-excitation
ventricular premature contraction
  couplets
ventricular pressure, right
ventricular pseudoperfusion beats
ventricular puncture
ventricular rate
ventricular reflux
ventricular refractoriness
ventricular refractory period
ventricular repolarization
ventricular reservoir
ventricular response

ventricular right-handedness
ventricular segmental contraction
ventricular sensed (VS) event
ventricular septal (VS)
ventricular septal aneurysm
ventricular septal defect (VSD), Swiss
    cheese
ventricular septal motion
ventricular septal summit
ventricular shift
ventricular single and double extra-
    stimulation
ventricular size
ventricular space
ventricular span
ventricular standstill
ventricular status
ventricular stiffness
ventricular synchrony
ventricular system
ventricular systole
ventricular tachycardia (VT, V tach)
ventricular transposition
ventricular wall motion
ventricularization of pressure
ventriculoarterial conduit
ventriculoarterial connections
ventriculoarterial discordance
ventriculoatrial (VA) conduction
ventriculoatrial effective refractory
    period
ventriculoatrial time-out
ventriculogram
    axial left anterior oblique
    bicycle exercise radionuclide
    biplane
    bubble
    digital subtraction
    dipyridamole thallium
    exercise radionuclide
    first pass radionuclide
    gated blood pool
    gated nuclear

ventriculogram *(cont.)*
    gated radionuclide
    intraoperative
    LAO (left anterior oblique)
        projection
    left (LVG)
    metrizamide
    radionuclide (RNV)
    RAO (right anterior oblique)
        projection
    retrograde left
    single plane left
    ventriculography
    xenon 133 (^{133}Xe)
ventriculogram
ventriculography
ventriculoinfundibular fold
ventriculomegaly
ventriculoperitoneal (VP)
ventriculoradial dysplasia
ventriculovenous shunt
ventriculus cordis
ventriculus terminalis
Venturi effect
venule (pl. venules)
Verbatim balloon catheter
Verbatim balloon probe
verge, anal
vergence, downward
Verluma (nofetumomab merpentan)
    imaging agent
vermian medulloblastoma
vermian veins
vermicular appendage
vermicular appendix
vermiform process
vermis
    cerebellar
    folium
vernix membrane
VERP (ventricular effective refractory
    period)
Versalab ultrasonic medical device

vertebra (pl. vertebrae)
  arch of
  articular process of
  basilar
  bullet-shaped
  caudal
  cervical (C1 through C7)
  coccygeal
  codfish
  cranial
  displaced
  dorsal (D)
  facet surface of
  false
  fish-mouth
  fractured
  fused
  last normal (LNV)
  lumbar (L1 through L5)
  midbody of
  olisthetic
  pancake
  pear-shaped
  picture-frame
  sacral (S1 through S5)
  scalloping of
  subluxed
  thoracic (T1 through T12)
  transitional
  transverse process of
  true
  wedging of olisthetic
vertebral ankylosis
vertebral arterial dissection
vertebral artery occlusion
vertebral artery syndrome
vertebral artery system
vertebral-basilar artery syndrome
vertebral-basilar ischemia
vertebral basilar insufficiency
vertebral body collapse
vertebral body endplate
vertebral collapse

vertebral column
vertebral endplate
vertebral involvement
vertebral pleural reflection
vertebral scalloping
vertebral segmentation anomaly
vertebral steal phenomenon
vertebral stripe
vertebral vein
vertebral venous plexus
vertebra plana fracture
vertebrobasilar circulation
vertebrobasilar disease
vertebrobasilar distribution stroke
vertebrobasilar insufficiency (VBI)
vertebrobasilar ischemia
vertebrobasilar occlusion
vertebrobasilar system
vertebrocostal rib
vertebroplasty
  percutaneous (PV)
  percutaneous polymethyl
    methacrylate
  unilateral transpedicular
    percutaneous
vertebrosternal rib
vertex, cube
vertex presentation
Vertex camera
vertex (pl. vertices)
vertical fracture
vertical heart
vertical long axial (VLA) images
vertical long axis slice
vertical plane
vertical shear fracture
vertical shear injury
vertical talus
vertigo, pressure-induced
VERT software
verumontanum
vesalianum of vertebral body
vesical (adj.)

vesical calculus, radiopaque
vesical distention
vesical diverticulum
vesical injury
vesical neck
vesical outlet obstruction
vesical stone
vesicle
 acoustic
 acrosomal
 air
 allantoic
 auditory
 cerebral
 cervical
 encephalic
 graafian
 malpighian
 pulmonary
 seminal
vesicle hernia
vesicoamniotic shunt
vesicocervicovaginal fistula
vesicocolic fistula
vesicocutaneous fistula
vesicoenteric fistula
vesicointestinal fistula
vesicorectal fistula
vesicosigmoidovaginal fistula
vesicostomy
vesicoureteral fistula
vesicoureteral reflux
vesicoureteral scintigram
vesicoureteral scintigraphy
vesicoureterogram
vesicoureterography (VCUG)
vesicoureterovaginal fistula
vesicourethral angle
vesicouterine fistula
vesicovaginal fistula
vesicovaginorectal fistula
vesicula (pl. vesiculae)
vesicular bronchiolitis

vesicular emphysema
vesiculography
vessel (pl. vessels)
 afferent
 afferent lymph
 angiographically occult
 anomalous
 arcuate
 atherectomized
 blood
 brachiocephalic
 caliber of
 capillary
 chyle
 circumflex
 codominant
 collateral
 collecting
 commencement of
 contralateral
 cranial
 crossing
 cross-pelvic collateral
 culprit
 curved
 deep lymph
 diminutive
 disease-free
 distal runoff
 dominant
 eccentric
 efferent
 efferent lymph
 end-on
 extracranial
 feeding
 gastroepiploic
 great
 heart and great
 in-plane
 infrapopliteal
 intercostal
 interlobular

vessel *(cont.)*
  internal pudendal
  intracranial
  intradural
  kidney
  lymph
  lymphatic
  musculophrenic
  nondominant
  occipital
  origin of a
  patent
  perforator
  peripelvic collateral
  peripheral
  peroneal
  pial
  plump
  pole of
  posterior lumbar
  renal
  retrograde filling of
  runoff
  splanchnic
  splenic
  superficial lymph
  superior gluteal
  takeoff of a
  tortuous
  transposition of
  vasospastic
  wraparound
vessel caliber
vessel closure, abrupt
vessel cutoff of contrast material
vessel loop
vessel rupture
vessel test-occluded
vessel topography
vessel tracing
vest, halo
vestibular apparatus

vestibular aqueduct syndrome (VAS)
vestibular canal
vestibular division of the eighth
  cranial nerve
vestibular schwannoma
vestibule
vestibulocochlear nerve
vestigial commissure
vestigial left sinoatrial node
VF, V fib (ventricular fibrillation)
V5 area
V5M Multiplane transducer
V5Ms shielded transducer
VFSS (videofluoroscopic swallowing
  study)
VFT (venous filling time)
VHL (von Hippel-Lindau) syndrome
VHP (Visible Human Project)
viable
viability
vibration frequency
vibratory motion
Vicq d'Azyr, band of (in brain)
VID (vitellointestinal duct)
VIDA 29 (Volumetric Image Display
  and Analysis)
Vidar scanner
videoangiography, digital
video-assisted thoracoscopic wedge
  resection
videoconferencing, teleradiology
videodensitometry (VD)
videodensity curves
videoendoscopic surgical equipment
videofluoroscopic imaging
videofluoroscopic swallowing study
  (VFSS)
videofluoroscopy
videoradiogram
videoradiography
videothoracoscopy
Viehweger 3-phase technique

Vieussens
  anulus of
  ansa of
  circle of
  isthmus of
  limbus of
  loop of
  ring of
  valve of
view (see also *position, projection*)
  abdominal
  Adams modification of Hermods-
    son
  afferent
  Ahlback
  air-contrast
  Albers-Schonberg
  Alexander
  Alexander stress
  Altschul
  anterior
  Anthonson subtalar joint
  AP (anteroposterior)
  AP inversion stress vagina
  AP lordotic
  AP supine
  apical
  apical and subcostal four-cham-
    bered
  apical four-chamber (echocardio-
    gram)
  apical lordotic
  apical two-chamber
  Arcelin
  axial plantodorsal
  axial sesamoid
  axillary
  axiolateral inferosuperior
  Ball AP (pelvimetry)
  ball catchers'
  Ball lateral (pelvimetry)
  baseline
  beam's-eye

view *(cont.)*
  Beath
  Beclere
  Berquist
  Bertel
  Bett trapezium
  Bigliani
  biplane orthogonal
  bird's-eye
  Blackett-Healy
  Blondeau
  Bloom and Obata
  Boehler (Böhler) angle
  Boehler (Böhler) calcaneal
  Boehler lumbosacral
  Broden
  Brattstrom
  Brewerton
  Bridgeman
  Broden subtalar joint (I and II)
  brow-down skull
  brow-up skull
  Buck modification of Cobey
  Bucky
  butterfly (AP, LPO, PA, RAO)
  Cahoon
  Caldwell
  Camp-Coventry
  capitellum
  cardiac long axis
  cardiac short axis
  carpal boss
  carpal bridge
  carpal canal
  carpal tunnel
  Carter-Rowe
  caudal
  Causton
  Chamberlain-Towne
  Chassard
  Chassard-Lapiné
  Chausse II
  Chausse III

view *(cont.)*

    Chausse IV
    chest (CXR)
    Cincinnati
    cine
    cineradiographic
    Clements-Nakayama
    clenched fist
    close-up
    coalition
    Cobey
    Cobey Saltzman
    comparison
    cone
    coned
    coned-down
    coronal
    coronal bending
    couch
    Coyle coronoid process
    Coyle radial head
    cranial angled
    craniocaudad, craniocaudal
    craniodorsal head
    cranioventral head
    cross-table lateral
    cross-table
    CTLV (cross-table lateral view)
    Danelius-Miller
    decubitus
    Deneer
    dens
    Didiee shoulder
    dorsiflexion
    dorsoplantar
    Duncan Howe
    Dutt
    efferent
    en face
    equilibrium
    erect
    expiration
    false profile

view *(cont.)*

    faux profil ("foh pro-fccl") (FP)
    FCS (full cervical spine)
    Ferguson
    first pass
    five-view
    flamingo
    flexion
    fluoroscopic
    flying angel (lateral thoracic inlet)
    follow-through
    four chamber apical
    Friedman
    frogleg
    frontal
    frontal oblique
    Fuchs
    full length
    Fürmaier
    Garth apical axial oblique (of
       shoulder)
    gated
    Gaynor-Hart
    Grandy lateral cervical spine
    Granger
    Grashey
    Haas
    Harris
    Harris-Beath axial hindfoot
    Hayes
    heavily penetrated
    Heinig
    hemiaxial
    Henschen
    hepatoclavicular
    Hermodsson internal rotation
    Hermodsson tangential
    Hickey (hip)
    Hickey (profile of mastoid region)
    Hill-Sachs
    hip to ankle
    Hirtz submentovertex (SMV)
    Hobbs

view *(cont.)*
  Holmblad knee
  Hughston patella
  ice-pick M-mode echocardiogram
  ileocecal spots
  infrapatellar
  inlet and outlet (pelvis)
  inspiration
  intraoperative
  inversion ankle stress
  Johner shoulder
  Johnson and Dutt
  Jones
  Judet oblique (of acetabulum)
  Judet pelvic
  jug handle
  kidneys, ureters, bladder (KUB)
  Kisch (hip)
  Knutson
  KUB (kidney, ureters, bladder)
  LAO (left anterior oblique)
  lateral
  lateral anterior drawer stress
  lateral bending view of spine
  lateral decubitus
  lateral medial
  lateral oblique
  lateral tilt stress ankle
  Lauenstein and Hickey
  Laurin x-ray
  Law
  Lawrence
  left anterior oblique (LAO)
  Leonard-George
  Lequesne
  Letournel iliac wing
  Lewis
  Lilienfeld coalition
  limited
  Lindblom AP lordotic chest
  long axial oblique
  long axis
  long axis parasternal

view *(cont.)*
  lordotic
  Lorenz
  Low-Beers
  Lysholm
  MacNab
  May
  Mayer
  medial lateral
  mediolateral
  mediolateral oblique
  Merchant
  Miller
  modified Cleaves
  mortise
  multiplanar reformatting (MPR)
  navicular
  Neer lateral
  Neer transscapular
  nonforeshortened angiographic
  nonstanding lateral oblique
  nonweightbearing
  notch
  oblique
  occipital
  odontoid
  open-mouth
  optimally positioned
  orthogonal
  outlet
  outlet (pelvis)
  over couch
  overhead
  overhead oblique
  Owen
  PA (posteroanterior)
  parasternal long axis
  parasternal short axis
  parietocanthal
  patellar skyline
  Pawlow
  pelvic inlet and outlet
  Pennal

view *(cont.)*
   pillar
   Pirie sinus
   plain
   planar
   plantar axial
   plantarflexion
   plantarflexion stress
   Porcher-Porot
   portable
   postvoid
   postevacuation
   postoperative
   preliminary
   preoperative
   prereduction
   prone
   prone lateral
   push-pull ankle stress
   push-pull hip
   RAO (right anterior oblique)
   ray-sum
   recumbent
   retromammary space
   reverse Towne
   reverse Waters
   Rhese
   right anterior oblique (RAO)
   right lateral decubitus
   right ventricular inflow
   Rippstein
   Robert
   Rocher
   Rockwood serendipity
   Rosenberg weightbearing
   routine magnification
   Sansregret modification of
      Chausse III
   scapular Y
   Schatzki
   Schneider
   Schüller (Schueller)
   scout

view *(cont.)*
   selective coronary arteriography
   semiflexed, anteroposterior
      (SF-AP)
   serendipity
   Settegast
   SF-AP
   short axis
   short axis parasternal
   Simmons
   single breath
   sitting-up
   skijump
   skyline
   SMV (submentovertex or sub-
      mentovertical)
   spider
   spot
   standing
   standing dorsoplantar
   standing lateral
   standing postvoid
   standing weightbearing
   static
   Stecher
   steep LAO oblique
   steep left anterior oblique
   Stenver
   stereoscopic
   Stockholm
   stork
   stress
   stress Broden
   stress eversion
   stress inversion
   Stryker notch
   subcostal four-chamber
   subcostal long axis
   subcostal short axis
   submental vertex
   submentovertex (SMV)
   submentovertical
   subxiphoid

view *(cont.)*
  sunrise
  sunset
  supine
  supine full
  supraspinatus outlet
  suprasternal notch
  Swanson
  swimmer's
  talar neck
  tangential
  tangential scapular
  Tarrant
  Templeton and Zim
  Tile
  tomographic
  Towne
  transaxillary lateral
  transcranial lateral
  transorbital
  transpharyngeal
  transscapular
  true lateral
  tunnel
  two-plane
  upright
  upright postvoid
  upright weightbearing
  Urist
  Valdini
  Velpeau axillary lateral
  Viehweger
  von Rosen
  Wallace-Hellier
  washout
  Waters
  weeping willow
  weightbearing
  weightbearing dorsoplantar
  West Point axillary lateral
  White leg-length
  window
  x-ray

view *(cont.)*
  Y
  Zanca
  Ziter scaphoid
viewbox, virtual reality
viewing
  cine-based
  film-based
  group
  PVR fly-through
view microtomography
view shadow projection micro-
  tomographic system
view sharing
view tray, Bucky
Viewnex software
Villaret-Mackenzie syndrome
villoglandular polyp
villous adenoma
villous atrophy
villous fronds
villous proliferation
villus (pl. villi)
  anchoring
  arachnoidal
  chorionic
  duodenal
  fingerlike
  floating
  gallbladder
  intestinal
  leaflike
  placental
  ridged-convoluted
  tongue-shaped
vinculum breve
vinculum longum
VingMed ultrasound system
VIPER PTA catheter
vipoma (or VIPoma)
VIPoma (vasoactive intestinal polypep-
  tide)
viral pneumonia

Virchow law of skull growth
Virchow perivascular space
Virchow psammoma
Virchow-Robin space
Virchow sentinel node
Virchow thrombosis triad
Virchow triad
Virchow-Troisier node
virilization
virilizing tumor
virtual angioscopy
virtual bronchoscopy
virtual colonsocopy
virtual CT bronchoscopy
virtual cystoscopy
virtual endoscopy
virtual gastroscopy
Virtual Institute for Computer
     Assistance in Clinical Radiology
virtual labor monitor (VLM)
virtual reality imaging
virtual reality simulator
virtual reality viewbox
Virtuoso portable three-dimensional
     imaging system
virus
VisCath fiberoptic imaging
viscera (pl. of viscus)
     abdominal
     abdominopelvic
     hollow
     intra-abdominal
     intraperitoneal
     pelvic
visceral angiogram
visceral cholesterol embolization
     syndrome
visceral embolus
visceral involvement
visceral layer
visceral pericardium
visceral peritoneum
visceral pleura

visceral pleurisy
visceral situs solitus
visceromegaly
visceroptosis
viscid
viscous (adj.)
viscus (pl. viscera)
     hollow
     perforated
     strangulated
VISI (volarflexed intercalated segment
     instability) deformity
visible anterior motion
Visible Human Project (VHP)
Vision camera
Vision MRI scanner
Vision 1.5-T Siemens MRI scanner
Vision Ten V-scan scanner
Visipaque (iodixanol) intravascular
     injection
Visipaque 270 (iodixanol) imaging
     agent
Visipaque 320 (iodixanol) imaging
     agent
Vistaflex biliary stent
Vistec x-ray detectable sponge
visual
visual cortex
visualization
     delayed
     inadequate
     optimal
     passive tracking and
     poor
     suboptimal
visualization and quantification
vital capacity (VC)
Vitalcor venous catheter
Vital-Port vascular access port
vitelline duct
vitellointestinal duct (VID)
Viterbi decoding
Vitrea 3-D system

VIVENDI virtual endoscopy system
VJ (ventriculojugular) shunt
VLA (vertical-long axial) images
VLM (virtual labor monitor)
VMO (vastus medialis obliquus)
vocal cords
  true
  false
VOD (veno-occlusive disease)
Voda catheter
Vogt bone-free projection for localization of foreign bodies in the orbit
VoiceRAD clinical reporting system
void (verb)
void (noun)
  flow
  signal
void determination
voiding cystogram
voiding cystourethrogram (VCUG)
voiding cystourethrography
voiding sequence
voiding study
volar angulation
volar capsule
volar carpal ligament
volar displacement
volarly
volar perilunate dislocation
volar wrist
volarward
Volkmann deformity
volume
  adequate stroke
  alveolar
  articular cartilage
  atrial emptying
  augmented stroke
  blood
  blood flow (BFV)
  carotid wall
  cavity
  central blood

volume *(cont.)*
  chamber
  circulating blood
  circulation
  clinical target
  closing
  controlled lung
  decreased stroke
  decreased tidal
  determination of lung
  diastolic atrial
  diminished lung
  Dodge area-length method for
    ventricular
  EDV
  end diastolic (EDV)
  end expiratory lung
  end systolic (ESV)
  end systolic residual
  endocardial
  epicardial
  ESV
  expiratory reserve (ERV)
  extracellular fluid
  fetal lung
  flow
  forward stroke (FSV)
  fractional moving blood
  gland
  hippocampal
  image
  increased extracellular fluid
  inspiratory reserve (IRV)
  left ventricular chamber
  left ventricular end diastolic
  left ventricular inflow (LVIV)
  left ventricular outflow (LVOV)
  left ventricular stroke
  LV (left ventricular) cavity
  minute
  pericardial reserve
  plasma
  prism method for ventricular

volume *(cont.)*
  pulmonary blood
  pyramid method for ventricular
  radionuclide stroke
  reduced plasma
  reduced stroke
  regional brain parenchymal
    (RBPV)
  regurgitant
  regurgitant stroke (RSV)
  residual (RV)
  respiratory
  right ventricular
  right ventricular end diastolic
  right ventricular end systolic
  scan
  Simpson rule method for
    ventricular
  slice
  stroke (SV)
  SV (stroke)
  systolic atrial
  Teichholz equation for left
    ventricular
  thermodilution stroke
  thin cylindrical uniform field
  total stroke (TSV)
  TSV (total stroke)
  ventricular end diastolic
volume acquisition
volume analysis
volume averaging
volume depletion, intravascular
volume element (voxel)
volume estimation
volume in abstract stereotactic space
volume loss
volume measurement, blood flow
volume overload
volume regulation
volume replacement
volume-rendered image
volumetric analysis

volumetric computed tomography
volumetric data
volumetric dataset
volumetric image (imaging)
volumetric image data
volumetric interpolated breathing-hold
  technique
volumetric mapping technique
volumetric minimally invasive stereotaxis
volumetric multiplexed transmission
  holography
volumetric resampling
volumetric scan
volumetric stereotaxis
volumetry
  hippocampal magnetic resonance
  tumor
voluming artifact
Voluson ultrasound system
volvulus
  cecal
  colonic
  midgut
  sigmoid
vomer bone
von Gierke disease
von Hippel-Lindau (VHL) syndrome
von Hippel tumor
von Meyenburg complex
von Recklinghausen syndrome
von Rosen view
Von Rokitansky syndrome
Vostal classification of radial fracture
voxel (volume element) (pl. voxels)
  adjacent
  cubic
  isotropic
  seed
voxel array
voxel-based morphometric findings
voxel-based morphometry
voxel gradient rendering

Voxel-Man software
VoxelView software
Voxgram multiple exposure hologram
VP (ventriculoperitoneal) shunt
VPB (ventricular premature beat)
VPC (ventricular premature complex)
VPC (ventricular premature
    contraction)
VPD (ventricular premature
    depolarization)
V peak of jugular venous pulse
VQ or V-Q (ventilation-perfusion)
    ratio (Q = quotient)
V-Q mismatch
VRT (venous refill time)
VRT (venous return time)
VS (ventricular septal)
VScore with AutoGate high quality
    cardiac imaging

VSD (ventricular septal defect)
VSD and absent pulmonary valve
    syndrome
V-shaped fracture
VTED (venous thromboembolic
    disease)
vulvar abscess
vulvar endometriosis
vulvar hematoma
vulvar hypertrophy
vulvar malignancy
vulvar stricture
vulvar tumor
vulvovaginal inflammation
VUSE, variable-angle uniform signal
    excitation
VUV (vacuum ultraviolet light).
v wave (on cardiac catheterization)
VWFs (velocity waveforms), Doppler

W, w

wafer, carmustine
wafer of endocardium
wagon wheel fracture
Wagstaffe fracture
waist (of anatomical structure)
Walcher position
Waldenström disease
Waldeyer fascia
walking pneumonia
wall
  abdominal
  aneurysmal
  anterior abdominal
  anterolateral
  apical
  axial
  bladder
  body
  bowel
  carotid
  cavity
  chest
  cyst
  cystic
  gallbladder
  inferior
  inferoapical

wall *(cont.)*
  intestinal
  left anterior chest wall
  luminal
  midabdominal
  nasal cavity
  posterior
  posterior abdominal
  posterolateral
  septal
  stomach
  thickened gallbladder
  thoracic
  vaginal
  variceal
  ventricular
Wallace-Hellier view of shoulder
wall akinesis
wall echo shadow (WES) sign
walled-off esophageal perforation
Wallenberg lateral medullary
  syndrome
wallerian degeneration
wall filter
wall hypokinesis
wall motion study
wall motion abnormalities (WMA)

wall, ruptured colonic
wall shear stress
Wallstent
wall thickening
wall thickness
Wanderer microcatheter
wandering pneumonia
wandering spleen
Ward triangle
warm nodule
washboard effect on myelography in
   cervical spondylosis
wash-in phase
washout
   delayed
   lung
   multibreath
   nitrogen
   perchlorate
   peripheral
   rapid contrast
   regional
   retrograde colonic
   teboroxime resting (TRW)
   xenon
washout curve
washout gradient
washout kinetics
washout phase
washout view
Wassel classification of thumb
   polydactyly
wasting
   muscle
   muscle fiber
wasting syndrome
Watanabe classification of discoid
   meniscus
water
   doped
   purified (contrast)
water bath
water bolus

water-bottle kidney
water contrast computed tomography
water density
waterfall stomach
Waterhouse-Friderichsen syndrome
water path
water perfusable tissue index
water range
water relaxation effect
water retention
water selective SE imaging sequence
water signal on magnetic resonance
   imaging scan
water specific three-point Dixon
   gradient echo
watershed infarct (infarction)
water soluble contrast media
Waters projection
Waterston groove
Waters view
Watson-Jones classification of spinal
   fractures
wave
   A
   abdominal fluid
   aperiodic
   C
   constant tilt
   continuous (CW)
   excitation
   fluid
   insonifying
   juvenile T
   low frequency shear
   non-Q
   non-single harmonic
   P
   peak regurgitant
   peristaltic
   primary peristaltic
   pulsed
   R/S
   rapid filling (RFW)

wave *(cont.)*
  rectangular non-single harmonic
  secondary
  secondary peristaltic
  shock
  single harmonic
  sinusoidal non-single harmonic
  slow filling
  systolic S
  T
  tertiary
  tidal
  triangular non-single harmonic
  V
  v
  Y
waveform
  apiculate
  dampened
  Doppler spectral
  exponential simultaneous
  flow velocity
  gradient
  monophasic
  monophasic shock
  monophasic truncated exponential
    simultaneous
  pressure
  pulse volume
  right atrial
  segmental renal artery
  truncated exponential simultaneous
    monophasic
  velocity (VWFs)
  venous
wavelength
  de Broglie
  readout
wavelet
  HARC-C (compression technique)
  lossy
wavelet compression
wavelet-encoded

wavelet scalar quantization (WSQ)
wavelet sub-band (or subband)
wave pattern, hepatic venous Doppler
WaveWire high performance angioplasty guidewire
waxy kidney
WBCS (white blood cell scintigraphy)
  with indium-111 [^{111}In])
weak carotid upstroke
weak signal
weaver's bottom
web
  duodenal
  esophageal
  fibrous
  finger
  hepatic
  intestinal
  laryngeal
  postcricoid
  terminal
  thumb
  venous
Web browser (World Wide Web in
  teleradiology)
Weber C fracture
Weber, circle of
Weber-Osler-Rendu syndrome
web space
wedge
  dynamic
  match-line
  mediastinal
wedge bonds
wedge compression fracture
wedged beam
wedged hepatic venography
wedge factors
wedge flexion-compression fracture
wedge fracture
wedge isodose angle
wedge pair beam
wedge position, pulmonary capillary

wedge pressure
wedge resection of kidney
wedge resection, video-assisted
  thoracoscopic
wedge-shaped mass
wedge-shaped density
wedge-shaped lobe
wedge-shaped perilesional enhancement
wedge-shaped vertebra
wedge-shaped zone
wedging deformity
wedging of olisthetic vertebra
wedging of vertebral interspace
weeping willow appearance on
  venogram
weeping willow view
Wegener granulomatosis
weightbearing (also weight-bearing)
weightbearing dome of acetabulum
weightbearing rotational injury
weightbearing films
weighted spin echo column (MRI)
weight, estimated fetal
weighting
  half scan fan-beam
  human visual sensitivity
weight loading, axial
Weil disease or syndrome (Adolf Weil)
Weill sign of pneumonia in infant
  (Edmond Weill)
Weinberg-Himelfarb syndrome
Weingarten syndrome
Weinstein-Boriani-Biagini spinal tumor
  classification
Weisenburg syndrome
Weiss-Baker syndrome
Weitbrecht ligament
welder's lung
well-differentiated tumor
well-inflated lung
well, posterior pericardial
well-preserved ejection fraction

well-type ionization chamber
Wenckebach AV (atrioventricular)
  block
Wenckebach phenomenon
Werner syndrome
Wernicke-Korsakoff syndrome
Wernicke region
WES (wall echo shadow) sign
Westermark sign
Westphal-Strümpell disease
West Point axillary lateral view
West Point shoulder view
wet lung syndrome
wet pleurisy
wet reading of x-ray film
wet swallow (on esophageal
  manometry)
Wexler catheter
Wharton tumor
wheelchair artifact
whettle bone
whiplash injury
whiplash technique
Whipple disease
whirlpool sign
whirl sign
whistle catheter tip
whistle-tip ureteral catheter
Whitacre spinal needle
Whitaker test
white-appearing blood pool
white blood cell scintigraphy (WBCS)
  with indium-111
white cerebellum sign
white clot syndrome
white commissure of spinal cord
white echo writing
white gaussian noise distortion
Whitehead deformity
White leg-length view
white light pattern projector
white lung syndrome
white matter, dysplastic

white matter infarct
white matter signal hyperintensity
white matter tract
white metastasis
white noise
white-out of lungs
white pneumonia
white point
white noise artifact
whitlow, melanotic
whole blood monoclonal antibody
whole body bone scintigraphy
whole body imaging
whole body imaging with magnified
  views
whole body 1.5T Siemens Vision
  MRI scanner
whole body PET scan
whole body staging
whole body 3T MRI system scanner
whole body 29FDG scanning
whole brain mean CBF
whole brain radiation therapy
whorl, coccygeal
whorled appearance
WHVP (wedged hepatic venous
  pressure)
Wiberg center edge (CE) angle
Wiberg classification of patellar types
wide beam scanning
widemouthed mucosal diverticulum
widemouth sac
wide neck bifurcation aneurysm
widened heart shadow
widened mediastinum
widened sulci
widened teardrop distance
widened thoracic outlet
widening
  aneurysmal
  ankle mortise
  crural cistern
  fusiform

widening *(cont.)*
  growth plate
  interpedicular distance
  interspinous
  joint
  mediastinal
  scapholunate
wide pulse
widespread metastases
wide window setting
width
  collimation
  isodose
  joint space (JSW)
  pulse
  window
Wiener MRI filter
Wigby-Taylor open-mouth oblique
  projection
Wiktor stent
Wilcoxon signed-rank test
Wilkins classification of radial
  fracture
Williams-Beuren syndrome
Williams-Campbell syndrome
Williamson sign
Williams projection to demonstrate the
  costovertebral and costotransverse
  joints
Williams syndrome
Willis
  antrum of
  arterial circle of
  artery of
  circle of
Willis pancreas
Willis pouch
willow fracture
Wilmad reference standards
Wilms tumor
Wilson cloud chamber
Wilson disease
Wilson-Mikity syndrome

Wiltse angle
winding, zero-pitch solenoidal
windmill artifact
window
  acquisition
  acoustic
  aorticopulmonary
  apical
  bone
  brain
  cortical
  esophageal
  gastric
  parasternal
  pericardial
  pulmonary parenchymal
  reconstruction
  soft tissue
  subcostal
  subdural
  suprasternal
window ductus
windowed
windowing
  histogram-based intensity
  intensity
  manual intensity
  mixture model intensity
window/level settings
window settings
window view
window width
windsock aneurysm
windup injury
wing
  iliac
  sphenoidal
winged scapula
Winiwarter-Buerger disease
Winiwarter-Manteuffel-Buerger
  disease
Winprint imaging laser printer

Winquist-Hansen classification of
  femoral fracture
Winslow, foramen of
Winslow pancreas
Winston-Lutz for LINAC-based
  radiosurgery
Winter-King-Moe scoliosis
Winter shunt
Wintrich sign
wire
  calibrated guide
  encircling
  figure of 8
  guide
  Ilizarov
  interfragment
  intracoronary Doppler flow
  intravascular guide
  lead
  Litespeed
  monitoring
wire fixation
wire localization
wire-related defect
Wirsung duct
Wishard catheter
Wiskott-Aldrich syndrome
wispy connection
Wits cephalometric measurement
WMA (wall motion abnormalities)
Wolfe breast carcinoma classification
Wolfe mammographic parenchymal
  patterns
wolffian duct
Wolff law (bone structure)
Wolff-Chaikoff effect
Wolff-Parkinson-White (WPW)
  syndrome
Wolf-Hirschhorn syndrome
Wolin meniscoid lesion
Wolman xanthomatosis
womb

woody mass
woolsorter's inhalation disease
woolsorter's pneumonia
word segmentation algorithm
workstation
  imaging
  ISG medical imaging
  MacSpect real-time NMR
  Radstation radiology
  Shebele physician reporting
  stacked-metaphor
  Sun
  Unix/X11
workup (n.), work up (v.)
wormian bone
wound
  exit
  gunshot (GSW)
  missile
  penetrating
  perforating
  puncture
  stab
wound cavity

WPW (Wolff-Parkinson-White)
  syndrome
wrap, fundoplication
wrap-around ghosting artifact
wrestler's elbow
wrinkle artifact
wrinkled pleura
Wrisberg cardiac ganglion
Wrisberg, intermediate nerve of
Wrisberg ligament
wrist
  gymnast's
  palmar
  SLAC (scapholunate arthritic
    collapse)
  volar
  Volz
wrist capsule
wristdrop
wryneck (torticollis)
W-shaped ileal pouch
WSQ (wavelet scalar quantization)
Wyburg-Mason arteriovenous
  malformation

X, x

x ("by" or "times")
xanthelasma
xanthoastrocytoma, pleomorphic
xanthogranulomatosis, necrobiotic
xanthogranulomatous cholecystitis
xanthoma
   gastric
   malignant fibrous
xanthomatosis, cerebrotendinous
xanthomatosis of long bones with
   spontaneous fracture
xanthomatosis, Wolman
XCT (x-ray computed tomography)
Xe (xenon)
XeCT (xenon computed tomography)
xenograft valve
xenon (Xe)
   ^{127}Xe imaging agent
   ^{133}Xe clearance technique
   ^{133}Xe imaging agent
xenon chloride (XeCl) excimer
xenon computed tomography (XeCT)
xenon energy window
xenon trap system
xenon washout studies
xenotransplantation
xerography

xeromammogram
xeromammography
xeroradiogram
xeroradiographic selenium plate
xeroradiography
x-height
Xillix LIFE-GI fluorescence
   endoscopy system
Ximatron simulator
XIP (x-ray in plaster)
xiphisternal joint
xiphoid angle
xiphoid bone
xiphoid cartilage
xiphoid process syndrome
xiphopubic area
x-irradiation
XKnife stereotactic radiosurgery
   system
XMG (x-ray mammogram)
XOP (x-ray out of plaster)
Xpeedior catheter
Xplorer 1000 digital x-ray imaging
Xplorer digital radiography
Xplorer filmless high resolution digital
   radiography imaging system
X-Prep bowel prep

746

Xpress/SX helical CT scanner
XRA (x-ray arteriography)
x-ray (pl. x-rays) (see *imaging*;
    position; *projection*; *view*)
  baseline
  portable
x-ray beam equalization
x-ray C-arm
x-ray detector, Si (Li)
x-ray film jacket
x-ray in plaster (XIP)
x-ray out of plaster (XOP)
x-ray penetration

x-ray sensitive vidicon
x-ray topography
X-Sept catheter
X-Sept sheath
Xtent catheter
Xtent probe
Xtent vascular access port
X-terminal
XT radiopaque coronary stent
X trough
X, Y, and Z coordinates for target
  lesion
Xylocaine

Y, y

Y (yttrium)
YAG (yttrium, aluminum, garnet) laser
Yb (ytterbium)
Y bone plate
Y configuration, inverted
Yergason test of shoulder subluxation
Y fracture
yield comparison
yoke
yokelike
yolk sac (YS) diameter
Young-Burgess classification of pelvic ring fractures

Young-Burgess modification of the Tile-Pennal classification system
Y plate
YS (yolk sac)
Y-shaped distortion
Y-T fracture
Y trough
"yuro radiology" (uroradiology)
ytterbium (Yb) (an element)
^{169}Yb (Yb-169) brachytherapy
yttrium radioactive source
yttrium-90 microspheres
Y view

Z, z

Zahn
  lines of
  pockets of
Zanca view of acromioclavicular joint
Zanelli projection to demonstrate
  TMJs
Zang space
Z axis
Z-dependent computed tomography
Z disk
zebra artifact
Zeek syndrome
Zellweger syndrome
Zener diode
Zenker diverticulum
Zenker pouch
zero-field splitting
zero-fill artifact
zero-pitch solenoidal winding
zeugmatography, Fourier
  transformation
zFFS (z-flying focal spot)
z-flying focal spot (zFFS)
Z interpolation algorithms
Zickel fracture classification system
Ziegler syndrome
Zielke derotation level

zinc, irradiated
Zingg fracture of zygomaticomaxillary
  complex
Zinn, tendon of
zipper artifact
Zipper balloon catheter
Ziter scaphoid view
ZK44012 imaging agent
Z-line of esophagus
ZMC (zygomaticomaxillary complex)
Z-Med balloon catheter
Zollinger-Ellison syndrome (ZES)
zonal gastritis
zone
  fracture
  junctional
  myometrial
  Rolando
  slow conduction (ZSC)
  sonolucent
  translucent
  Westphal
z point pressure
ZSC (zone of slow conduction)
Z-score on bone densitometry
Zucker catheter
Zuckerkandl bodies

749

Zuckerkandl convolution
ZY plane
zygapophyseal articulation
zygapophyseal joint
zygoma
zygomatic arch

zygomatic bone
zygomaticomaxillary complex (ZMC)
  fracture
zygomatic process
zygomaticomalar area
zygomaticomaxillary fracture